Patient Studies in Valvular, Congenital, and Rarer Forms of Cardiovascular Disease

To my wife Kathleen, my children Gordon and Marian, and my grandchildren Caroline, Ellen, Audrey, and Bridget.

PATIENT STUDIES IN VALVULAR, CONGENITAL, AND RARER FORMS OF CARDIOVASCULAR DISEASE

AN INTEGRATIVE APPROACH

Franklin B. Saksena, MD, CM, FACC, FACP, FRCP(C), FAHA

Senior Attending Physician 1973–2005,
Currently Voluntary Attending Physician,
Division of Adult Cardiology,
John H. Stroger, Jr. Hospital of Cook County,
Chicago, Illinois

Associate Professor of Clinical Medicine,
Feinberg School of Medicine,
Northwestern University &
Assistant Professor of Medicine,
Rush Medical School, Chicago, Illinois

Attending Physician, Swedish Covenant Hospital,
Chicago, Illinois

Attending Physician, St Mary of Nazareth Hospital,
Chicago, Illinois

WILEY Blackwell

Registered Office
John Wiley & Sons, Ltd, The Atrium, Southern Gate, Chichester, West Sussex, PO19 8SQ, UK

Editorial Offices
9600 Garsington Road, Oxford, OX4 2DQ, UK
The Atrium, Southern Gate, Chichester, West Sussex, PO19 8SQ, UK
111 River Street, Hoboken, NJ 07030-5774, USA

For details of our global editorial offices, for customer services and for information about how to apply for permission to reuse the copyright material in this book please see our website at www.wiley.com/wiley-blackwell

Library of Congress Cataloging-in-Publication Data

Saksena, Franklin B., author.
Patient studies in valvular, congenital, and rarer forms of cardiovascular disease: an integrative approach / Franklin B. Saksena.
p. ; cm.
Includes indexes.
ISBN 978-1-118-46979-8 (pbk.)
I. Title.
[DNLM: 1. Cardiovascular Diseases–diagnosis–Case Reports. 2. Diagnosis, Differential–Case Reports. WG 141]
RC670
616.1′075–dc23

2014049380

A catalogue record for this book is available from the British Library.

Wiley also publishes its books in a variety of electronic formats. Some content that appears in print may not be available in electronic books.

Cover images repeated from figures within the book. See figure captions for more details. Top left-hand image: Figure 6.5. Bottom left-hand image: Figure 57.1. Middle image: Figure 36.8. Right-hand image: Figure 28.8.

Set in 9/12pt Meridien by SPi Publisher Services, Pondicherry, India
Printed and bound in Singapore by Markono Print Media Pte Ltd

1 2015

CONTENTS

The year the patient was first seen is shown in brackets

The year the patient was first seen is shown in brackets

ABOUT THE AUTHOR

Franklin B. Saksena, MD, CM, FACP, FRCP(C), FACC, FAHA and member of the American society of Echocardiography.

Dr Saksena served as a Senior Attending Physician in the Department of Cardiology at Stroger Hospital of Cook County, Chicago for over 32 years. He remains active at Stroger Hospital of Cook County as a Voluntary Attending Physician in Adult Cardiology. While working for Stroger Hospital of Cook County he was Director of the Cardiac Catheterization laboratory and for a period was Acting Chief of Cardiology.

Dr Saksena is currently an Associate Professor of Clinical Medicine at Northwestern University and an Assistant Professor of Medicine at Rush Medical School. He also maintains a part-time private practice in Cardiology and Internal Medicine at the Swedish Covenant Hospital and St Mary of Nazareth hospital.

Educated in England, Canada and the USA, Dr Saksena obtained his medical degree at Queen's University, Kingston, Ontario, Canada. He spent a total of 6 months in Pathology (Queen's University and University of Chicago). He was a Pulmonary Fellow at the University of Chicago for 2 years and spent 3 years as a Cardiology fellow (Northwestern Medical school and Toronto University hospitals).

Dr Saksena enjoys teaching physical diagnosis to medical students and residents and endeavors to apply deductions to bedside diagnosis that draw upon the reasoning and observation skills made famous by the well-known character of Sherlock Holmes. He has won a number of awards for excellence in teaching cardiology and physical diagnosis to medical students and residents and is much sought after by medical students and those in the MD PhD program.

Dr Saksena authored a monograph entitled *Hemodynamics in Cardiology: Calculations and Interpretations* (Praeger Scientific, New York, 1983), and a second monograph entitled *Color Atlas of Local and Systemic Signs of Cardiovascular Disease* (Blackwell Publishing, 2008). A medical textbook, *The Art and Science of Cardiac Physical Diagnosis* by Drs Ranganathan, Sivacyan and Saksena was published in 2006 (Humana Press, Totowa, NJ).

As a Sherlock Holmes enthusiast and a member of the highly regarded Baker Street Irregulars, he has published Sherlock Holmes crossword puzzle books: *101 Sherlock Holmes Crossword Puzzles* in 2000, and *101 More Sherlock Holmes Crossword Puzzles* in 2011, both of which were published by the Battered Silicon Dispatch Box in Canada.

PREFACE

A number of cardiology training programs emphasize coronary artery disease and tend to neglect other aspects of cardiology, such as valvular, congenital heart, or vascular disease. I would like to redress this imbalance by reiterating the importance of history and physical findings in detecting valvular, congenital, or vascular disease, and to correlate the clinical findings to invasive and non-invasive studies. I believe that this approach will be useful to cardiologists in training as well as to cardiologists interested in problem solving. Recognition of auscultatory findings is now one of the requirements for candidates sitting for the Cardiology Board examinations.

Each patient study consists of the following sections: history, physical examination, phonocardiography (whenever possible), ECG, chest X ray, echocardiography, hemodynamics, and sometimes angiography. In order to challenge the reader, these sections may or may not be randomized. Readers should write an interpretation for each section as well as answering the questions posed. They may then compare their results with my comments, which are given at the end of each chapter. At the beginning of the book is a worked example giving a step-by-step solution.

This method of teaching has been used by many clinicians, including Dr Willis Hurst [1, 2], as it allows the reader to fit the data together and come to a conclusion. The reader is less likely to sift the data carefully if the diagnosis is revealed as a chapter heading or on the same page as the clinical information. Giving the diagnosis away at the start of the presentation is analogous to reading the last chapter of a mystery novel first, and what challenge is that to the problem solver?

The patient studies have been arranged in approximately chronological order from 1966 to 2013, with emphasis on establishing a likely diagnosis based on the tools available at that time. The approximate dates when a test became generally available in the Chicago area are as follows:

Coronary angiography:	late 1960s
M-mode echocardiography:	early 1970s
two-dimensional echocardiography:	late 1970s
Doppler echocardiography:	1980s
Transesophageal echocardiography:	late 1980s
CT angiography of chest, single slice:	early 1990s
CT angiography of chest, multislice:	late 1990s

The latter part of the book contains several studies in which the ECG, chest X ray, and echocardiography provide diagnostic information that was undetected by physical examination.

References

[1] Hurst JW, Lutz JF. Clinical essays on the heart. Volume 4 Correlative Cardiology, New York, McGraw Hill, 1984.

[2] Hurst JW. Cardiac Puzzles Parts 1 and 2. St Louis, Mosby-Yearbook Inc,1995.

ACKNOWLEDGMENTS

I would like to thank the following Physicians for supplying data on their patients:

- Dr D. Deano: patient 51
- Dr K. Duque: patients 52, 53, 64
- Dr Goritsas and Dr Curran: patient 63
- Dr M. Klodnycky : patients 20, 13w, 56, 64
- Dr R. Reddy: patient 13w
- Dr O'Campo, Dr Imman, Dr Jolly, and Dr Yadav: patient 62
- Dr J. Shapiro and Dr S. S. Kim: patient 46
- Dr Z. Naheed for pediatric echocardiograms (Figures 9–11, 43a–11, and 47–22).

I would like to thank Dr M. Bhorade, Dr V. Vedam, and Dr B. Deal for their comments on some portions of the manuscript as well as the radiological advice of Dr J. Connolly. I would also like to thank Dr Ian Carr for past advice on patients with congenital heart disease. I remain responsible for any errors in the text and images in this book. I thank all the physicians and technicians who were involved in the invasive and noninvasive procedures.

I would like to thank my son, Gordon, for computer assistance. He saved my data when the computer crashed and rebuilt a computer with double its usual memory capacity. I would like to thank my wife, Kathleen, and my daughter, Marian, for doing some of the proofreading. My wife Kathleen was very supportive throughout the writing of this book. She tolerated the mounds of journals that were several feet high and having the house turned once again into a mini Library of Congress.

I owe a debt of gratitude to the librarians, Lizabeth Giese and Mary Lasquety, for finding important references for me. I also appreciate the invaluable help of Eric Basir in the preparation of the images for publication.

I am very thankful for the cordial and patient cooperation of the staff members at Wiley Blackwell, especially Claire Bonnett and Andrew Hallam, as well as Elisabeth Dodds, Julie Elliott, and Thomas Hartman.

I am also grateful to Patty Donovan and Lesley Montford.

ABBREVIATIONS

5HIAA hydroxyindolacetic acid

AA ascending aorta
AAA abdominal aortic aneurysm
AAW anterior aortic wall
AC aortic cusps
ACG apex cardiogram
AD aortic dissection
ALA accessory left atrium
Ao aorta
AP anteroposterior (chest X ray view)
AR aortic regurgitation
ASD atrial septal defect
ASH asymmetric septal hypertrophy
AV arterio-venous *or* atrio-ventricular
AVA aortic valve area

B/F black/female or African –American female (the latter term is in more common use now)
BP blood pressure
BSA body surface area
BUN blood urea nitrogen

CABG coronary artery bypass graft
CAD coronary artery disease
Cao arterial oxygen content
CCP chronic constrictive pericarditis
CCU critical care unit
CHD congenital heart disease
CI cardiac index
CNS central nervous system
CO cardiac output
COPD chronic obstructive pulmonary disease
Cpa pulmonary artery oxygen content
CPK creatine phosphokinase
CR carotid pulse
CT computed tomography
C/T cardiothoracic ratio
CVA cerebral vascular accident

D dicrotic notch
DE the slope DE is the opening mitral diastolic velocity (M-mode echocardiography)
dfp diastolic filling period

ECG electrocardiogram
EF the slope EF is the closing mitral valve velocity (M-mode echocardiography)
EKG electrocardiogram
E&O onset of ejection and mitral valve opening respectively (in ACG)
ER emergency room
ESR erythrocyte sedimentation rate
EVR endovascular graft repair

FA femoral artery

G1 gravida 1
GI gastrointestinal

Hb hemoglobin
HCM hypertrophic cardiomyopathy
HEENT head-ears-eyes –nose -throat
HR heart rate

ic intercostal space
ICD implantable cardioverter defibrillator
IF intimal flap
IRBBB incomplete right bundle branch block
IV intravenous
IVC inferior vena cava
IVCD intraventricular conduction delay
IVDA IV drug abuser
IVS interventricular septum

LA left atrium
LAD left anterior descending coronary artery
LAE left atrial enlargement
LAO left anterior oblique
LCFA left common femoral artery
LDPA left dorsalis pedis artery
LIMA left internal mammary artery
LLL left lower lobe
LLSB left lower sternal border
LPOPA left popliteal artery
LPTA left posterior tibial artery
LUSB left upper sternal border
LV left ventricle
LVEDP left ventricular end-diastolic pressure

LVEF LV ejection fraction
LVH left ventricular hypertrophy
LVOT left ventricular outflow tract

MDG mean mitral diastolic gradient
MFH malignant fibrous histiocytoma
MI myocardial infarction
MR mitral regurgitation
MRA magnetic resonance angiography
MRI magnetic resonance imaging
msg mean systolic gradient
MUGA multiple-gated acquisition
MV mitral valve
MVA mitral valve area
MVP mitral valve prolapse

P percussion wave
P1 para 1
PA pulmonary artery *or* postero-anterior (chest X ray)
PAC premature atrial contraction
PADP PA diastolic pressure
PAW pulmonary artery wedge
PDA persistent ductus arteriosus
PKD polycystic kidney disease
PPD purified protein derivative
PR pulmonary regurgitation
PS pulmonary stenosis
PTCA percutaneous transluminal coronary angioplasty
PV pulmonary vein
PVC premature ventricular contraction
PVD peripheral vascular disease
PVR pulmonary vascular resistance

Q_p pulmonary blood flow
Q_s systemic blood flow

R respiratory rate
RA right atrium
RAE right atrial enlargement
RAO right anterior oblique
RBBB right bundle branch block
RBC red blood cell
RCA right coronary artery
RCFA right common femoral artery
RCT cardiac resynchronization therapy
RDPA right dorsalis pedis artery
RFP rapid filling phase (seen in ACG)
RLL right lower lobe
RLSB right lower sternal border
RPOPA right popliteal artery
RPTA right posterior tibial artery
RR respiratory rate
RSV ruptured sinus of valsalva
RUSB right upper sternal border
RV right ventricle
RVEDP right ventricular end-diastolic pressure
RVH right ventricular hypertrophy
RVOT right ventricular outflow tract
RVSP RV systolic pressure

S1 first heart sound
S2 second heart sound
S3 third heart sound
SAI systolic area index
SAM systolic anterior motion of the mitral valve
SEM systolic ejection murmur
sep systolic ejection period
SLP slow filling phase
SV stroke volume
SVC superior vena cava
SVR systemic vascular resistance

T temperature
T tidal wave
TA tricuspid atresia
TA Takayasu's arteritis
TB tuberculosis
TC Tako-tsubo cardiomyopathy
TEE Transesophageal echocardiography
TIBC total iron binding capacity
TOF Tetralogy of Fallot
t-PA tissue plasminogen activator
TR tricuspid regurgitation
TSH thyroid stimulating hormone

U/S ultrasound

VA ventricular aneurysm
VDRL Venereal Disease Research Laboratory
VO_2 oxygen consumption
V/Q ventilation /blood flow
VSD ventricular septal defect
VT ventricular tachycardia

WBC white blood count
WPW Wolff–Parkinson–White

Orientation symbols

A anterior
I inferior
L left
P posterior
R right
S superior

WORKED EXAMPLE

The following worked example shows how the author envisages that readers shall work through each patient case.

The author's comments are shown in **bold** type.

Example answers that the reader might give are shown in *italics*.

Questions and action points are shown in *red italics*.

Numbers within square brackets refer to the references at the end of each chapter.

The reader should review and interpret the data sequentially, and compare their answers to mine, which are given at the end of each chapter.

15-year-old man admitted with chest pain and a chest deformity in 1977.

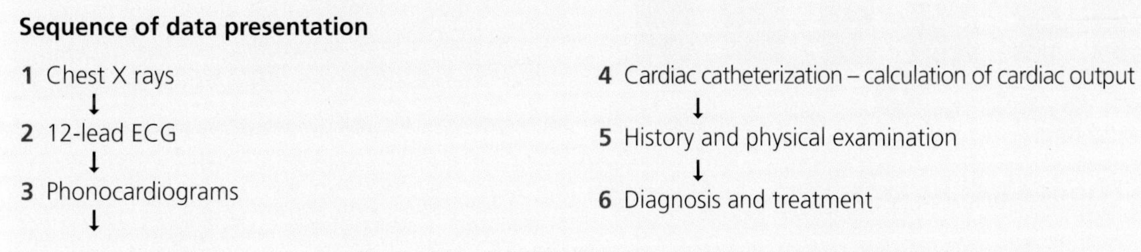

Sequence of data presentation

1 Chest X rays
↓
2 12-lead ECG
↓
3 Phonocardiograms
↓
4 Cardiac catheterization – calculation of cardiac output
↓
5 History and physical examination
↓
6 Diagnosis and treatment

1 Chest X rays

PA chest X ray (Figure WE.1a)

This shows a very large left PA, which probably represents post-stenotic dilatation of the left PA, as seen in pulmonic stenosis. The C/T ratio is normal (0.42). As the LA is not well seen mitral stenosis cannot be excluded. The clear lung fields tend to exclude a significant left to right shunt or any pulmonary congestion.

Most patients with pulmonary stenosis have a left-sided aortic arch, as in this patient. A right-sided arch might suggest a coexistent TOF.

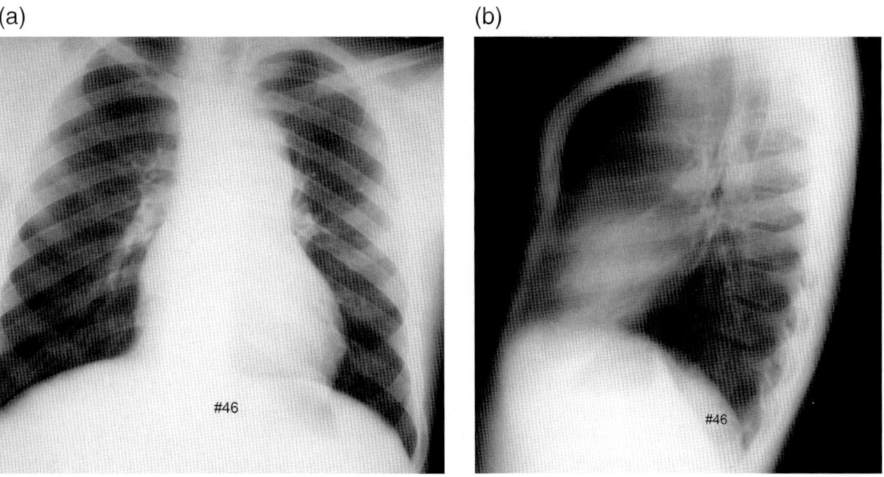

Figure WE.1 (a) PA chest X-ray. (b) Lateral chest X-ray.

Lateral chest X ray (Figure WE.1b)

There is anterior bulging of the upper sternum, which could be an isolated phenomenon but is known to be associated with long standing RVH. No dilatation is seen of the RV in this view. So far the diagnosis points to pulmonary stenosis with severe RVH.

2 12-lead ECG

The patient has severe RVH and right atrial enlargement.

There are tall pointed P waves in 2, 3, F due to right atrial enlargement.

There is marked right-axis deviation (+130°).

The R wave height in lead V1 in a normal 15-year-old male is usually about 0.6 mv (range 0–1.6 mv). The R wave in V1 in our 15-year-old patient is monophasic and very tall (3 mv). R waves of this height, along with inverted T waves in V1–4, are often associated with suprasystemic RV systolic pressures.

R waves this tall in V1 are commonly seen in severe pulmonic stenosis and in my experience are unusual in mitral stenosis or pulmonary embolism.

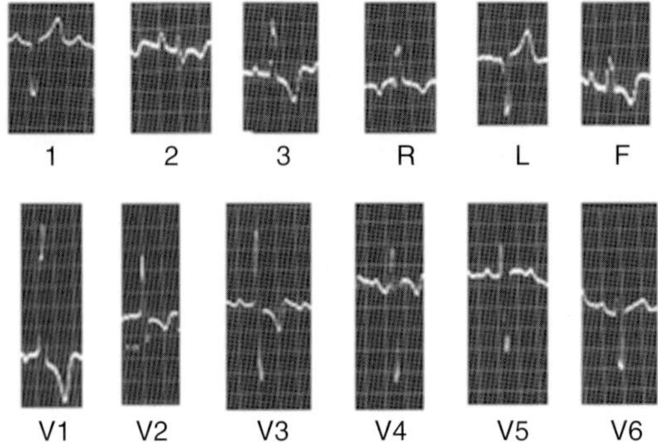

Figure WE.2 12-lead ECG rate 100/min. Normal standardization in limb leads, V1, V3–6. Half standardization in V2.

3 Phonocardiograms

Phonocardiogram at apex and simultaneous RV and aortic pressures

There is a prominent S4, which has a similar amplitude to the S1. S2 has a smaller amplitude than S1. Splitting of S2 is not well seen. The RV pressure greatly exceeds the aortic pressure, which correlates well with the tall R wave in V1 (Figure WE.2).

These findings indicate severe RV hypertension and a non-compliant ventricle (most likely RV). The systolic murmur is not well recorded at the apex.

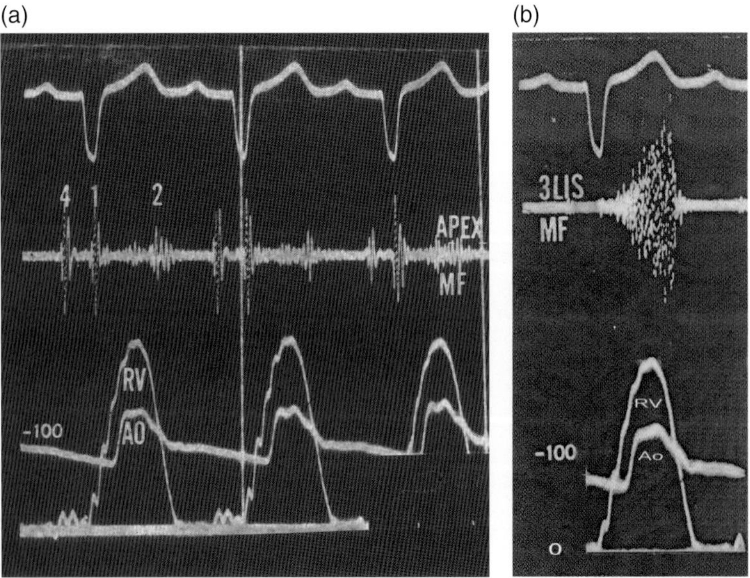

Figure WE.3 (a) Phonocardiogram at apex and simultaneous RV and aortic pressures. 0–100 mmHg scale. (b) Phonocardiogram at left 3rd interspace parasternally and simultaneous RV and aortic pressures. 0–100 mmHg scale.

Phonocardiogram at left 3rd interspace parasternally and simultaneous RV and aortic pressures

The systolic murmur shows late peaking in the left 3rd interspace, indicating severe pulmonic stenosis.

4 Cardiac catheterization – calculation of cardiac output

There is a peak gradient in systole across the pulmonic valve of 183 mmHg, indicative of severe pulmonic stenosis. The a wave in the RA pressure tracing is slightly elevated to 9 mmHg. Left heart pressures are normal **(LA had been entered via a patent foramen ovale)**. *Simultaneous samples of blood from the RA, PA, and ascending aorta were within normal limits and thus tend to rule out a cardiac shunt.*

Calculation of the cardiac output

Data

Hemoglobin 12 gm%, SvO_2 70%, SaO_2 96%, VO_2 174 mL/min (from the legend of Figure WE.4)

Hints

1 Find the oxyhemoglobin carrying capacity.
2 Convert the PA and aortic oxygen saturations to oxygen contents.
3 Obtain the AV O_2 difference.
4 Calculate the cardiac output from the O_2 consumption and the AV O_2 difference.

Step 1: Find the oxyhemoglobin carrying capacity
1 g of hemoglobin combines with 1.36 m of O_2, so we have 12 g of hemoglobin combining with 12 × 1.36 or 17.6 vol% (or mL oxygen per 100 mL of blood).

Step 2: Convert oxygen saturations to oxygen content
oxygen content = percentage saturation × oxyhemoglobin carrying capacity
Thus PA O_2 content = 70% of 17.6 vol% = 12.4 vol%
Aortic O_2 content = 96% of 17.6 vol% = 16.9 vol%

Step 3: Calculate the AV oxygen content difference
16.9–12.4 - 4.5 vol%, i.e. 45 volumes per liter of blood

Step 4: Calculate the Fick cardiac output (CO)

$$CO = \frac{\text{oxygen consumption}}{\text{AV oxygen difference}} = \frac{174 \text{ mL/min}}{45 \text{ mL/L}} = 3.86 \text{ L/min}$$

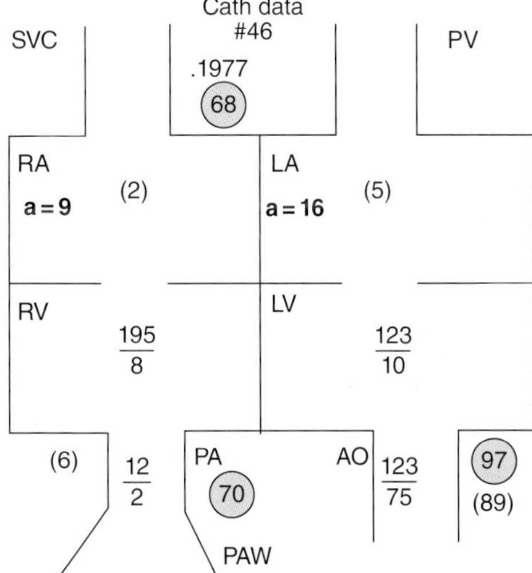

Figure WE.4 Cardiac catheterization data. Numbers in brackets are mean pressures (mmHg). Numerators in RV and LV are systolic pressures, denominators in the ventricles are end-diastolic pressures, and denominators in the aortic and pulmonary arteries are diastolic pressures (mmHg). Numbers in circles are percentage oxygen saturations. RV angiography confirmed the presence of valvular pulmonic stenosis.

What is the cardiac output if the hemogloblin is 13 g%, the oxygen consumption is 174 mL/min, the PA saturation is 70%, and the aortic oxygen saturation is 96%?

5 History and physical examination

15-year-old male with a history of chest pain and easy fatiguability. The chest pain was unrelated to exertion. No history of rheumatic fever. He had a long-standing chest deformity.

Physical examination revealed a 58 inches tall youth weighing 75 lb. BP 107/63. HR 100/min regular.

There were prominent 'a' waves in the neck, pectus carinatum.

Prominent RV lift (2+ out of 3+).

S1 normal. P2 not heard. No ejection click.

Grade 4/6 systolic murmur best heart at the 2nd left interspace with radiation over most of the precordium.

Lungs clear. Normal peripheral pulses. No cyanosis or clubbing.

The patient had a prominent 'a' wave in the jugular venous pulse, which could be due to pulmonary stenosis, pulmonary hypertension, or tricuspid stenosis. The RV lift reflects RV hypertension or possibly pulmonary hypertension. Pulmonary hypertension is unlikely as the P2 is barely audible.

A systolic murmur heard best in the 3rd left interspace parasternally could be due to an ASD or pulmonic stenosis. An ASD is unlikely as there was no wide fixed splitting of the second sound, no pulmonary vascular congestion, and severe RV hypertension is quite unusual.

The late peaking of the pulmonary systolic murmur along with an inaudible P2 favor severe pulmonic stenosis.

6 Diagnosis and treatment

Severe pulmonic stenosis.

Pulmonary valve surgery.

Once readers have analysed the patient data and performed the necessary calculations they can compare their answers to mine given at the end of the book. Often the answers are followed by a discussion, key points, and references.

Key points

1. A prominent 'a' wave in the neck veins, RV lift, late peaking of a pulmonary systolic murmur, and absent P2 are features of severe pulmonary stenosis.
2. A tall monophasic R wave in V1, right-axis deviation, and right atrial enlargement also favor significant pulmonary stenosis.

COMPANION WEBSITE

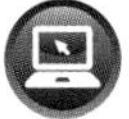 A companion website for this book is available at **www.wiley.com/go/saksena/patientstudies**

The website contains a further 24 Online Patient Studies. Some of these are linked to Patient Studies in the printed book and are noted as such. Below is the full contents list for the Online Patient Studies.

- Online Patient Study 1 24-year-old female with dyspnea and jaundice after surgery (1970)
- Online Patient Study 2 41-year-old man with dyspnea and dark urine after surgery (1970)
- Online Patient Study 3 66-year-old female with recurrent heart failure (1970)
- Online Patient Study 4 39-year-old man with hemoptysis and dyspnea (1974)
- Online Patient Study 5 46-year-old man and the perils of walking in the street (1974)
- Online Patient Studies 6–8 47-year-old man with left-sided chest pain (1975); 51-year-old man with chest pain and hypertension (1984); 52-year-old man with dyspnea and mental confusion (2004)
- Online Patient Study 9 72-year-old female with dyspnea and anasarca (1977)
- Online Patient Study 10 61-year-old man with chest pain and syncope (1976)
- Online Patient Study 11 17-year-old female with dyspnea, a heart murmur, and cardiomegaly (1992)
- Online Patient Study 12 24-year-old man with a heart murmur (1970)
- Online Patient Study 13 19-year-old female with leg pain and headaches (1985)
- Online Patient Study 14 43-year-old female with dyspnea, palpitations, and syncope (1989)
- Online Patient Study 15 18-year-old female with fatigue and a life-long murmur (1999)
- Online Patient Study 16 56-year-old female with abdominal pain and an abnormal ECG (2009)
- Online Patient Study 17 69-year-old man with lower extremity pain (2003)
- Online Patient Study 18 Asymptomatic young man with an unusual chest X ray (1960s)
- Online Patient Study 19 68-year-old man with chest pain and bradycardia (1994)
- Online Patient Study 20 73-year-old man with an ischemic cardiomyopathy (2013)
- Online Patient Study 21 89-year-old man with a non-functioning pacemaker (1997)
- Online Patient Study 22 Elderly man with a VVI pacemaker (1978)
- Online Patient Studies 23–24 56-year-old man who has a pacemaker unattached to the heart (2009); 50-year-old man with two pacemakers (2010)

The year the patient was first seen is shown in brackets

1 PATIENT STUDY 1

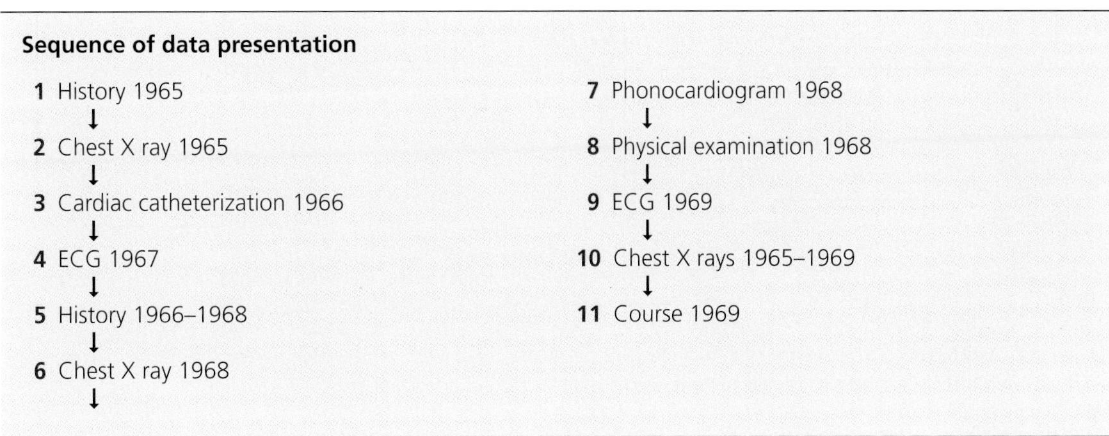

Sequence of data presentation

1 History 1965
↓
2 Chest X ray 1965
↓
3 Cardiac catheterization 1966
↓
4 ECG 1967
↓
5 History 1966–1968
↓
6 Chest X ray 1968
↓
7 Phonocardiogram 1968
↓
8 Physical examination 1968
↓
9 ECG 1969
↓
10 Chest X rays 1965–1969
↓
11 Course 1969

1 History 1965

This patient is a chronic alcoholic. He was told of a heart murmur at age 20 in 1939 and has had dyspnea on exertion since that time. He has had two admissions for heart failure, in 1962 and 1964.

2 Chest X ray 1965

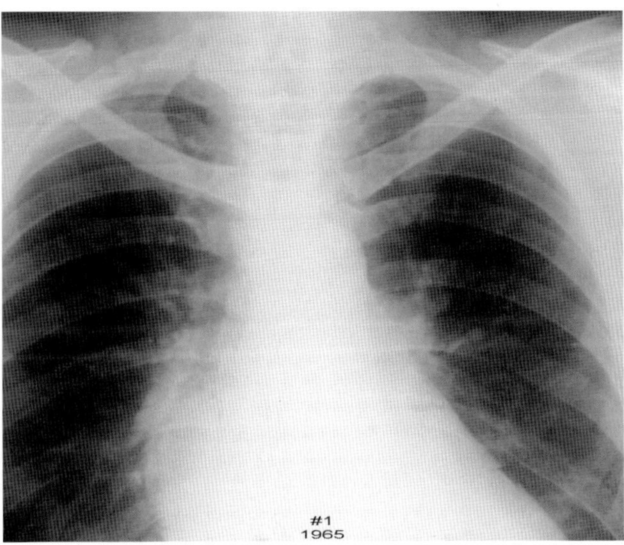

Figure 1.1 Chest X ray 1965.

Patient Studies in Valvular, Congenital, and Rarer Forms of Cardiovascular Disease: An Integrative Approach, First Edition. Franklin B. Saksena.

Companion Website: www.wiley.com/go/saksena/patientstudies

3 Cardiac catheterization 1966

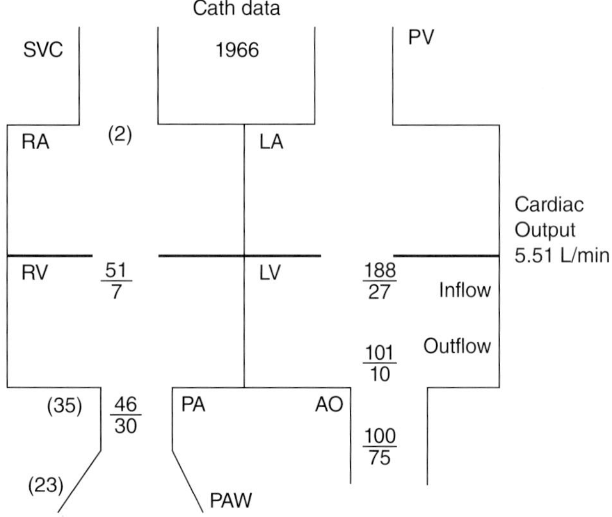

Figure 1.2 Cardiac catheterization data 1966. Numbers in brackets are mean pressures (mmHg), numbers in the denominators are end-diastolic pressures in the ventricles and diastolic pressures in the pulmonary artery and aorta.

Table 1.1 Additional cardiac catheterization data 1966
LVH, left atrial enlargement, subaortic chamber, MR
Normal aortic root angiogram

4 ECG 1967

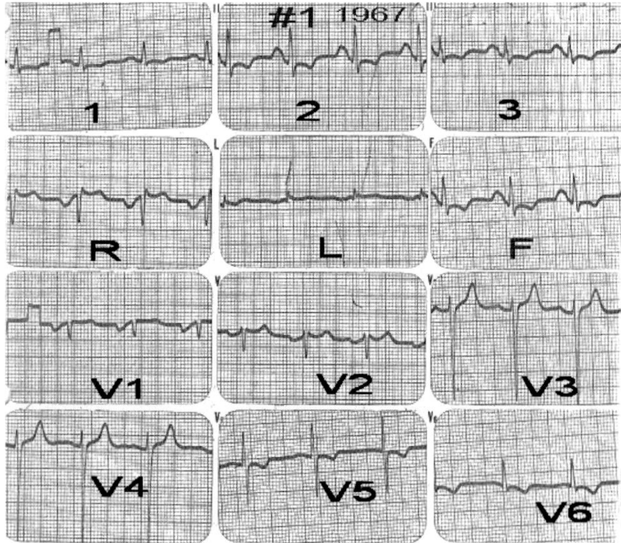

Figure 1.3 ECG 1967.

5 History 1966–1968

The patient was offered surgery in 1966 for hypertrophic subaortic stenosis but refused. He was treated with diuretics warfarin and digoxin, and advised to stop drinking alcohol. He was diagnosed as having schizophrenia in 1967.

The patient has had intermittent atrial fibrillation since 1966.

In 1968 he returned to hospital with exertional dyspnea.

6 Chest X ray 1968

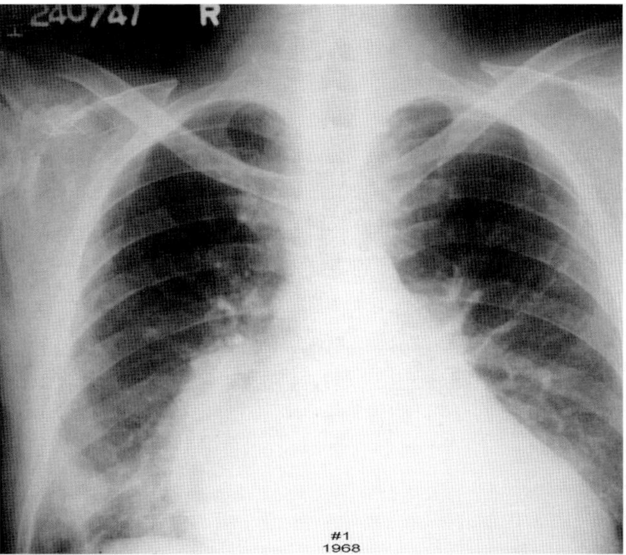

Figure 1.4 Chest X ray 1968.

7 Phonocardiogram 1968

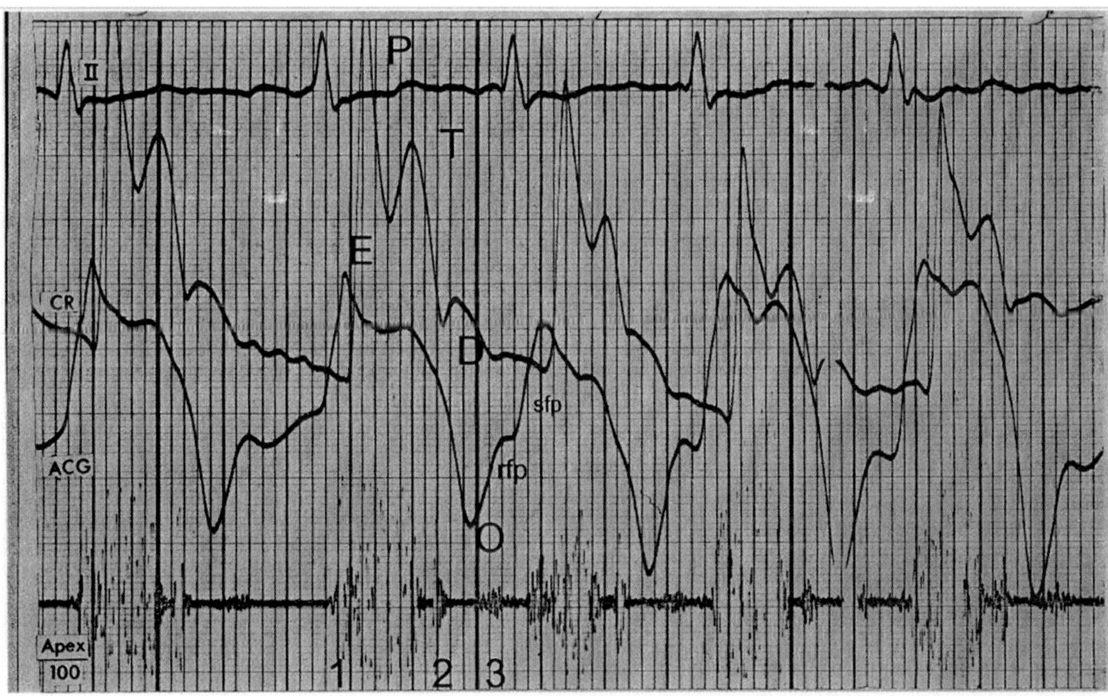

Figure 1.5 Phonocardiogram of carotid pulse and apexcardiogram 1968. Carotid pulse: D = dicrotic notch; P = percussion wave; T = tidal wave. Apex cardiogram (ACG): rfp = rapid filling phase; sfp = slow filling phase; E&O correspond to onset of ejection & mitral valve opening respectively.

8 Physical examination 1968

BP 160/90, HR 100/min.
No increase in jugular venous pressure. Prominent 'a' wave in neck veins.
Pulsus bisferiens.
Apex was in the 6th interspace in the anterior axillary line. RV lift 1+.

S1–1 decreased. S2 paradoxically split. S3 and S4 at apex.
Grade 4/6 systolic murmur with ejection/pansystolic quality, best heard at LLSB, radiating to apex and axilla.
The murmur increased in intensity with a valsalva maneuver.
No edema or clubbing.
A few rhonchi were heard in the lung fields.

9 ECG 1969

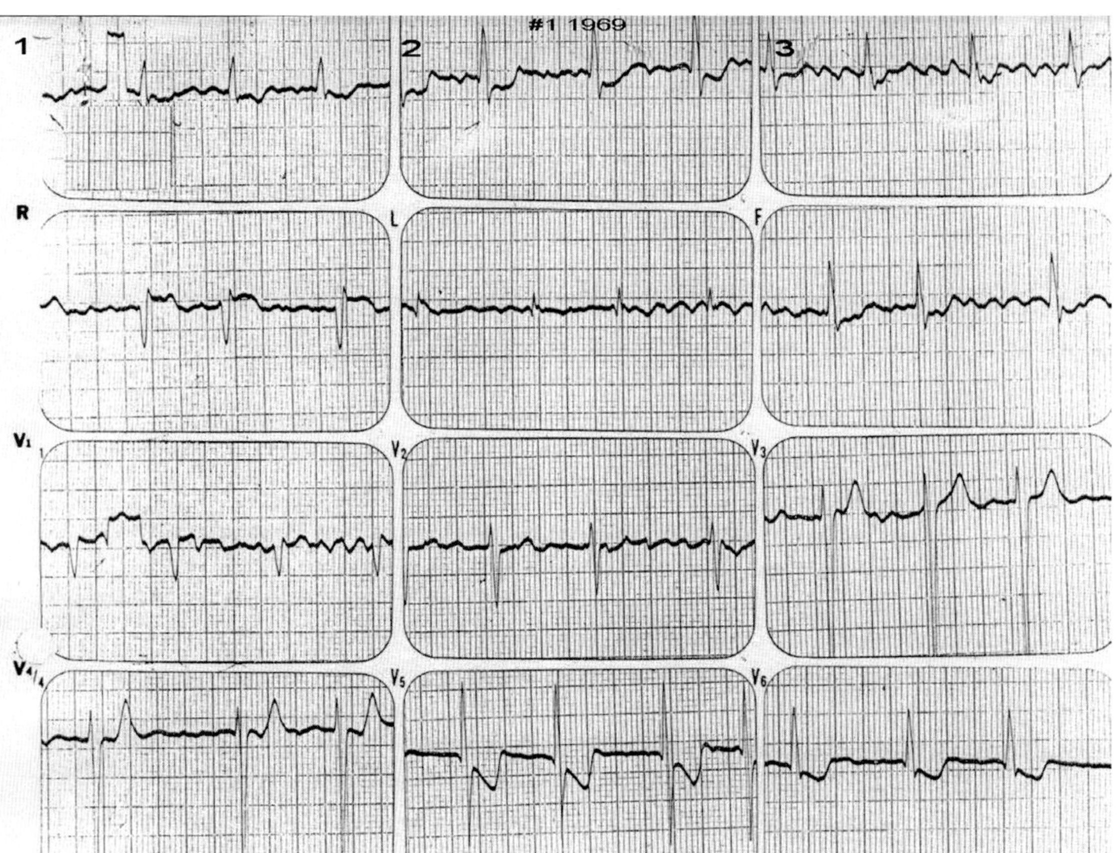

Figure 1.6 ECG 1969.

10 Chest X rays 1965–1969

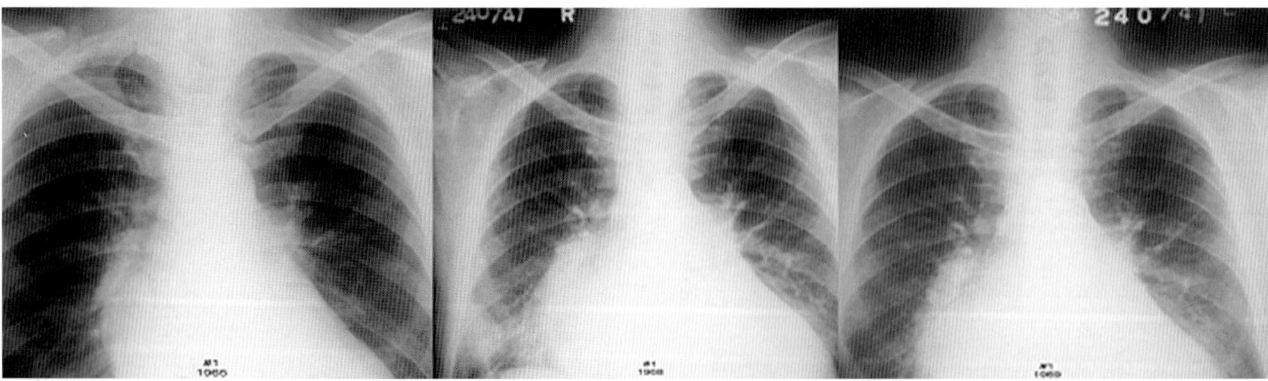

Figure 1.7 Chest X rays 1965–1969.

11 Course 1969

The patient had recurrent heart failure and atrial fibrillation, and died suddenly in 1969.

What would you expect to find at autopsy?

Answers and commentary

1 History 1965

The patient had a heart murmur and heart failure, which could be due to valvular heart disease. Alcoholic cardiomyopathy might also account for his symptoms of heart failure.

2 Chest X ray 1965

The heart is probably enlarged and there are increased lung markings. The entire lung fields are not fully seen for technical reasons.

3 Cardiac catheterization 1966

This showed moderately severe pulmonary hypertension (PA mean of 35 mmHg), a systolic gradient of 87 mmHg between LV inflow and LV outflow tracts, and no gradient in systolic across the aortic valve. The cardiac index was normal. There was LVH, LAE, and mitral regurgitation. Coronary angiography was not available at this time.

Impression: hypertrophic subaortic stenosis.

4 ECG 1967

The ECG shows sinus rhythm. Rate 78/min. PR 0.16 s. QRS 0.09 s. QRS axis +50°, LVH with repolarization abnormalities and left atrial enlargement.

5 History 1966–1968

The patient continues to have evidence of heart failure. As he had refused surgery he was treated with anti-congestive measures and anticoagulants.

6 Chest X ray 1968

There is now cardiomegaly with enlargement of the proximal PAs and some pulmonary congestion, which would account for his dyspnea.

7 Phonocardiogram 1968

The carotid pulse shows a rapid upstroke, a bisferiens pulse with the percussion (P) wave being much taller than the tidal (T) wave. There is a diamond-shaped systolic murmur recorded at the apex and an apical S3.

A bisferiens pulse with a taller percussion wave than the tidal wave is characteristic of HCM. The other cause of a bisferiens pulse is seen in aortic regurgitation, but in that case the P wave and T wave are about equal. The presence of a systolic murmur rather than a diastolic murmur (of aortic regurgitation) makes it even more likely that HCM is the correct diagnosis.

The rapid carotid upstroke is also characteristic of LV outflow obstruction rather than aortic stenosis. In aortic stenosis the carotid upstroke is delayed and is of decreased amplitude (pulsus parvus et tardus).

The presence of an S3 is unusual in HCM, but in this case is probably due to LV dysfunction.

8 Physical examination 1968

The history of alcoholism and heart failure could represent an alcoholic cardiomyopathy. The physical examination, however, is more in favor of HCM in view of the apical systolic murmur that increases with stage 2 valsalva maneuver and the bisferiens carotid pulse detected on phonocardiography.

The presence of moderate cardiomegaly is unusual in HCM but may be seen in advanced cases.

9 ECG 1969

Ventricular rate: 70–80/min. QRS 0.08 s. QRS axis +50°. Further ST depression and sagging noted due to LVH and digoxin effect.

Atrial fibrillation is now seen.

10 Chest X rays 1965–1969

There is a progressive increase in cardiac size and pulmonary congestion.

11 Course 1969

The loss of the atrial contribution to cardiac output in a patient with a stiff LV (due to LVH) led to progressive heart failure. His sudden death in 1969 was probably due to a ventricular arrhythmia.

At autopsy the heart weighed 850 g. He had HCM with a dilated LA full of thrombi. There was evidence of peripheral emboli (kidneys, left temporal area), possibly because he was not taking anticoagulants on a regular basis (alcoholism, schizophrenia). There was pulmonary congestion but no pulmonary embolism. There was no significant coronary artery disease.

Key points

1. The presence of a rapid carotid upstroke and an aortic systolic murmur that increases during the valsalva maneuver is suggestive of HCM.
2. The loss of the atrial contribution to cardiac output (due to atrial fibrillation) may precipitate LV failure.
3. Patients with HCM may die suddenly from ventricular arrhythmias.
4. Anticoagulants are indicated in patients with atrial fibrillation, but may not be advisable if the patient is an alcoholic and has a mental disorder.

Further reading

Ommen SR, Nishimura RA. Hypertrophic cardiomyopathy. *Curr Probl Cardiol* 2004; 29: 235–289 (270 references).

2 PATIENT STUDY 2

Sequence of data presentation

1 History 1973 and 1984
↓
2 ECG 1973
↓
3 Chest X ray 1973
↓
4 LV and aortic pressure curves 1973
↓
5 Intracardiac pressures 1973 and 1984
↓
6 Additional hemodynamic data 1973 and 1984
↓
7 Right and left heart catheters 1973
↓
8 Oxygen saturation sample run 1973 and 1984
↓
9 Cardiogreen dye curves 1973
↓
10 LAO aortogram 1973
↓
11 Physical examination 1973
↓
12 Physical examination 1984
↓
13 Echocardiogram 1984
↓
14 ECG 1984
↓
15 Chest X ray 1984
↓
16 Coronary angiography 1984
↓
17 Aortography 1984
↓
18 Follow-up 1984–2003

1 History 1973 and 1984

24-year-old man first seen in 1973 because of a heart murmur found on a pre-employment physical examination. He had mild dyspnea on playing basketball. No history of rheumatic fever, chest pain, or syncope.

He underwent a diagnostic work-up in 1973 but was lost to follow-up for 11 years.

In 1984 he returned to hospital with dyspnea and leg edema.

2 ECG 1973

Heart rate 125/min. PR interval 0.18 s. QRS interval 0.08 s. QRS axis +75°. R in V1 + S in V6 = 5.3 mv.

Patient Studies in Valvular, Congenital, and Rarer Forms of Cardiovascular Disease: An Integrative Approach, First Edition. Franklin B. Saksena.

Companion Website: www.wiley.com/go/saksena/patientstudies

3 Chest X ray 1973

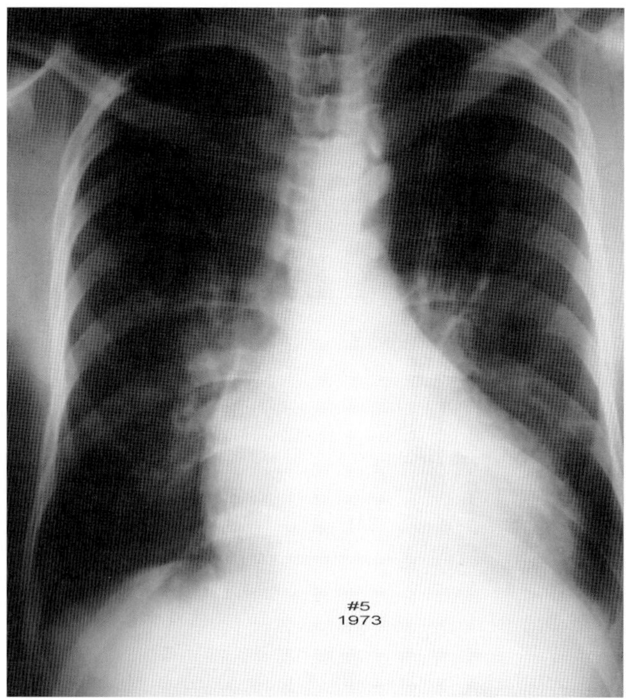

Figure 2.1 Chest X ray 1973.

4 LV and aortic pressure curves 1973

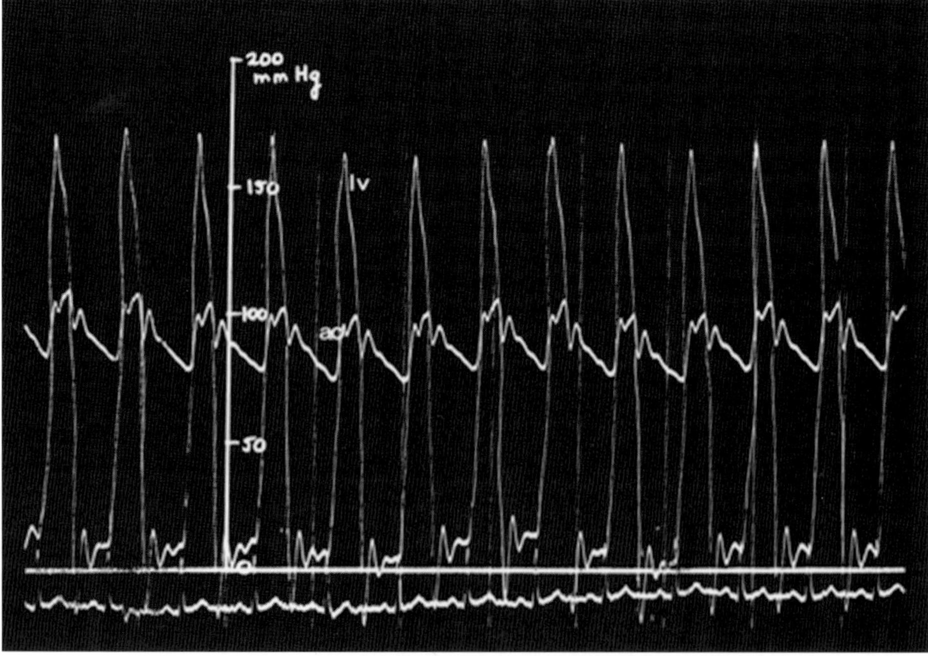

Figure 2.2 Simultaneous LV and aortic pressures.

5 Intracardiac pressures 1973 and 1984

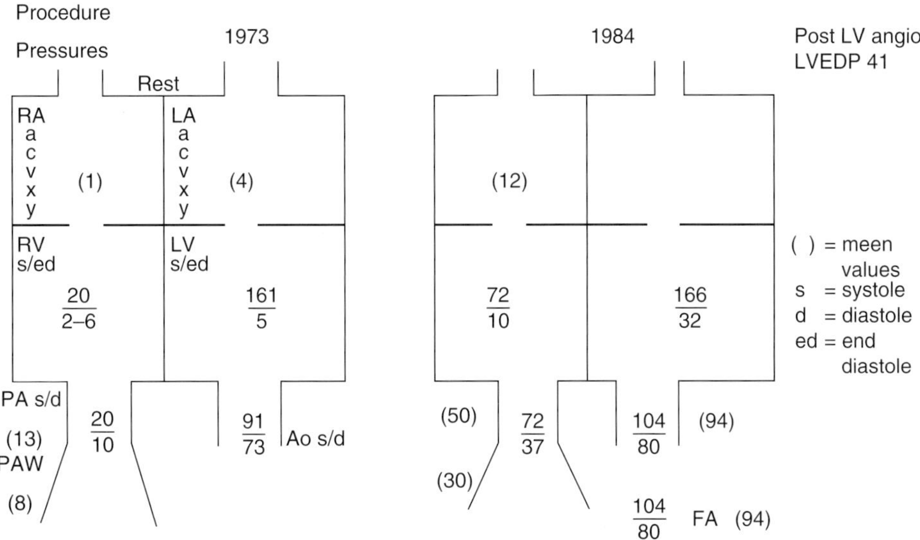

Figure 2.3 Pressures 1973 and 1984.

6 Additional hemodynamic data 1973 and 1984

Table 2.1 Pressure and flow and valve area measurements 1973 and 1984

	1973	1984
Cardiac index (L/min/m^2)	4.75	2.56
Mean systolic aortic gradient (mmHg)	42	50
Aortic valve area (cm^2)	1.5	0.5
LV ejection fraction	Normal	0.35

7 Right and left heart catheters 1973

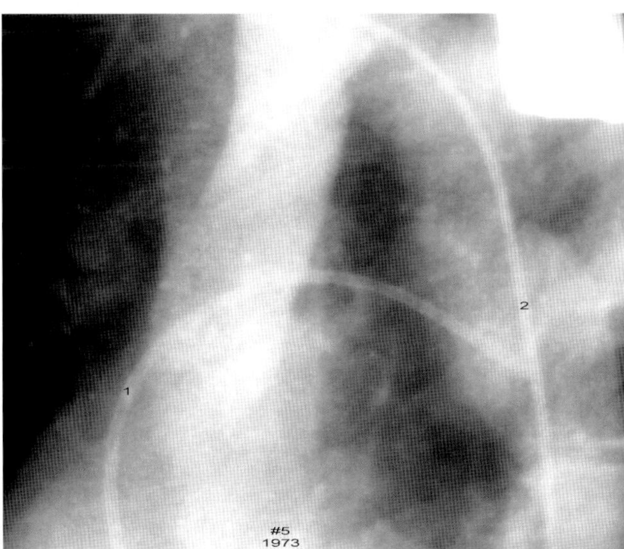

Figure 2.4 Pulmonary and aortic catheters 1973.

8 Oxygen saturation sample run 1973 and 1984

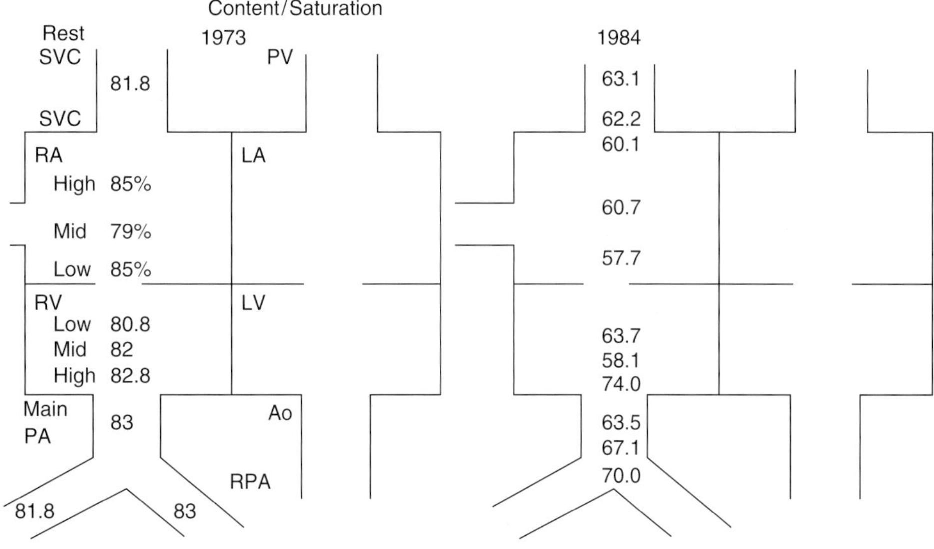

Figure 2.5 Oxygen sample run 1973 and 1984.

9 Cardiogreen dye curves 1973

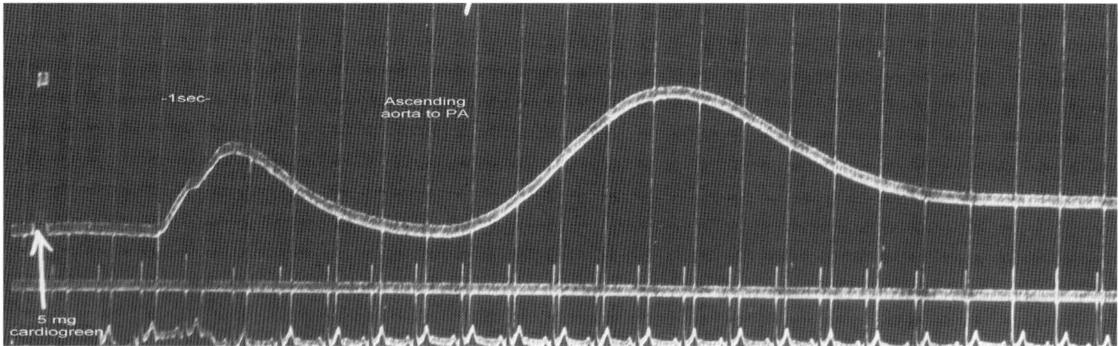

Figure 2.6 Aortic arch to pulmonary dye curve 1973. Time (s) vs concentration of dye (mg/L). Vertical lines are l s apart. Injection site of cardiogreeen: aortic arch. Sampling site: PA. Corrected appearance time takes into account the time it takes for the dye to traverse a 125 cm catheter (~0 s).

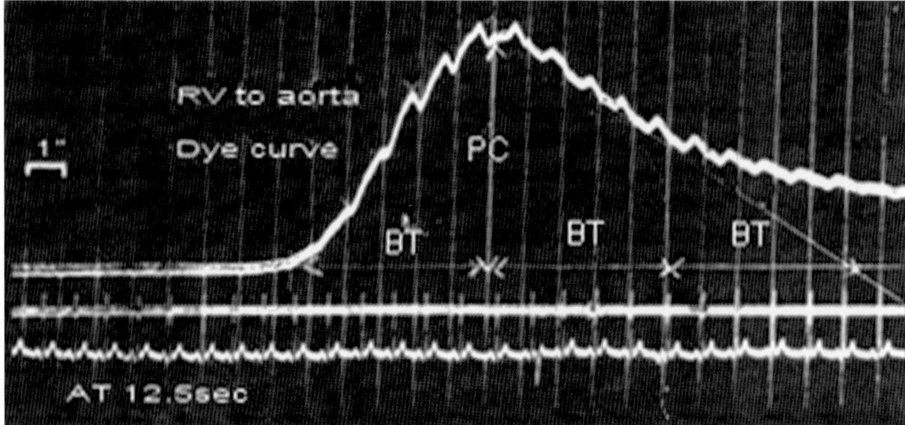

Figure 2.7 RV to aortic dye curve 1973. Calculate the pulmonary/systemic flow ratio from the data derived from Figures 2.6 and 2.7. Peak concentration (*Pc*) = 4 units. Concentration of dye one build-up time after peak concentration (*Pc* + BT) = 2.2 units. Concentration of dye two build-up times after peak concentration (*Pc* +2BT) = 1.3 units. AT, appearance time; BT, build-up time' PC, peak concentration of dye.

10 LAO aortogram 1973

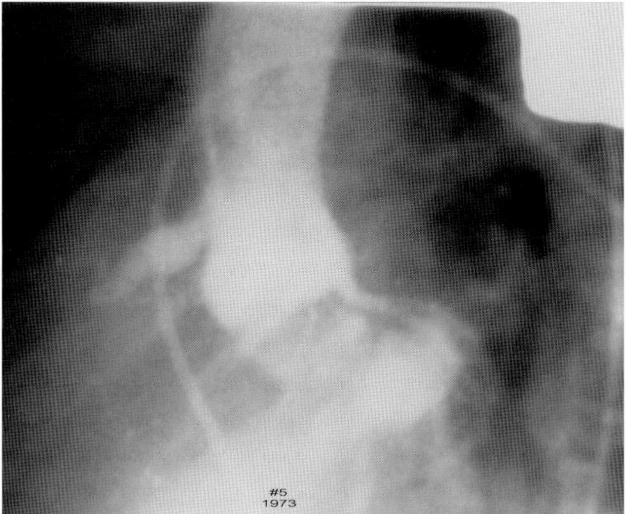

Figure 2.8 Aortic root angiogram LAO view.

11 Physical examination 1973

68 inches tall, 128 lb male. BP 110/80. P 70/min. Regular rhythm.

There was mild jugular venous pressure elevation.

The apex beat was in the 5th interspace in the mid-clavicular line. 1+ LV lift.

There was a systolic thrill felt in the suprasternal notch.

S1 was decreased.

S2 is maximum in the left 3rd interspace parasternally. Narrow physiological splitting of S2.

No S3 or S4.

Grade 3/6 ejection systolic murmur heard at LLSB and RLSB with radiation to the right.

Side of the neck. The intensity of the murmur was not affected by isometric exercise using a standardized hand grip.

Lungs clear.

No abdominal findings.

Good peripheral pulses.

12 Physical examination 1984

Patient was lost to follow-up for 11 years. He returned in 1984 with dyspnea and edema for the previous month.

68 inches tall, 146 lb, anxious male. BP 104/80.

Some decrease in carotid amplitude.

LV sustained lift at apex. RV 1+ lift LLSB.

Apex beat 5th interspace just outside the mid-clavicular line.

S1 normal. S2 single. A2=P2. S3 1+ at apex.

Grade 3/6 aortic systolic murmur.

Grade 3/6 aortic regurgitant murmur.

All pulses in legs and arms present but with some decrease in amplitude.

Lungs clear.

13 Echocardiogram 1984

LV and LA were enlarged. LVH, aortic valve thickening.

14 ECG 1984

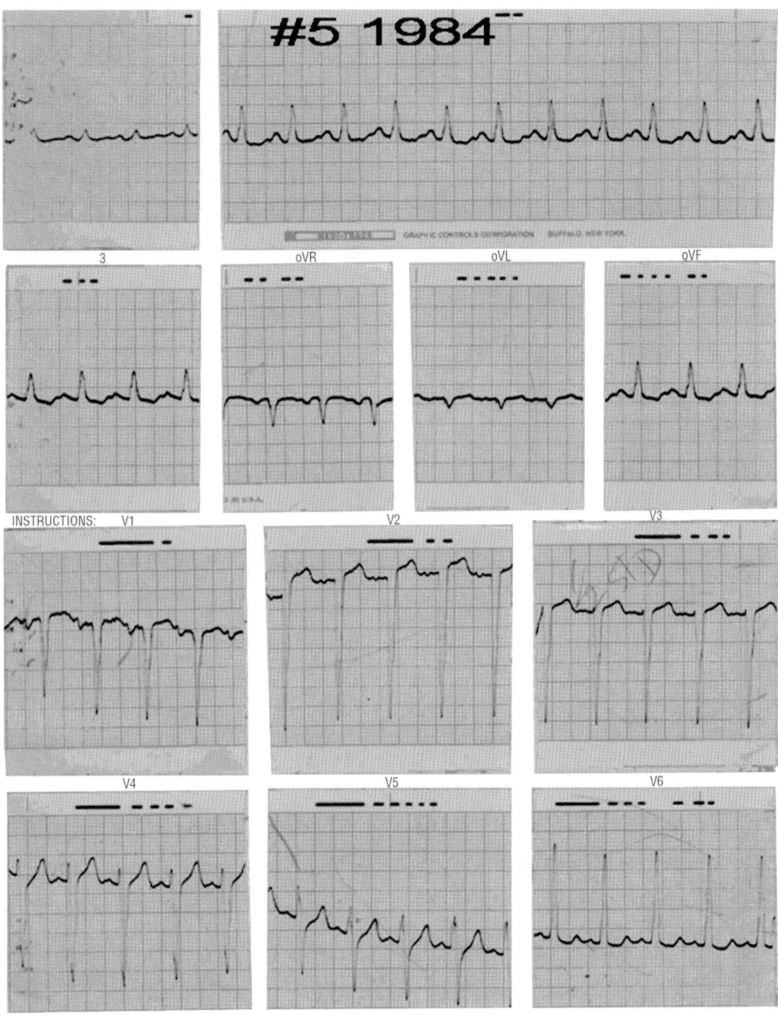

Figure 2.9 ECG 1984.

15 Chest X ray 1984

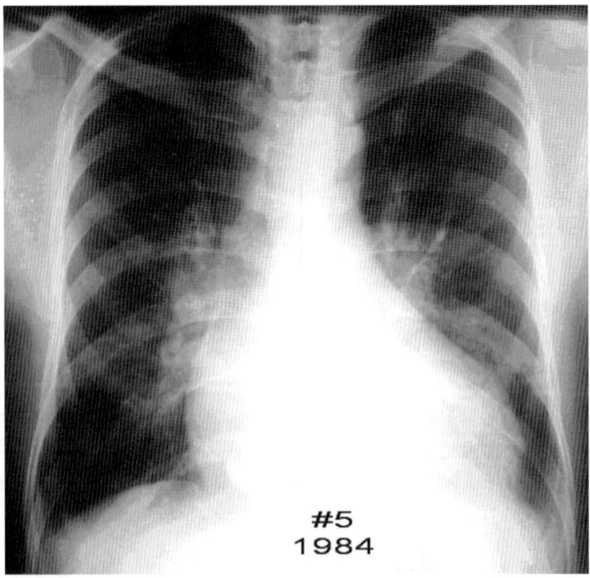

Figure 2.10 Chest X ray 1984.

16 Coronary angiography 1984

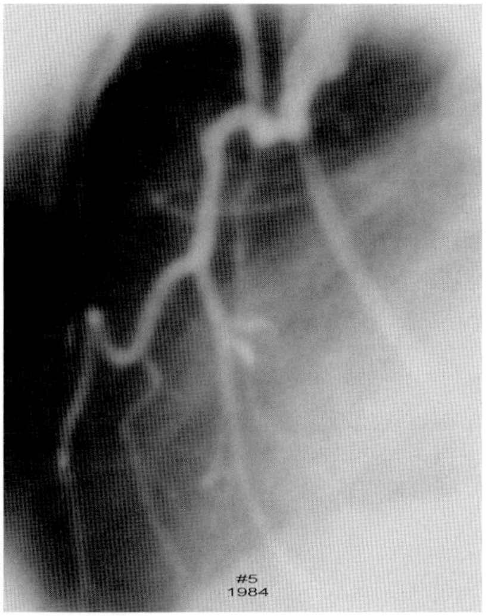

Figure 2.11 Right coronary angiogram LAO view 1984.

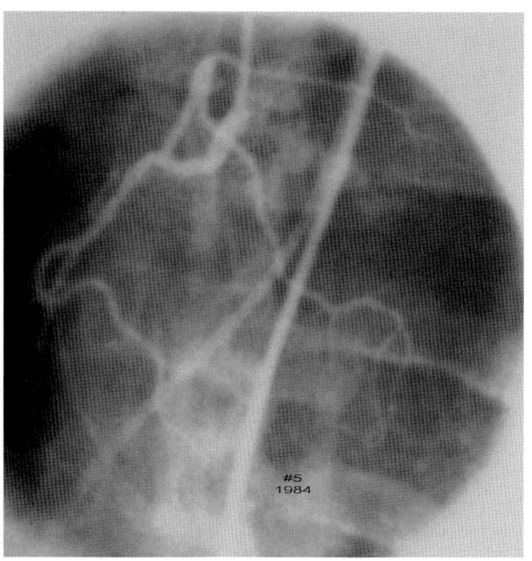

Figure 2.12 Right coronary angiogram RAO view 1984.

17 Aortography 1984

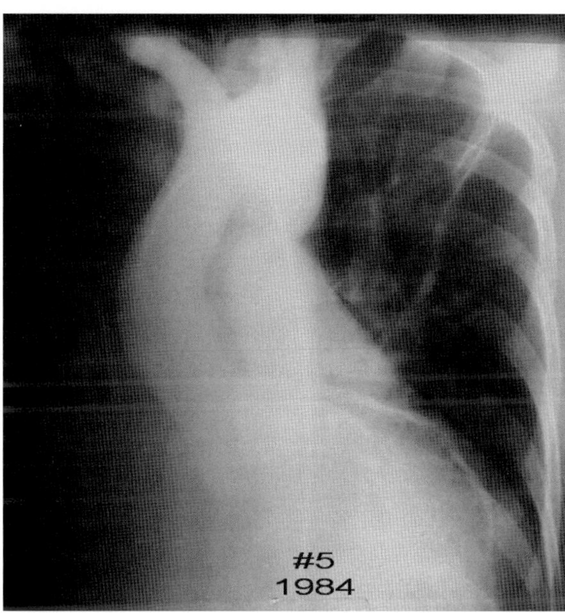

Figure 2.13 Aortogram AP view 1984.

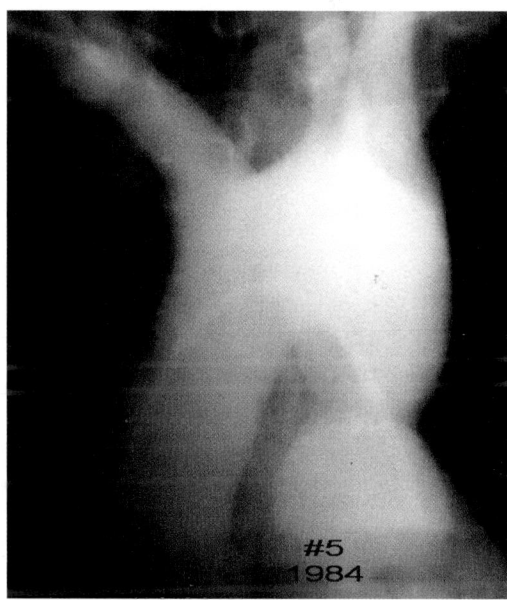

Figure 2.14 Aortogram lateral view 1984.

18 Follow-up 1984–2003

Table 2.2 Echocardiographic data 1996 and 2002

	ECG dimensions (cm)	
	1996	**2002**
Left atrium	4.2	4.6
LV end-diastolic dimension	4.0	4.9
LV end-systolic dimension	3.0	3.5
LV septal thickness	1.4	1.7
LV posterior wall thickness	1.0	1.7
LV systolic function	Normal	Normal
Peak flow velocity across aortic valve prosthesis (m/s)	2.25	2.95

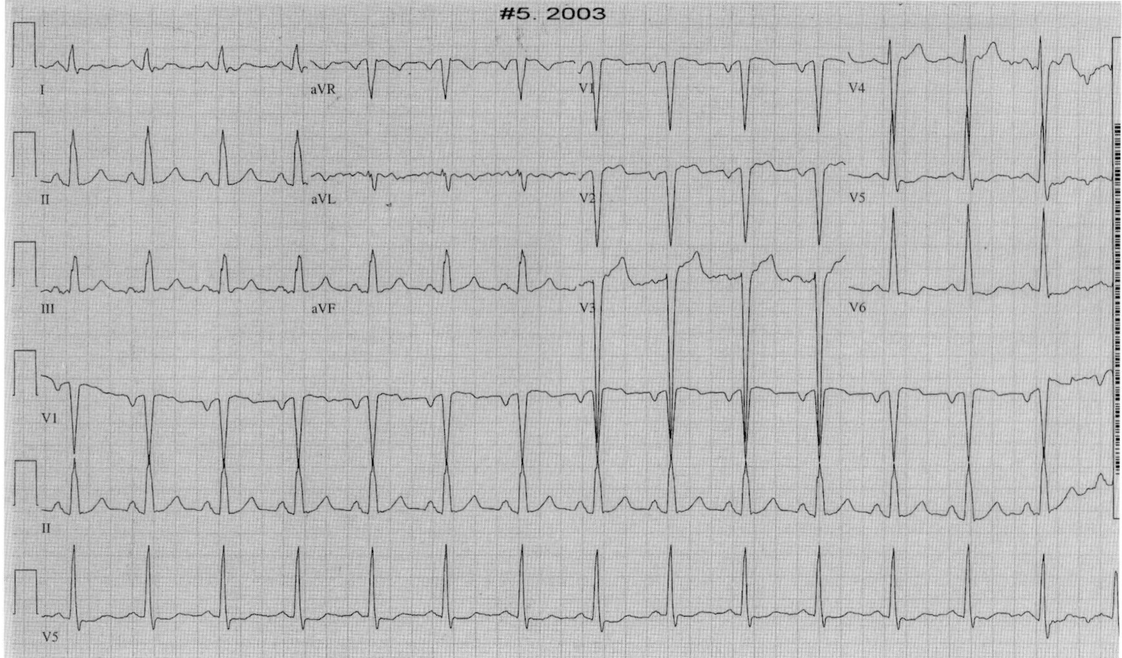

Figure 2.15 ECG 2003.

What is the diagnosis?

Answers and commentary

1 History

A heart murmur and dyspnea may suggest aortic or mitral valvular disease.

2 ECG 1973

At 24 years old, the patient had sufficient voltage criteria for LV hypertrophy according to the Manning criteria (SV1 + RV6 > 5.3 mv in 20–29-year-old age group [1]).

3 Chest X ray 1973

The heart is enlarged with a rounded and inferiorly displaced apex suggestive of LV enlargement. The aortic knob is not enlarged and is located more superiorly than normal. The proximal pulmonary arteries are enlarged.

4 LV and aortic pressure curves 1973

The LV pressure contour was obtained using the trans-septal approach. The aortic pressure contour shows a rapid upstroke and a bisferiens pulse wave. There is a large gradient in systole across the aortic valve.

These findings may be seen in aortic valvular stenosis or LV outflow obstruction. The former diagnosis is most likely as fluoroscopy showed a calcified aortic valve. The rapid upstroke of the aortic pressure may be seen in younger patients with aortic stenosis, especially in the presence of a high cardiac index (4.75 L/min/m^2).

5 and 6 Intracardiac pressures and additional hemodynamic data 1973 and 1984

In 1973 the right heart pressures were normal. There was a mean gradient in systole of 42 mmHg across the aortic valve. At this time the cardiac index was increased and the aortic valve area was only mildly reduced to 1.5 cm^2. Angiography (Figure 2.8) confirmed the presence of a bicuspid aortic valve.

In 1984 the patient had severe pulmonary hypertension (mean PA = 50 mmHg).The gradient in systole across the aortic valve had increased to 50 from 42 mmHg, but the calculated aortic valve area had become critically narrowed (0.5 cm^2). The cardiac index had fallen from 4.75 to 2.56 L/min/m^2. The patient's LV function had also deteriorated since 1973 as the LVEDP had increased from 5 to 32 mmHg and the LV ejection fraction had fallen to only 0.35.

7 Right and left heart catheters 1973

The right heart catheter (on the left-hand side of Figure 2.4) has traversed the PA and entered the descending aorta via a PDA.

The tip of the left heart catheter (on the right-hand side of Figure 2.4) is in the ascending aorta. The aortic arch is much more superior than usual to the pulmonary arterial catheter due to buckling or a pseudocoarctation of the aorta. 1 = PA, catheter 2 = aortic catheter (see labelling on Figure 2.4).

8 Oxygen sample run 1973 and 1984

The 1973 venous samples show an elevated oxygen saturation throughout the right heart, probably due to a high output (cardiac index 4.75 L/min/m^2). No definite step up is seen in this sample oxygen run.

In 1984 there is a fall in oxygen saturation in the right heart, reflecting a fall in cardiac index (2.56 L/min/m^2). No definite step up in oxygen saturation is seen (mean RV O_2 saturation = 65.2%, mean PA O_2 saturation = 66.9%).

A normal O_2 sample run tends to rule out all but the smallest of left to right shunts ($Q_p/Q_s \leq 1.3/1$) [2].

9 Cardiogreen dye curves 1973

The early appearance of dye in the PA when injected into the aortic arch is indicative of a left to right shunt from either a ductus or an aorto-pulmonary window. The latter has an occurrence 1/200 of that of a ductus so ductus is the most likely diagnosis.

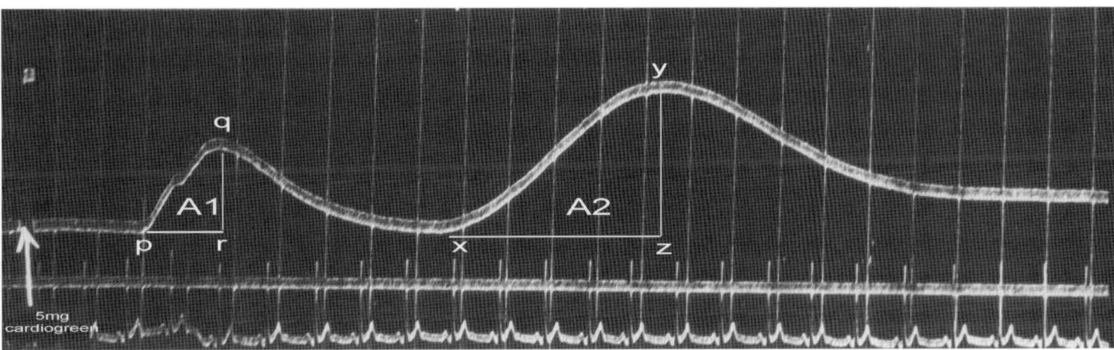

Figure 2.16 Calculation of left to right shunt from aortic–PA dye curve. A1, area of forward 'triangle' pqr = 0.5 (pr × qr) ≡ left to right shunt. A2, area of forward 'triangle' xyz = 0.5 (xz × yz) ≡ systemic blood flow.

In Figures 2.5 and 2.16 the initial smaller curve represents the left to right shunt and the larger second curve the systemic flow.

Using the forward triangle method the Q_p/Q_s ratio is 1.22/1:

Area A1 = 1 × 1.2 Area A2 = 2.8 × 1.9
Q_{L-R}/Q_S = Area 1/Area 2 = 0.22
or $(Q_p - Q_s)/Q_s = 0.22$
or $Q_p/Q_s = 1.22/1$

In Figure 2.7 the forward dye curve from the RV to the aorta shows a prolonged disappearance time due to the left to right shunt. This is the basis for the empirically derived Carter formulae [3] to calculate the Q_p/Q_s ratio. In this patient the Q_p/Q_s ratio is 1.52/1.

Carter's equations

$$\frac{QL-R}{Q_p} \times 100 = 141 \times \frac{C_{p+bt}}{C_p} - 42 \qquad (1)$$

$$\frac{QL-R}{Q_p} \times 100 = 135 \times \frac{C_{p+2bt}}{C_p} - 14 \qquad (2)$$

Substituting $C_p = 4$ $C_{p+bt} = 2.2$ and $C_{p+2bt} = 1.4$ we get:

in equation 1: $\frac{QL-R}{Q_p} \times 100 = 35.55$

and in equation 2: $\frac{QL - R}{Q_p} \times 100 = 33.25$

Average results of equations 1 and 2 = 34.4

$Q_{l\text{–}r} = Q_p \times 0.34.4$
$Q_p - Q_s = Q_p \times 0.344$
$1 - Q_s/Q_p = 0.344$
$Q_p/Q_s = 1.52$

In conclusion there is a small left to right shunt at ductus level. The average of the two methods above yields a Q_p/Q_s ratio of 1.37/1.

10 LAO artiogram 1973

The aortic valve is bicuspid. The right coronary artery is only about 3 cm long. It is dilated proximally due to Kawasaki's disease and then tapers off distally.

11 and 12 Physical examinations 1973 and 1984

The patient has mild to moderate aortic stenosis, based on the diamond-shaped systolic murmur and the voltage criteria for LVH in 1973.

In 1984 the patient has evidence of pulmonary hypertension (based on RV lift). He has LV failure due to a combination of aortic stenosis and aortic regurgitation. The pulses have a decreased amplitude compared to 1973, reflecting a low output state.

13 Echocardiogram 1984

The echocardiogram provides some additional information, i.e., LV and LA enlargement.

14 ECG 1984

The rhythm is sinus tachycardia. Rate 110/min. PR 0.16. QRS 0.08. QRS axis +75°.

P wave is biphasic in V1 with a larger negative deflection due to LA enlargement. There is voltage criteria for LVH. There is poor R wave progression in V1–3 due to LVH.

15 Chest X ray 1984

There is mild cardiomegaly with rounding and inferior displacement of the apex suggestive of LV enlargement, unchanged from 1973. The proximal pulmonary vessels are more prominent than in 1973.

16 Coronary angiography 1984

The right coronary artery shows about a 1 cm proximal fusiform dilatation but now extends to the inferior surface of the heart. Left coronary angiography (not shown) normal.

17 Aortogram 1984

The ascending aorta appear normal. There is redundancy or buckling of the arch and descending aorta with mild narrowing of descending aorta just distal to the left subclavian artery. There is no gradient in systole across this narrowed site.

18 Follow-up 1984–2003

At operation (1984) the patient had a severely calcified bicuspid aortic valve and a small PDA. The aortic valve was replaced with a #19 Bjork–Shiley aortic valve and the ductus ligated. He was placed on long-term warfarin.

His aortic valve prosthesis continued to function well over the next 19 years and he remained normotensive throughout this time.

Echocardiography (Table 2.2)

In 1996 the echocardiogram showed mild LA enlargement, LVH and normal systolic LV function. In 2002 the echocardiogram showed some increase in LVH and normal LV systolic function. The peak flow velocity across the Bjork–Shiley valve increased from 2.25 m/s in 1996 to 2.95 m/s in 2002, which is within the accepted range for this type of valve in the presence of normal LV systolic function [4].

ECG 2003 (Figure 2.15)

The rhythm was sinus with a rate of 87/min. PR 0.160 s. QRS 0.106 s. Axis +70°.

SV1 + RV5 = 3.5 mv. P biphasic V1. Poor R wave progression V1–3 due to LVH or anteroseptal myocardial infarction.

Impression: (i) LVH with increase in repolarization abnormalities since 1984, (ii) LA enlargement, (iii) anteroseptal wall infarction cannot be excluded.

In 2003 the patient was diagnosed with three-vessel coronary artery disease. He had 80% stenoses of the left anterior descending coronary artery and the circumflex coronary artery. The right coronary artery was occluded at its origin, most likely due to atherosclerotic disease rather than Kawasaki disease. Coronary artery bypass surgery was planned but the patient was lost to follow-up.

Final diagnoses

1. Calcific bicuspid aortic valve stenosis
2. Mild aortic regurgitation
3. LV failure
4. Pulmonary hypertension
5. Regression of Kawasaki's disease
6. Pseudocoarctation of aorta
7. Three-vessel coronary artery disease

Discussion

Aortic valve disease

A bicuspid aortic valve occurs in about 2% of the general population [5–7]. About 50% of those with a bicuspid valve will have complications, namely aortic stenosis, aortic regurgitation or endocarditis [5].

Aortic stenosis is most commonly due to a calcified bicuspid aortic valve in patients between 35 and 70 years old [5–10]. In this patient the aortic valve became progressively more calcified over an 11-year period, leading to critical narrowing of the aortic valve.

He had a systolic ejection murmur radiating to the neck consistent with aortic stenosis. The absence of an ejection click reflects the severity of the valve calcification. The presence of LVH, pulmonary hypertension and a reduced carotid artery amplitude indicates severe aortic stenosis. The degree of aortic valve calcification on fluoroscopy has also been correlated with significant aortic stenosis [11].

A bicuspid aortic valve was diagnosed in 1973 on aortic root angiography (Figure 2.9) by detecting two unequal sized cusps and doming of the valve leaflets in systole. However, nowadays a bicuspid aortic valve would be diagnosed non-invasively by two-dimensional echocardiography [12].

This patient underwent aortic valve replacement because his aortic stenosis was severe enough to produce symptoms and signs of heart failure. He was placed on warfarin.

Persistent ductus arteriosus

PDA occurs in about 10% of all cases of congenital heart disease with an incidence of 2–4 per 1000 term births [13, 14].

The patient has a small clinically silent PDA that was ligated at operation in 1984, incidental to his aortic valve surgery.

As a rule a ductus should be closed to prevent LV failure, eliminate the risk of endarteritis and reduce the risk of pulmonary vascular disease [15]. A controversy exists about whether or not to close a very small ductus [13].

Kawasaki syndrome (mucocutaneous lymph node syndrome)

This syndrome is an acute systemic inflammatory illness of young children often resulting in coronary artery aneurysms, rarely myocardial infarction and sudden death [16–18]. Coronary artery aneurysms occur in 15–20% of patients [19]. These aneurysms usually involve the proximal coronary arteries and may be fusiform or saccular [19, 20].

This patient had clinically silent Kawasaki disease, characterized by fusiform dilatation of the proximal right coronary artery, which had partially resolved 11 years later. Spontaneous regression of coronary artery aneurysms due to Kawasaki syndrome has been reported [14, 16, 19] but in patients much younger than in this one.

Pseudocoarctation of aorta

This rare entity consists of redundancy or kinking of the aorta such that the arch and descending aorta occupies a more superior position in the mediastinum. It has been misdiagnosed on plain PA chest X ray as a left upper mediastinal mass [21, 22].

Pseudocoarctation of the aorta must be distinguished from coarctation of the aorta by the absence of systemic hypertension, femoral pulse delay, collateral circulation, and a systolic gradient across the narrowed site [21].

In this patient pseudocoarctation was diagnosed by aortography and the absence of a gradient across the narrowed portion of the descending aorta. Multisection CT [23] is another way of diagnosing pseudocoarctation of the aorta.

Pseudocoarctation is usually a benign condition but aneurysmal formation may develop beyond the kinked aorta [23]. Pseudocoarctation has been associated with congenital aortic stenosis [21], as in this patient.

Key points

- The most common cause of aortic stenosis is a calcified bicuspid aortic valve.
- Other complications of a calcified bicuspid aortic valve are aortic regurgitation and endocarditis.
- The indications for surgery in aortic stenosis can be remembered using the AAA mnemonic: **A**sthma of cardiac origin, **A**ttacks of Unconsciousness, and **A**ngina.
- Kawasaki's disease may be clinically silent and on occasion may regress spontaneously.
- Pseudocoarctation of the aorta is usually benign and is often associated with a bicuspid aortic valve.

References

[1] Manning GW, Smiley JR. QRS voltage criteria for left ventricular hypertrophy in a normal male population. *Circulation* 1964; 29: 224–230.

[2] Antman EM, Marsh JD, Green LH et al. Blood oxygen measurements in the assessment of intracardiac left to right shunts: A critical appraisal of methodology. *Am J Cardiol* 1980; 46: 265–271.

[3] Carter SA, Bajec DF, Yannecelli E et al. Estimation of left to right shunt from arterial dilution curves. *J. Clin Lab Med* 1960; 55: 77–88.

[4] Zabalgoita M. Echocardiographic assessment of prosthetic heart valves. *Curr Probl Card* 1992; 17: 267–325.

[5] Roberts WC. In: Levine HJ (ed.) *Clinical Cardiovascular Physiology*. Grune and Stratton, New York, 1974, pp 1–56.

[6] Roberts WC, Jong M Ko. Frequency by decades of unicuspid, bicuspid and tricuspid aortic valves in adults having isolated aortic valve replacement for aortic stenosis with or without associated aortic regurgitation. *Circulation* 2005; 111: 920–925.

[7] Siu SC, Silversides CK. Bicuspid aortic valve disease. *J Am Coll Cardiol* 2010; 55: 2789–2800.

[8] Passik CS, Ackermann DM, Pluth FR et al. Temporal changes in the causes of aortic stenosis: A surgical pathologic study of 646 cases. *Mayo Clin Proc* 1987; 62: 119–123.

[9] Sabet HY, Edwards WD, Tazelaar HD et al. Congenitally bicuspid aortic valves: a surgical pathology study of 542 cases (1991–1996) and a literature review of 2715 additional cases. *Mayo Clin Proc* 1999; 74: 14–26.

[10] Subramanian R, Olson LJ, Edwards WD. Surgical pathology in pure aortic stenosis. A study of 374 cases. *Mayo Clin Proc* 1984; 59: 683–690.

[11] Glancy L, Freed TA, Kevin P et al. Calcium in the aortic valve. Roentgenologic and hemodynamic correlations in 148 patients. *Ann Int Med* 1969; 71: 245–250.

[12] Brandenburg RO, Tajik AJ, Edwards WD et al. Accuracy of 2 dimensional echocardiographic diagnosis of congenital bicuspid aortic valve: echocardiographic-anatomic correlation in 115 patients. *Am J Cardiol* 1983; 51: 1469–1473.

[13] Fortescue EB, Lock JE, Galvin T et al. To close or not to close: The very small patent ductus arteriosus. *Congenit Heart Dis.* 2010; 5: 354–365.

[14] Schneider KJ, Moore JW. Patent ductus arteriosus. *Circulation* 2006; 114: 1873–1882.

[15] Wu JC, Child JS. Common congenital heart disorders. *Curr Probl Cardiol* 2004; 29: 641–696.

[16] Burns JC, Shike H, Gordon JB et al. Sequelae of Kawasaki disease in adolescents and young adults. *J Am Coll Cardiol* 1996; 28: 253–247.

[17] Kawasaki T, Kosaki F, Okawa S et al. A new infantile acute febrile mucocutaneous lymph node syndrome (MLNS) prevailing in Japan. *Pediatrics* 1974; 54: 271–276.

[18] Rowley AH. Kawasaki disease: Novel insights into etiology and genetic susceptibility. *Ann Rev Med* 2011; 62: 69–77.

[19] Takahashi M, Mason W, Lewis AB. Regression of coronary aneurysms in patients with Kawasaki syndrome. *Circulation* 1987; 75: 387–394.

[20] Satou GM, Giamelli J, Gewitz MH. Kawasaki disease. Diagnosis, management, and long term implications. *Cardiol Rev* 2007; 15: 163–169.

[21] Nasser WK, Helmen C. Kinking of the aortic arch (pseudocoarctation) Clinical, radiographic, hemodynamic and angiographic findings in eight cases. *Ann Int Med* 1966; 64: 971–978.

[22] Pattinson JN, Grainger RG. Congenital kinking of the aortic arch. *Br Heart J* 1959; 21: 555–561.

[23] Sebastia C, Quiroga S, Boye R et al. Aortic stenosis: Spectrum of diseases depicted at multi-section CT. *Radiographics* 2003; 23: 579–591.

3 PATIENT STUDY 3

Sequence of data presentation

1 History
↓
2 ECG
↓
3 Chest X ray PA and lateral views
↓
4 Hemodynamics
↓
5 Physical examination
↓
6 Course

1 and 2 History and ECG

This 27-year-old man was admitted to hospital in 1973 with hemoptysis for 5 days. He had a past history of rheumatic fever and had had exertional dyspnea since 1968.

His ECG in 1973 showed atrial fibrillation and right-axis deviation.

3 Chest X ray PA and lateral views

(a) (b)

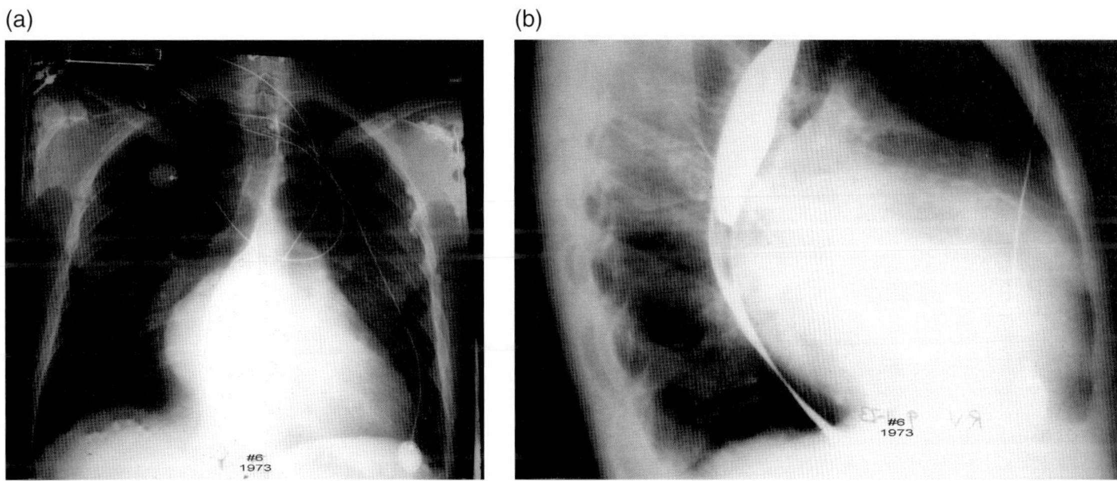

Figure 3.1 (a) Chest x-ray PA view. (b) Chest X ray lateral view.

Patient Studies in Valvular, Congenital, and Rarer Forms of Cardiovascular Disease: An Integrative Approach, First Edition. Franklin B. Saksena.

Companion Website: www.wiley.com/go/saksena/patientstudies

4 Hemodynamics

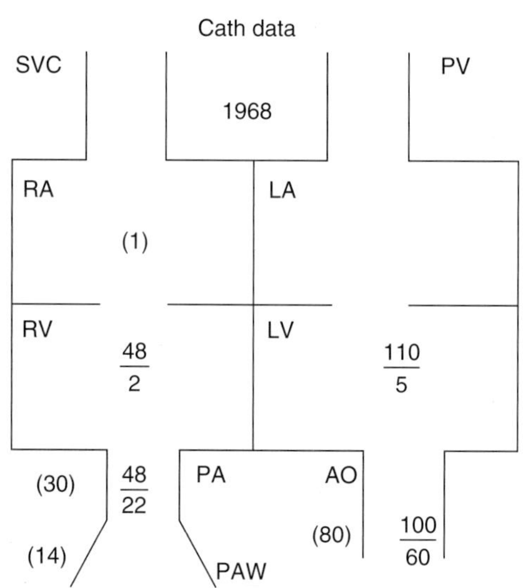

Figure 3.2 Cardiac catheterization data 1968.

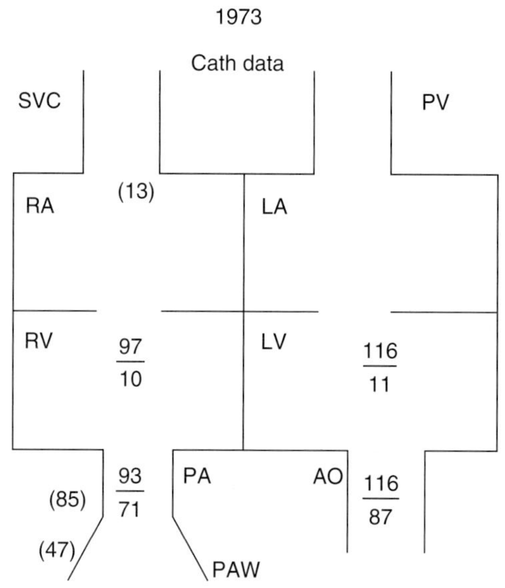

Figure 3.3 Cardiac catheterization data 1973.

	1968	1973
Cardiac index	1.8 L/min/m^2	1.5 L/min/m^2
Mitral diastolic gradient	12 mm Hg	23 mm Hg
P.V.R	480 d.s.cm^{-5}	1280 d.s.cm^{-5}
Mitral valve area	0.7 cm^2	0.6 cm^2
Heart rate	78/min	110–160/min

Figure 3.4 Mitral valve data 1968 and 1973.

5 Physical examination

67 inches tall, 116 lb male. BP 110/70, HR 110–160/min.
RV lift.
Systolic and diastolic thrills at apex.
Apex 6th intercostal space just outside the mid-clavicular line.
S1+1, S2+2, P2 increased, S3 apex.
Grade 4/6 apical diastolic murmur.
Grade 2/6 pansystolic apical murmur.
Grade 4/6 diamond-shaped systolic murmur at LLSB.

6 Course

After the pressures and cardiac output had been obtained the patient suddenly became hypotensive and developed ventricular fibrillation requiring DC shock and intubation. No angiograms were obtained.
He had an uneventful recovery in the coronary care unit a few hours later.

What might have caused this hypotensive episode?

Answers and commentary

1 and 2 History and ECG

The history of rheumatic fever, dyspnea, and hemoptysis is suggestive of mitral valvular disease. The patient was now in atrial fibrillation.

3 Chest X ray

The chest X rays show a large LA and dilated RV. The former is best seen in the lateral view, in which the large LA has pushed the esophagus posteriorly. Pulmonary vascular congestion could not be reliably assessed as the lung fields were over-exposed.

4 Hemodynamics

The cardiac catheterization data of 1968 showed moderately severe mitral stenosis with only mild pulmonary hypertension (PA mean 30 mmHg). However, by 1973 the patient had developed severe pulmonary hypertension (PA mean 85 mmHg).

A satisfactory wedge position of the right heart catheter was verified by obtaining an oxygen saturation of 99%. The gradient across the mitral valve had increased from 12 to 23 mmHg along with a rise in pulmonary vascular resistance.

5 Physical examination

Physical examination confirmed the presence of severe mitral stenosis, severe pulmonary hypertension, and probable tricuspid regurgitation, as well as right heart failure.

6 Course

The episode of hypotension in the cardiac catheterization laboratory could have been due to a combination of acute stress-related right heart failure and a temporary obstruction of the mitral valve by the large LA thrombus.

At surgery the mitral valve was thickened and its orifice had a fish mouth deformity due to commissural fusion. The valve orifice area was severely reduced to 0.6 cm^2 (using the known dimensions of the background grid) and corresponded closely to the calculated area obtained by the Gorlin formula (Figure 3.5). The normal mitral valve orifice area is 4–5 cm^2.

A large clot was evacuated from the LA. The mitral valve was replaced with a Starr–Edward prosthesis. The patient also underwent tricuspid valvuloplasty. He was discharged on warfarin and did well over the next year.

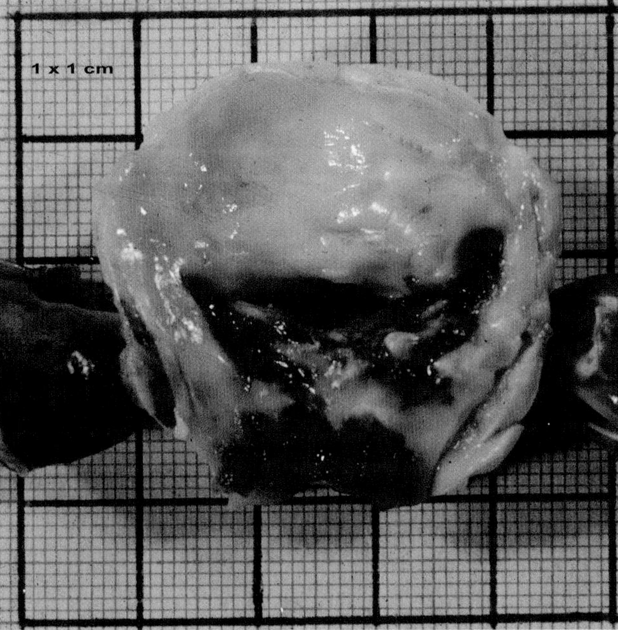

Figure 3.5 Mitral valve removed at surgery.

Key points

1. Untreated patients with mitral stenosis can rapidly develop severe pulmonary hypertension and severe tricuspid regurgitation.
2. The pansystolic murmur at the apex in patients with mitral stenosis may be due to MR but may not be easily distinguished from tricuspid regurgitation.
3. The combination of LA and RV enlargement on chest X ray is a common feature of mitral stenosis.
4. A large LA clot can temporarily obstruct the mitral valve completely and lead to sudden death.
5. The wedge pressure is best validated if one obtains a fully saturated blood sample, especially in the setting of severe pulmonary hypertension.

Further reading

Bruce CJ, Nishimura RA. Newer advances in the diagnosis and treatment of mitral stenosis. *Curr Probl Cardiol* 1998; 23: 130–192 (111 references).

4 PATIENT STUDY 4

Sequence of data presentation

1 History
↓
2 Chest X ray 1974
↓
3 ECG 1974
↓
4 Pressures
↓
5 Angiograms
↓
6 Physical examination

1 History

22-year-old female P1 G1 admitted to hospital with dyspnea on walking one block or up one flight of stairs. She has had no PND or syncope. She has had exertional chest pain for the last 7 years.

She does not drink alcohol or smoke. Family history is unremarkable.

2 Chest X ray 1974

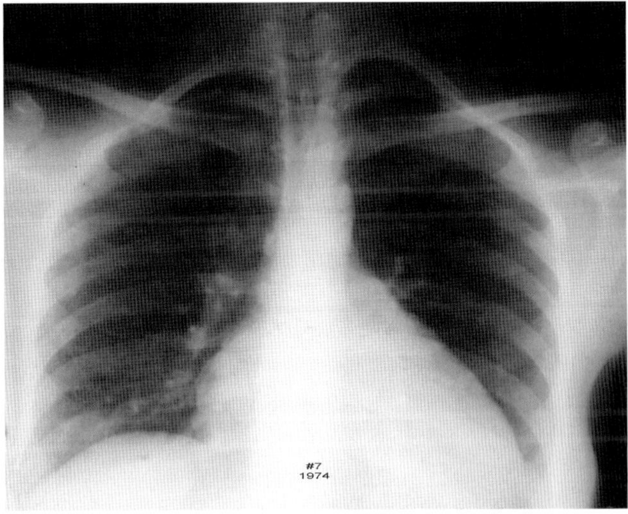

Figure 4.1 Chest X ray PA view.

Patient Studies in Valvular, Congenital, and Rarer Forms of Cardiovascular Disease: An Integrative Approach, First Edition. Franklin B. Saksena.

Companion Website: www.wiley.com/go/saksena/patientstudies

3 ECG 1974

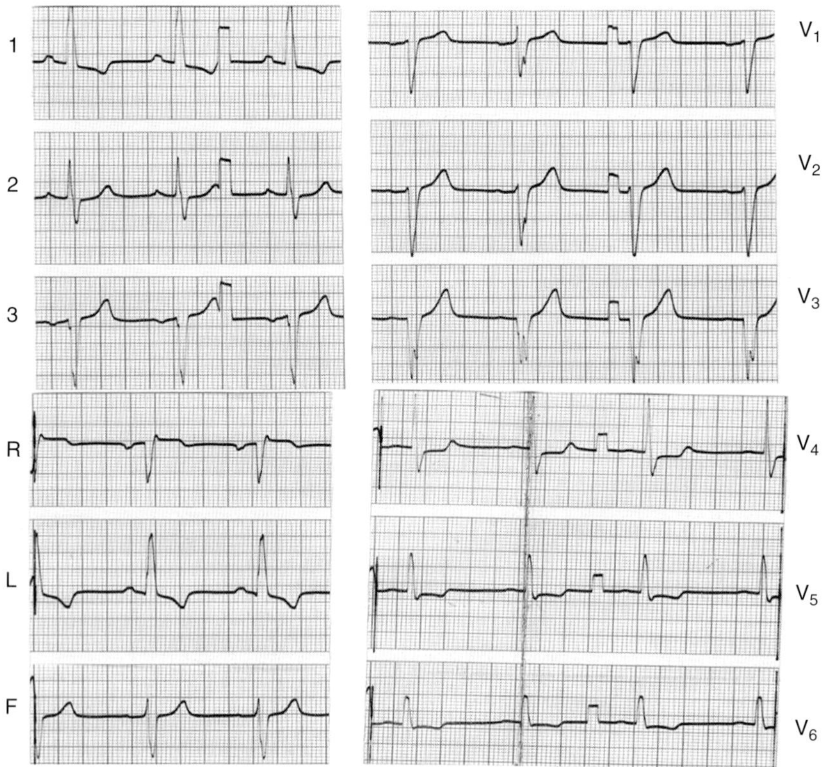

Figure 4.2 12-lead ECG. All leads are half standard.

4 Pressures

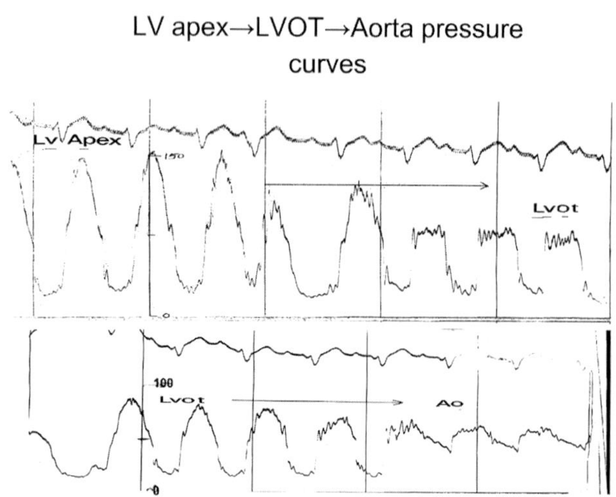

Figure 4.3 Upper panel: catheter was withdrawn from apex to LV outflow tract (0–150 mmHg scale). Lower panel: LV catheter being withdrawn from LV outflow tract to aorta (0–100 mmHg scale).

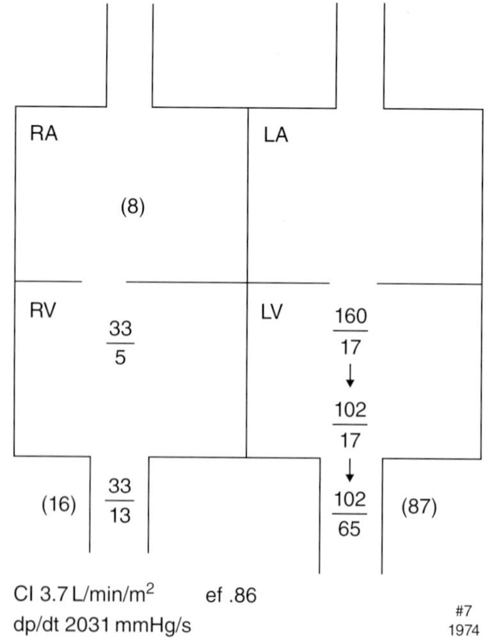

Figure 4.4 Cardiac catheterization. Cardiac index 3.7 L/min/m², LV ejection fraction 0.86, LV dp/dt 2031 mmHg/s.

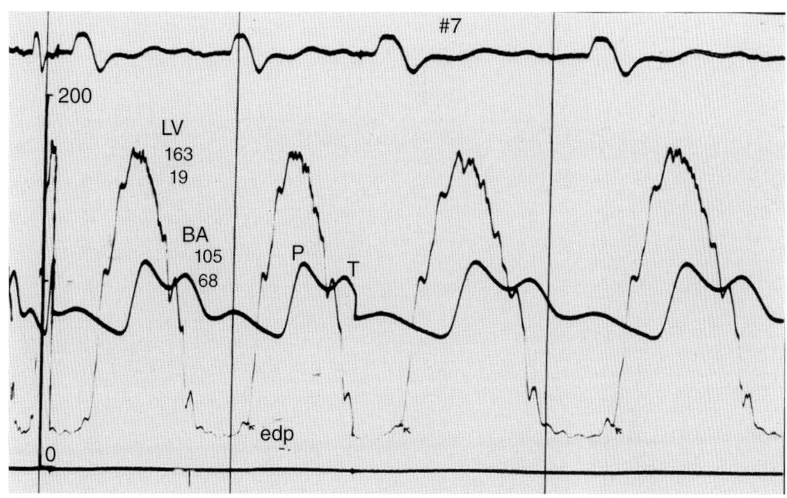

Figure 4.5 LV and brachial artery pressures. 0–200 mmHg scale.

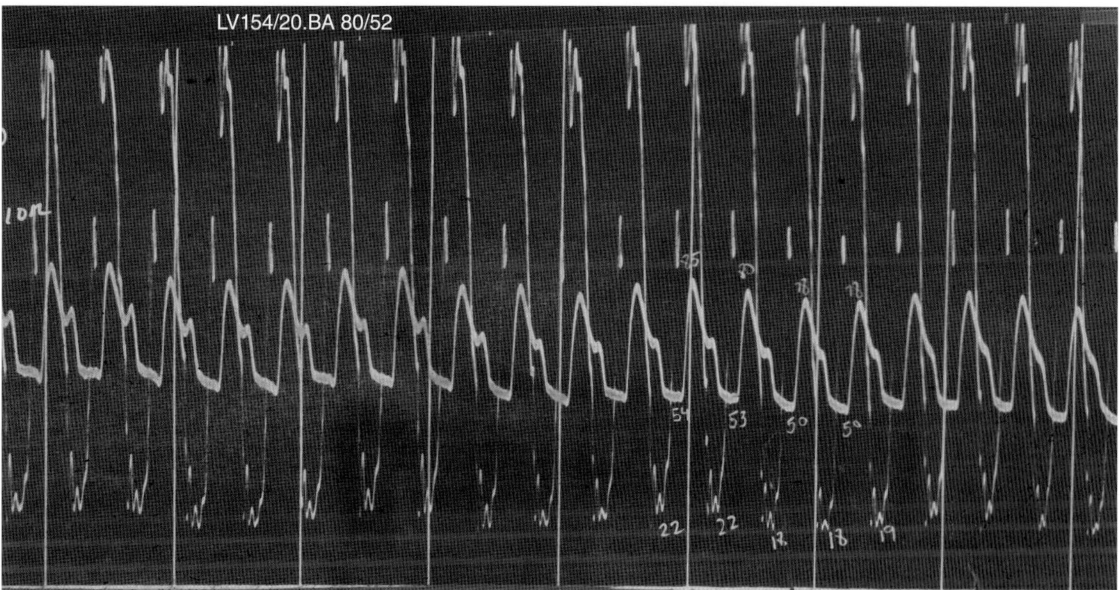

Figure 4.6 LV and brachial artery pressures during isoproterenol (isuprel) infusion.

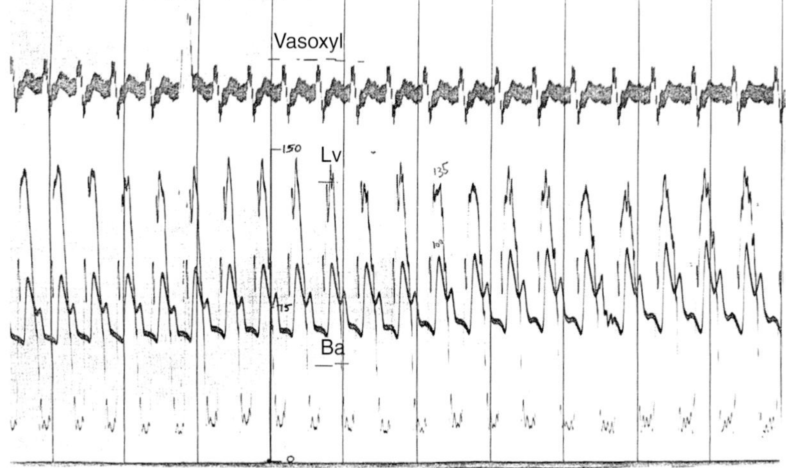

Figure 4.7 LV and brachial artery pressures during methoxamine (vasoxyl) infusion.

5 Angiograms

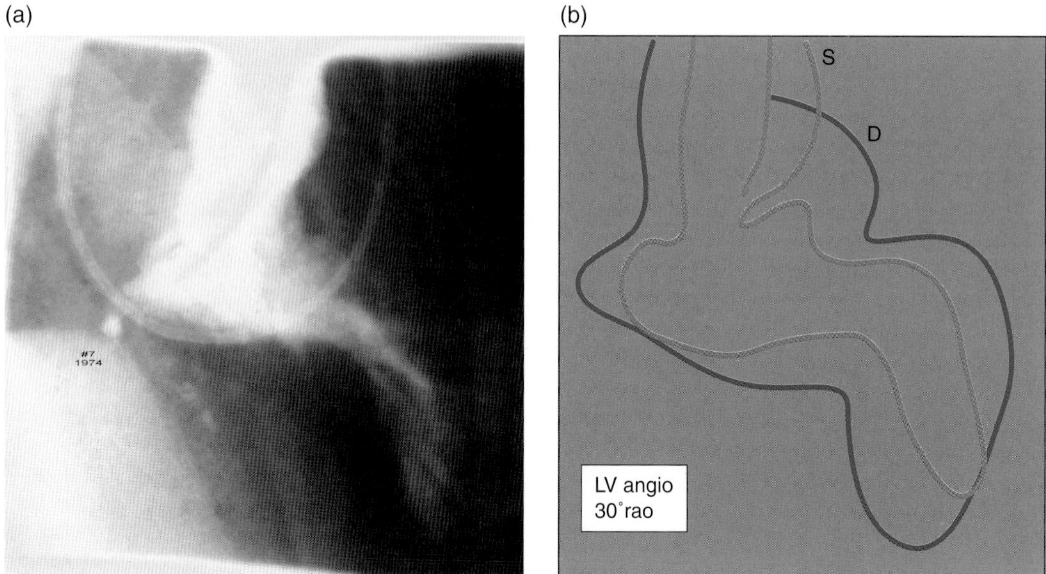

Figure 4.8 (a) LV angiogram 30°, RAO view. (b) Diagram of LV angiogram in (a). S, end systole; D, end diastole.

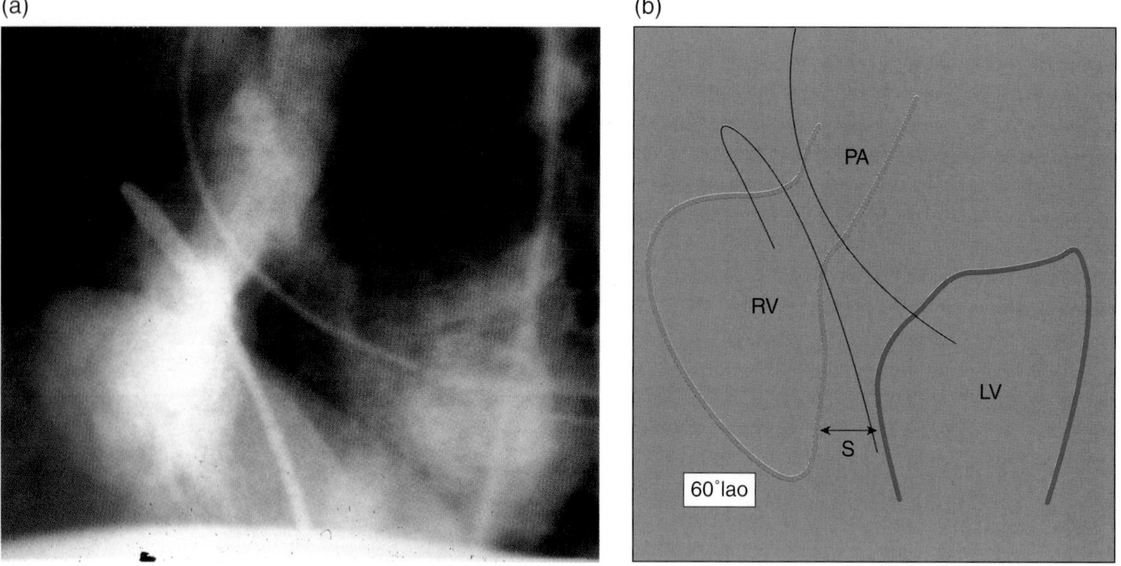

Figure 4.9 (a) Biventricular angiogram 60°, LAO view. (b) Diagram of biventricular angiogram in (a).

6 Physical examination

63 inches tall, 104 lb alert female. BP 96/70, HR 72/min regular. R 18, T 98 °F.
No elevation of jugular venous pressure. Rapid carotid artery upstroke with a bisferiens pulse.
Apex beat 5th interspace just inside the mid-clavicular line.
S1 normal. S2 normal. S4 at apex (palpable).
Grade 4/6 systolic ejection murmur at LLSB and apex.
The murmur decreased with squatting and is increased during valsalva maneuver.
Lungs are clear to percussion and auscultation.
No hepatomegaly.
No clubbing, cyanosis, or edema.

What is the diagnosis?

Answers and commentary

1 History

A young woman with exertional chest pain could have an anomalous coronary artery arising from pulmonary artery, coronary vasculitis, or aortic valvular or subvalvular disease. Coronary atherosclerosis would be unusual in this young patient.

2 Chest X ray 1974

There is cardiomegaly with probable LV and RV enlargement. There is some increase in the pulmonary vascular markings. A lateral view (not shown) provided no further information.

3 ECG 1974

The rhythm is sinus. Rate 68/min. PR interval 0.21 s. QRS interval 0.08 s. QRS axis −20°.

The P is biphasic in V1 due to LA enlargement. S in V1 + R in V5 = 5.2 mv, indicative of LVH.

The findings so far point to aortic or subaortic valvular disease.

4 Pressures

Pressure withdrawal curves from LV apex to LV outflow tract to aorta

There is a gradient in systolic across the LV outflow tract, which is indicative of subaortic stenosis.

Intracardiac pressures

There is a peak systolic gradient of 58 mmHg between the LV apex and LV outflow tract, but no gradient in systole across the aortic valve.

Diagnosis: subaortic stenosis.

LV (apex) – brachial artery pressures

There is a gradient in systole across the brachial artery and the LV apex. The brachial pressure contour shows a bisferiens pulse with a prominent percussion wave exceeding the height of the tidal wave in systole. These findings are characteristic of HCM.

LV–brachial artery pressures during isoproterenol (isuprel) infusion

The gradient between the LV apex and brachial artery gradually increases during the infusion. Isuprel decreases the peripheral vascular resistance, promotes narrowing of the LV outflow tract (the pinch-cock effect), and thus increases the systolic gradient.

LV–brachial artery pressure after IV methoxamine (vasoxyl)

The gradient between the LV apex and brachial artery decreased progressively. Methoxamine is a pure vasoconstrictor. It increases the peripheral vascular reisistance and nullifies the pinch-cock effect of the LV outflow tract, thus reducing the systolic gradient (Figure 4.10).

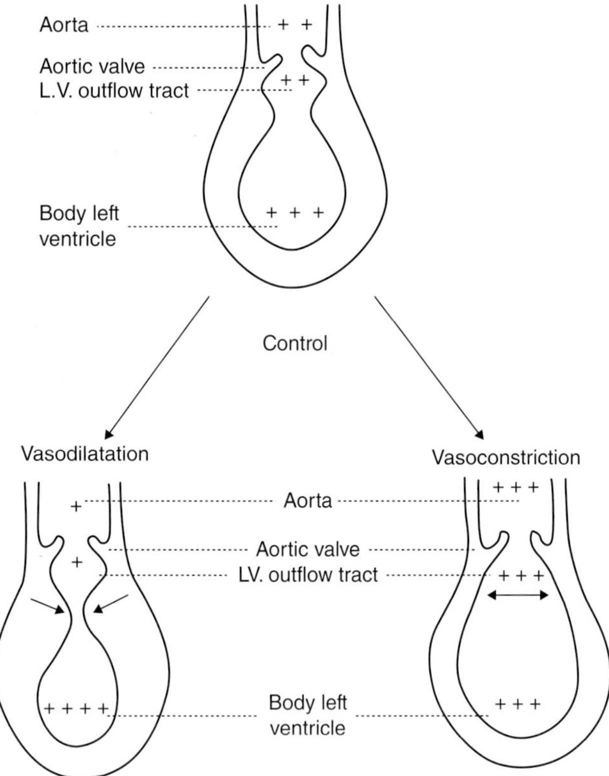

Figure 4.10 The effect of vasodilatation and vasoconstriction on the LV outflow tract. Vasodilatation decreases the LVOT 'distending pressure' and increases the subaortic gradient (++++ vs +). Conversely, vasoconstriction increases the LVOT 'distending pressure' and decreases the subaortic gradient (+++ vs +++) (11). Source: Wigle ED, Rakowski H, Kimball BP et al. (1995). Reproduced with permission of Elsevier.

5 Angiograms

LV angiogram

This shows a hypercontractile LV (LV ejection fraction 0.85) with almost complete obliteration of the LV cavity in systole. The shape of the LV in systole has been likened to a ballarina's foot. No MR.

Biventricular angiography

This showed a thickened interventricular septum.

6 Physical examination

The presence of a rapid carotid upstroke, a bisferiens pulse, and a systolic murmur that decreases during squatting and increases during a valsalva maneuver are diagnostic of HCM.

Discussion

HCM is a disease of unknown etiology, occurring in 1:500 of the population, usually inherited as a Mendelian autosomal dominant trait [1, 2]. It is characterized as an asymmetric hypertrophy of LV or RV and associated microscopically with myocyte disarray [10]. Myocyte disarray often affects over 20% of the ventricle [2, 3].

LV outflow tract obstruction occurs in at least 25% of patients [2, 4]. This obstruction is usually due to systolic anterior motion of the mitral valve along with mitral leaflet–septal contact. The obstruction in HCM may be absent at rest (but inducible), labile, or persistent [5].

The sequence of events in HCM is ejection–obstruction–leak [5]. The rapid ejection in the first half of systolic gives rise to the percussion wave in the aortic pressure contour. Next the sphincter-like action of the LVOT leads to reduced flow, as seen in the tidal wave (see Figure 4.5). The leak refers to the late systolic onset of MR, which occurs in most patients with HCM [6].

HCM with LVOT obstruction should be considered in a patient with a diamond-shaped systolic murmur at LLSB with a bifid carotid pulse in the absence of aortic regurgitation or a high output state [6]. A systolic thrill in HCM has been associated with a subaortic gradient of 75 mmHg [7].

The murmur (and hence the subaortic gradient) increases whenever the LV volume is decreased (e.g. during the strain phase of the valsalva maneuver, when moving from a squatting to a standing position, during exercise, or with vasodilator drugs). The murmur may be intensified by an increase in LV contractility (e.g. post PVC, digitalis, isoprotenolol). An increase in LV volume will decrease the murmur's intensity (squatting, vasoconstrictor drugs) (Figure 4.10) [8].

Two-dimensional and continuous wave Doppler echocardiography has almost completely replaced the need for cardiac catheterization [5] as these noninvasive studies can show the site of the asymmetric septum (ASH), the systolic anterior motion of the mitral valve (SAM), measure the LV thickness and the subaortic gradient, and demonstrate mitral regurgitation [9]. If there is no subaortic gradient at rest it may be induced by having the patient do a valsalva maneuver, giving a vasodilator such as amyl nitrate, or doing exercise [6].

Cardiac catheterization, including an isoproterenol challenge, may be required to induce a significant subaortic gradient if the results of echocardiography in highly symptomatic patients are inconclusive [10].

The use of isoproterenol to induce a significant subaortic gradient allows the selection of those symptomatic patients that might benefit from LV septal myomectomy [4]. Isoproterenol challenge can also be used following a septal myomectomy to determine the efficacy of surgery in abolishing the subaortic gradient [4, 10, 11].

Magnetic resonance imaging has a role in defining the site and extent of HCM [5, 6] as well as assessing the results of LV septal myomectomy [1].

Key points

1. The diagnostic features of HCM are a rapid carotid upstroke, a bisferiens pulse, and a hemodynamically significant aortic systolic murmur.
2. The aortic systolic murmur in HCM decreases during squatting and increases during a valsalva maneuver.
3. Echocardiography will detect the three phases of HCM: ejection, obstruction, and leak.
4. Isoproterenol infusion is diagnostically useful to provoke an LV outflow gradient if the echocardiogram is inconclusive in the symptomatic patient.
5. Isoproterenol infusion is also useful to decide which patients may benefit from septal myomectomy and to assess its efficacy postoperatively.

References

[1] Andrew CYT, Dhillon A, Desai MY. Cardiac magnetic resonance in hypertrophic cardiomyopathy. *J Am Coll Cardiol Img* 2011; 4: 1123–1137.
[2] Maron BJ. Hypertrophic cardiomyopathy. A systematic review. *JAMA* 2002; 287: 1308–1320.
[3] Marian AJ. Contemporary treatment of hypertrophic cardiomyopathy. *Tex Heart Instit J* 2009; 36: 194–204.
[4] Schaff HV, Dearani JA, Ommen SR et al .Expanding the indications for septal myectomy in patients with hypertrophic cardiomyopathy: Results of operation in patients with latent obstruction. *J Thorac Cardiovasc Surg* 2012; 143: 303–309.
[5] Wigle ED, Rakowski H, Kimball BP et al. Hypertrophic cardiomyopathy. Clinical spectrum and treatment. *Circulation* 1995; 92: 1680–1692.
[6] Ommen SR, Nishimura RA. Hypertrophic cardiomyopathy. *Curr Prob Card* 2004; 29: 239–289.
[7] Frank S, Braunwald E. Idiopathic hypertrophic subaortic stenosis. Clinical analysis of 126 patients with emphasis on the natural history. *Circulation* 1968; 37: 759–787.
[8] Wigle ED, David PR, Labrosse CJ et al. Muscular subaortic stenosis. The interrelation of wall tension, outflow tract 'distending pressure' and orifice radius. *Am J Cardiol* 1965; 15: 761–772.
[9] Maron BJ, Maron MS, Wigle ED, Braunwald E. The 50 year history, controversy, and clinical implications of left ventricular outflow tract obstruction in hypertrophic cardiomyopathy. *J Am Coll Cardiol* 2009; 54: 191–200.
[10] Elesber A, Nishimura RA, Rihal CS et al. Utility of isoproterenol to provoke outflow tract gradients in patients with hypertrophic cardiomyopathy. *Am J Cardiol* 2008; 101: 516–520.
[11] Stewart WJ, Schiavone WA, Salcedo EE et al. Intraoperative Doppler echocardiography in hypertrophic cardiomyopathy: Correlations with the obstructive gradient. *J Am Coll Cardiol* 1987; 10: 327–335.

5 PATIENT STUDY 5

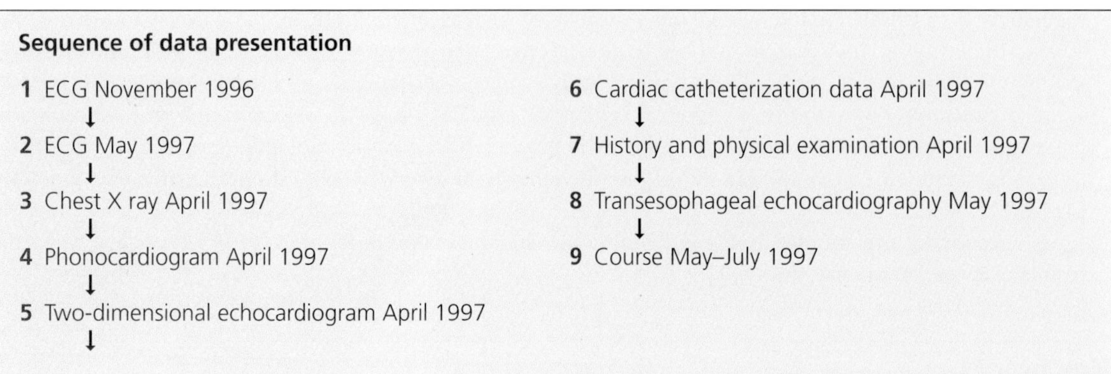

Sequence of data presentation

1 ECG November 1996
↓
2 ECG May 1997
↓
3 Chest X ray April 1997
↓
4 Phonocardiogram April 1997
↓
5 Two-dimensional echocardiogram April 1997
↓
6 Cardiac catheterization data April 1997
↓
7 History and physical examination April 1997
↓
8 Transesophageal echocardiography May 1997
↓
9 Course May–July 1997

1 ECG November 1996

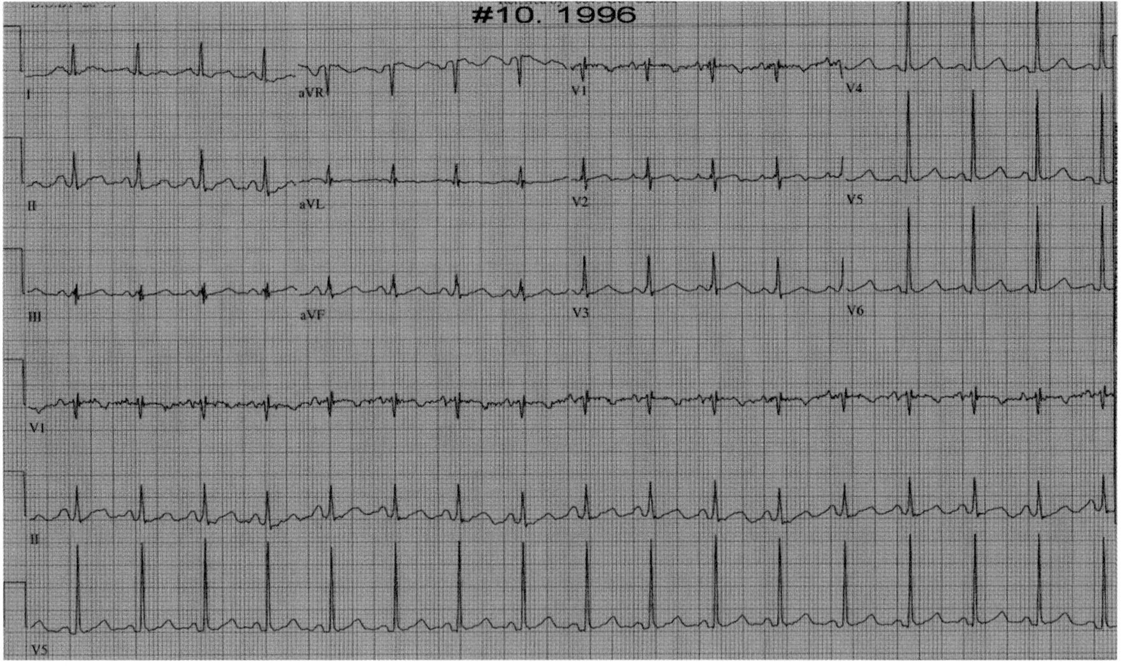

Figure 5.1 ECG November 1996. Comment on rhythm, rate, QRS axis, PR, QRS. Readers should note the rate, rhythm, PR, QRS intervals, QRS axis, and their impression.

Patient Studies in Valvular, Congenital, and Rarer Forms of Cardiovascular Disease: An Integrative Approach, First Edition. Franklin B. Saksena.

Companion Website: www.wiley.com/go/saksena/patientstudies

2 ECG May 1997

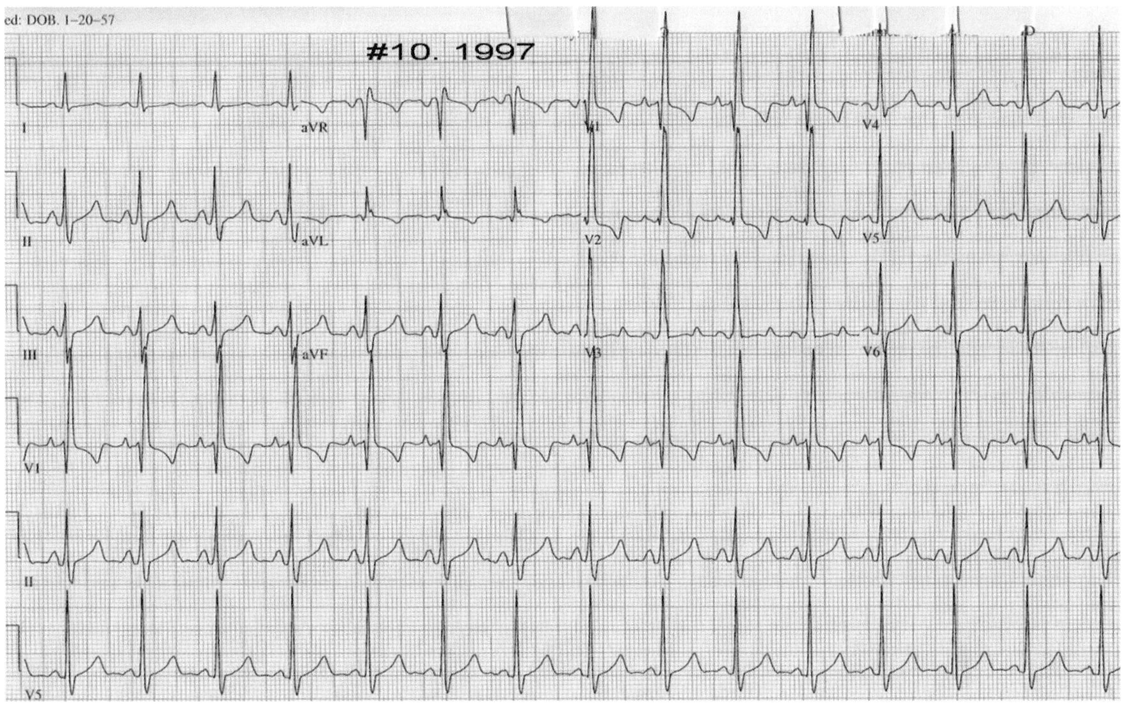

Figure 5.2 ECG April 1997. Comment on rhythm, rate, QRS axis, PR, QRS. Impression:

3 Chest X ray April 1997

(a) (b)

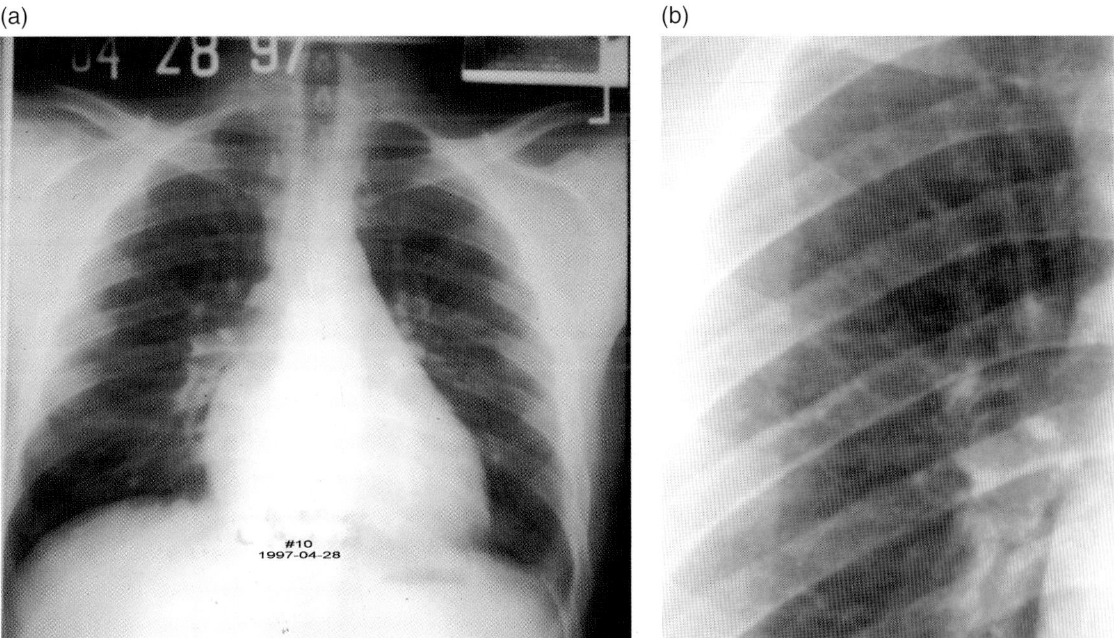

Figure 5.3 (a) Chest X ray PA view April 1997. (b) Enlargement of right lung field area.

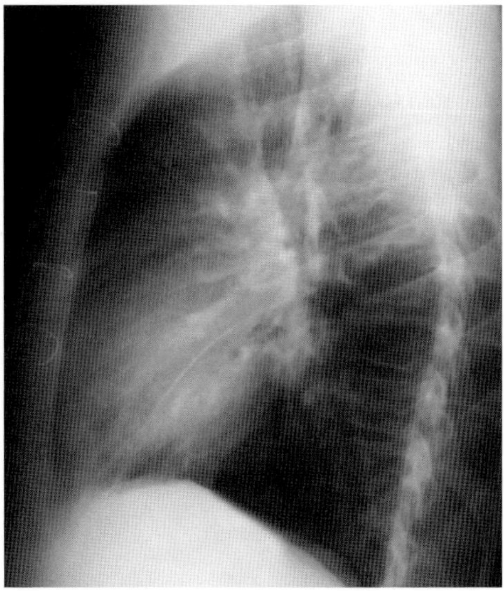

Figure 5.4 Lateral chest X ray April 1997.

4 Phonocardiogram April 1997

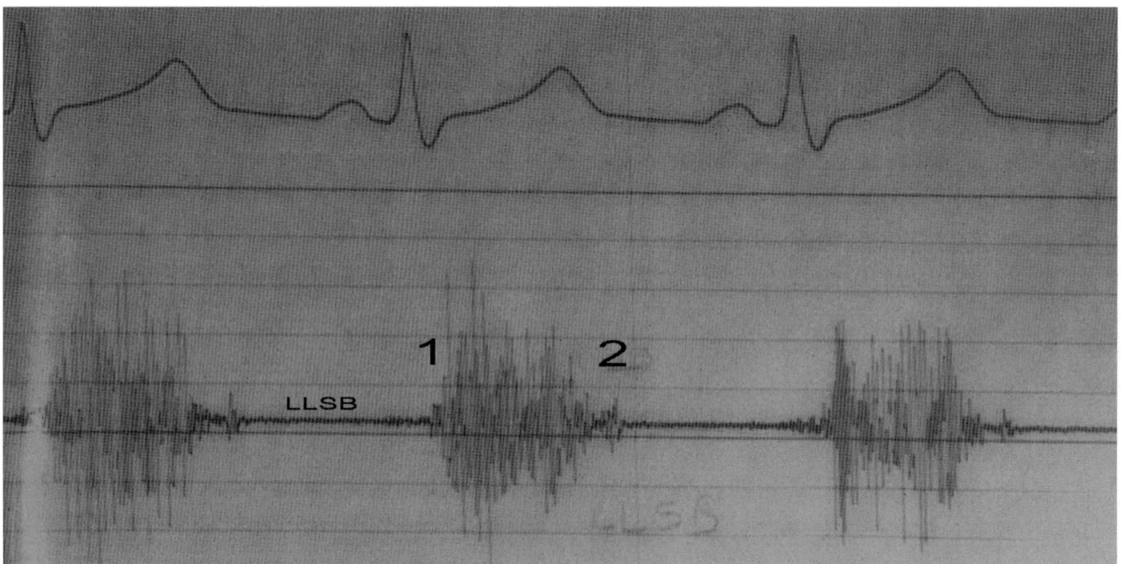

Figure 5.5 Phonocardiogram recorded at LLSB April 1997.

5 Two-dimensional echocardiogram April 1997

a. Chamber measurements (cm)
Aortic root diameter 3.2:
Left atrium 4.2:
LV end diastolic dimension 5.0
LV end systolic dimension 3.4.
LV septum 1.1;
LV posterior wall 1.1
RA 5.3

b. Peak velocity across the tricuspid valve 3.5 m/sec

c. Normal LV systolic contractility

Figure 5.6 Two-dimensional echocardiogram April 1997 (some of the data).

Calculate the RV systolic pressure, assuming a RA mean pressure of 10 mmHg. Compare the results of RV systolic pressure with cardiac catheterization data from 2 days later.

6 Cardiac catheterization data April 1997

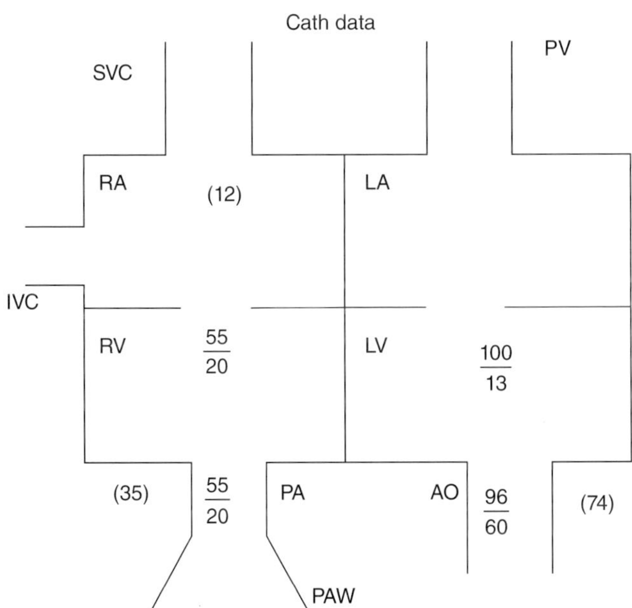

Figure 5.7 Intracardiac pressures and additional data. LV end-diastolic volume index 96 mL/m^2. LV end-systolic volume index 29 mL/m^2.

What is the LV ejection fraction? What would you expect the LV angiogram to show? The aortic root angiogram was normal and there was a small coronary–LV fistula (not shown).

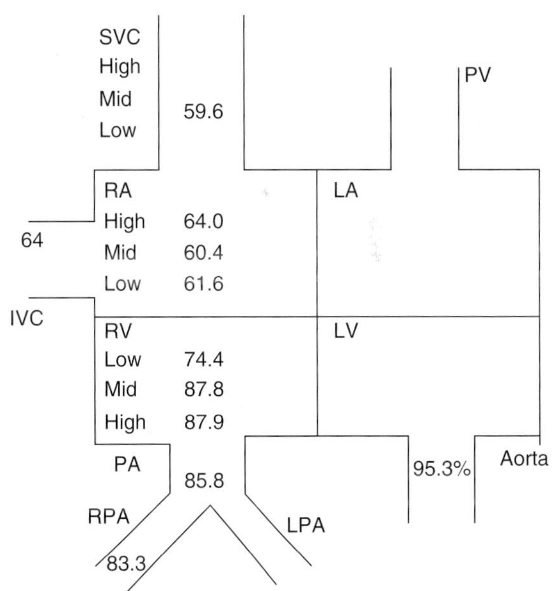

Figure 5.8 Oxygen saturation sample run.

What is the pulmonary/systemic flow ratio?

7 History and physical examination April 1997

History

The patient was a 40-year-old man who was stabbed in the chest in the left 4th interspace parasternally.

He was admitted to hospital in November 1996 in shock. He underwent successful pericardial and RV repair.

A systolic murmur was noted about 1 week later. A VSD and tricuspid regurgitation were found on echocardiography in November 1996. Surgical repair of VSD was delayed to allow full recovery from his emergency sternotomy and to allow the inflammation to subside before re-entering the chest.

He was readmitted to hospital in April 1997 with symptoms of wheezing and edema. Patient was a chronic alcoholic and cocaine user.

Physical examination

5 feet 9 inches tall, 153 lb male. BP 90/70. HR 88/min regular. There was a lateral chest wound scar and a well-healed median sternotomy incision.

The carotid amplitude was diminished. There was a prominent 'v' wave in the neck veins. The apex beat was in the 6th interspace 9 cm from the mid-sternal line.

S1 normal. S2 normal splitting. There was a grade 5/6 diamond-shaped systolic murmur maximum at the 3rd left interspace parasternally. This murmur radiated to the left 4th interspace parasternally and faded towards the apex.

Lungs were clear to percussion and auscultation.

No clubbing, cyanosis, or edema.

Comment on the history and physical examination. What is your diagnosis?

8 Transesophageal echocardiography May 1997

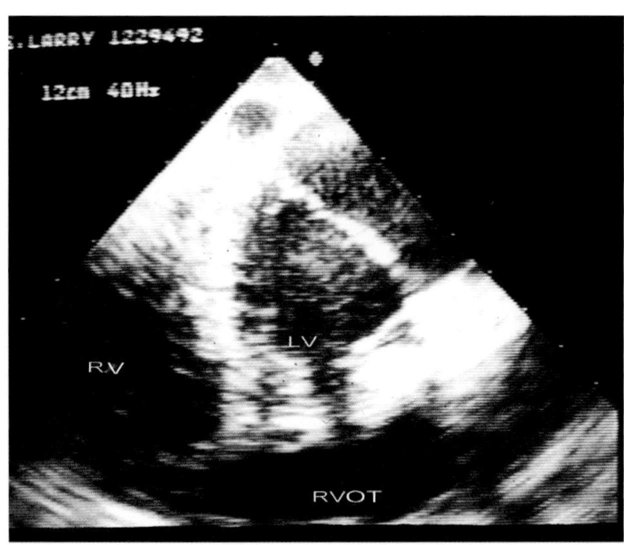

Figure 5.9 Transesophageal echocardiogram May 1997.

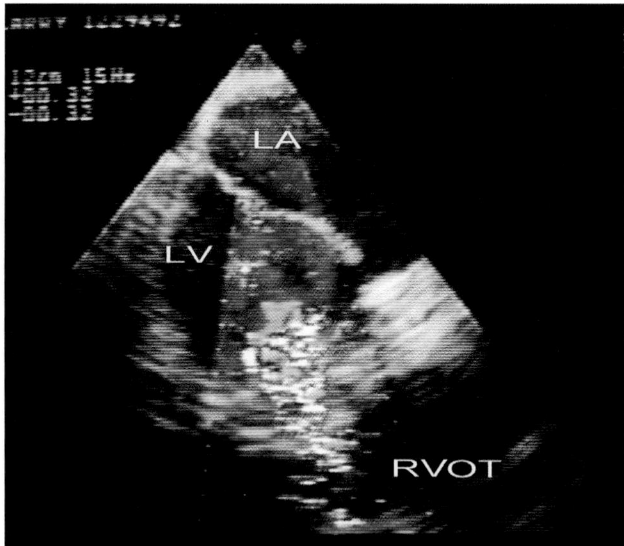

Figure 5.10 Transesophageal echocardiogram with color flow Doppler May 1997.

9 Course May–July 1997

At surgery the tricuspid valve appeared intact. Two septal defects were seen, a small one in the muscular septum and a larger one in the RV outflow tract. Both septal defects were closed with 0.6 mm size Gore-tex patches. Correction of the small coronary–LV fistula was not considered necessary. The patient had an uneventful recovery.

Answers and commentary

1 ECG November 1996

The rhythm is sinus. Rate 102/min. PR 0.15 s. QRS 0.08 s. QRS axis +40°.
Impression: sinus tachycardia.

2 ECG April 1997

The rhythm is sinus. Rate 90/min. PR 0.13 s. QRS 0.100 s. QRS axis +40°.
P waves are 3 mm tall in 2, 3, F, suggestive of RA enlargement. R′ in V1 = 10 mm may indicate RVH.
Impression: incomplete RBBB has appeared since November 1996. RVH and RAE may also be present.

3 Chest X ray April 1997

The PA view shows cardiomegaly with possible LV enlargement. The pulmonary vasculature is prominent, with vessels extending almost to the edge of the lung fields.
The lateral view shows sternal suture wires and possible RV enlargement.

4 Phonocardiogram April 1997

There is a pansystolic murmur, which tends to be diamond shaped, recorded at the LLSB. This could be due to a VSD or tricuspid regurgitation or both.

5 Two-dimensional echocardiogram April 1997

There was bi-atrial enlargement. LV size and function were normal.
The RV systolic pressure may be calculated as follows [2]:
RV systolic pressure $= 4v^2 +$ RA mean pressure = 60 mmHg
where v is the peak velocity across the tricuspid valve, i.e. 3.5 m/s, and RA mean pressure is 10 mmHg (assumed).
This is very similar to the RV systolic pressure of 55 mmHg found at cardiac catheterization 2 days later.
A single VSD 1 cm in diameter was also seen on two-dimensional echocardiography.

6 Cardiac catheterization April 1997

Cardiac catheterization

The RA pressure is moderately elevated. The RVEDP pressure is 20, indicative of RV dysfunction (? prior knife injury, ? secondary to VSD). There is moderately severe pulmonary hypertension. The RVEDP and the PA diastolic pressure are identical, probably due to pulmonary regurgitation.
There is some LV dysfunction as the LVEDP is slightly raised (13 mmHg).
The LV end-diastolic volume is increased slightly (normal 70 ± 20 mL/m²).
The LV ejection fraction is $\frac{96 - 29}{96}$ or 69%, which is normal.
The LV angiogram showed a subpulmonic VSD.

Oxygen saturation sample run

There is a step up in oxygen saturation on entering the RV from the RA, indicative of a VSD. The arterial oxygen saturation is normal (95.3%).
The average oxygen saturations in the RA and PA are 62% and 84.6%, respectively.
The pulmonary/systemic flow ratio (Q_p/Q_s) may then be calculated:

$$\frac{Q_p}{Q_s} = \frac{S_a - S_{ra}}{S_a - S_{pa}} = \frac{95.3 - 62.0}{95.3 - 84.6} = \frac{3.1}{1}$$

This is a significant left to right shunt.

7 History and physical examination

The patient had a high VSD produced by a knife wound. As noted previously there may be a time delay before the VSD becomes apparent after a cardiac contusion [1].
The systolic murmur was grade 5 in intensity, implying that this was a small VSD. As the VSD had been present for at least 6 months the patient had developed LV enlargement, moderate pulmonary hypertension, and secondary tricuspid regurgitation. However, as the tricuspid regurgitation was detected in November 1996 on echocardiography, some injury to this valve may have occurred secondary to the knife wound. It is likely that the diamond shaped murmur and the prolonged systolic duration of the murmur may have been due to both a VSD and a TR. The presence of a prominent 'v' wave in the neck veins supports the clinical

diagnosis of tricuspid regurgitation. As no injury to the tricuspid valve was seen at surgery, it is reasonable to assume that tricuspid regurgitation was secondary to pulmonary hypertension. Cardiac catheterization was useful in quantifying the size of the left to right shunt as well detecting a small coronary–LV fistula.

The echocardiogram in April failed to detect the increased LV end-diastolic volume noted on cardiac catheterization. Neither the echocardiogram nor the LV angiogram detected a small second VSD in the muscular septum.

8 Tranesesophagral echocardiography May 1997

This procedure was carried out just prior to cardiac surgery. It confirmed that there was a narrow passage between the LV and RV at the level of the RV outflow tract.

9 Course May-June 1997

As the left-to-right shunt was significant (Q_p/Q_s over 2/1), the patient was sent to surgery, where he underwent successful repair of the muscular and subpulmonic VSDs using a Gore-tex patch 0.6 mm in diameter for each of the VSDs.

Key points

1. Patients admitted in shock following a chest stabbing need careful follow-up to exclude other latent cardiac injuries once they have recovered from emergency surgery.
2. A VSD produced by a stabbing can involve the muscular and membranous portion of the septum.
3. TEE is an excellent way of detecting where the septum was injured but can miss smaller defects involving the muscular septum (as did the LV angiogram).

References

[1] Rollins MD, Koehler RP, Stevens MH, et al. Traumatic ventricular septal defect: Case report and review of the English literature since 1970. *J Trauma* 2005; 58: 175–180.

[2] Yock PG, Popp RL. Noninvasive estimation of right ventricular systolic pressure by Doppler ultrasound in patients with tricuspid regurgitation. *Circulation* 1984; 70: 657–662.

6 PATIENT STUDY 6

Sequence of data presentation

1 History
↓
2 ECG
↓
3 Chest X ray
↓
4 Pressures
↓
5 Oxygen sample run
↓
6 Catheter positions
↓
7 Angiography
↓
8 Cardiogreen dye curves
↓
9 Physical examination
↓
10 Operation

1 History

54-year-old black male admitted to hospital in 1975 with dyspnea for 2 months.
He had a life-long history of a heart murmur. No history of rheumatic fever or hypertension.
He drank 1 pint of whiskey a day for 15 years. Occasional smoker.

2 ECG

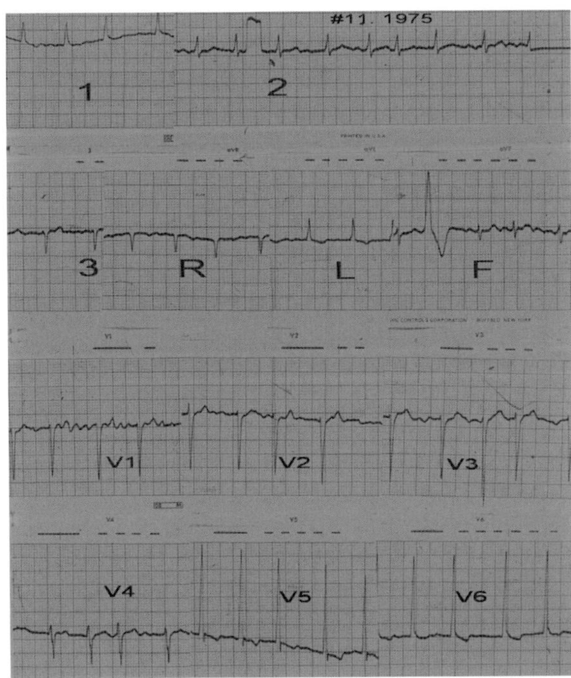

Figure 6.1 12-lead ECG 1975.

Patient Studies in Valvular, Congenital, and Rarer Forms of Cardiovascular Disease: An Integrative Approach, First Edition. Franklin B. Saksena.

Companion Website: www.wiley.com/go/saksena/patientstudies

3 Chest X ray

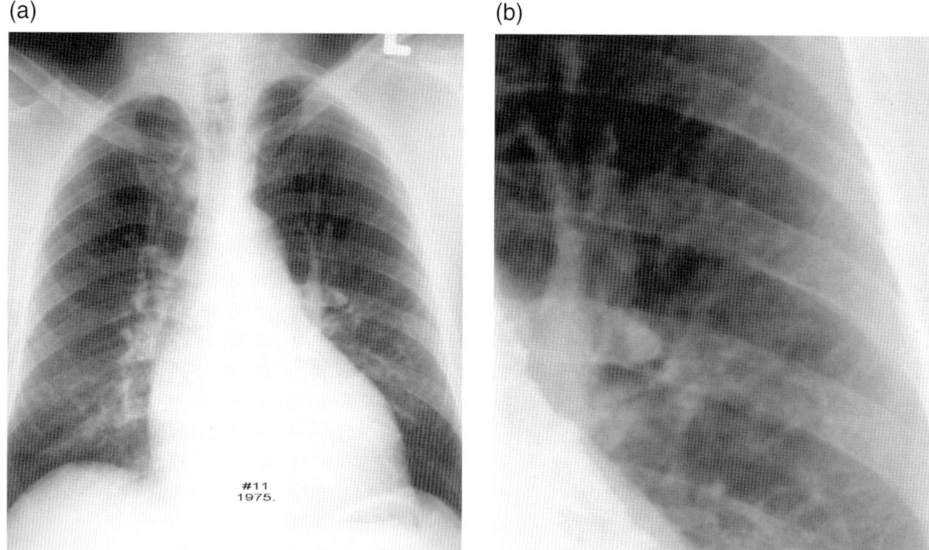

Figure 6.2 PA chest X ray.

4 Pressures

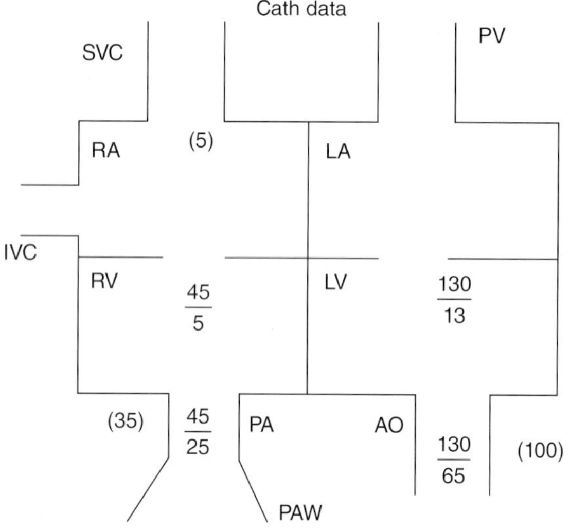

Figure 6.3 Right and left heart catheterization. Addendum: M-mode echocardiogram showed LV and LA enlargement.

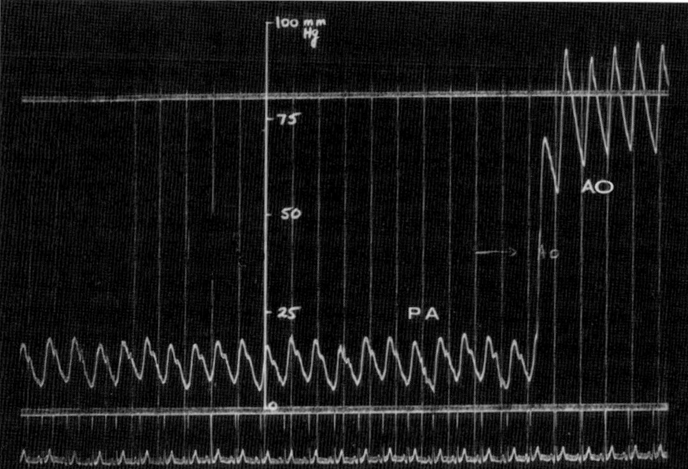

Figure 6.4 Pulmonary and aortic pressures. 0–100 mmHg scale.

5 Oxygen saturation run

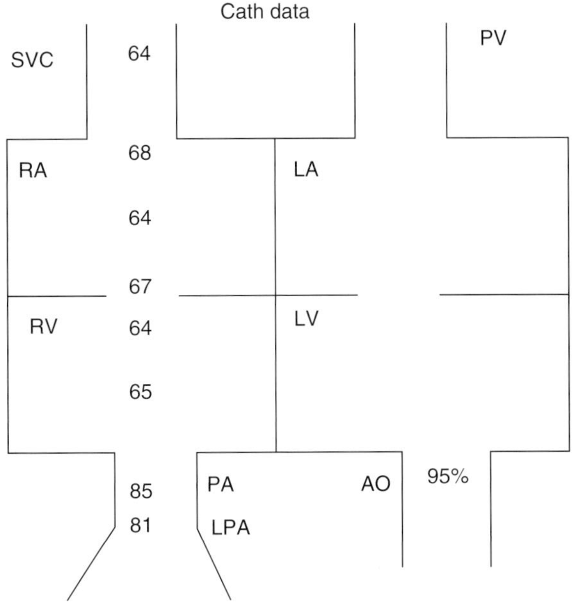

Figure 6.5 Oxygen saturation sample run. Hemoglobin 14.6 gm%. Estimated oxygen consumption 250 mL/min.
Calculate the blood flow.

6 Catheter positions

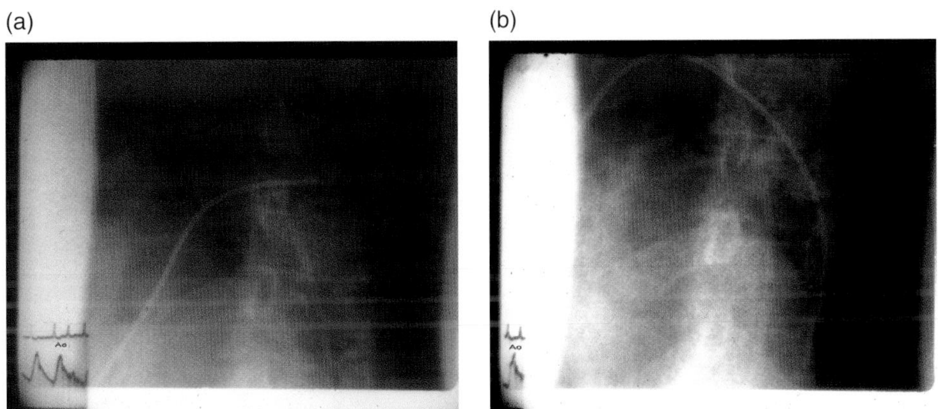

Figure 6.6 Catheters in PA and aorta.
Comment on the significance of the positions of the PA and aortic catheters.

7 Angiography

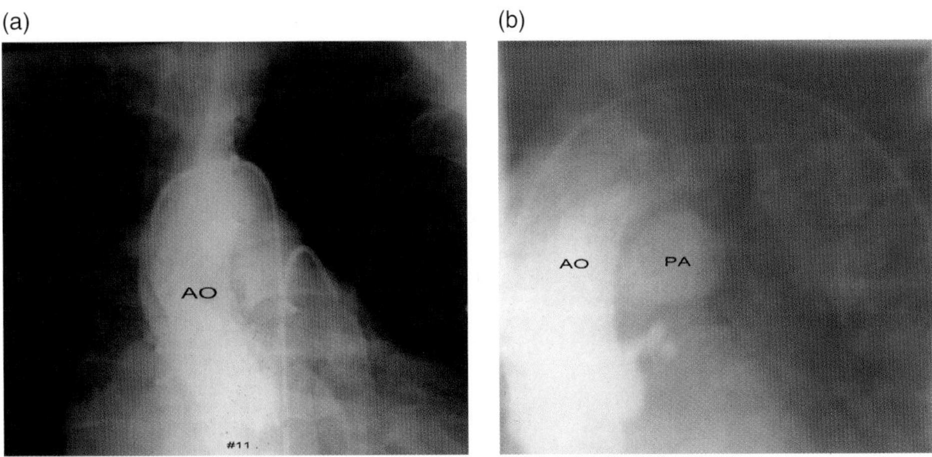

Figure 6.7 (a) AP view of aortogram. (b) Lateral view of aortogram.

8 Cardiogreen dye curves

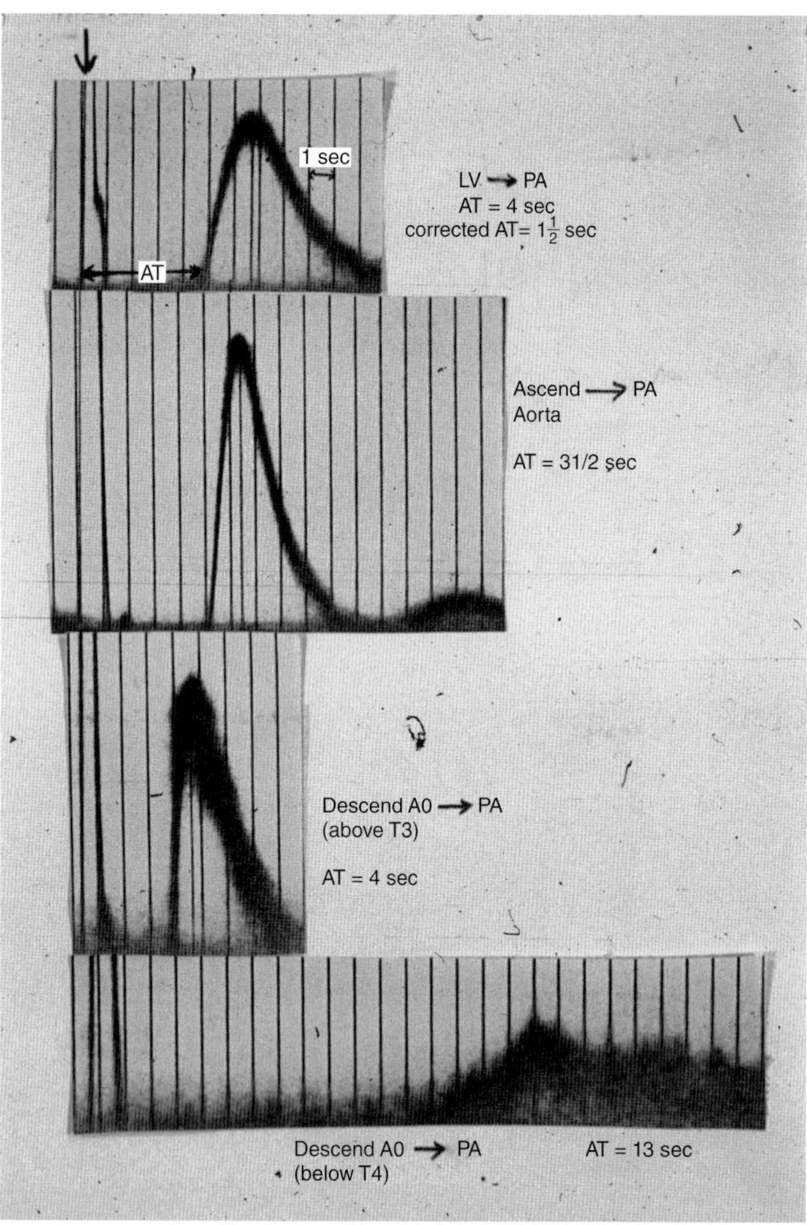

Figure 6.8 Cardiogreen dye curves. Arrow indicates where dye was injected. Vertical lines are l s apart. AT, appearance time.

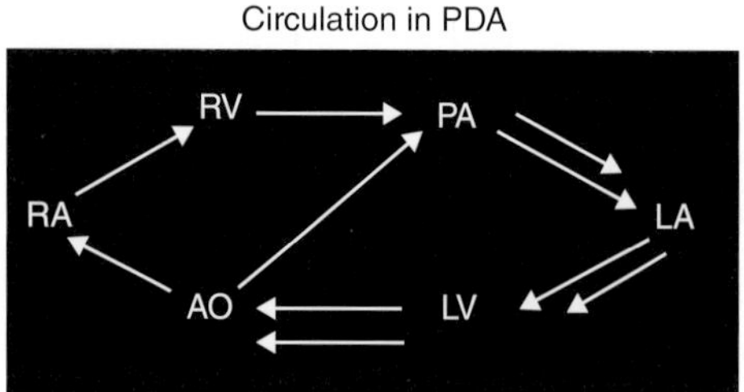

Figure 6.9 Circulation in PDA. Blood flows from the Ao to the PA via a PDA, resulting in pulmonary arterial, left atrial, and left ventricular enlargement.

9 Physical examination

BP 130/70. Pulse 86/min. The pulse was hyperdynamic and irregular.
R 16/min. T 97.4 °F.
Prominent carotid pulsations.
Apex beat was in the 6th interspace 2 cm outside the mid-clavicular line.
Sustained LV impulse.
S1 normal. S2 showed an increase in P2.
Grade 4/6 pansystolic murmur that continued into mid diastole, loudest in the left 2nd and 3rd interspaces parasternally.
No leg edema, cyanosis, or clubbing. Normal peripheral pulses.
Lungs were clear.
No hepatomegaly.

What is the diagnosis and treatment?

Answers and commentary

1 History

A life-long heart murmur could be due to valvular or congenital heart disease. The absence of a history of rheumatic fever does not exclude rheumatic heart disease. His dyspnea could be due to early heart failure from valvular or congenital heart disease, or possibly from an alcoholic cardiomyopathy.

2 ECG

Rate 75–100/min. Rhythm: atrial fibrillation with rare PVC. PR QRS 0.06 s. QRS axis 0°. S in V1+. R in V6 = 5 mv. Impression: LVH with repolarization abnormalities and atrial fibrillation.

3 Chest X ray

There is mild cardiomegaly (C/T ratio 0.53) and possibly LV enlargement. The proximal pulmonary arteries are enlarged and there is some pulmonary vascular congestion. The panel on the right shows plethoric vessels extending to the periphery of the left lung field.

4 Oxygen sample run

There is a step up in the oxygen saturation on entering the PA from the RV. This is most likely due to a PDA.
Less common causes of such a step up are an aorto-pulmonary window or an anomalous coronary artery arising from the PA [1].
The PA oxygen saturation in PDA may not reflect a true mixed venous sample because a catheter in the left pulmonary artery will sample blood taken from both the ductus and the blood ejected by the RV [1].
Thus the calculation of the Q_p/Q_s ratio (shown below) in PDA is an approximation at best.
As the arterial oxygen saturation is normal, the shunt is most likely only a left to right one.
The pulmonary/systemic flow ratio is 2.5/1, as shown below:

pulmonary blood flow (Q_p) = oxygen consumption/pulmonary AV O_2 difference
systemic blood flow (Q_s) = oxygen consumption/systemic AV O_2 difference

Therefore Q_p/Q_s = systemic AV O_2 difference/pulmonary AV O_2 difference
= (Cao – Crv)/(Cao – Cpa), where C is oxygen content and Crv is pre-shunt sample
= (Sao – Srv)/(Sao – Spa), where S is oxygen saturation
= (95 – 65)/(95 – 83)
= 2.5/1

5 Pressure measurements

There is moderately severe pulmonary hypertension (PA mean 35 mmHg).
There is a slight increase in the LVEDP to 13 mmHg, which could be due to LV failure or a noncompliant LV. The pulse pressure is wider than usual, which may be seen in several conditions, for example aortic regurgitation, an A–V shunt (e.g. PDA), or a high output state.

6 Catheter positions

The pressures indicate that the catheter was advanced from the PA to the aorta. Such findings are indicative of a connection between the PA and the aorta, such as a PDA or an aortopulmonary window. An aortic pulmonary window is very rare and occurs in 1/200 the incidence of a PDA.

In the left-hand panel of Figure 6.6 the catheter is in the PA and has advanced to the aorta, as shown by the arterial pressure in the cine trace at the lower left-hand corner. In the right-hand panel the PA catheter has been advanced to the descending aorta, which is indicative of a ductus rather than an aortopulmonary window. If the catheter had advanced up the ascending aorta rather than the descending aorta then an aortopulmonary window would have been proven.

Thus the catheter positioning shows that we are dealing with a ductus and not an aortopulmonary window.

7 Aortogram

Injection of contrast media into the ascending aorta shows early filling of the PA due to a ductus. While the ductus is not well seen in the lateral view, the PA is seen to be separate from the ascending aorta, thus making an aortopulmonary window unlikely.

8 Cardiogreen dye curves

The early appearance of cardiogreen when it was injected into the LV or the ascending aorta and sampled from the PA also indicates an aortic to pulmonary connection. This connection is between T3 and T4 on the basis of the descending aorta to PA dye curve (below T4) and the ascending aorta to PA dye curve (above T3).

Figure 6.9 describes the circulation with a PDA that can make it easier to visualize the course of the dye when injected in the aorta and sampled from the PA.

9 Physical examination

The presence of a continuous murmur maximum at the left 2nd interspace parasternally is highly suggestive of a PDA. Usually there is late peaking of the systolic component of the murmur, but this was not mentioned in this physical examination. A continuous murmur starts in systolic and spills over into diastole, but is not necessarily pan diastolic. The heart was enlarged and there was evidence of pulmonary hypertension. The absence of cyanosis or clubbing favors a left to right shunt.

Other causes of a continuous murmur need to be excluded. In the absence of any chest deformity a continuous murmur heard in the 3rd or 4th left interspace favors a ruptured sinus of valvsalva or a coronary AV fistula. A VSD with aortic regurgitation may also simulate a continuous murmur but is usually best heard in the 3rd or 4th left interspace without late peaking of the systolic component of the VSD [2].

10 Diagnosis and treatment

The patient had a moderate-sized PDA with moderately severe pulmonary hypertension, left heart enlargement, and a pulmonary/systemic flow ratio of 2.5/1.

At operation in December 1975 the ductus was surrounded by fibrous tissue. During dissection around the ductus, the ductus was perforated. The patient was placed on carotid pulmonary bypass. The ductus was transected and the pulmonary side sutured closed. The aortic side was sutured closed and a Dacron graft wrapped around the aorta to reinforce the aortic stitch. He did well postoperatively.

Discussion

PDA occurs about 1 in 2000 births and accounts for 5–10% of all congenital heart diseases [3]. In the presence of a normal position of the aortic arch the ductus connects the left PA near its origin to the descending aorta just inferior to the left subclavian artery.

A PDA usually manifests itself early in life as a left to right shunt. The size of the shunt depends on the level of the pulmonary vascular resistance [3], the width and length of the ductus [4] as well as the ability of the LV to tolerate the volume overload. Once the pulmonary resistance rises the left to right shunt diminishes and eventually a right to left shunt occurs. Eisenmenger syndrome develops when the PA pressure exceeds the systemic BP, often associated with a ductal diameter of 0.7–1.6 cm [4].

This patient developed LV failure late in life as his left to right shunt flow was not that high. His LV failure was aggravated by the existence of atrial fibrillation.

The natural history of a PDA is for death to occur usually from heart failure at the age of 35 [5]. By age 60 about 60% of patients with PDA are dead [5].

There are occasional patients with PDA reported in the literature surviving to old age [4, 6], presumably because they only have a mild to moderate left to right shunt. Echocardiography is considered the pre-eminent diagnostic tool in PDA [7], but it should not replace a careful physical examination of the patient.

In 1975 surgical closure of the PDA was the only available treatment for this patient. It is common now to close the PDA with Gianturco or Ni-occlud coils in children [3] or an Amplatzer ductal occluder I for adults [8]. A case can still be made for surgical closure of the ductus, especially if it is very large [3] or is heavily calcified.

Key points

1. A patient with a PDA can present late in life with heart failure (given that 60% of PDA patients are dead by age 60).
2. Patients with a left to right shunt from a PDA have a continuous murmur best heard at the 2nd or 3rd interspace parasternally. The diastolic component of the murmur can shorten with progressive pulmonary hypertension.
3. A calcified ductus can make surgical closure more hazardous.

References

[1] Rudolph AM. *Congenital diseases of the heart. Clinical-Physiological Considerations*, 2nd edn. Armonk, NY, Futura, 2001, p 97 and pp184–190.

[2] Constant J. *Continuous murmurs*. In: Bedside Cardiology, 5th edn. Philadelphia, Lippinocott Williams & Wilkins, 1999, pp 267–282.

[3] Schneider KJ, Moore JW. Patent ductus arteriosus. *Circulation* 2006; 114: 1873–1882.

[4] Tikoff G, Echegaray HM, Schmidt AM et al. Patent ductus arteriosus complicated by heart failure. Classification based on clinical and serial hemodynamic studies. *Am J Med* 1969; 46: 43–51.

[5] Campbell M. Natural history of persistent ductus arteriosus. *Brit Heart J* 1968; 30: 4–13.

[6] Ong K, Madan R. Patent ductus arteriosus diagnosed in old age. *Am J Geriatr Card* 1998; 7: 14–16.

[7] Shyu KG, Lai LP, Lin SC et al. Diagnostic accuracy of transesophageal echocardiography for detecting patient ductus arteriosus in adolescents and adults. *Chest* 1995; 108: 1201–1205.

[8] Meadows J, Landzberg MJ. Advances in transcatheter interventions in adults with congenital heart disease. *Prog Cardiovasc Dis* 2011; 53: 265–273.

7 PATIENT STUDY 7

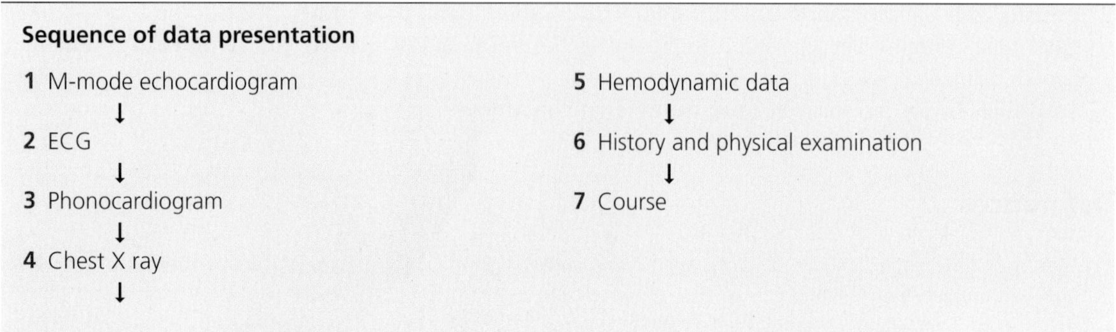

Sequence of data presentation

1 M-mode echocardiogram
↓
2 ECG
↓
3 Phonocardiogram
↓
4 Chest X ray
↓
5 Hemodynamic data
↓
6 History and physical examination
↓
7 Course

1 M-mode echocardiogram

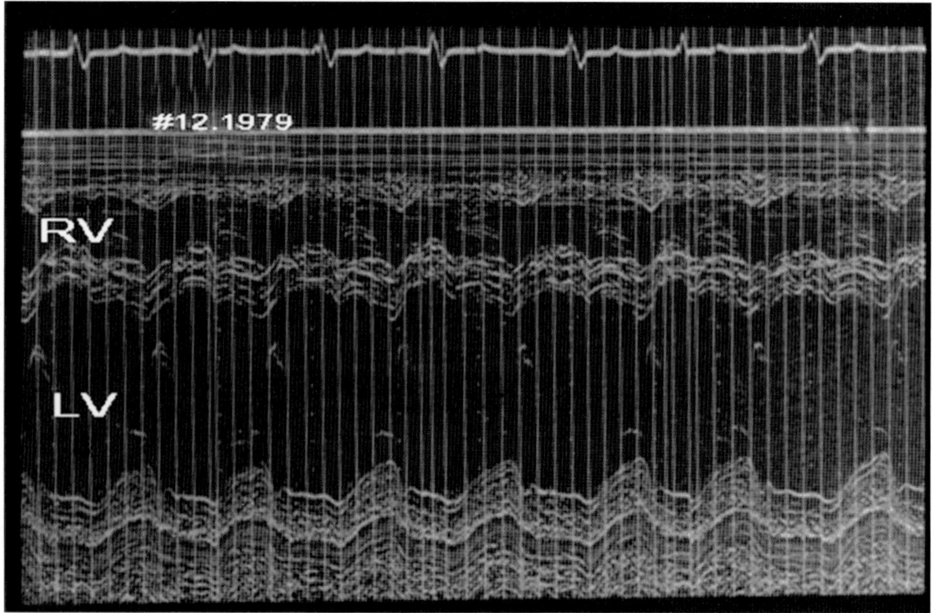

Figure 7.1 M-mode echocardiogram. The dots are 1 cm apart.

Patient Studies in Valvular, Congenital, and Rarer Forms of Cardiovascular Disease: An Integrative Approach, First Edition. Franklin B. Saksena.

Companion Website: www.wiley.com/go/saksena/patientstudies

2 ECG

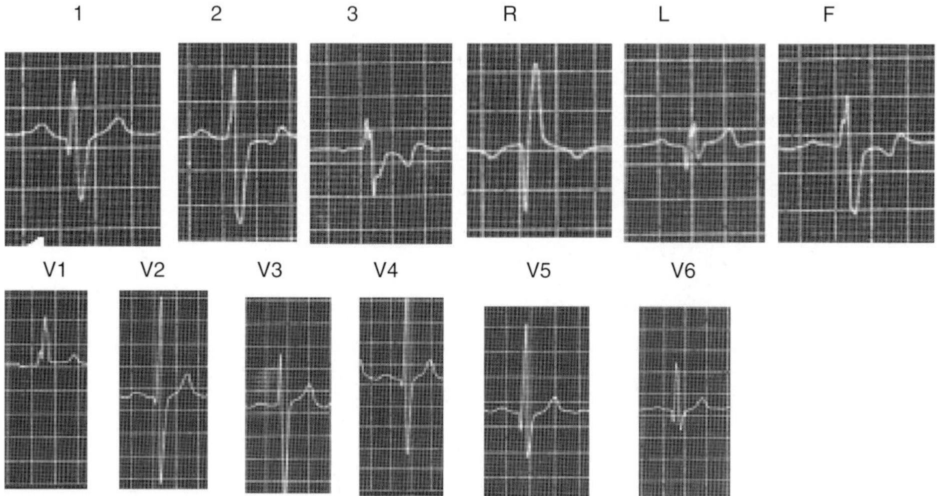

Figure 7.2 12-lead ECG.

3 Phonocardiogram

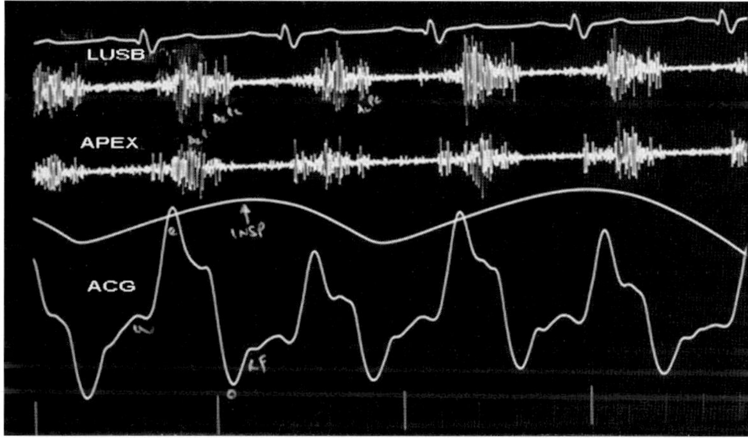

Figure 7.3 Phonocardiogram showing, from the top, ECG, phonocardiograms recording at the left 3rd interspace parasternally (LUSB), recording at apex, respiratometer, and ACG.

4 Chest X ray

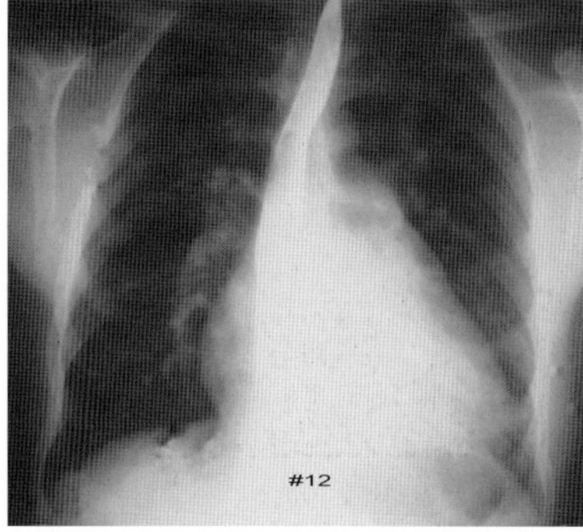

Figure 7.4 Chest X ray PA view with barium swallow.

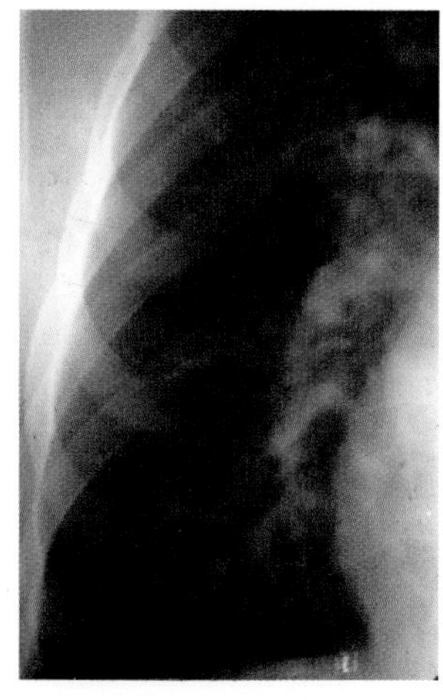

Figure 7.5 Right lung field. PA view.

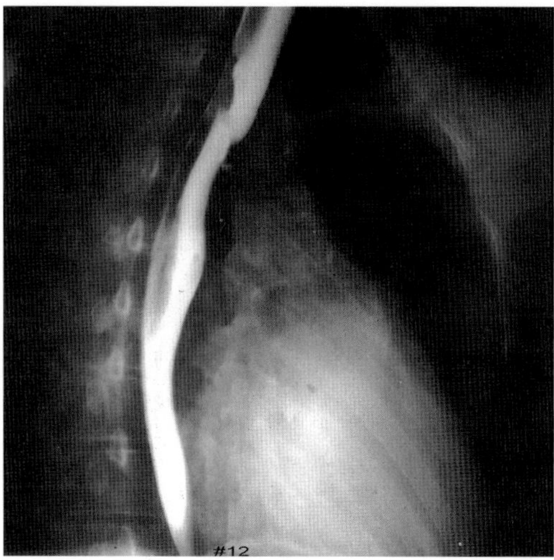

Figure 7.6 Chest X ray in RAO projection with barium swallow.

5 Hemodynamic data

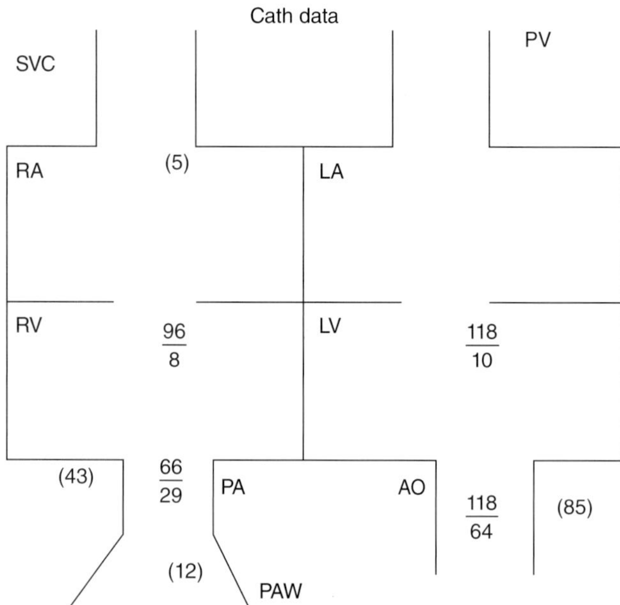

Figure 7.7 Intracardiac pressures.

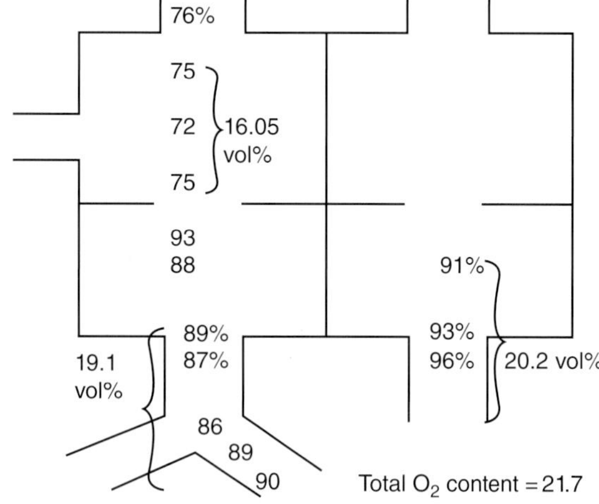

Figure 7.8 Oxygen content sample run.

Calculate the blood flow measurements given that the oxygen consumption is 344 mL/min. Calculate the pulmonary and systemic vascular resistances.

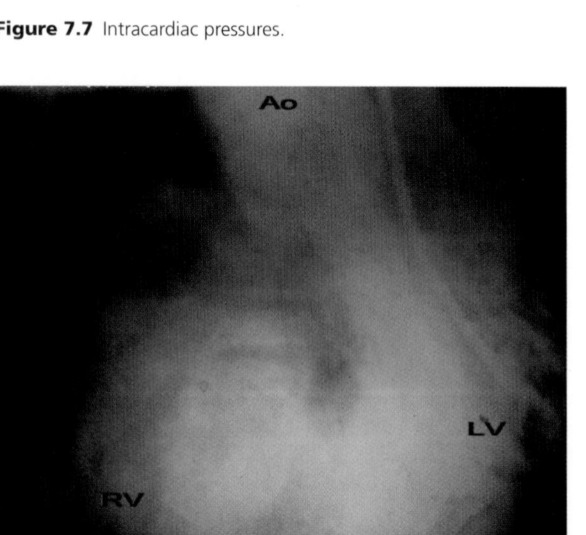

Figure 7.9 LV angiogram in 60° LAO view.

6 History and physical examination

History

21-year-old Hispanic male admitted to hospital in 1979 with dyspnea on exertion for 2 months. He denies any history of rheumatic heart disease or difficulty in playing soccer as a youth. He came to the USA 6 months ago and whilst working on the railroad developed dyspnea on moderate activity.

No history of paroxysmal nocturnal dyspnea, orthopnea, or hemoptysis.

Physical examination

63 inches tall, 114 lb male. BP 110/70. HR 90/min. RR 15/min.

There was a pectus excavatum. No cyanosis or clubbing.

Apex beat at the 6th interspace in the mid-clavicular line. Right parasternal lift.

S1 normal. S2 showed a loud P2. S3 apex.

Grade 4/6 systolic murmur that extended to all of systole and had crescendo–decrescendo features. The murmur was maximal at the 4th left interspace parasternally.

Grade 2/6 apical diastolic rumble.

7 Course

Comment on the likely course.

Answers and commentary

1 M-mode echocardiogram

LV end-diastolic dimension = 7.0 cm, LV septum = 1.8 cm

LV end-systolic dimension = 5.0 cm, LV posterior wall = 1.8 cm

RV end-diastolic dimension = 2.0 cm

Impression: (i) moderately enlarged LV, (ii) moderately severe LVH.

2 ECG

Rhythm sinus. Rate 86/min. PR 0.20 s. QRS 0.06 s. QRS axis indeterminate.

R wave in V1 = 2 mv (as chest leads are half standard). T inverted 3, F.

Impression: (i) RVH, (ii) nonspecific T wave abnormalities.

3 Phonocardiogram

There is a crescendo–decrescendo systolic murmur recorded at the LUSB and at the apex. The 4th beat shows a slight increase in the murmur (LUSB) on inspiration, suggestive of a flow murmur across the pulmonic valve.

The murmur at the apex could be of left-sided or right-sided origin, depending on whether the apex is occupied by the RV or the LV. A left-sided lesion has to be present to account for the LVH and LV enlargement (e.g. MR or VSD).

4 Chest X ray

There is cardiomegaly in the PA film mostly due to LV enlargement (C/T ratio 0.63). RV, LA, and main PAs are enlarged. There is pulmonary plethora (Figure 7.5).

Figure 7.6 shows an enlarged PA and LA enlargement (as the LA has pushed the barium-filled esophagus posteriorly).

5 Hemodynamic data

Intracardiac pressures

There is a small gradient in systole across the pulmonic valve suggestive of mild pulmonic stenosis or a high flow across the pulmonary valve in systole. There is moderately severe pulmonary hypertension. Left heart pressures are normal.

Oxygen sample run

There is a step up in oxygen saturation on entering the RV from the RA, indicative of a VSD.

Calculation of left to right shunt

Data

Oxygen consumption = 344 mL/min (Vo_2)
Aortic oxygen content = 202 mL/L (Cao)
Pulmonary artery oxygen content = 191 mL/L (Cpa)
RA oxygen content = 160.5 mL/L (Cx)

$$Q_p = \frac{344}{202-191} = 31.2 \text{ L/min} \quad Q_s = \frac{344}{202-160.5} = 8.3 \text{ L/min}$$

$$Q_p/Q_s = 3.8/1$$

where Q_p is pulmonary blood flow and Q_s is systemic blood flow, as defined below:

$$Q_p = \frac{Vo_2}{Cao - Cpa} \quad Q_s = \frac{Vo_2}{Cao - Cra}$$

Calculation of pulmonary and systemic resistances

$$\text{Pulmonary vascular resistance } (PVR) = \frac{PA - PAW}{Q_p} \times 80$$

$$= \frac{43-12}{31.2} \times 80 = 79 \; dyn.\text{sec}.cm-5$$

$$\text{Systemic vascular resistance } = \frac{Ao - RA}{Q_s} \times 80$$

$$\text{SVR} = \frac{85-5}{8.3} \times 80 = 771 \text{ dyn.sec.cm} - 5$$

where Ao, PA, PAW, and RA are mean pressures (mmHg).
The PVR is normal and the SVR mildly reduced.

LV angiogram in 60° LAO view

LV angiography shows filling of the RV via a large VSD in the subaortic position.

6 History and physical examination

The patient has evidence of pulmonary hypertension (RV lift, loud P2).

The pansystolic murmur is due to both a VSD and increased flow across the pulmonic valve. The diastolic murmur is due to increased flow across the mitral valve from the left to right shunt, producing relative mitral stenosis. This diastolic murmur often occurs when the Q_p/Q_s ratio exceeds 2/1 (in this patient it was 3.8/1).

7 Course

The patient underwent successful closure of the VSD with a Teflon patch as well as pulmonary valvotomy.

Discussion

VSDs occur in about 2 out of 1000 new births and comprise 20% of all cases of congenital heart disease [1].

This patient had a large left to right shunt at VSD level with a pulmonary/systemic ratio of 3.8/1, a pulmonary/systemic systolic pressure ratio of 0.55, and a normal pulmonary vascular resistance. This left to right shunt led to LV enlargement and pulmonary hypertension.

The usual indications for surgical closure of a VSD include a symptomatic patient, $Q_p/Q_s > 1.5/1$, pulmonary systolic pressure > 50 mmHg, and LV volume overload [1]. This patient was thus a suitable candidate for surgical closure of the VSD, which he underwent successfully.

Patients with pulmonary/systemic systolic pressure > 0.66 may still be considered for surgery provided the Q_p/Q_s ratio is at least 1.5/1 [2]. Those patients with irreversible pulmonary hypertension, especially if their pulmonary vascular resistance > 560 dyn.sec cm^{-5}, have a high operative risk [1, 2].

Transcatheter closure devices are best suited for treating a muscular VSD with an adequate rim, rather than a perimembraneous VSD, as there is a risk of aortic valve damage if closure devices are used for perimembranous VSDs [2, 3].

Several echocardiographic methods are now available to show the location of a VSD and detect any associated anomalies. Doppler flow studies can readily calculate the RV systolic pressure, the Q_p/Q_s ratio and the size of the VSD [4].

1. RV systolic pressure (RVSP)
   a. RVSP = systolic blood pressure – $(4v^2)$
      where v is the peak velocity across the VSD.
   b. RVSP = $(4v^2_{TV})$ + RA mean pressure
      where v_{TV} is the peak velocity across the tricuspid valve in those patients with significant tricuspid regurgitation.
2. Calculation of Q_p/Q_s

$$\frac{Q_p}{Q_s} = \frac{SV_{rvot}}{SV_{lvot}}$$

where SV_{rvot} = stroke volume via RV outflow tract = area of RVOT × mean velocity across RVOT × time.
SV_{lvot} = stroke volume via LV outflow tract = area of LVOT × mean velocity across LVOT × time
Errors may occur if the outflow area is incorrectly measured or there is an arrhythmia.

3. The size of the VSD may be assessed by the proximal isovelocity surface area (PISA) method and the continuity principle [5].

$$A_{vsd} \times VTI = 2\Pi r^2 \times v_a$$

where A_{vsd} = area of VSD cm^2, VTI = velocity time integral across VSD (cm), $2\Pi r^2$ = surface area of a hemisphere of radius r (cm^2), and V_a = aliasing velocity (cm/s) at a distance r from the VSD.

Key points

1. VSD is the most common form of congenital heart disease.
2. Surgical closure is recommended in the symptomatic VSD patient who has $Q_p/Q_s > 1.5/1$, pulmonary systolic pressure >50 mmHg, and LV volume overload.
3. Cardiac catheterization and echo Doppler studies can measure the size of the defect, the pulmonary/systemic flow ratio, and the RV pressures. Measurement of the pulmonary/systemic resistance can also be obtained at cardiac catheterization.
4. Patients with a VSD who have a high pulmonary vascular resistance (>560 dyne.sec.cm^{-5}) and $Q_p/Q_s < 1.5/1$ pose a high surgical risk for closure.

References

[1] Ammash NM, Warnes CA. Ventricular septal defects in adults. *Ann Int Med* 2001; 135: 812–824.
[2] Minette MS, Sahn DJ. Ventricular septal defects. *Circulation* 2006; 114: 2190–2197.
[3] Webb GD et al. *Ventricular septal defect.* In: Braunwald's heart disease, A textbook of Cardiovascular Medicine, 9th edn, Bonow RO (ed.). WB Saunders, Philadelphia, 2011, p 1432.
[4] Pai RG, Shah PM. Echocardiographic and other noninvasive measurements of cardiac hemodynamics and ventricular function. *Curr Probl Cardiol.* 1995; 20: 681–772.
[5] Moises VA, Maciel BC, Hornberger LK et al. A new method for noninvasive estimation of ventricular septal defect shunt flow by Doppler color Fflow mapping: Imaging of the laminar flow convergence region on the left septal surface. *J. Am Coll Cardiol* 1991; 18: 824–832.

8 PATIENT STUDY 8

Sequence of data presentation

1 Physical examination
↓
2 Phonocardiogram
↓
3 M-mode echocardiogram
↓
4 ECG
↓
5 Chest X ray 1979
↓
6 Cardiac catheterization 1979
↓
7 Additional hemodynamic data 1979
↓
8 Angiography
↓
9 Chest X ray 1980
↓
10 Cardiac catheterization 1980
↓
11 Additional hemodynamic data 1980
↓
12 History and course

1 Physical examination

67 inches tall, 148 lb male. BP 110/70. Pulse 78/min regular.
No cardiomegaly. S1 normal intensity. S2 single.
Grade 4/6 continuous murmur heard at the LUSB.
Grade 3/6 early diastolic blowing murmur heard at the RUSB.
Lungs clear.
Good peripheral pulses. No cyanosis or clubbing.

2 Phonocardiogram

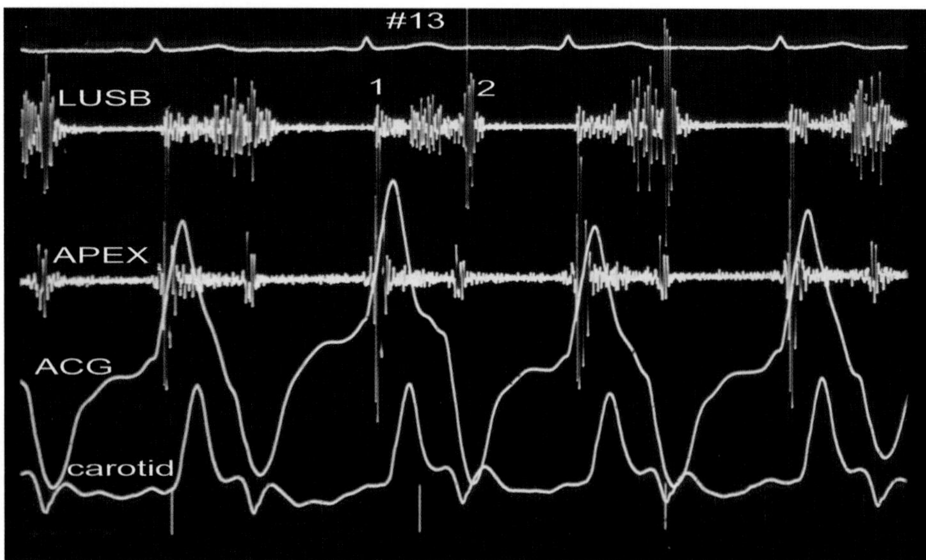

Figure 8.1 Phonocardiogram 1979. From above downwards are the ECG, phonocardiograms (LUSB, apex), ACG, and carotid pulse tracings.

Patient Studies in Valvular, Congenital, and Rarer Forms of Cardiovascular Disease: An Integrative Approach, First Edition. Franklin B. Saksena.

Companion Website: www.wiley.com/go/saksena/patientstudies

3 M-mode echocardiogram

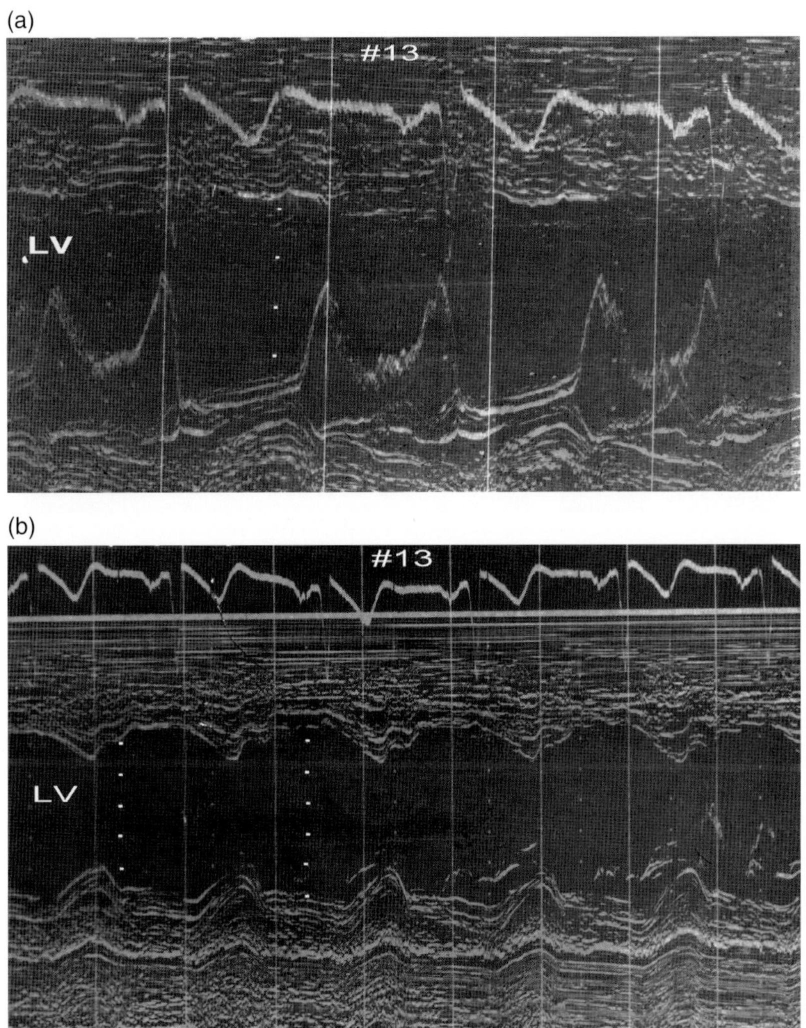

Figure 8.2 (a) M-mode echocardiogram of the mitral valve 1979. (b) M-mode echocardiogram of the LV cavity 1979. The distance between each vertical dot is 1 cm.

4 ECG

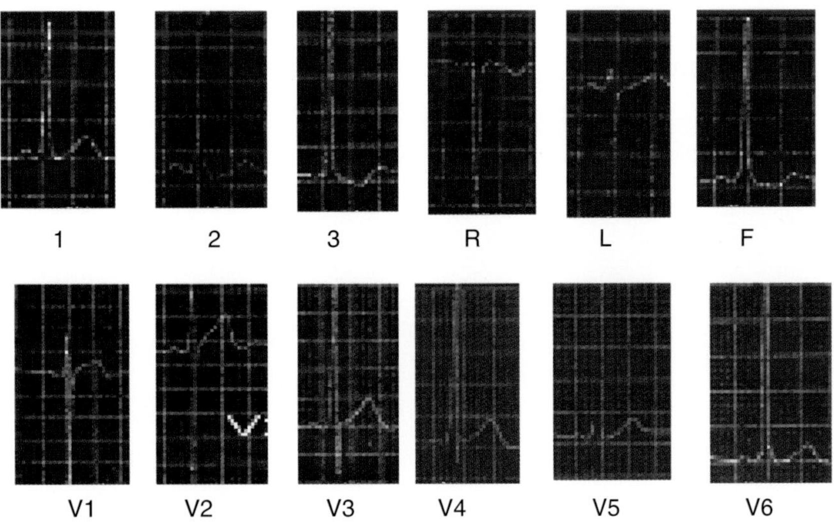

Figure 8.3 12-lead ECG 1979.

5 Chest X ray 1979

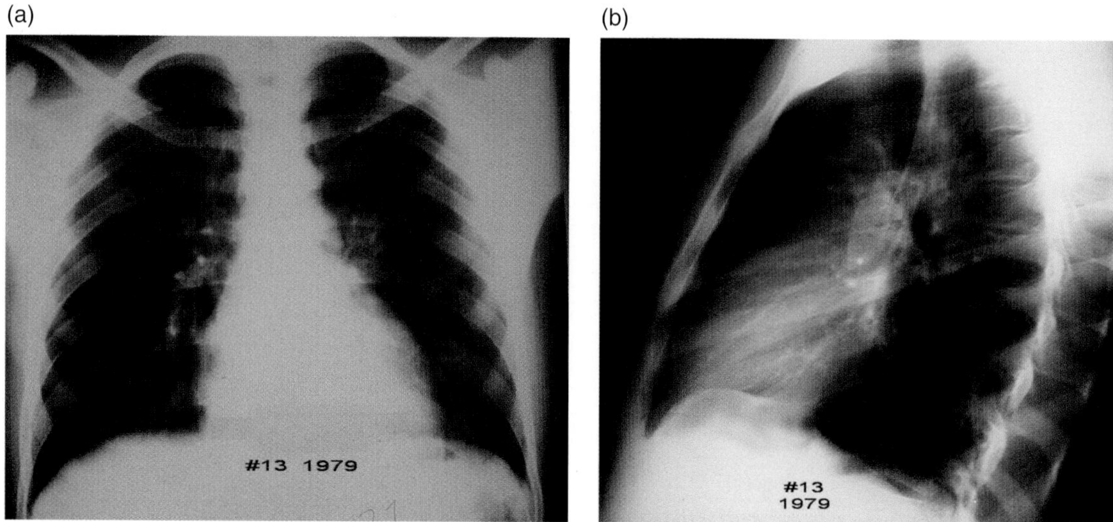

Figure 8.4 Chest X ray 1979. (a) PA view. (b) Lateral view.

6 Cardiac catheterization 1979

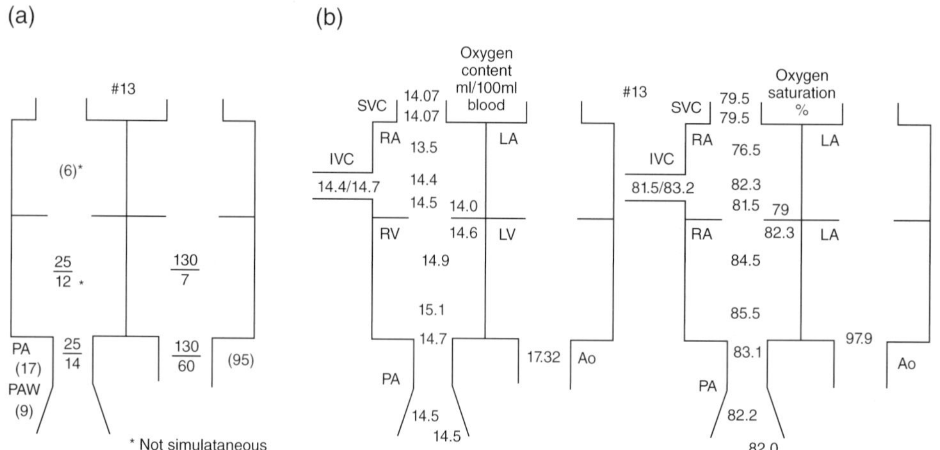

Figure 8.5 (a) Hemodynamic data 1979. (b) Oxygen sample run 1979 (O_2 content and corresponding O_2 saturation).

Table 8.1 Additional hemodynamic data (respiratory gas analysis, LV–PA dye curve) 1979

Respiratory gas analysis	Hemoglobin 13.2 g%
Minute ventilation	9.4 L/min
O_2 consumption	150 mL/min
O_2 consumption index	82 mL/min/m^2
CO_2 production	113 mL/min
Respiratory quotient	0.76
Body surface area	1.82 m^2

LV to PA cardiogreen dye curves

Injecting cardiogreen dye into the LV and sampling from the PA showed an appearance time of 4.4 seconds. The corrected appearance time, taking into account the catheter transit time of the green dye is l.4 seconds.

Comment on the respiratory gas analysis data.
What are the cardiac output and the cardiac index using data from Figure 8.5b and the oxygen consumption given above?

7 Additional hemodynamic data 1979

Table 8.2 Additional hemodynamic data (LV volumes)

LV end-diastolic volume index	110 mL/m^2
LV end-systolic volume index	43 mL/m^2
HR	90/min

What is the LV ejection fraction?
What is the regurgitant fraction using the cardiac output data from Table 8.1?

8 Angiography

(a) (b)

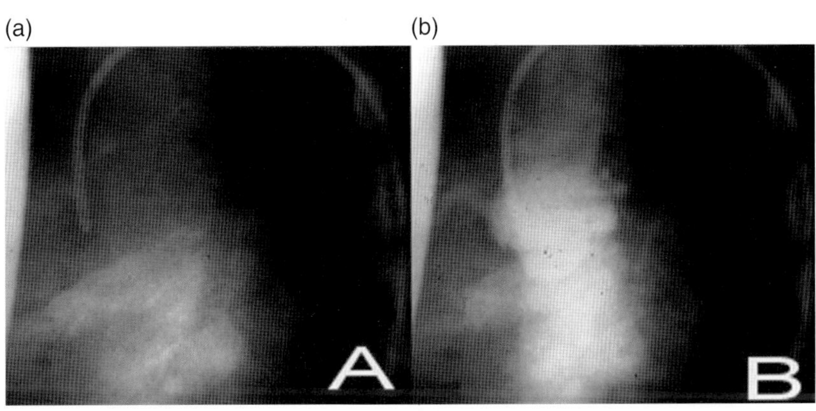

(c)

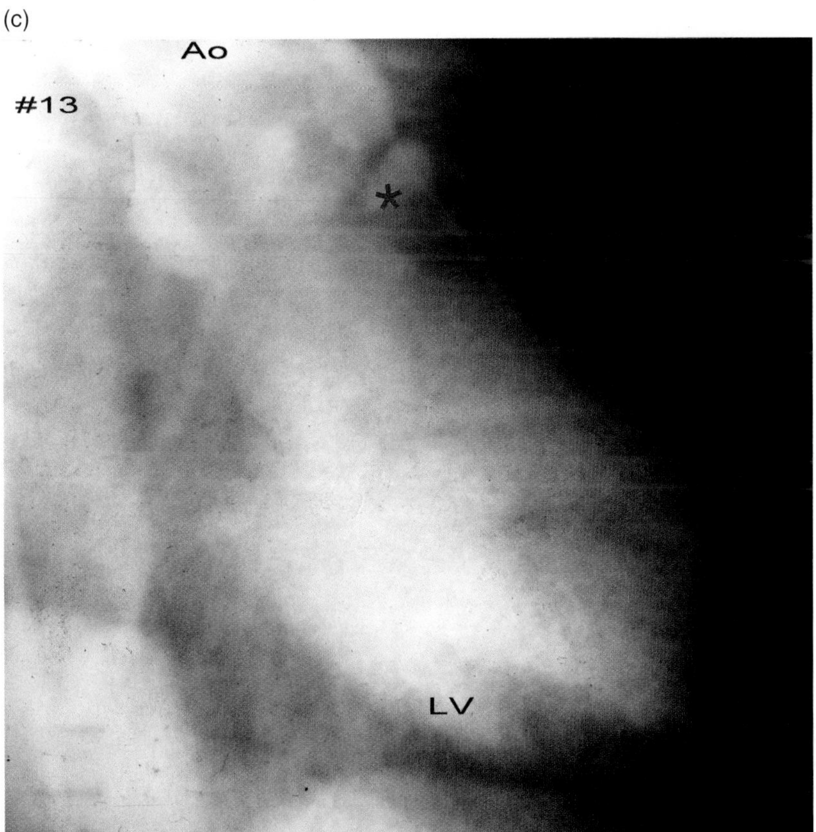

Figure 8.6 Aortic root angiography 1979 in 60° LAO position, before and during angiography. In panel (a) the arterial catheter is positioned just superior to the aortic valve. Panel (b) shows an aortogram with the catheter in the same position as in panel (a). (c) LV angiogram 1979 in 30° RAO position.

What structure has been labeled with a red star (*)?

9 Chest X ray 1980

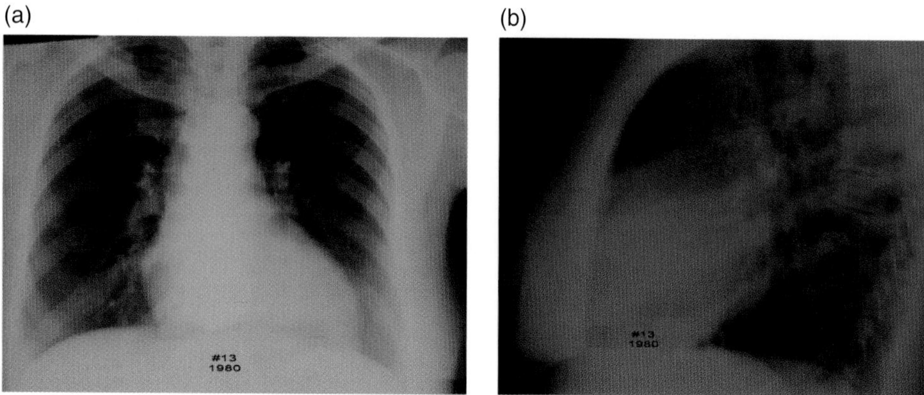

Figure 8.7 Chest X ray 1980. (a) PA view. (b) Lateral view.

10 Cardiac catheterization 1980

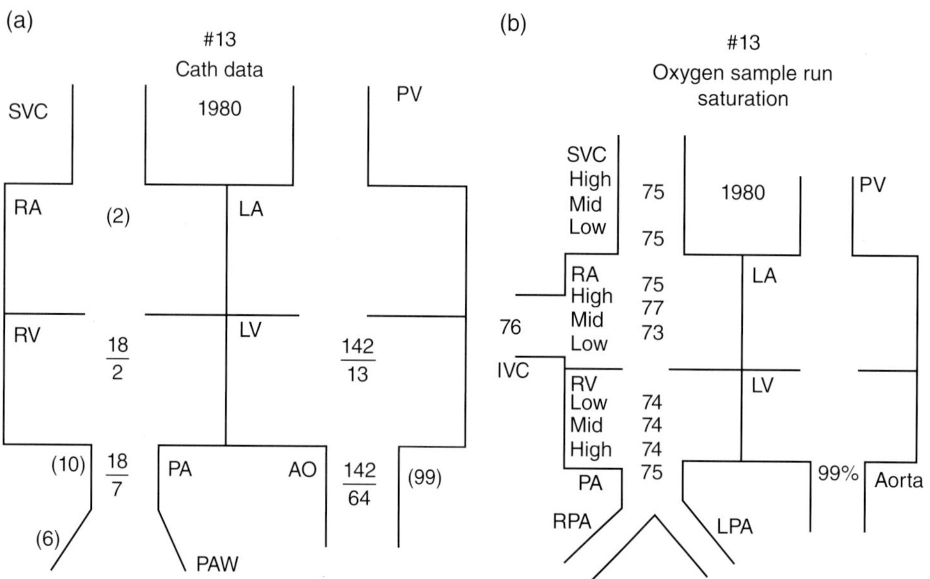

Figure 8.8 (a) Hemodynamic data 1980. (b) Oxygen sample run 1980.

Table 8.3 Additional hemodynamic data (volumes and blood flow) 1980

Cardiac output	6.8 L/min
Cardiac index	3.7 L/min/m^2
LV end-diastolic volume index	167 mL/m^2
LV end-systolic volume index	77 mL/m^2
HR	70/min

What is the LV ejection fraction?
What is the regurgitant fraction?

11 Additional hemodynamic data 1980

See Table 8.3.

12 History and course

20-year-old man admitted to hospital with atypical chest pain. He has had a known heart murmur since childhood.

At age 3, he had a small VSD with a pulmonary/systemic ratio of 1.9/1. The mean PA pressure was 20 mmHg.

At age 12, the pulmonary/systemic ratio was 1.3/1 with a mean PA pressure of 10 mmHg.

At age 20, in 1979, he had a VSD detectable by LV to PA dye curve but not by oximetry. The mean PA pressure was 17 mmHg. There was now 4+ aortic regurgitation (Figure 8.6a).

At surgery in 1979 the patient had a large VSD that was partially occluded by a prolapsed right coronary cusp of the aortic valve. The cusp was torn and elongated.

The VSD was closed with a Teflon velour patch graft and the aortic valve was repaired.

At age 21, the VSD was closed but 4+ aortic regurgitation was still present.

Answers and commentary

1 Physical examination

A continuous murmur at the LUSB (presumed to be at the left 2nd interspace parasternally) would suggest a PDA. Usually the murmur of a PDA has a late systolic accentuation and then spills into diastole [1], but this was not mentioned on this patient's examination.

A continuous murmur may also be heard in ruptured sinus of valsalva or coronary AV fistula, but these are usually heard in the left 3rd interspace parasternally.

Other conditions that can simulate a continuous murmur are aortic stenosis with aortic regurgitation, mitral stenosis with an atrial septal defect, or VSD with aortic regurgitation.

The diastolic blowing murmur heard at the RUSB is due to aortic regurgitation. If the murmur was in fact heard best at the RUSB then coexistent aortic root involvement is likely.

The lack of cardiomegaly or a wide pulse pressure would imply that aortic regurgitation is either of recent onset or is mild.

2 Phonocardiogram

There is a mid-to-late systolic murmur recorded at the left 2nd interspace, which tends to fade in the apical area. No obvious diastolic murmur is seen. High-frequency murmurs of aortic regurgitation are often difficult to record. Luisada (personal communication) has successfully recorded such murmurs by converting the phonocardiographic signal to a 3rd derivative, but this was not done in this patient.

The systolic murmur at the left 2nd interspace could be due to increased pulmonary flow or a high VSD [2].

The apex cardiogram and carotid pulse are normal.

3 M-mode echocardiogram

There is diastolic fluttering of the anterior mitral valve leaflet, suggestive of aortic regurgitation (Figure 8.2a).

The LV end-diastolic dimension is 5.2 cm and the LV end-systolic dimension is 3.2 cm (Figure 8.2b). Thus the LV diameter is normal in this one plane. The LV septum is not well seen. The LV posterior wall thickness is probably increased.

4 ECG

The rhythm is sinus. Rate 72/min. PR 0.16 s. QRS 0.05 s. frontal QRS axis +75°.

SV1 + RV6 = 5.2 mv.

Impression: borderline evidence for LVH in a 20-year-old man.

5 Chest X ray 1979

The heart size is normal, with a cardio-thoracic ratio of 0.45. The aortic knob is not enlarged. The proximal pulmonary arteries are enlarged. In the lateral view the RV does not appear enlarged.

6 Cardiac catheterization 1979

Right heart pressures are normal (Figure 8.5a). The aortic pulse pressure is slightly widened. The latter may be seen in aortic regurgitation or a high output state.

The averages for the oxygen content of RA, RV, PA, and aorta are 14.1, 14.9, 14.56, and 17.32 mL%, implying a slight step up in oxygen content on entering the RV from the RA (Figure 8.5b). This finding, in conjunction with the early appearance of an LV to PA dye curve, indicates a small VSD is present.

Table 8.1 shows normal respiratory gas analysis data with the measured oxygen consumption closely matching the corresponding expected value.

Given:

oxygen consumption (V_{O_2}) = 150 mL/min

arterial oxygen content (Cao) = 17.32 mL/100 mL blood

pulmonary artery content (Cpa) = 14.56 mL/100 mL blood

we can get an approximate value for the systemic blood flow, as the left to right shunt is small, using the following formula:

$$Q_s = \frac{V_{O_2}}{\text{Cao} - \text{Cpa}}$$

$$= \frac{150}{(17.32 - 14.56)10}$$

$$= 5.43\ \text{L/min}$$

Systemic flow index = 5.4/1.82 = 2.97 L/min/m^2

7 Additional hemodynamic data 1979

Given:

LV end-diastolic volume index is increased to 110 mL/m^2 (normal = 70 ± 20 mL/m^2)

LV end-diastolic volume index (LVEDVI) = 110 mL/m^2

LV end-systolic volume index (LVESVI) = 43 mL/m^2 (normal 24 ± 10 mL/m^2)

∴ angiographic stroke volume index (SVI) = 110 − 43 = 67 mL/m^2

$$\text{LV ejection fraction} = \frac{\text{LVEDVI} - \text{LVESVI}}{\text{LVEDVI}} = \frac{67}{110} = 60\%$$

The LV end-diastolic volume is increased but the LV ejection fraction is normal.

Given:

angiographic stroke volume index = 67 mL/m^2

heart rate = 90/min

angiographic cardiac output index = 67 × 90 = 6.030 L/min/m^2

systemic flow index = 2.97 L/min/m^2

$$\text{regurgitant fraction} = \frac{\text{angiographic.output} - \text{systemic.output}}{\text{angiographic.output}}$$

$$= \frac{6.03 - 2.97}{6.03} = 0.51$$

This represents a moderately severe degree of regurgitation.

8 Angiography

Aortic root angiography

In Figure 8.6a, the aortic catheter is positioned just superior to the aortic valve. Figure 8.6b shows an aortic root injection of contrast media showing severe aortic regurgitation (4+/4+) and a small puff of contrast material entering a high (subarterial) VSD.

LV angiography

The aortic cusps are prominent and appear distorted (Figure 8.6c). The red star (*) is a prolapsed right coronary cusp.

9 Chest X ray 1980

The C/T ratio has increased slightly from 0.45 to 0.5. The pulmonary arteries remain prominent. In the lateral view the RV appears enlarged.

10 Cardiac catheterization 1980

Right heart pressures remain normal. LVEDP has increased slightly to 13 mmHg, implying minimal LV dysfunction. There is a wide pulse pressure (aorta 142/64) as before.

The sample run (Figure 8.8b) is normal.

11 Additional hemodynamic data 1980

The LV end-diastolic volume has increased from 110 to 167 mL/m^2 (normal 70 ± 20 mL/m^2).

The LV end-systolic volume index has also increased from 43 to 77 mL/m^2 (normal 24 ± 10 mL/m^2).

∴ LV stroke volume index = 167 − 77 = 90 mL/mL/m^2.

LV ejection fraction = (167 − 77)/167 = 0.54

Given:

HR = 90/min

stroke volume index = 90 mL/min/m^2

cardiac index = 3.7 L/min/m^2

body surface area = 1.82 m^2

then the angiographic cardiac index = heart rate × stroke volume index

= 90 × 90 = 8.1 L/min/m^2

$$\text{regurgitant.fraction} = \frac{\text{angiographic.cardiac index} - \text{cardiac.index}}{\text{angiographic.cardiac.index}}$$

$$= \frac{8.1-3.7}{8.1} = 0.54$$

This degree of regurgitation is similar to the preoperative value in 1979.

12 History and course

The patient has had a small VSD since age 3 and developed aortic regurgitation at age 20, with a moderately elevated regurgitant fraction of 51%. At surgery in 1979 the VSD was in fact large but was partially occluded by a prolapsed right coronary cusp. The right cusp was elongated, torn, and had a perforation in it. The VSD was closed with a Teflon patch and an aortic valvuloplasty was performed.

In 1980 the VSD was confirmed as closed but the patient had recurrence of severe aortic regurgitation with slight deterioration of LV function. He will need to have aortic valve replacement.

Discussion

The patient had a subarterial VSD, which would account for the diamond-shaped systolic murmur at the LUSB as the shunted blood enters directly into the main PA [2, 3].

Between 3 and 12 years of age the VSD was small based on $Q_p/Q_s < 2$ and normal PA pressures.

The 'continuous murmur' heard at LUSB was due to a subarterial VSD and the development of aortic regurgitation. Perloff [2] has noted that unlike a PDA the systolic murmur of the subarterial VSD does not have a late systolic accentuation or envelop the 2nd sound.

The patient had developed moderately severe aortic regurgitation by the age of 20 based on the increased LV volumes and high regurgitant fraction.

Aortic regurgitation developed as a result of a prolapse of one or more cusps into the subarterial VSD because of the Venturi effect of the left to right shunt [4] on the cusps (see Figure 8.9).

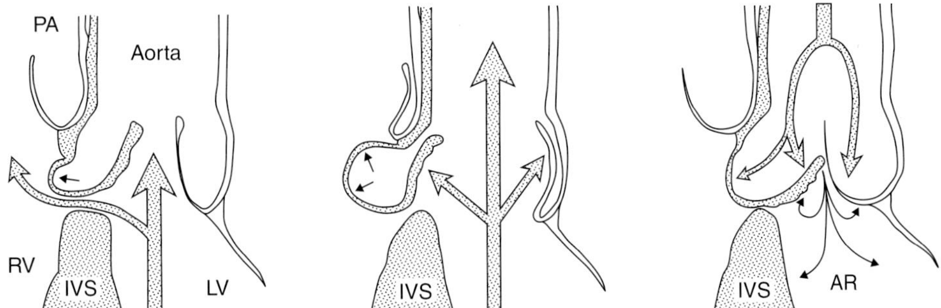

Figure 8.9 In the left-hand panel blood is being ejected in early systole across the VSD. In the middle panel the aortic cusp is sucked into the VSD because of the Venturi effect of the left to right shunt. In the right-hand panel during diastole the aortic cusp is pushed further into the VSD, preventing coaptation of the aortic leaflets and leading to aortic regurgitation [4]. Source: Tatsuno K, Konno S, Ando M et al. (1973). Reproduced with permission from Wolters Kluwer Health.

Aortic regurgitation may develop in 5% of VSD patients in the USA [2]. Early surgery is necessary as aortic regurgitation worsens over time [2, 5].

The VSD was detected only by the LV to PA dye curve and appeared to be very small based on the oximetry and aortogram. At surgery the VSD was large as its orifice was mostly covered by a prolapsed coronary cusp, making it appear that the VSD was small.

The LV has to bear the brunt of the left to right shunt as well as the new onset of aortic regurgitation. The LV volumes were moderately increased. Sometimes the M-mode echocardiogram may not reflect the increase in LV volume if only one dimension, namely the LV end-diastolic dimension, is being used.

The patient underwent aortic valvuloplasty, which seemed to be a reasonable approach in view of his young age. However, the results were short-lived as the aortic regurgitation was present a year later with a further increase in LV volume, a severely elevated regurgitant fraction, and early LV dysfunction (reduced ejection fraction and some increase in LVEDP).

This patient will need to have aortic valve replacement with long-term anticoagulants if a mechanical valve is used.

Key points

1. Patients with a VSD and aortic regurgitation may mimic a continuous murmur on physical examination.
2. Prolapse of an aortic cusp is associated with a subarterial VSD, resulting in aortic regurgitation.
3. The size of the left to right shunt is underestimated because the aortic cusp partially blocks the VSD.
4. The aortic regurgitation becomes worse over time.
5. Early surgery is required to treat aortic regurgitation, with either valvuloplasty or valve replacement as well as closing the VSD.

References

[1] Perloff JK. *Ventricular septal defect. The Clinical Recognition of Congenital Heart Disease,* 5th edn. WB Saunders, Philadelphia, 2003, p 335.

[2] Rudolph AM. *Venticular septal defect. Congenital diseases of the heart: Clinical–physiological considerations,* 2nd edn. Futura, Armonk, NY, 2001, pp 197–244.

[3] Ammash NM, Warnes CA. Ventricular septal defects in adults. *Ann Int Med* 2001; 135: 812–824.

[4] Tatsuno K, Konno S, Ando M et al. Pathogenetic mechanisms of prolapsing aortic valve and aortic regurgitation associated with ventricular septal defect. Anatomical, angiographic and surgical considerations. *Circulation* 1973; 48: 1028–1037.

[5] Yacoub MH, Knan H, Stavri G et al. Anatomic correction of the syndrome of prolapsing right coronary aortic cusp, dilatation of the sinus of Valsalva and ventricular septal defect. *J Thorac Cardiovasc Surg* 1997; 113: 253–260.

9 PATIENT STUDY 9

Sequence of data presentation

1 History 1975
↓
2 ECGs 1975 and 1976
↓
3 Vectorcardiogram 1976
↓
4 Chest X ray January 1975
↓
5 Hemodynamic data January 1975
↓
6 Fluoroscopy and angiography January 1975
↓
7 Physical examination January 1975
↓
8 Initial diagnosis and treatment
↓
9 Chest X rays March 1975
(6 weeks post operation)
↓
10 Chest X ray February 1976
↓
11 History and physical examination 1976
↓
12 Hemodynamic data 1976
↓
13 Echocardiograms 1976
↓
14 Chest X rays and follow-up 1976

1 History

23-year-old black female nullipara, admitted to hospital with a 3-week history of progressive dyspnea on exertion, paroxysmal nocturnal dyspnea, and leg edema.

She was told that she had had a heart murmur and scarlet fever at age 11.

No history of hypertension, diabetes, or alcoholism.

No known heart problems in her nine siblings.

2 ECGs 1975 and 1976

Sinus rhythm with first-degree heart block, left-axis deviation (–90°) and RVH.

The 1976 ECG is shown in Figure 9.1.

Patient Studies in Valvular, Congenital, and Rarer Forms of Cardiovascular Disease: An Integrative Approach, First Edition. Franklin B. Saksena.

Companion Website: www.wiley.com/go/saksena/patientstudies

(a)

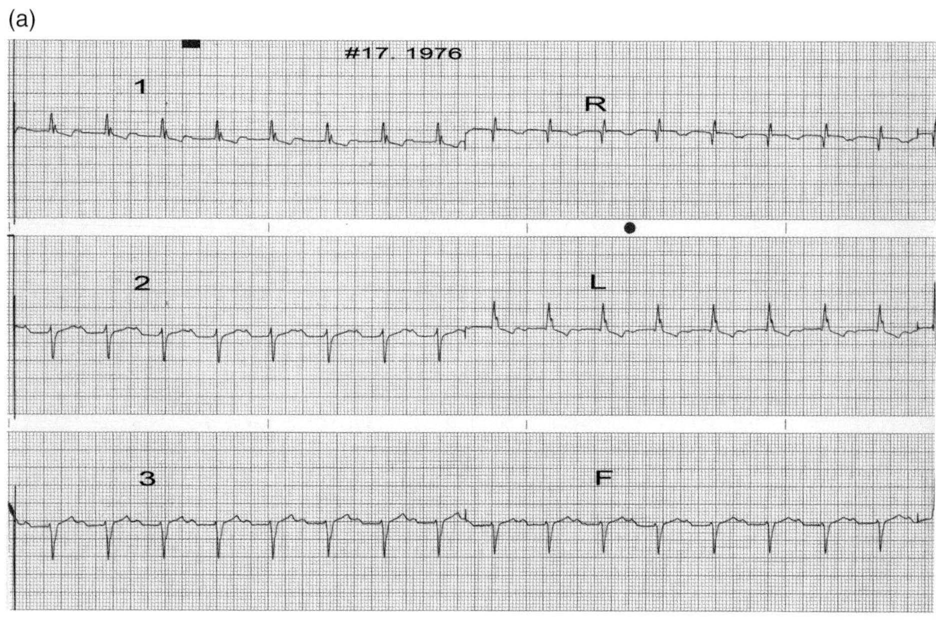

(b)

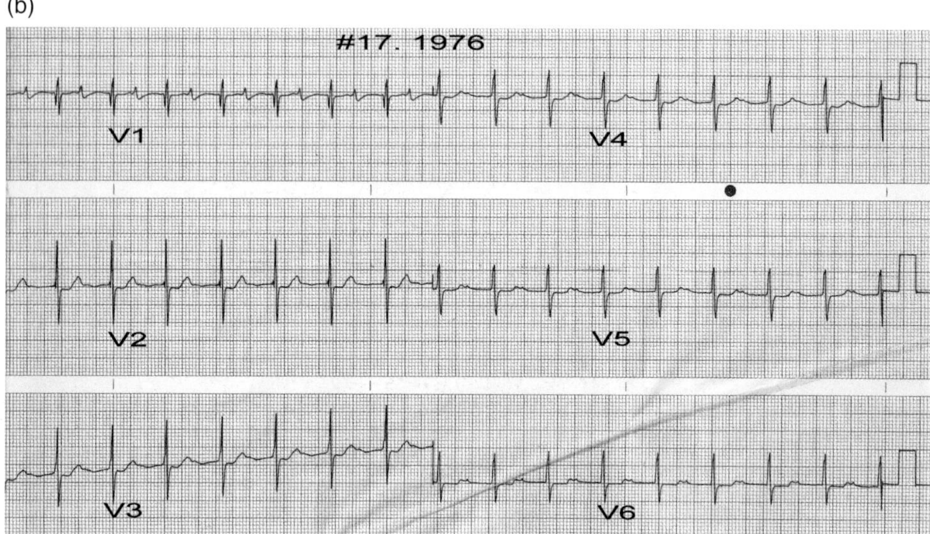

Figure 9.1 12-lead ECG 1976. Sinus rhythm. Rate 100/min.

3 Vectorcardiogram 1976

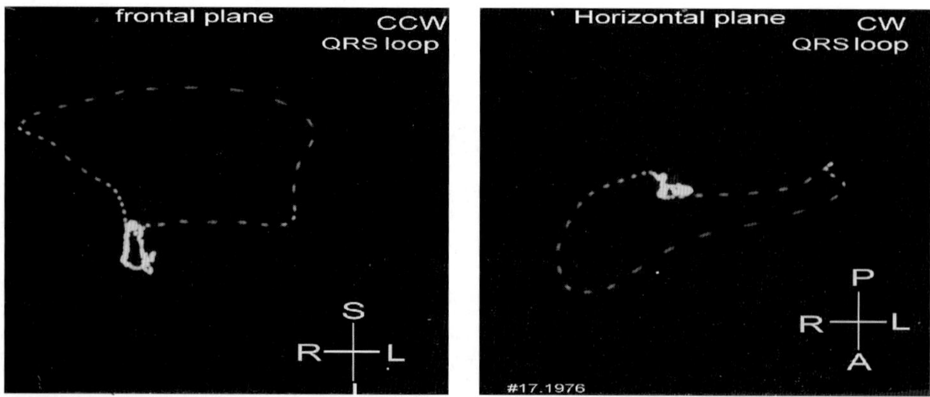

Figure 9.2 Vectorcardiogram 1976. The left panel shows the QRS loop in the frontal plane, activated in a counterclockwise direction. The right panel shows the QRS loop in the horizontal plane, activated in a clockwise direction. In both panels each dot is 4 ms apart. I, inferior; A, anterior; L, left; P, posterior; R, right; S, superior.

4 Chest X ray January 1975

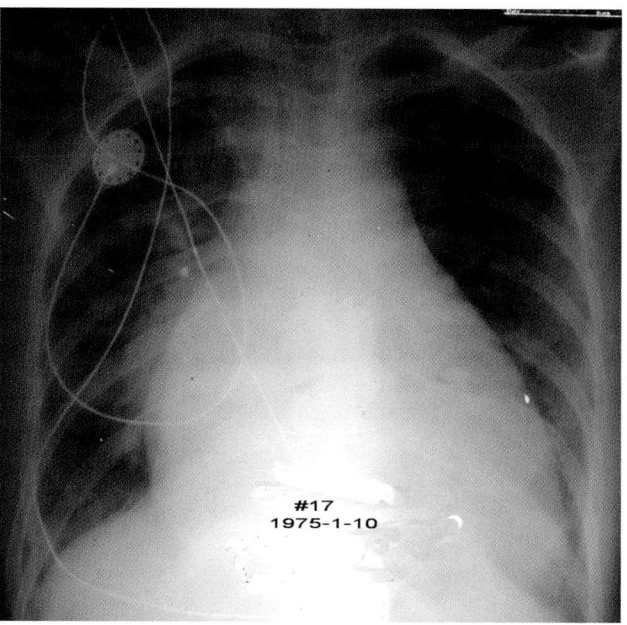

Figure 9.3 Portable chest X ray January 1975, taken in CCU.

5 Hemodynamic data January 1975

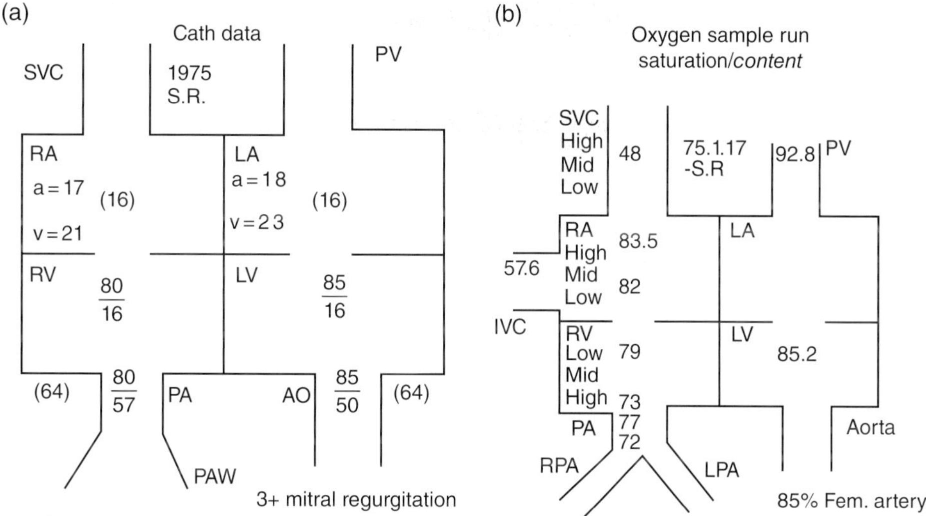

Figure 9.4 (a) Intracardiac pressures January 1975. (b) Oxygen sample run using oxygen saturations January 1975.

Table 9.1 Shunt calculations January 1975

Hemoglobin	15.7 g %
Oxygen consumption	164 mL/min
Oxygen content (mL/100 mL blood)	
SVC	10.1
PA	15.6
PV	19.5
FA	17.9

Calculate the left to right and the right to left shunts.

6 Fluoroscopy and angiography January 1975

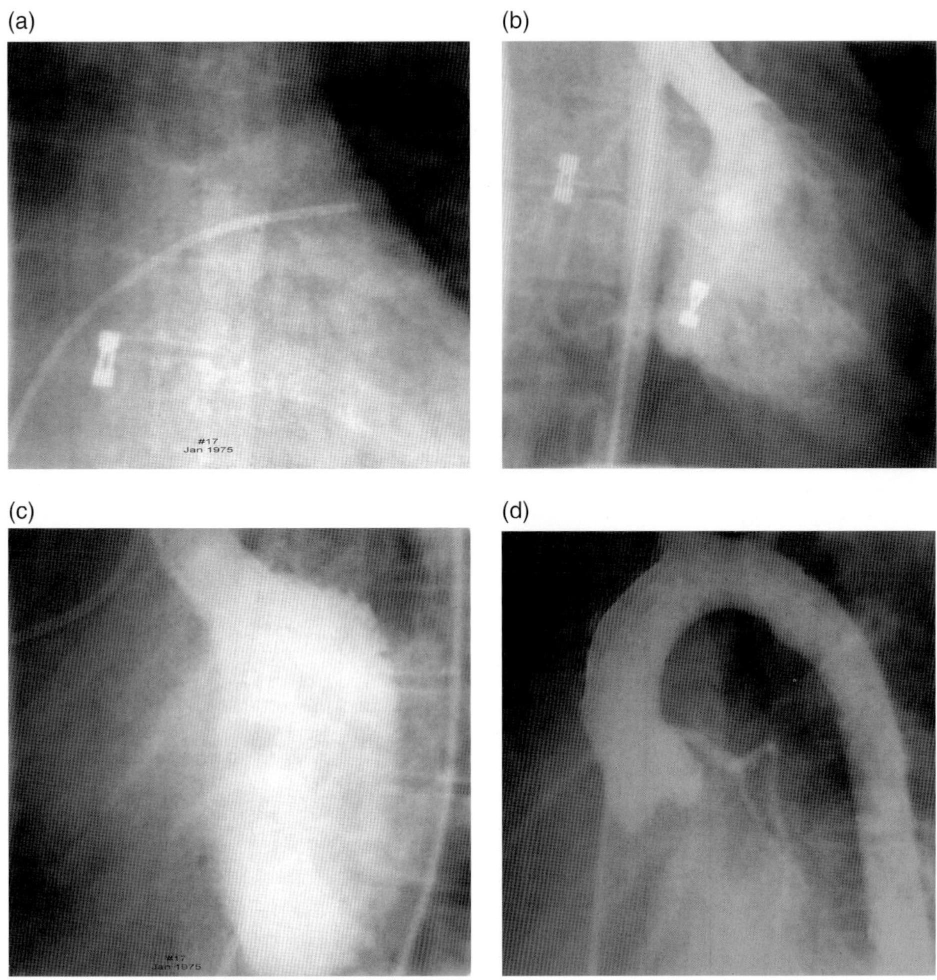

Figure 9.5 (a) Right heart catheter AP view January 1975. (b) LV angiogram AP view January 1975. (c) LV angiogram 60° LAO view January 1975. (d) Aortic root angiogram 60° LAO view January 1975.

Where is the right heart catheter located (refers to Figure 9.5a)?

7 Physical examination January 1975

62 inches tall female weighing 91 lb. BP 160/80. P 100/min regular. R 30/min. Early clubbing.
Increased jugular venous pressure.
Apex beat is in the 5th interspace, 0.5 cm outside the mid-clavicular line.
RV lift 2+ out of 3+.
S1 decreased. S2 showed a loud P2. S3 2+ at apex.
Grade 4/6 harsh ejection systolic murmur, maximum at LLSB with radiation to the apex.
The next day this murmur became holosystolic.
Grade 3/6 diastolic rumble maximum at LLSB radiating to the apex.
Anterior bowing of sternum. Lung fields showed decreased air entry bilaterally. No rales.
Liver span 15 cm.
Leg edema 2+.

8 Initial diagnosis and treatment

The patient underwent a surgical procedure in January 1975.

What is the likely diagnosis?
What was the surgical procedure?

9 Chest X rays March 1975 (6 weeks post operation)

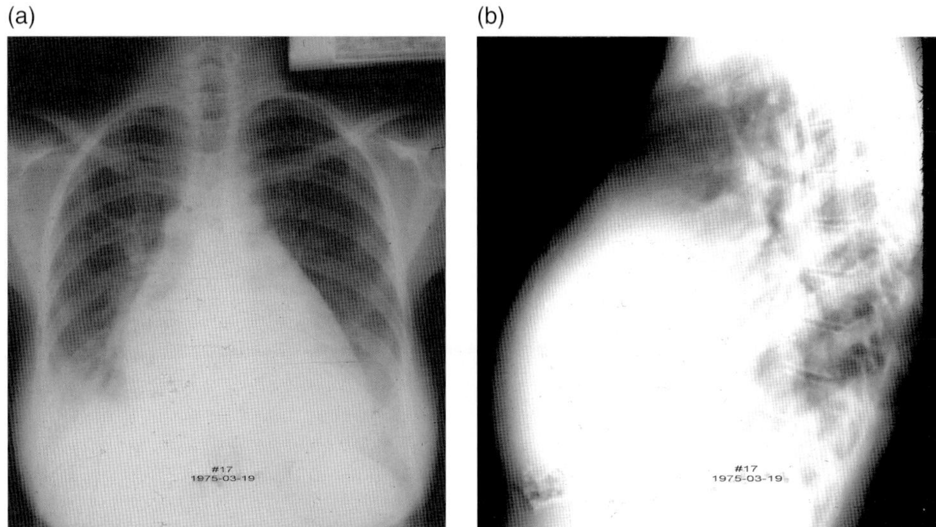

Figure 9.6 (a) Chest X ray PA view March 1975. (b) Chest X ray lateral view March 1975.

10 Chest X ray February 1976

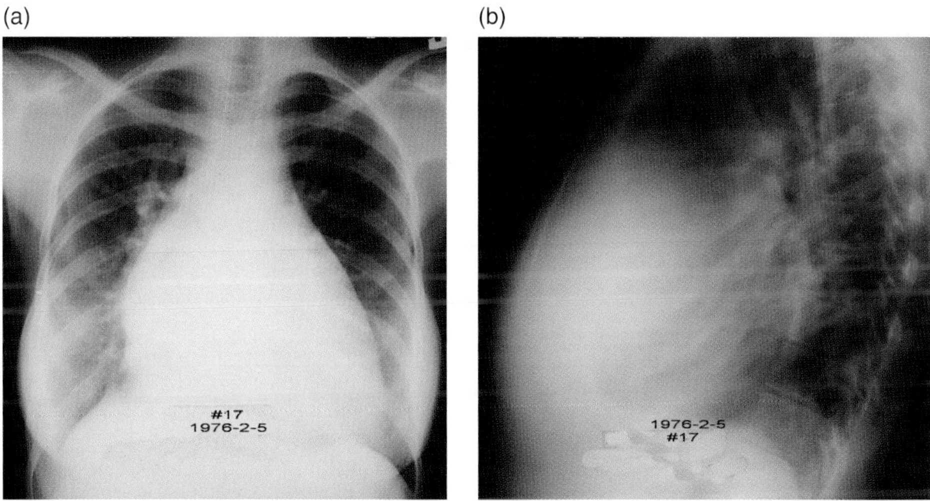

Figure 9.7 (a) PA chest X ray February 1976. (b) Lateral chest X ray February 1976.

11 History and physical examination 1976

History

The patient was readmitted to assess the efficacy of open-heart surgery done a year ago. She was able to walk several blocks slowly without dyspnea and do light housework. No paroxysmal nocturnal dyspnea, leg edema, or syncope.

Physical examination

62 inches tall, 101 lb female. BP 110/80. P 80/min, sinus rhythm.
Patient had clubbing.
A prominent cv wave in the neck was seen along with a pulsatile liver.
RV lift 2+. Apex beat in the 5th interspace, 15 cm from the mid-sternal line.

Median sternotomy scar.
S1 loud. S2 loud P2.
Grade 4/6 pansystolic murmur at LLSB.
Grade 2/6 diastolic rumble at LLSB.
Grade 2/6 pansystolic apical murmur.
Grade 3/6 ejection systolic murmur at the left 3rd interspace parasternally.
Lungs showed decreased air entry on left side.
No crepitations.
No leg edema.

12 Hemodynamic data 1976

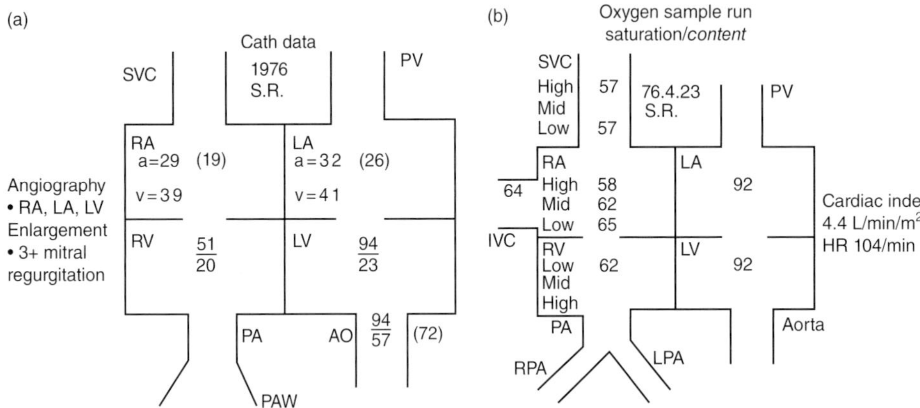

Figure 9.8 (a) Intracardiac pressures April 1976. (b) Oxygen sample run using oxygen saturations April 1976.

Table 9.2 LV volume and cardiac output data April 1976

LV end-diastolic volume	281 mL
LV end-systolic volume	122 mL
Cardiac output	6.12 L/min
Heart rate	104/min

Calculate the LV ejection fraction.
Calculate the regurgitant fraction.

13 Echocardiograms 1976

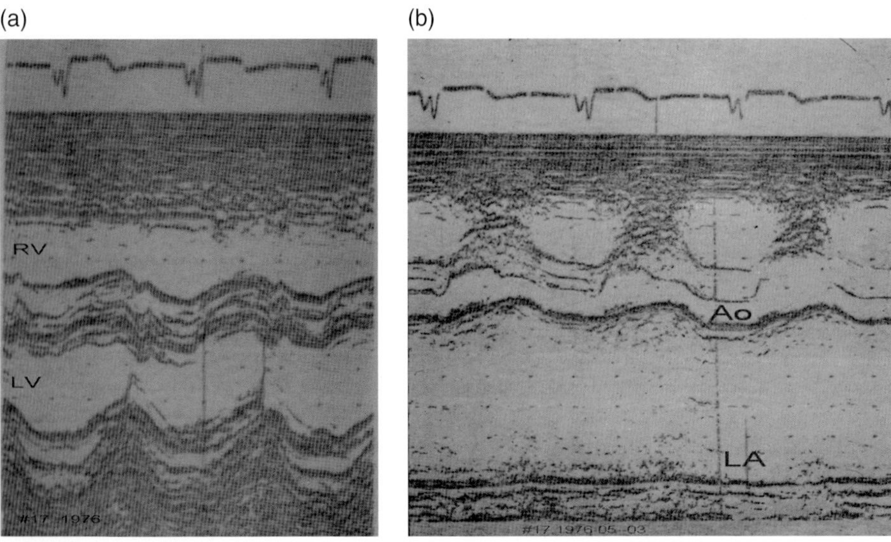

Figure 9.9 (a) M-mode echocardiogram showing right and left ventricles. (b) M-mode echocardiogram showing aorta (Ao) and LA.

14 Chest X rays and follow-up 1976

She had two further admissions in 1976 for congestive heart failure.

(a)

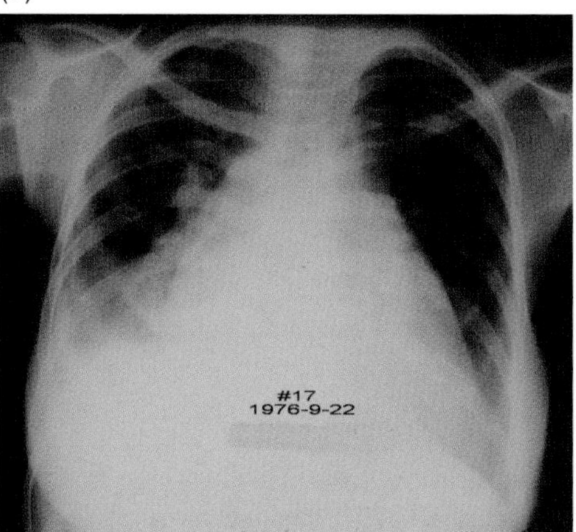

(b)

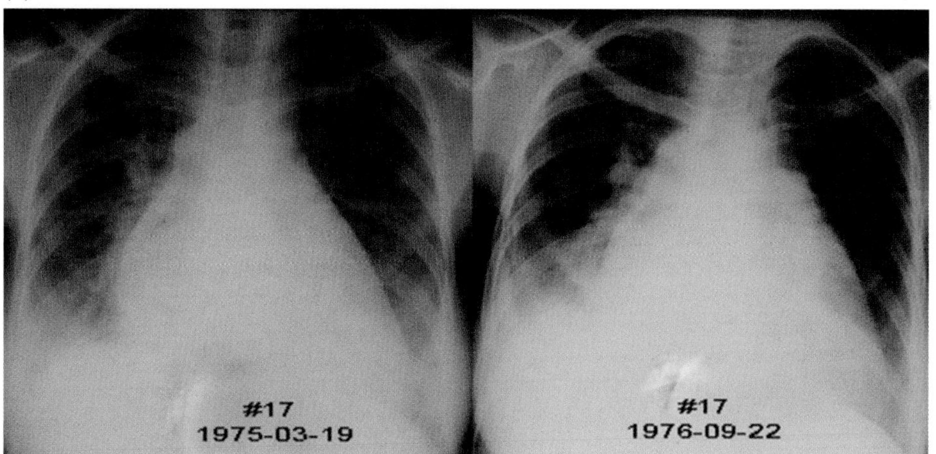

Figure 9.10 (a) PA chest X ray September 1976. (b) Comparison of March 1975 and September 1976 chest X rays.

Answers and commentary

1 History

The patient was admitted to hospital in heart failure. The history of a heart murmur and scarlet fever is suggestive of rheumatic fever.

2 ECG 1975 and 1976

The rhythm is sinus with first-degree heart block. Rate 100/min. PR 0.38 s. QRS 0.05 s. QRS axis is –80°. qR in V1. Biphasic P in V1. Deep S in V5.

Impression: there is RVH, LA enlargement, and left-axis deviation.

Similar findings were seen in 1975, namely RVH and left-axis deviation.

Patients with mitral stenosis may have RVH and right-axis deviation but not left-axis deviation. Left-axis deviation in a young patient is usually seen if there is a primum ASD. Less common causes of left-axis deviation are a common atrium, tricuspid atresia, transposition of the great vessels, or double outlet RV [17].

3 Vectorcardiogram 1976

In the left panel of Figure 9.2 the frontal QRS loop is directed counterclockwise with a mean QRS vector of +280° or –80°. These vectorcardiographic findings suggest one of the diagnoses mentioned above, the most common being a primum ASD. The normal QRS loop in the frontal plane is clockwise with a mean QRS vector of +60°.

In the right panel the horizontal QRS loop shows mostly anterior forces suggestive of RVH. The mean QRS vector is +90°. The normal horizontal QRS loop is directed slightly more posteriorly with a mean QRS vector of +350° or −10°.

4 Chest X ray January 1975

There is generalized cardiomegaly with prominent proximal right PA as well as pulmonary vascular congestion.

5 Hemodynamic data January1975

In Figure 9.4a the RA and LA pressures are moderately elevated and equal. Patients with a large ASD often have equal pressures in RA and LA [2].

TR might be inferred because of v wave > a wave in RA, especially in the presence of severe pulmonary hypertension.

There is biventricular dysfunction based on the high filling pressures (16 mmHg).

Moderately severe MR would also account for the high LA pressure.

There is systemic hypotension.

Figure 9.4b shows the oxygen sample run. There is a significant step up in oxygen saturation on entering RA from the SVC, which is indicative of an ASD. There is arterial desaturation suggestive of a right to left shunt.

Blood flow measurements are given in Table 9.1.

Data:

oxygen consumption 164 mL/min

SVC 10.1 mL/100 mL blood or 10.1 mL%

PA 15.6 mL/100 mL blood or 15.6 mL%

PV 19.5 mL/100 mL blood or 19.5 mL%

FA 17.9 mL/100 mL blood or 17.9 mL%

Q_p = pulmonary blood flow, Q_s = systemic blood flow, and Q_{ep} = effective pulmonary blood flow (L/min)

$$Q_p = \frac{V_{O_2}}{C_{pv} - C_{pa}} = \frac{164}{10(19.5 - 15.6)} = 4.20 \text{ L/min}$$

$$Q_s = \frac{V_{O_2}}{C_{ao} - C_x} = \frac{164}{10(17.9 - 10.1)} = 2.1 \text{ L/min}$$

$$Q_{ep} = \frac{V_{O_2}}{C_{pv} - C_x} = \frac{164}{10(19.5 - 10.1)} = 1.74 \text{ L/min}$$

where Q_{ep} is the effective pulmonary blood flow, i.e. the actual venous blood that reaches the lungs to be oxygenated and Cx is the SVC sample.

$$\therefore Q_{l \to r} = Q_p - Q_{ep} = 4.20 - 1.74 = 2.46 \text{ L/min}$$

$$Q_{r \to l} = Qs - Q_{ep} = 2.10 - 1.74 = 0.36 \text{ L/min}$$

Thus the shunt is predominantly left to right with a small right to left component.

6 Fluoroscopy and angiography January 1975

In Figure 9.5a the right heart catheter has entered the LA from the RA because of an ASD. In Figure 9.5b there is partial filling of the LV with contrast material in the AP view. There is scalloping of the right border of the LV and a suggestion of a mitral valve cleft. No swan neck deformity is seen.

In Figure 9.5c the LV is seen in a 60° LAO view. No VSD seen.

In Figure 9.5d the aorta is seen in the 60° LAO view. No persistent ductus seen.

7 Physical examination January 1975

The patient had early clubbing, which should suggest a right to left shunt in the differential diagnosis.

She had pulmonary hypertension on the basis of an RV lift and loud P2.

She was in biventricular failure as evidenced by her tachypnea, cardiomegaly, elevated jugular venous pressure, an apical S3, hepatomegaly, and leg edema.

The systolic murmur at LLSB and apex could be due to MR and/or TR.

The LLSB diastolic rumble probably reflects increased flow across the tricuspid valve, producing relative tricuspid stenosis. On the basis of hemodynamic data there was no tricuspid stenosis.

Anterior bowing of the sternum seen on physical examination and chest X ray (Figure 9.6b) is indicative of chronic RV overload from early childhood.

8 Initial diagnosis and treatment

Primum ASD (later modified to common atrium with atrioventricular septal defect).

Cleft mitral valve with MR.

TR.

Severe pulmonary hypertension.

Bidirectional shunting across an ASD.

At surgery on 4 Febraury1975 the patient was found to have a common atrium, cleft mitral, and tricuspid leaflets. The atria were partitioned with a 7.5 × 7.5 cm patch and the mitral and tricuspid valves were repaired. She had atrial tachyarrhythmias post operatively.

9 Chest X rays March 1975 (6 weeks post operation)

There may be slightly less cardiomegaly compared to January 1975. The right PA remains enlarged.

The lateral view shows anterior bowing of the sternum and RV enlargement.

10 Chest X ray February 1976

There has been a further increase in size in the RV based on the right sided bulge in PA view and further encroachment of upper sternal space in lateral chest X ray.

C/T ratio 0.67.

11 History and physical examination 1976

Her exercise tolerance has improved since surgery done in February 1975, but she now has severe TR and MR on physical examination.

12 Hemodynamic data 1976

Hemodynamic data are seen in Fig 9.8a. There has been a further increase in RA pressure with a 'v' wave that now greatly exceeds the 'a' wave indicative of severe TR. The RV systolic pressure has fallen from 80 to 51 mmHg. There is still significant biventricular dysfunction with elevated RV and LV filling pressures of 20 and 23 mmHg, respectively. The PA could not be entered via the femoral vein approach because of severe TR and a huge RA. The LA pressure has increased to 26 mmHg, possibly due to LV dysfunction and MR.

In Figure 9.8b the LV end-diastolic volume has markedly increased (to 281 mL) as has the LV end-systolic volume (122 mL). Stroke volume = 281 − 122 = 159 mL.

$$\text{LV ejection.fraction} = \frac{281 - 122}{281} = 0.57$$

LV angiographic or total cardiac output = 159 × 104 = 16.54 L/min

Cardiac output = 6.12 L/min

Regurgitant fraction (includes mitral regurgitation) $= \frac{16.54 - 6.12}{16.65} = 0.63$

Thus, while the LV ejection fraction is normal, the regurgitant fraction is severely elevated. Systolic function is probably impaired as the LVEF should be increased above normal as the LV is unloaded in severe MR.

Figure 9.8b shows the oxygen saturation sample run. The right heart catheter did enter the LA via the RA, which is indicative of an ASD. However, the ASD was small as no significant step up was seen in RA compared to SVC, therefore arterial saturation has improved from 85% to near normal (92%).

13 Echocardiograms 1976

Figure 9.9a shows RVH and a normal size LV.

Figure 9.9b shows a normal sized aortic root and a moderately enlarged LA. LA enlargement and RVH were also seen on the ECG.

14 Chest X rays and follow-up 1976

The patient had two further admissions between April and September 1976 for congestive heart failure.

A chest X ray in September 1976 showed a further increase in heart size since February 1976. There was now a right-sided pleural effusion.

Mitral valve replacement and possible tricuspid valvuloplasty were recommended. The patient refused to have surgery and died in December 1976 of intractable heart failure.

Postmortem showed huge atria each measuring 8–9 cm in diameter, RV hypertrophy (RV 0.9 cm, LV 1.1cm) and LV dilatation. A residual ASD measuring 0.5 cm was seen adjacent to the 7.5 cm ×7.5 cm atrial patch. The tricuspid valve was thin and pliable, and showed a repaired cleft of its posterior leaflet. The mitral valve was also thin and pliable, and showed a repaired cleft of its anterior leaflet.

The coronary arteries were normal.

The patient also had a large hydrothorax (1000 mL) and ascites (1500 mL).

Discussion

The patient had a common atrium and associated cleft mitral and tricuspid leaflets.

A common atrium occurs in less than 1% of all congenital heart diseases [2]. It may very rarely occur as an isolated entity [3, 4].

The SVC blood and pulmonary venous blood may intermingle so a bidirectional shunt may occur, especially in the face of a high pulmonary vascular resistance [5]. This bidirectional leads in turn to arterial desaturation [5] (as in this patient).

It has been suggested that patients with a common atrium are more liable to develop pulmonary hypertension at an earlier age than patients with a large secondum ASD [2].

A single atrial structure seen in the levophase of a PA angiogram is suggestive of a common atrium [6].

The auscultatory features of a common atrium are similar to a secondum ASD, i.e. a wide fixed split S2, a pulmonary flow murmur, and RV overload. Unlike the typical secundum ASD, cyanosis [5, 7] and clubbing may be seen in patients with a common atrium.

Usually patients with a common atrium are associated with an endocardial cushion defect (atrioventricular septal defect) [6–8]. The defect may be partial or complete: a partial defect usually just involves a cleft mitral valve leaflet, whereas a complete defect involves cleft mitral and tricuspid leaflets [7] (as in this patient).

The absence of the atrioventricular septum leads to anterior displacement of the mitral valve, positioning it on the same anatomical plane as the tricuspid valve (best seen in the four-chamber view on two-dimensional echocardiography) [9] (Figure 9.12). The cleft in the mitral valve leaflet divides it into an upper portion and a lower portion. The lower portion is attached to the septum and the upper portion is attached to the septum and aortic annulus [10].

Patients with an atrioventricular septal defect may have MR and TR, left-axis deviation, and a counterclockwise rotation of the frontal QRS loop.

The characteristic angiographic features of an atrioventricular septal defect are (i) a swan neck deformity of the LV outflow tract in diastole, (ii) scalloping of right border of the LV in systole, and (iii) a cleft mitral valve in systole [8, 10, 11]. Another example of a swan neck deformity is seen in Figure 9.11.

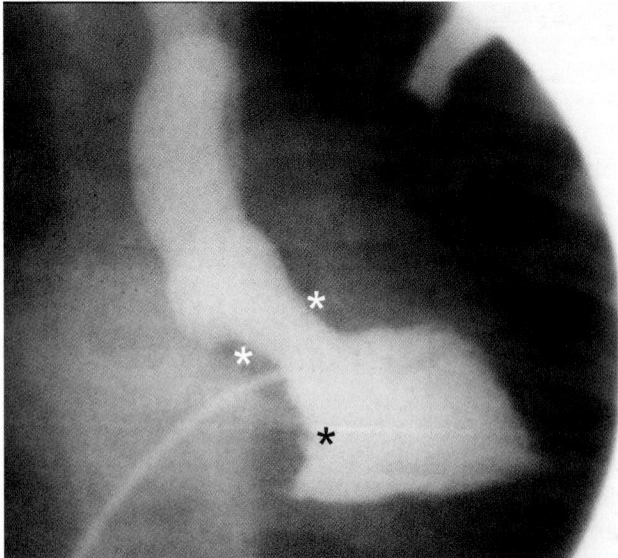

Figure 9.11 AP LV angiogram in another patient, an infant with an endocardial cushion defect, showing the goose neck deformity of the LV outflow tract (between two white stars), scalloping of the right border of the LV, and a cleft mitral valve (to the left of the red star). Mild mitral valve regurgitation is also seen.

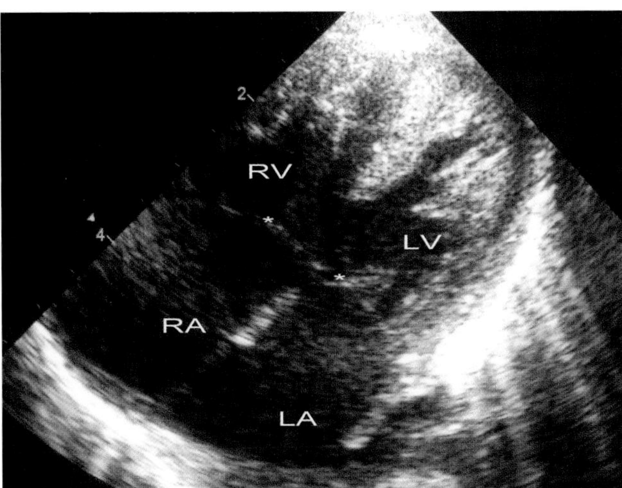

Figure 9.12 Two-dimensional echocardiogram showing the four-chamber view of a 33-week-old 1500 g premature infant with Down syndrome (4 March 2011). There is a 7 mm common AV canal. The mitral and tricuspid valves are on the same anatomical plane (marked with *), a characteristic feature of an AV canal defect. Normal RV and LV sizes. Not shown is a patent foramen ovale and a PDA.

The swan or goose neck deformity of the LV outflow tract has been attributed to the abnormal attachment of the upper segment of the mitral valve swinging upwards in the LV cavity, causing an apparent narrowing of the LV outflow tract [1], but not all authors agree with this explanation [12].

Two-dimensional echocardiography will also provide accurate information about the AV valves and the narrowing of the LV outflow tract [13, 14] but this was not available to this patient in 1976. Now the echocardiographic diagnosis of an AV canal defect can be made in infancy (Figure 9.12).

Surgical treatment of a common atrium consists of partitioning the atrium using an Ivalon sponge, a Teflon patch [15, 16], or an autologous pericardial patch [3].

Mitral cleft repair can lead to an increase in MR [11], as in this patient. However, other studies [7, 17, 16] have been more successful in doing mitral cleft repair. Mitral valve replacement may be required in some patients [17], but this patient refused to undergo mitral valve replacement.

Key points

1. A common atrium occurs in <1% of congenital heart defects.
2. A bidirectional shunt occurs in such patients, accounting for cyanosis and clubbing in a patient that otherwise has the findings of a secundum ASD (i.e. wide fixed splitting of S2, pulmonary flow murmur, and RV overload pattern).
3. A common atrium may be associated with cleft mitral and tricuspid leaflets.
4. Echocardiography is now able to diagnose an AV septal defect in infancy.
5. The cleft valve leaflets may be repaired or require valve replacement.
6. Attempts to repair the cleft leaflets may not be successful and result in an increase in TR and MR.

References

[1] Burke RP, Horvath K, Landzberg M et al. Long term follow-up after surgical repair of ostium primum atrial septal defect in adults. *J Am Coll Cardiol* 1996; 27: 696–699.

[2] Hung J-S, Feldt RH, Owings W et al. Electrocardiographic and angiocardiographic features of common atrium. *Circulation* 1970; 26: 639 (abstract).

[3] Blanchard DG, Scott ED. Single atrium. *Circulation* 1997; 95: 273.

[4] Somerville J. Atrioventricular defects. *Mod Conc CVS Dis* 1971; 40: 33–38.

[5] Ellis Jr FH, Kirlin JW, Swan HJC, DuShane JW, Edwards JE. Diagnosis and surgical treatment of common atrium (Cor triloculare-biventriculare). *Surgery* 1959; 45: 160–172.

[6] Baron MG. Abnormalities of the mitral valve in endocardial cushion defects. *Circulation* 1972; 45: 672–680.

[7] Gasul B, Arcilla RA, Lev M. *Heart Disease in Children.* Philadelphia, Lippincott, 1966, pp 391–396.

[8] Munoz-Armas S, Diaz Gorrin JR, Anselmi G et al. Single atrium. Embryologic, anatomic, electrocardiographic and other diagnostic features. *Am J Cardiol* 1968; 21: 639–652.

[9] Ferdman DJ, Bradey D, Rosenzweig EB. Common atrium and pulmonary vascular disease. *Pedriatr Cardiol* 2011; 32: 595–598.

[10] Te-Chuan Chou. *Electrocardiography in Clinical Practice. Adult and Pediatric*, 4th edn, Philadelphia, WB Saunders, 1996, p 106.

[11] Rastelli GC, Rahimtoola SH, Ongley PA et al. Common atrium: Anatomy hemodynamics and surgery. *J Thorac Cardiovasc Surg* 1968; 55: 834–841.

[12] Hirai S, Hamanaka Y, Mitsui N et al. Surgical repair of a common atrium in an adult. *Ann Thorac Cardiovasc Surg* 2003; 9: 130–133.

[13] Somerville J, Jefferson K. Left ventricular angiography in atrioventricular defects. *Br Heart J* 1968; 30: 446–457.

[14] Sittiwangkul R, Ma RY, McCrindle BW et al. Echocardiographic assessment of obstructive lesions in atrioventricular septal defects. *J Am Col Cardiol* 2001; 38: 253–261.

[15] Blieden LC, Randall PA, Castaneda AR Lucas RV, Edwards JE. The 'goose neck' of the endocardial cushion defect. *Anatomic Basis Chest* 1974; 65: 13–17.

[16] Geva T, Ayres NA, Pignatelli RH. Echocardiographic evaluation of common atrioventricular canal defects: a study of 206 consecutive patients. *Echocardiography* 1996; 13: 387–99.

[17] Levy MJ, Salomon J, Vidne BA. Correction of single and common atrium with reference to simplified terminology. *Chest* 1974; 66: 444–446.

10 PATIENT STUDY 10

Sequence of data presentation

1 History, physical examination, laboratory data, and course (February to March)
↓
2 Echocardiogram (March)
↓
3 Additional physical findings (March)
↓
4 Echocardiogram (April)
↓
5 Cardiac catheterizations (April)
↓
6 LV angiography
↓
7 Course (May)
↓
8 Angiography
↓
9 Physical examination (August)
↓
10 ECG (August)
↓
11 Chest X ray (August)
↓
12 Cardiac catheterization (August)
↓
13 LV angiography (August)
↓
14 Echocardiogram (August)
↓
15 Echocardiogram (September)
↓
16 Course 1976 onwards

1 History, physical examination, laboratory data, and course (February to March)

History

17-year-old black male admitted with fever and myalgias. Five days prior to admission he had sustained blunt trauma to right thigh, resulting in persistent pain and swelling.

No prior history of cardiovascular disease, rheumatic fever, or drug abuse.

Physical examination

76 inches tall, 155 lb lethargic male. BP 110/70. P 90/min regular. T 102.8 °F.

Normal heart size. Grade 2/6 pulmonary flow murmur.

Laboratory data

WBC 8600/mm^3. CPK 3370 I.U. (normal 0–50 I.U.).

ECG nonspecific ST changes.

Chest X ray normal.

Blood cultures grew *Staphylococcus aureus*.

Course (February to March)

He was treated with intravenous antibiotics over the next month. He developed Janeway lesions, subconjunctival hemorrhages, and micro-infarcts in the retina.

Patient Studies in Valvular, Congenital, and Rarer Forms of Cardiovascular Disease: An Integrative Approach, First Edition. Franklin B. Saksena.

Companion Website: www.wiley.com/go/saksena/patientstudies

2 Echocardiogram (March)

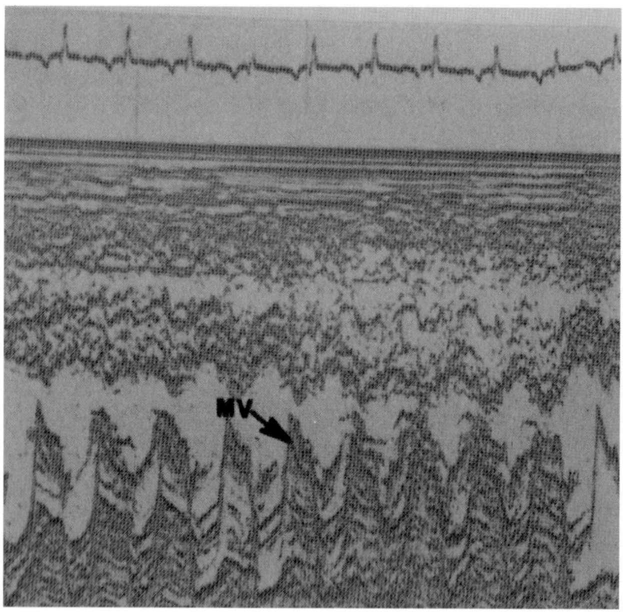

Figure 10.1 M-mode echocardiogram (6 March). Source: Saksena FB, Kramer NE, Towne WD et al. (1978). Reproduced with permission of Elsevier.

3 Additional physical findings (March)

On 22 March an intermittent pericardial friction rub was heard.

On 31 March a 3/6 apical pansystolic murmur was detected. The patient was still running a low-grade fever but the blood cultures were negative.

A gallium scan showed multiple areas of muscle abscesses.

4 Echocardiogram (April)

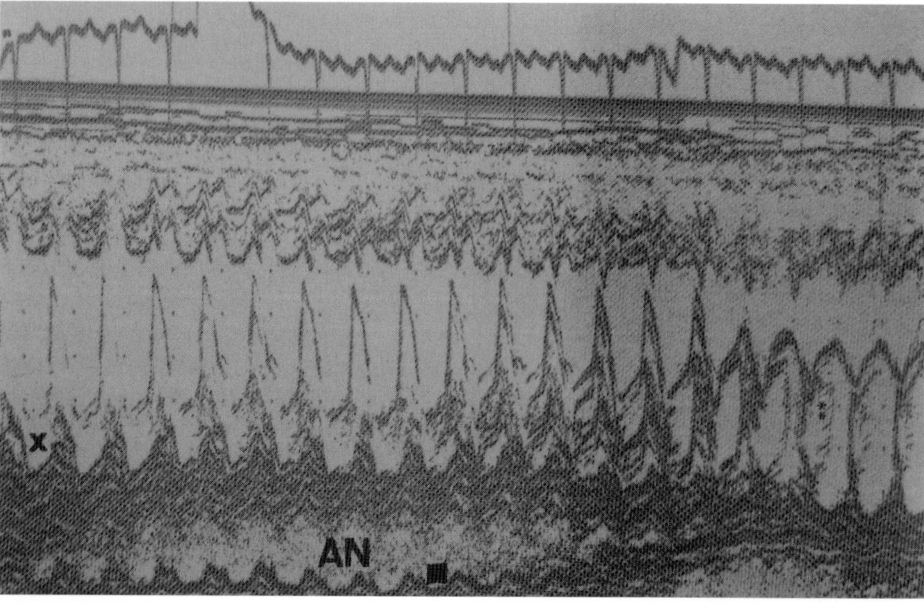

Figure 10.2 M-mode echocardiogram. AN, echo free space. Source: Saksena FB, Kramer NE, Towne WD et al. (1978). Reproduced with permission of Elsevier.

5 Cardiac catheterizations (April)

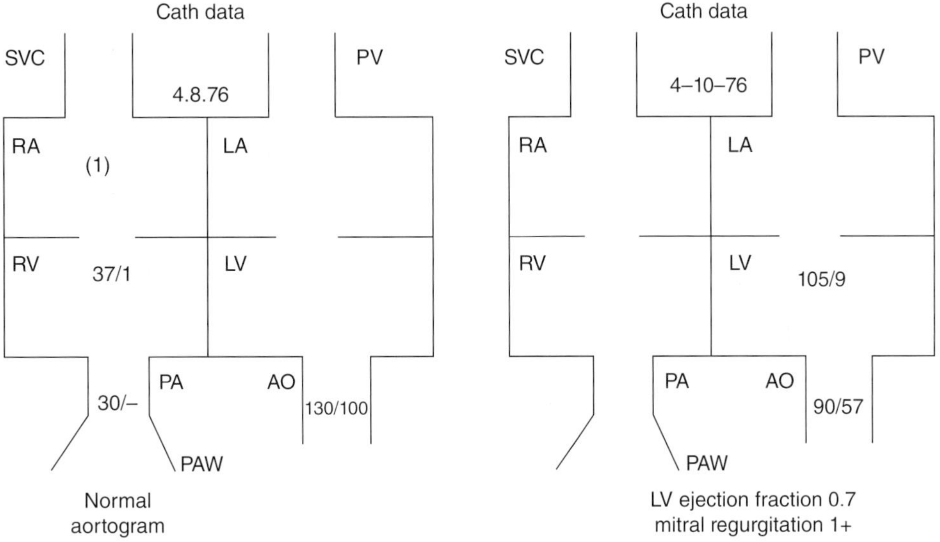

Figure 10.3 Cardiac catheterization data (8 April and 10 April).

6 LV angiography

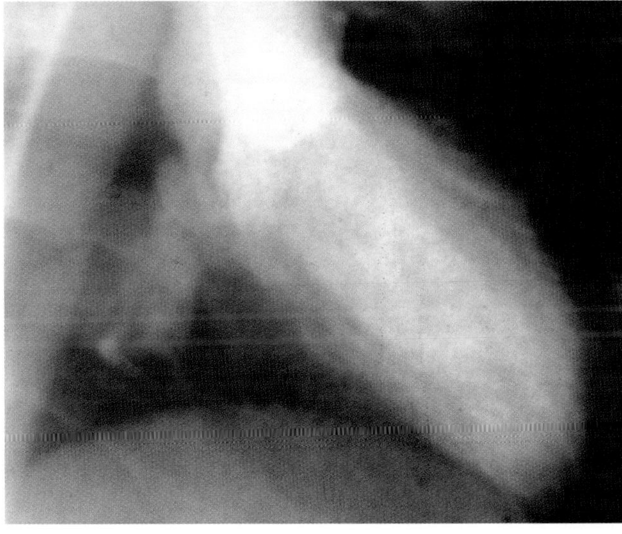

Figure 10.4 LV angiogram. 30° RAO projection (10 April). Source: Saksena FB, Kramer NE, Towne WD et al. (1978). Reproduced with permission of Elsevier.

7 Course (May)

The patient developed abdominal pain and obstructive jaundice. Bilirubin 8.2 mg%. Alkaline phosphatase 1606 I.U. Liver scan showed decreased uptake in right lobe.

8 Angiography

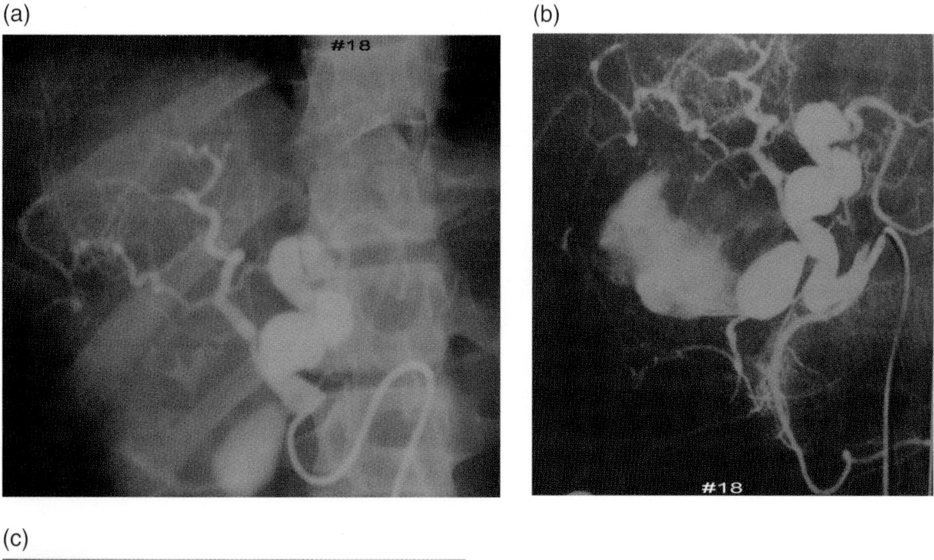

(c)

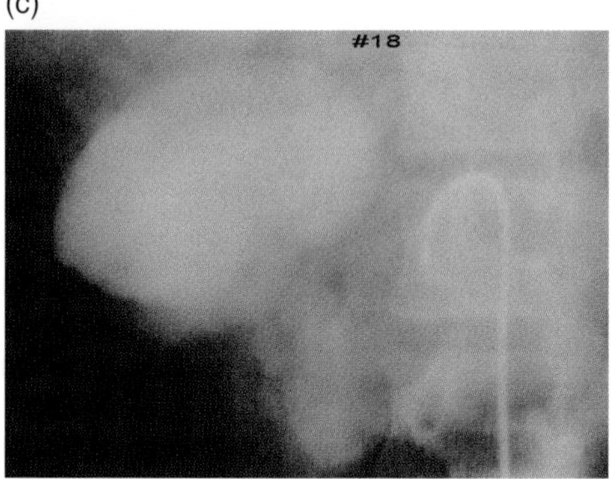

Figure 10.5 (a) Hepatic artery angiogram – early phase AP projection. (b) Hepatic artery angiogram – mid-phase AP projection. (c) Hepatic artery angiogram – late phase AP projection. Source: Mojab K, Lim L, Esfahani F et al. (1977). Reproduced with permission of the American Roentgen Ray Society.

What is the diagnosis and treatment?

9 Physical examination (August)

There was mild elevation of jugular venous pressure.
Apex beat was in the 5th left interspace 4 cm lateral to the mid-clavicular line.
There was a hyperdynamic systolic pulsation noted along the left sternal border.
S1 was loud, S2 was also loud and palpable. A2 = P2. S3 and S4 were heard at the apex.
Grade 3/6 apical systolic murmur.
Grade 2/6 ejection systolic murmur best heard at LLSB, increasing on inspiration.
The liver was mildly enlarged.

10 Electrocardiogram (August)

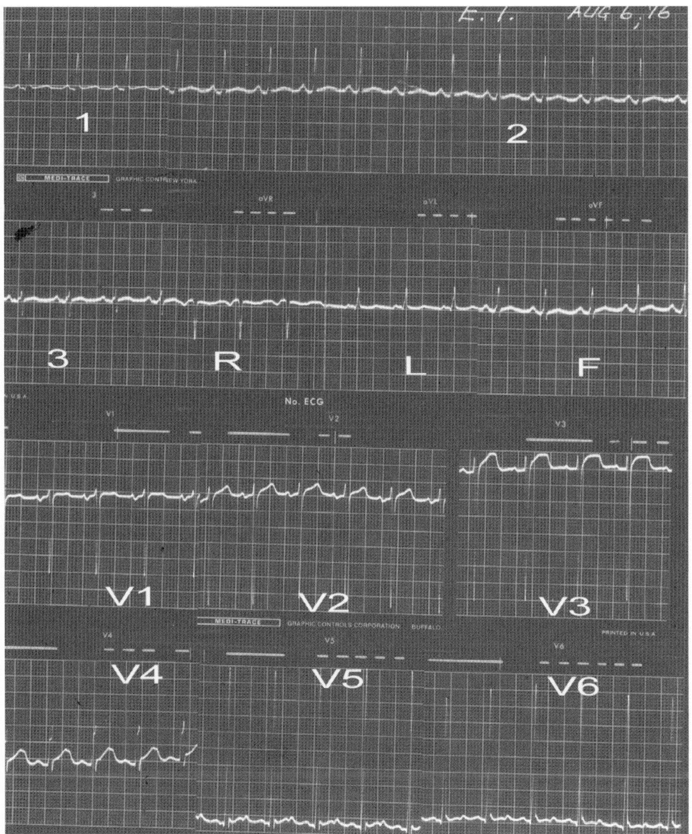

Figure 10.6 ECG (August).

11 Chest X ray (August)

Chest x-ray report: Cardiomegaly with normal pulmonary vasculature.

12 Cardiac catheterization (August)

Table 10.1 Cardiac catheterization data (April and August)

	Pressures (mmHg)		
	8 April 1976	10 April 1976	6 August 1976
RA	1		
RV s/ed	37/1		
PA s/d	30/–		
LV s/ed		105/9	128/14
Ao s/d	130/100	90/57	122/80
Cardiac index	2.28 L/min/m^2		
Ejection fraction		0.7	
Mitral regurgitation		1+	3+

d, diastole; ed, end diastole; s, systole.

13 LV angiography (August)

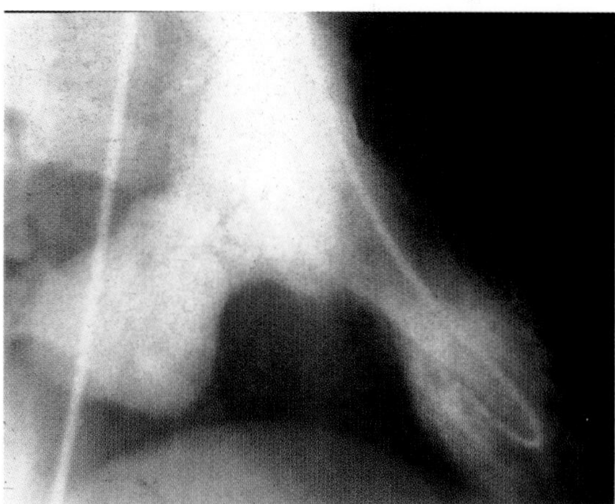

Figure 10.7 LV angiogram 30° RAO projection (August). Source: Saksena FB, Kramer NE, Towne WD et al. (1978). Reproduced with permission of Elsevier.

14 Echocardiogram (August)

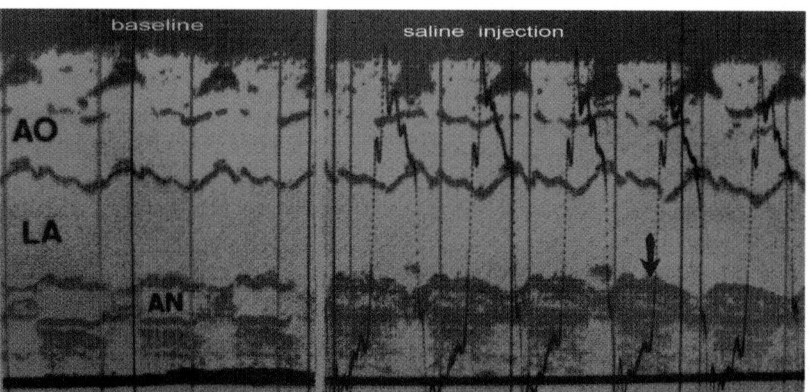

Figure 10.8 M-mode echocardiogram before and after saline injection (↓) into AN. Source: Saksena FB, Kramer NE, Towne WD et al. (1978). Reproduced with permission of Elsevier.

15 Echocardiogram (September)

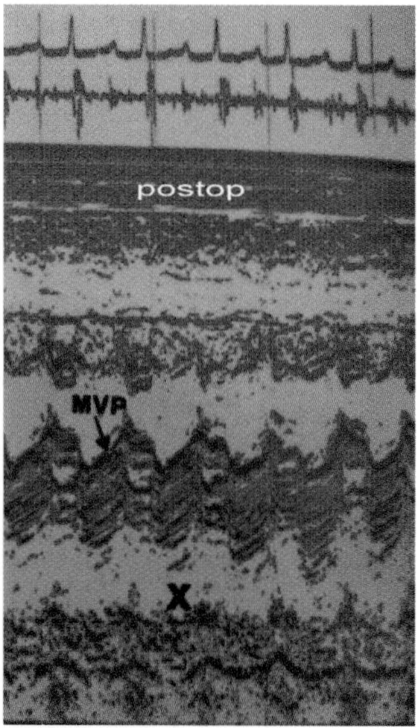

Figure 10.9 M-mode echocardiogram postoperatively (September). Source: Saksena FB, Kramer NE, Towne WD et al. (1978). Reproduced with permission of Elsevier.

16 Course 1976 onwards

Comment on the diagnosis, treatment, and likely course.

Answers and commentary

1 History, physical examination, laboratory data, and course (February to March)

The patient presents with fever, myositis, and a pulmonary flow murmur. He has a staphylococcal septicemia with septic emboli to the eye and skin.

2 Echocardiogram (March)

On 6 March the M-mode echocardiogram shows shaggy densities of the anterior mitral valve leaflet (marked with an arrow), suggestive of vegetations. The LV does not appear enlarged. Diagnosis: staphylococcal endocarditis.

3 Additional physical findings (March)

The patient developed a transient pericarditis and now has a murmur of MR along with muscle abscesses.

4 Echocardiogram (April)

There is a localized echo-free space posterior to the posterior LV wall showing systolic expansion (black rectangle). This echo-free space could be a localized pericardial effusion or a myocardial abscess (labeled AN in diagram).

5 Cardiac catheterizations (April)

On 8 April 1976 the cardiac catheterization showed diastolic hypertension. A RA angiogram showed no abnormalities but in the levophase there appeared to be a LV aneurysm. A repeat cardiac catheterization on 10 April 1976 showed normal LV pressures and mild MR.

6 LV angiogram

LV angiography showed a posterobasal aneurysm at the level of the mitral valve ring.

7 and 8 Course (May) and angiography

The patient's staphylococcal infection lead to aneurysmal dilatation of the right and left hepatic arteries with a large pseudo-aneurysm of the right antero-inferior branch. At surgery this pseudo-aneurysm had ruptured and compressed the cystic and biliary ducts, and was the cause of the patient's obstructive jaundice.

The right hepatic artery branch was ligated, the pseudo-aneurysm evacuated, and cholecystectomy performed. The patient had an uneventful recovery and his liver function tests returned to normal [1].

9 Physical examination (August)

The patient's heart size had increased, probably due to increasing MR and heart failure. The presence of a systolic pulsation adjacent to the LLSB and the gallop sounds are all compatible with a LV aneurysm. The loud P2 suggests pulmonary hypertension.

10 ECG (August)

The rhythm is sinus, 95/min. PR 0.20, QRS 0.07, QRS axis +50°.

Insufficient criteria for LVH in a 17-year-old man.

Impression: sinus rhythm with borderline first-degree heart block.

11 Chest X ray

Borderline cardiomegaly with clear lung fields.

12 Cardiac catheterization (August)

The LVEDP has increased from 9 to 14 mmHg, which is suggestive of LV dysfunction. MR has increased from 1+ to 3+.

13 LV angiography (August)

The posterobasal LV aneurysm has increased in size from 10 April.

14 Echocardiogram (August)

Injection of saline into the aneurysm (AN) led to obliteration of the echo-free space, indicating that the echo-free space represented the aneurysmal sac.

15 Diagnosis and treatment

At surgery the patient had a pseudo-aneurysm of the posterobasal wall of the LV. It was 2 cm wide at its neck, 10 cm long, and 0.2 cm thick, with an estimated volume of 50 mL. It was located just below the mitral valve and inferior to the circumflex coronary artery. There were no clots in the pseudo-aneurysm. Both mitral valve leaflets had perforations. No adhesive pericarditis.

The mouth of the pseudo-aneurysm was closed off with a Dacron patch and the mitral valve replaced with a stented porcine aortic valve.

16 Echocardiogram (September)

The echo-free space has been obliterated since surgical closure of the mouth of the pseudo-aneurysm. The mitral valve prosthesis appears to be functioning normally.

17 Course 1976 onwards

He remained asymptomatic over the next 2 years.

Discussion

The patient had a staphylococcal septicemia in February 1976 but did not have detectable mitral valve involvement until March 1976. Up to 15% of patients with bacterial endocarditis may have no detectible murmur initially [2].

Physical examination in August 1976 showed cardiomegaly, MR, and left sternal border pulsations. These pulsations probably were due to the RV being pressed anteriorly against the parasternal area by either a large LA (secondary to MR) or a posterior LV aneurysm [3].

M-mode echocardiography played an important role in the diagnosis of this patient, demonstrating vegetations on the mitral valve as well as detecting the mouth of the LV posterior pseudo-aneurysm [4].

LV angiography added to the M-mode echocardiographic data by locating the pseudo-aneurysm just below the mitral valve and showing that the pseudo-aneurysm had grown progressively larger over a 4-month period [4].

At surgery, the pseudo-aneurysm was located in the posterobasal free wall of the LV, inferior to the mitral valve and the circumflex artery. There was no involvement of the membraneous septum or the aorto-mitral intervalvular fibrosa by the aneurysm.

Mycotic aneurysms of the LV usually involve the membraneous septum or the mitral-aortic intervalvular fibrosa [5]. Unique to this patient was the burrowing of the mycotic aneurysm into the posterobasal free wall of the LV.

Similar angiographic findings for the LV have been described in African males with idiopathic mitral subannular left ventricular aneurysm, but unlike this case they had no underlying infection and were probably of congenital origin [6].

As these acute LV pseudo-aneurysms are liable to rupture [7], early operative closure is essential, as was carried out in this patient.

Mycotic aneurysms may occur in up to 15% of patients with infective endocarditis [8]. These result from bacterial seeding of the vessels, usually by Staphyloccoccus. Common sites of mycotic aneurysms include the proximal aorta and arteries supplying the visceral organs, the extremities, and the brain [8].

This patient had mycotic aneurysms involving a branch of the hepatic artery [1], leading to pseudo-aneurysm formation and rupture. Prompt surgical ligation of the hepatic artery branch and evacuation of the ruptured pseudo-aneurysm was accomplished without sequelae.

Key points

1. Staphylococcal septicemia resulted in mitral valve endocarditis, pseudo-aneurysm of posterobasal LV, mycotic aneurysms of the hepatic artery, and myositis.

2. Echocardiography played an important diagnostic role in this patient by detecting the mitral valve vegetations and the presence of a posterobasal LV pseudo-aneurysm.
3. Angiography was instrumental in detecting a progressively enlarging LV pseudo-aneurysm as well delineating hepatic mycotic aneurysms.
4. Surgery was successful in treating the LV pseudo-aneurysm and hepatic mycotic aneurysm.

References

[1] Mojab K, Lim L, Esfahani F et al. Mycotic aneurysm of the hepatic artery causing obstructive jaundice. *Am J Roentgenol* 1977; 128: 143–144 (same patient as in reference 4).

[2] Sande MA, Kartalija M, Anderson J. *Infective endocarditis*. In: Hurst's The Heart, 10th edn. New York, McGraw-Hill, 2001, p 2102.

[3] Ranganathan N, Sivaciyan V, Saksena FB. *The art and science of cardiac physical examination*. Totowa, New Jersey, Humana Press, 2006, p 133.

[4] Saksena FB, Kramer NE, Towne WD et al. Infective aneurysm of the left ventricle: angiographic and echocardiographic features. *Am Heart J* 1978; 96: 384–388.

[5] Sudhakar S, Sewani A, Agrawal M et al. Pseudoaneurysm of the mitral-aortic intervalvular fibrosa: A comprehensive review. *J Am Soc Echocardiogr* 2010; 23: 1009–1018.

[6] Beck W, Schrire V. Idiopathic mitral subannular left ventricular aneurysm in the Bantu. *Am Heart J* 1969; 78: 28–33.

[7] Hulton EA, Blankstein R. Pseudoaneurysms of the Heart. *Circulation* 2012; 125: 1920–1925.

[8] Bayer AS, Scheld WM. *Endocarditis and intravascular infections*. In: Principles and Practice of Infectious Diseases, 5th edn, Mandell GL, Bennett JE, Dolin R (eds). Philadelphia, Churchill Livingstone, 2000, pp 857–902.

11 PATIENT STUDY 11

Sequence of data presentation

1 History 24 November 1977
↓
2 M-mode echocardiogram
↓
3 ECG
↓
4 Cardiac catheterization and chest X ray
↓
5 Additional catheterization data
↓
6 Aortic root angiogram
↓
7 Physical examination 24 November 1977
↓
8 Diagnosis and treatment plan
↓
9 Follow-up chest X rays

1 History 24 November 1977

24-year-old man admitted to hospital with a 1-day history of fever and right leg pain then left leg pain following a recent tooth extraction.

He states that he has had a heart murmur for several years. He stopped using IV heroin 9 months ago.

2 M-mode echocardiogram

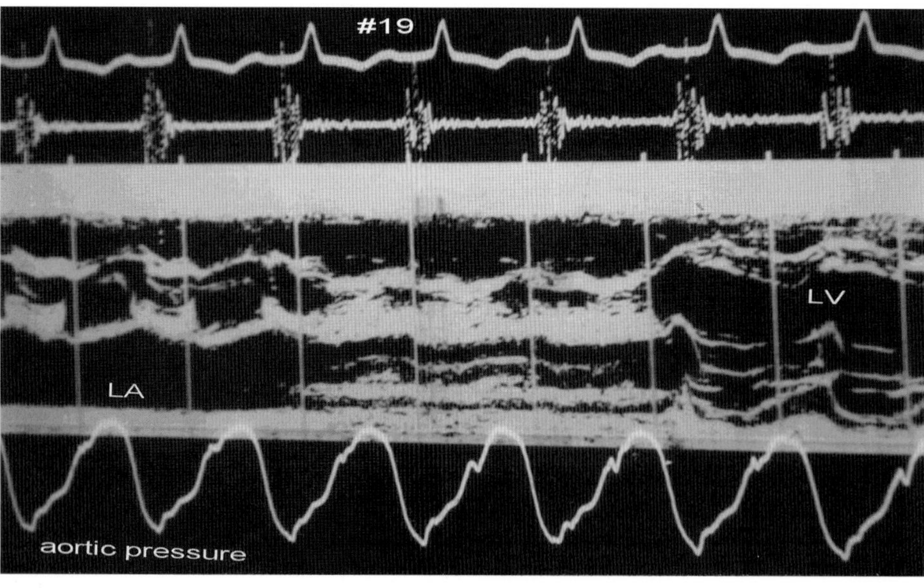

Figure 11.1 M-mode echocardiogram, along with ECG, phonocardiogram, and aortic pressure tracing 1977.

Patient Studies in Valvular, Congenital, and Rarer Forms of Cardiovascular Disease: An Integrative Approach, First Edition. Franklin B. Saksena.

Companion Website: www.wiley.com/go/saksena/patientstudies

3 ECG

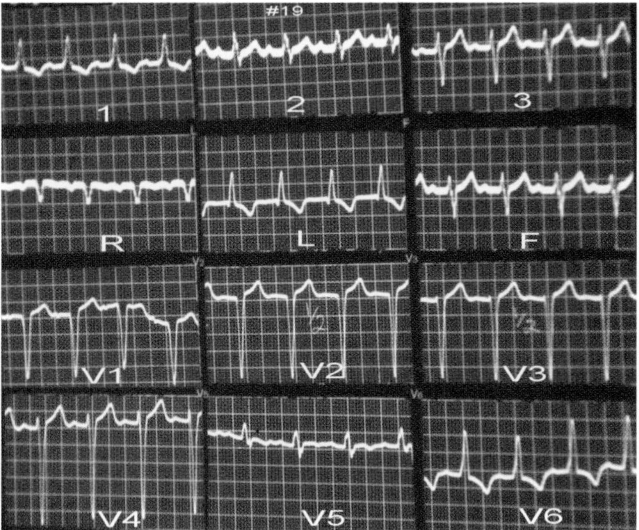

Figure 11.2 12-lead ECG 9 December 1977.

4 Cardiac catheterization and chest X ray 9 December 1977

C/T ratio was 0.5. Lung fields clear.

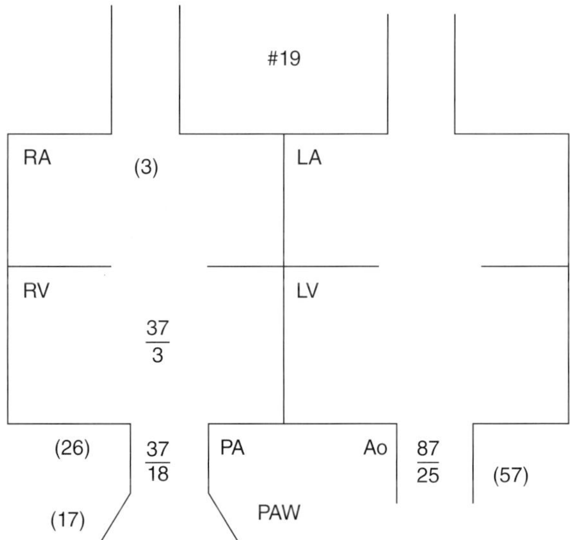

Figure 11.3 Cardiac catheterization and chest X ray report 9 December 1977.

5 Additional catheterization data

Table 11.1 LV volumes, cardiac output, and HR

LV end-diastolic volume	346 mL
LV end-systolic volume	106 mL
Fick cardiac output	9.2 L/min
HR	100/min
Body surface area	1.91 m^2

Calculate the pulmonary vascular resistance and the systemic vascular resistance.
Calculate the LV ejection fraction.
Calculate the regurgitant fraction.

6 Aortic root angiogram

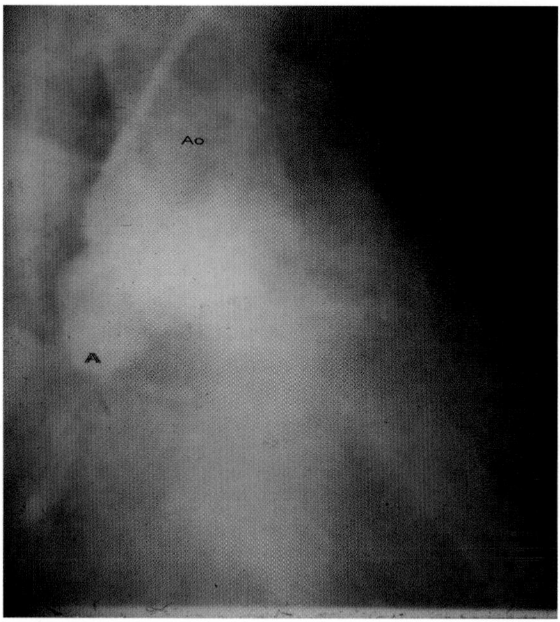

Figure 11.4 Catheter positioned a few centimetres superior to the aortic valve. RAO projection. Aortic root angiogram in 30° RAO projection 9 December 1977.

7 Physical examination 24 November 1977

70 inches tall, 163 lb. BP 100/40. HR 100/min regular, febrile.
Brisk carotid upstroke.
Apex beat is in the 6th interspace just outside the mid-clavicular line.
S1 normal. S2 increased P2. S3 0.
Grade 3/6 aortic systolic murmur.
Grade 3/6 diastolic blowing murmur heard down LLSB.
Lungs clear.
The right leg pulses were initially decreased on admission. Later the left leg and foot pulses were transiently reduced.

8 Diagnosis and treatment plan

What is the diagnosis and treatment plan?

Answers and commentary

1 History

The patient had a fever following tooth extraction, which could suggest a bacteremia. The leg pain has not been described adequately so no conclusions can be made. The presence of a heart murmur and prior IV drug use are risk factors for infective endocarditis. Blood cultures grew alpha hemolytic streptococcus.

2 M-mode echocardiogram

There is thickening of the non-coronary cusp of the aortic valve in the first two panels on the left. Panels 4–6 show an irregular thickening of the right and non-coronary cusps.
These findings indicate a vegetation on the aortic cusps.

The LA and LV are not enlarged. The aortic pressure contour shows absence of a dicrotic notch, suggestive of aortic regurgitation.

3 ECG

The rate is 100/min. The rhythm is sinus. PR 0.19 s. QRS 0.11 s. QRS axis –20°.

T inverted in 1, L, V6. SV1 + RV6 = 5.5 mv.

Impression: LVH with repolarization abnormalities.

Based on the above data (sections 1–3) the patient has aortic valve endocarditis, aortic regurgitation with LVH, and the endocarditis was due to *Streptococcus viridans*.

4 Cardiac catheterization and chest X ray

There was mild pulmonary hypertension (PA mean 26 mmHg). The wedge pressure was elevated to 17 mmHg, which could be due to either mitral valvular disease or LV dysfunction. Lacking an LV pressure, mitral valvular disease cannot be excluded.

The aortic pressure shows a wide pulse pressure compatible with aortic regurgitation or a high output state. The aortic systolic pressure is reduced.

A normal C/T ratio was seen on chest X ray despite the three-fold increase in LV volumes, as seen below.

5 Additional catheterization data

(a) LV ejection fraction

LV end-diastolic volume (LVEDV) = 346 mL

LV end-systolic volume (LVESV) = 106 mL

∴ stroke volume = LVEDV – LVESV = 240 mL

$$\text{LV ejection fraction} = \frac{\text{stroke.volume}}{\text{LVEDV}} = \frac{240}{346} = 0.69$$

The LV ejection fraction is at the upper limits of normal, implying normal LV systolic function in the face of significant aortic regurgitation.

(b) Regurgitant fraction

Angiographic stroke volume = 240 mL

Heart rate = 100/min

Fick cardiac output = 9.2 L/min

Total angiographic cardiac output = 240 mL ×100 = 24 L/min

Total forward cardiac output = 9.2 L/min

∴ regurgitant output = 24 – 9.2 = 14.8 L/min

$$\text{or regurgitant fraction} = \frac{14.8}{24} = 62\%$$

This indicates severe regurgitation.

(c) Resistance measurements

Pressures: Fick cardiac output = 9.2 L/min

PA mean = 26 mmHg

PAW mean = 17 mmHg

RA mean = 3 mmHg

Aortic mean = 57 mmHg

$$\text{Pulmonary vascular resistance} = \frac{\text{PA} - \text{PAW}}{\text{cardiac.output}} \times 80 = \frac{26-17}{9.2} \times 80 = 79 \text{ dyn.sec.cm}^{-5}.$$

$$\text{Systemic vascular resistance} = \frac{\text{Ao} - \text{RA}}{\text{cardiac.output}} \times 80 = \frac{57-3}{9.2} \times 80 \text{ or } 470 \text{ dyn.sec.cm}^{-5}.$$

The pulmonary vascular resistance is normal, whereas the systemic vascular resistance is low, compatible with aortic regurgitation.

6 Aortic root angiogram

In Figure 11.4 the aortic catheter is seen just above the aortic valve and there is filling of the LV, indicating aortic regurgitation. There is a saccular aneurysm of the aortic non-coronary cusp (A).

7 Physical examination 24 November 1977

There is moderately severe aortic regurgitation on the basis of a diastolic decrescendo blowing murmur heard down the LLSB, along with cardiomegaly, a wide pulse pressure, and a brisk carotid artery upstroke. The latter tends to rule out significant aortic stenosis. The murmur across the aortic valve in systole is most likely a flow murmur commonly seen in patients with significant aortic regurgitation.

The intermittent absence of the right leg pulses was due to a proven (R) femoral artery embolism on admission. The intermittent absence of the (L) leg and foot pulses later could have been due to an embolism (thrombus or vegetation) in the left leg.

8 Diagnosis and treatment plan

Diagnosis

Acute aortic regurgitation due to infective endocarditis.

Emboli to legs (thrombi or vegetation).

The patient had 3 weeks of antibiotic therapy and then underwent surgery.

At surgery on 16 December 1977 all three aortic cusps had friable vegetations destroying the valves, such that there was barely any attachment of the cusps to the aortic annulus.

The non-coronary cusp was destroyed and there was a sinus tract going into the myocardium from the region of the non-coronary cusp.

The aortic valve was replaced with a 27 mm porcine Hancock valve. The sinus tract was closed.

The patient did well following aortic valve replacement.

9 Follow-up chest X rays

Figure 11.5a shows a PA chest X ray taken 2 weeks after surgery in which the C/T ratio is 0.44 and lung fields are clear. The porcine valve is not visible in this view.

Figure 11.5b shows a lateral chest X ray with the aortic porcine ring seen in the upper half of the cardiac silhouette. The customary wires repairing the sternum are not seen as the sternum was closed with ethiflex sutures.

Figure 11.6 shows a PA chest X ray taken 7 months after surgery in which the C/T ratio remains within normal limits.

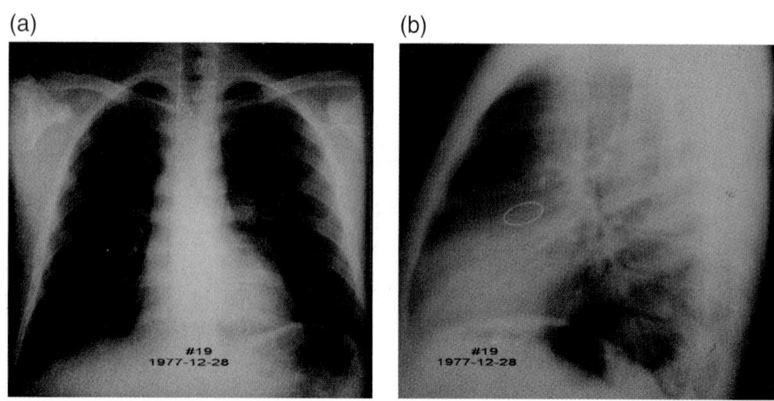

Figure 11.5 (a) Chest X ray PA view 28 December 1977. (b) Chest X ray lateral view 28 December 1977.

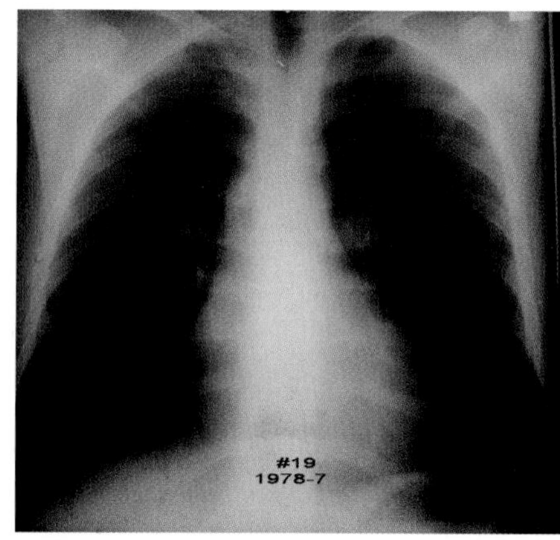

Figure 11.6 Chest X ray PA view 22 July 1978.

Discussion

The patient had aortic valve endocarditis with severe aortic regurgitation. There is a reluctance to do a valve replacement on IVDAs as they may return to their drug habit and be noncompliant with medications and medical follow-up.

He had been off drugs for 9 months and did undergo aortic valve replacement, but he was lost to long-term follow-up. At the present time only if the IVDA patient is enrolled in a drug rehabilitation program should valve surgery for endocarditis be a consideration [3].

The incidence of endocarditis in IVDAs is approximately two to four cases per 1000 years of drug abuse [3] or about 2–5% per patient year [1, 2].

The typical drug user with endocarditis is a male aged about 30 [1, 3, 5]. The most common organism causing endocarditis is staphylococcus. Other organisms causing endocarditis are streptococcus, enterococcus, fungi, and Gram-negative bacilli [3]. Polymicrobial endocarditis is occurring more frequently with a concomitant rise in mortality [4, 5].

IVDAs are at high risk for endocarditis, usually of the tricuspid valve, and may also have left-sided valvular involvement, which carries a much higher mortality rate than a right-sided lesion [1, 5]. Over 60% of IVDA patients with endocarditis have no pre-existing valvular disease [1, 5].

M-mode echocardiogram can detect these vegetations but two-dimensional echocardiography provides additional information as to their size and mobility [6]. In addition two-dimensional or TEE provides information as to the severity of the regurgitation, the extent of biventricular dysfunction, and the spread of the infection to the myocardium [1, 6] (see Figures 11.7 and 11.8). Patients will usually need to have TEE prior to and during valve surgery [1, 2].

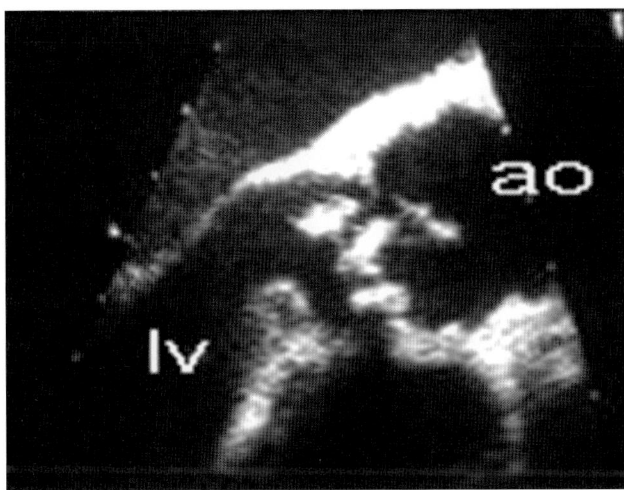

Figure 11.7 Two-dimensional echocardiogram showing a 0.5 × 1.2 cm mobile mass attached to the aortic valve (27 August 2011) in a 27-year-old man with a history of using crack cocaine and IV heroin. In 2009 he had a cadaver aortic valve replacement for endocarditis at another hospital but continued his IV heroin use. He was admitted to hospital in 2011 twice with severe aortic regurgitation (BP 135/35) due to a staphylococcal endocarditis. RV systolic pressure ~75 mmHg. LV ejection fraction 0.60. In 2011 two separate cardiovascular surgeons turned the patient down for a repeat aortic valve replacement.

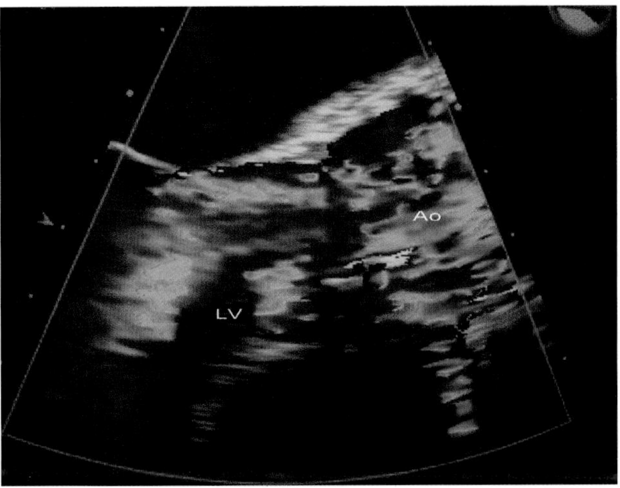

Figure 11.8 Doppler study of aortic valve (same patient as Figure 11.7) showing severe aortic regurgitation.

Key points

1. The patient, a former drug addict, had a streptococcal septicemia that lead to aortic valve endocarditis and a septic embolism to the leg.
2. M-mode echocardiography detected the aortic vegetations involving at least two cusps in this patient. Since the advent of two-dimensional echocardiography and TEE the size and mobility of the vegetations can also be assessed.
3. He had severe aortic regurgitation on the basis of physical findings, aortography, a dilated LV, and a high calculated regurgitant fraction.
4. Despite a high LV end-diastolic volume there was no cardiomegaly or LV failure on chest X ray in this patient.
5. Aortic valve replacement for aortic valve endocarditis is required if the patient is in heart failure.

References

[1] Mauri L, de Lemos JA, O'Gara PT. Infective endocarditis. *Curr Probl Cardiol* 2001; 26: 557–612 (detailed review article).

[2] Prendergast BD, Tornos P. Surgery for infective endocarditis. Who and when? *Circulation* 2010; 121: 1141–1152.

[3] Sexton DJ, Chu VH. *Infective endocarditis in injection drug users*. www.uptodate.com, 2013, pp 1–9.

[4] Sousa C, Botelho C, Rodrigues D et al. Infective endocarditis in intravenous drug abusers: an update. *Eur J Clin Microbiol Infect Dis* 2012; 31: 2905–2910.
[5] Starakis I, Mazokopakis EE. Injecting illicit substances epidemic and infective endocarditis. Infectious Disorder – Drug *Targets* 2010; 10: 22–26.
[6] Tornos P, Gonzalez-Alujas T, Thuny F et al. Infective endocarditis: the European viewpoint. *Curr Probl Cardiol* 2011; 36: 169–222 (covers antibiotic regimens in detail).

12 PATIENT STUDY 12

Sequence of data presentation

1 History 1976
↓
2 ECG 1976
↓
3 Chest X ray 1976
↓
4 M-mode echocardiogram 1976
↓
5 Cardiac catheterization data 1964–1980
↓
6 Additional cardiac catheterization data
↓
7 Diagnosis
↓
8 Physical examination
↓
9 Follow up data

1 History

48-year-old black female para 5 gravida 5 admitted to hospital in 1976 with an acute abdomen attributed to pelvic inflammatory disease. She was referred to cardiology because of dyspnea on walking one block.

She was diagnosed with heart disease during her first pregnancy in 1946. In 1950 she had a right hemiparesis.

She underwent diagnostic cardiac catheterizeation in 1964 followed by cardiac surgery.in 1965.

In 1970 she underwent a second cardiac catheterization and it was elected to follow the patient medically with medically with digoxin, diuretics, and warfarin.

She was readmitted in 1976 because of increasing exertional dyspnea over the previous few months.

No history of hypertension, diabetes, or syphilis. Patient does not smoke and only uses alcohol occasionally.

2 ECG 1976

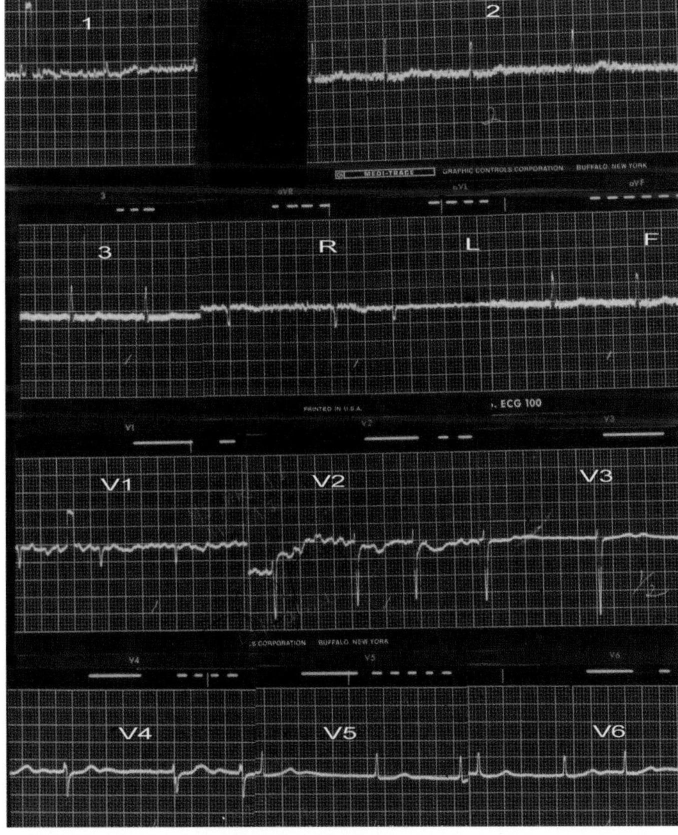

Figure 12.1 12-lead ECG 1976.

Patient Studies in Valvular, Congenital, and Rarer Forms of Cardiovascular Disease: An Integrative Approach, First Edition. Franklin B. Saksena.

Companion Website: www.wiley.com/go/saksena/patientstudies

3 Chest X ray 1976

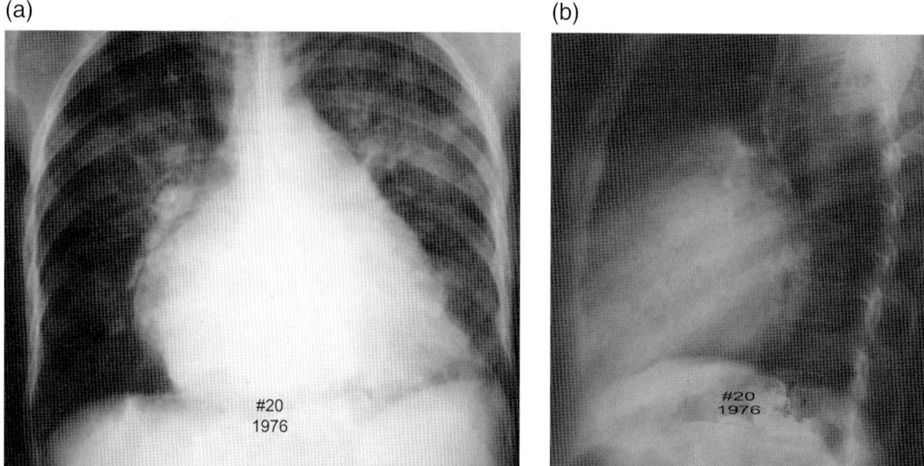

Figure 12.2 (a) PA chest X ray 1976. (b) Lateral chest X ray 1976.

4 M-mode echocardiography 1976

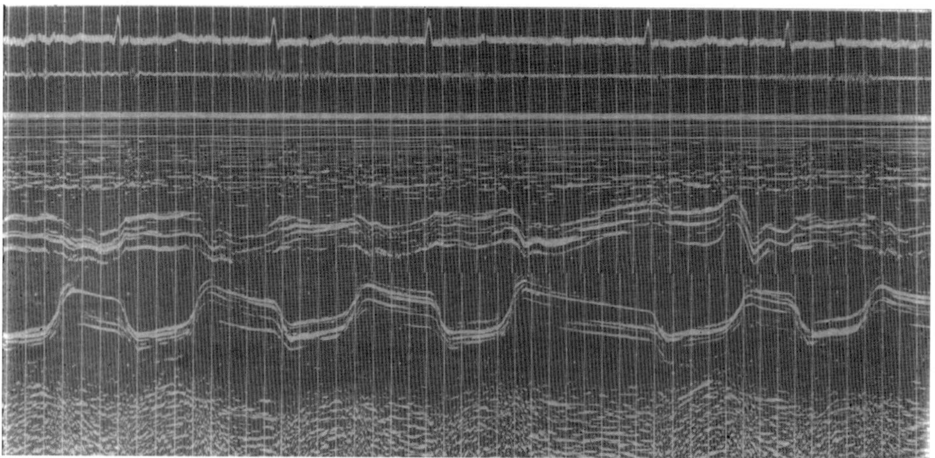

Figure 12.3 M-mode echocardiogram at mitral valve level 1976.

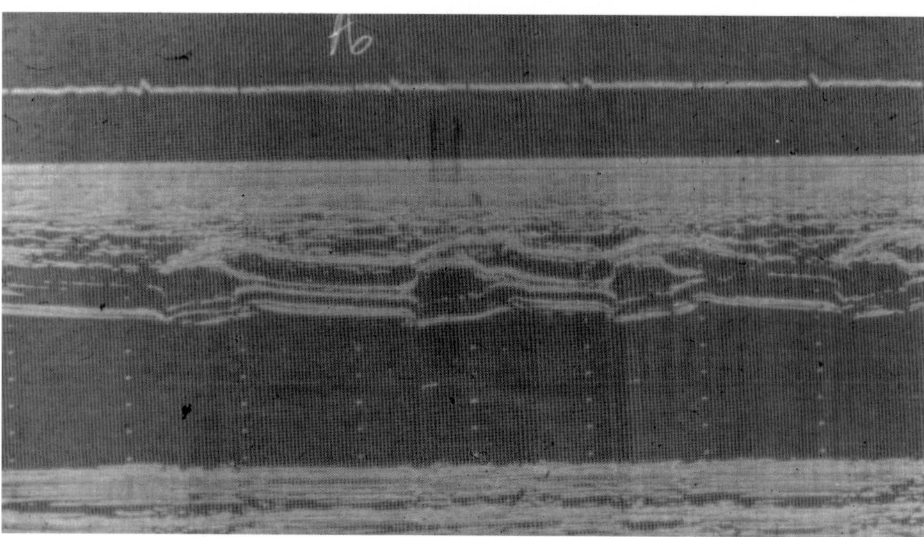

Figure 12.4 M-mode echocardiogram at aortic valve level 1976.

5 Cardiac catheterization data 1964–1980

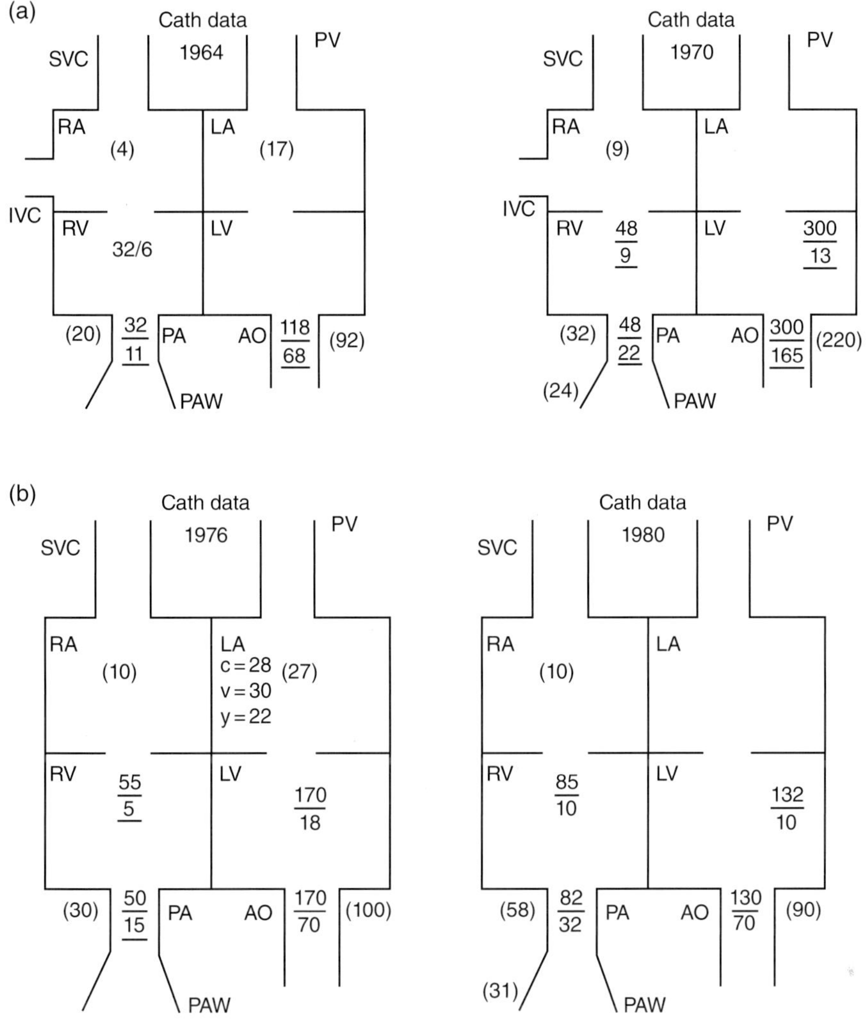

Figure 12.5 (a) Cardiac catheterization data 1964 and 1970. (b) Cardiac catheterization data 1976 and 1980.

6 Additional cardiac catheterization data

Table 12.1 Additional hemodynamic data 1964–1980.

	1964	1970	1976	1980
Cardiac output (L/min)	3.2	2.3	3.2	3.5
Mitral diastolic gradient (mm Hg)		15	11.3	21
Mitral valve area (cm^2)			0.4	0.7
Mitral regurgitation		Trace	Trace	0
Aortic regurgitation	1+	1+	2+	2+
LV ejection fraction				0.58
LV end diastolic volume (mL)				110
Coronary artery disease				25% stenosis right coronary

Body surface area = 1.3 m^2

7 Diagnosis and treatment?

Comment on the diagnosis and treatment.

8 Physical examination 1976

60 inches tall female weighing 88 lb. BP 100/60. HR 100/min irregular.
No elevation of jugular venous pressure. Normal carotid amplitude.
Apex beat was in the 5th left interspace in the anterior axillary line.
S1 was increased in intensity.
S2 revealed a loud P2 component.
Opening snap was heard at the apex.
Grade 2/6 apical diastolic rumble.
Grade 5/6 holosystolic apical murmur.
Grade 2/6 high-pitched diastolic murmur heard down LLSB.
Lungs clear to percussion and auscultation.
No hepatomegaly or pedal edema.

9 Follow up data

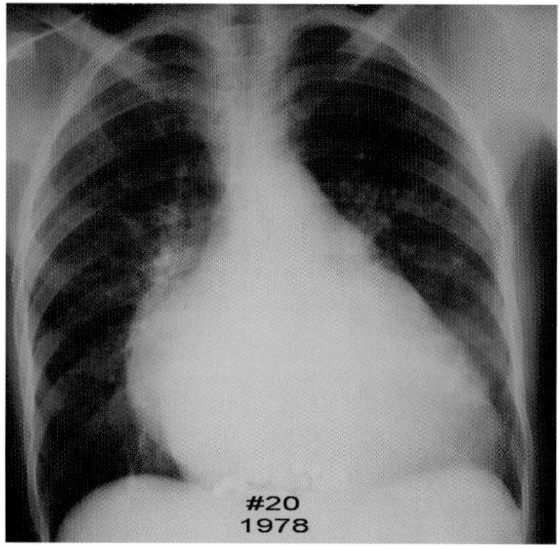

Figure 12.6 Chest X ray 1978.

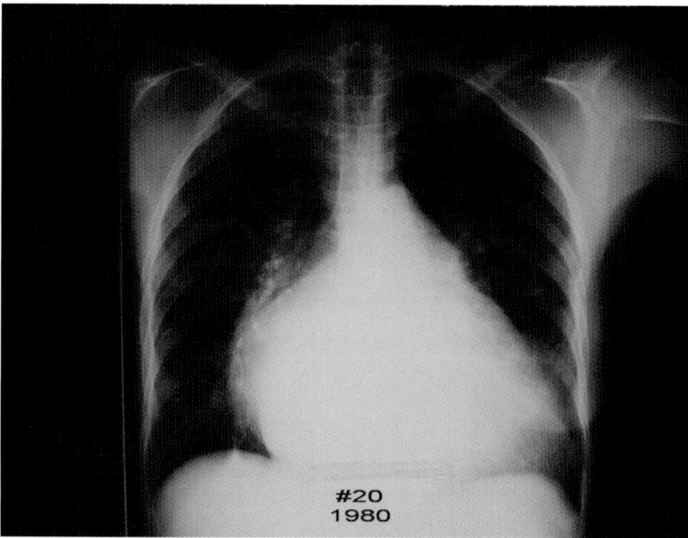

Figure 12.7 Comparison of 1976 and 1980 chest X rays.

Answers and commentary

1 History 1976

The patient had rheumatic heart disease diagnosed during her first pregnancy. She probably developed atrial fibrillation soon afterwards and had a cerebral embolus that resulted in a right hemiparesis.

Mitral stenosis was diagnosed in 1964 and she underwent mitral valve commissurotomy in 1965 (see Figure 12.5). She had mitral restenosis diagnosed in 1970 but was treated medically at that time with digoxin, diuretics, and warfarin.

As her mitral valve disease had progressed she was readmitted in 1976 for further evaluation.

2 ECG 1976

The rhythm is atrial fibrillation with an average ventricular rate of 65/min. QRS interval 0.04 s. QRS axis +60°.

3 Chest X ray 1976

The PA chest X ray (Figure 12.2a) shows an enlarged heart (C/T ratio = 0.64), mainly involving the right heart. There is straightening of the left heart border due to LA enlargement. The proximal pulmonary arteries are enlarged with distal tapering of the pulmonary vessels, suggesting pulmonary hypertension.

The RV is enlarged (Figure 12.2b) and occupies a large portion of the retrosternal space (at least three interspaces). The LA is also enlarged and pushes the esophagus posteriorly.

The findings of RV and LA enlargement along with pulmonary hypertension are highly suggestive of mitral stenosis.

4 M-mode echocardiogram 1976

The mitral valve echogram shows concordant movement of the anterior and posterior mitral valve leaflets (Figure 12.3). The EF slope is reduced and the mitral valve leaflets are thickened. These findings are indicative of mitral stenosis. The patient was in atrial fibrillation.

The LA is enlarged (Figure 12.4) to at least 5 cm or 3.8 cm/m^2 (normal 1.2–2.1 cm/m^2). The aortic valve opening excursion is reduced, possibly due to a low output state.

5 and 6 Cardiac catheterization data 1968–1980 and additional cardiac catheterization data

In 1964 right heart pressures were normal. The LA pressure (measured directly) was elevated to 17 mmHg. Data are lacking on the mitral diastolic gradient and mitral valve area. The cardiac output was low (3.2 L/min) and there was mild aortic regurgitation (1+).

In 1970 the mean PA pressure had risen to 32 mmHg from 20 mmHg in 1964. No data were mentioned on the mitral valve area or the mitral diastolic gradient. There was severe systemic hypertension. The cardiac output had fallen to 2.3 L/min.

In 1976 there was still a moderate degree of pulmonary hypertension (PA mean 30 mmHg). The LA pressure (obtained transseptally) had risen to 27 mmHg compared to 17 mmHg in 1964. There was critical mitral stenosis based on a mitral diastolic gradient of 11 mmHg and a mitral valve area of 0.4 cm^2.

Angiographically, there was insignificant mitral regurgitation and a slight increase in the severity of aortic regurgitation (2+).

In 1980 there was severe pulmonary hypertension (PA mean 58 mmHg) and a further rise in gradient across the mitral valve to 21 mmHg. The mitral area was still critically reduced (0.7 cm^2).

The LV end-diastolic volume was normal (110 cc or 79 cc/m^2), indicating that aortic regurgitation was at best mild. LV systolic function (based on the LV ejection fraction) was normal and there was no significant coronary artery disease.

7 Diagnosis

Severe mitral stenosis with pulmonary hypertension and atrial fibrillation.

Tricuspid regurgitation.

Mild aortic regurgitation.

8 Physical examination

The holosystolic murmur at the apex was attributed to tricuspid regurgitation rather than mitral regurgitation as it is likely that the apex was occupied by the RV and not the LV.

The patient had mitral stenosis based on the loud S1, the opening snap, and diastolic apical rumble.

The presence of a loud P2 would suggest pulmonary hypertension, confirmed at cardiac catheterization. Tricuspid regurgitation was deemed secondary to pulmonary hypertension.

The diastolic blowing murmur down the left sternal border was due to aortic regurgitation, which appeared to have been angiographically present for several years.

9 Follow-up data

There was a further increase in heart size in 1978 with a C/T ratio of 0.71.

In 1980 the C/T ratio had risen to 0.74.

The patient underwent successful mitral valve replacement in March 1980 and was doing well 3 months later.

Discussion

This patient had all the classic features of mitral stenosis complicated by atrial fibrillation, hemiparesis, mitral restenosis, pulmonary hypertension, and tricuspid regurgitation [1, 2].

The patient was a candidate for mitral valve replacement in 1976 as she had a mitral valve area of only 0.4 cm^2 and mild pulmonary hypertension, but she refused surgery.

In 4 years the pulmonary hypertension had become severe and her mitral valve area remained critically reduced. She did undergo successful mitral valve replacement in 1980.

Usually the PA pressure will fall after successful surgical relief of the mitral stenosis [3], but long-term follow-up of this patient was not available. At some future point she may require surgical treatment of her aortic regurgitant lesion.

Key points

1. The patient had progressive mitral stenosis complicated by atrial fibrillation, hemiparesis, mitral restenosis, pulmonary hypertension, and tricuspid regurgitation.
2. She finally agreed to have mitral valve replacement, but at this late stage (age 52) she may only attain a modest reduction in her pulmonary hypertension.

References

[1] Bruce CJ, Nishimura R. Newer advances in the diagnosis and treatment of mitral stenosis. *Curr Probl Cardiol* 1998; 23: 130–192.

[2] Wood P. An appreciation of mitral stenosis. Part 1 Clinical features. *Br Med J* 1954; 1: 1051–1063; Part 2 Investigations and results. *Br Med J* 1954; 1: 1113–1124 (a study of 300 cases of mitral stenosis).

[3] Abbo KM, Carroll JD. Hemodynamics of mitral stenosis: A review. *Cathet Cardiovasc Diagn* 1994; suppl 2: 16–25.

13 PATIENT STUDY 13

Patients 13 and 14 had similar findings. The discussion about these patients is given in Patient Study 14.

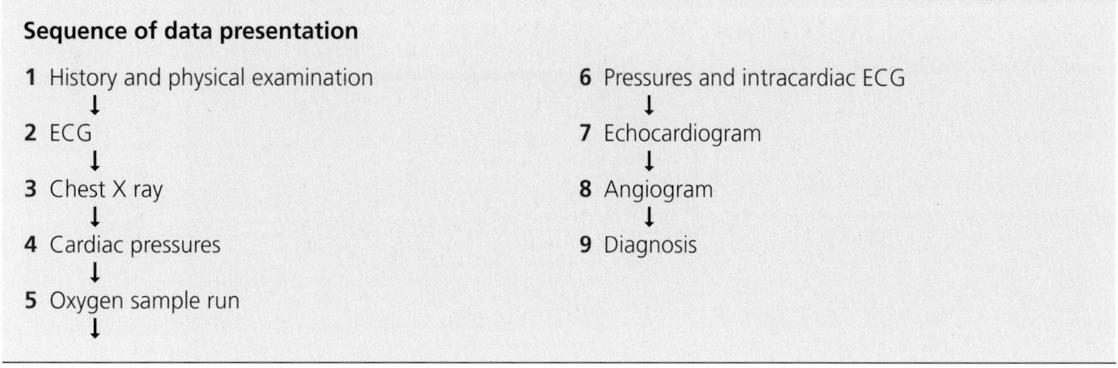

Sequence of data presentation

1 History and physical examination
↓
2 ECG
↓
3 Chest X ray
↓
4 Cardiac pressures
↓
5 Oxygen sample run
↓
6 Pressures and intracardiac ECG
↓
7 Echocardiogram
↓
8 Angiogram
↓
9 Diagnosis

1 History and physical examination

History

This 19-year-old man had a history of easy fatigue playing soccer. No dyspnea or palpitations. No history of heart disease, diabetes, or TB.

Physical examination

67 inches tall, 119 lb male. BP 102/80. Pulse 76/min regular. R 18/min. T 98 °F.
Cyanosis and clubbing.
No elevation of jugular venous pressure.
Apex beat was in the 5th left intercostal space 2 cm lateral to the mid-clavicular line.
There was a parasternal lift 2+.
S1 loud. S2 normal. S3 + 1.
There was a grade 2/6 diamond-shaped systolic murmur heard over the left 3rd and 4th interspace parasternally. No radiation to axilla or carotid arteries. The murmur decreased during valsalva maneuver.
No edema. Normal peripheral pulses.

Patient Studies in Valvular, Congenital, and Rarer Forms of Cardiovascular Disease: An Integrative Approach, First Edition. Franklin B. Saksena.

Companion Website: www.wiley.com/go/saksena/patientstudies

2 ECG

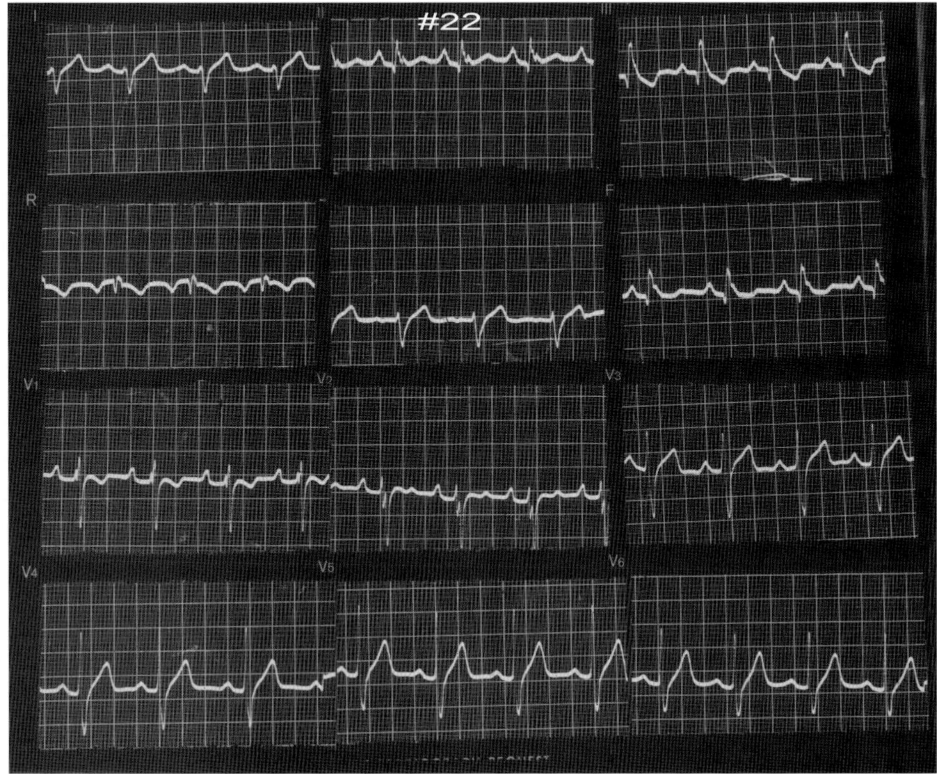

Figure 13.1 ECG

3 Chest X ray

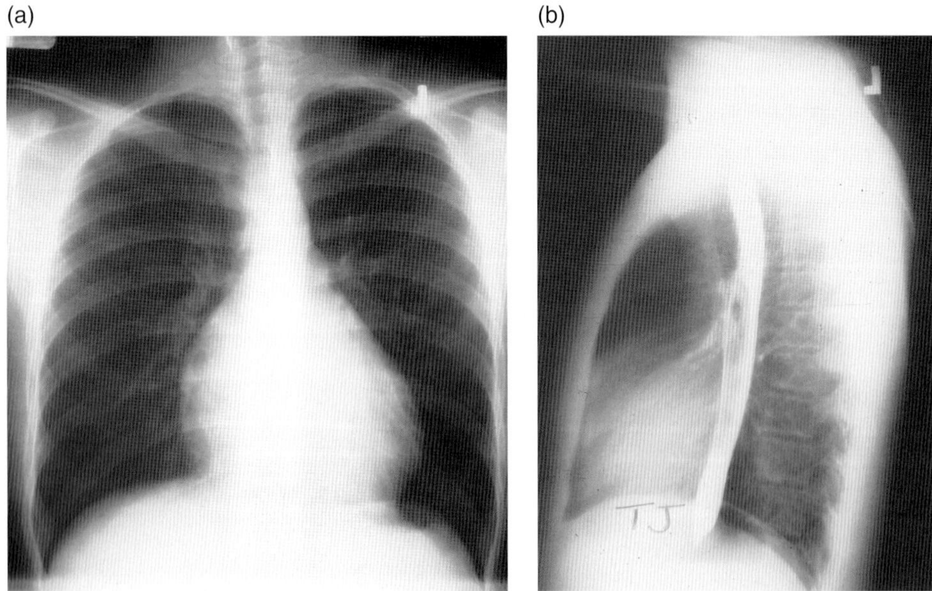

Figure 13.2 (a) Chest X ray PA view. (b) Chest X ray lateral view.

4 Cardiac pressures

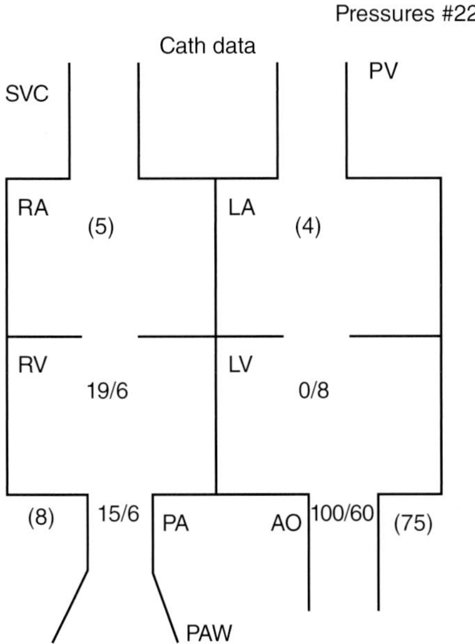

Figure 13.3 Cardiac pressures.

5 Oxygen sample run

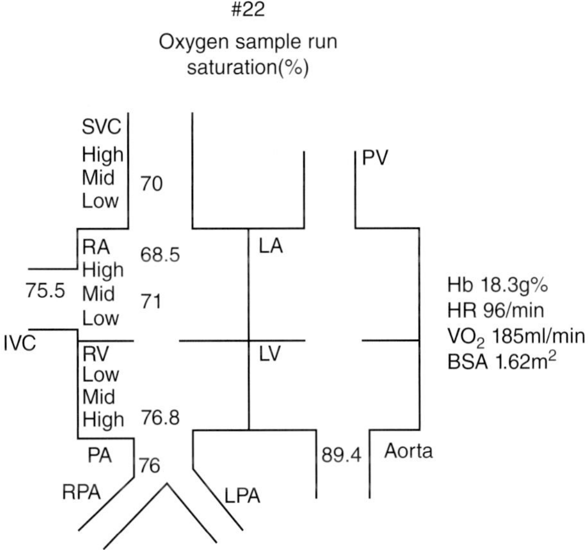

Figure 13.4 Oxygen sample run and additional data.

What is the pulmonary/systemic flow ratio?

6 Pressures and intracardiac ECG

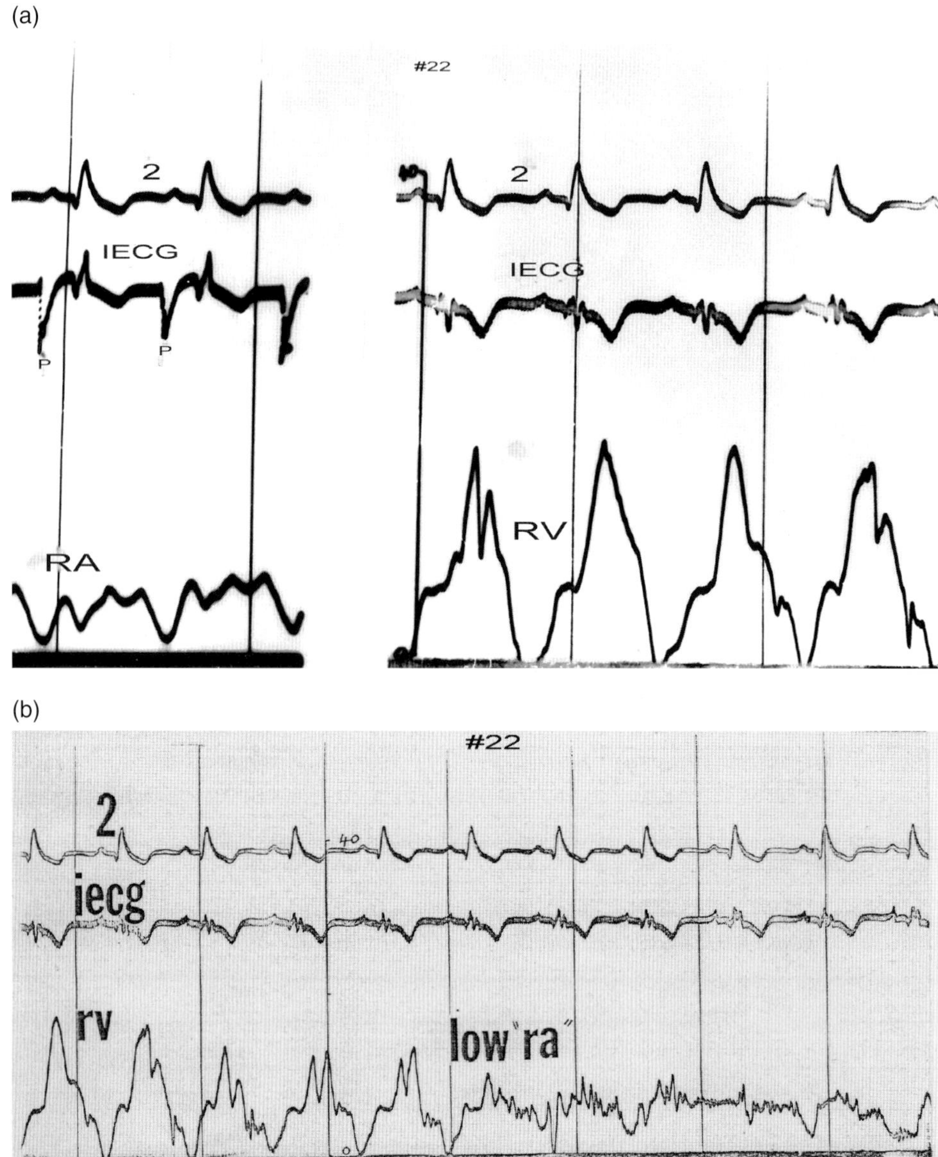

Figure 13.5 (a) Left panel: there is a large inverted P wave on the intracardiac ECG (iecg) when the catheter is in the RA. Right panel: the P wave is very small with a wider QRS on the intracardiac ECG when the catheter is in the RV. (b) Pullback from RV to RA with simultaneous intracardiac ECG and surface lead 2. The intracardiac ECG shows a ventricular QRS contour in RV and the low RA.

7 Echocardiogram

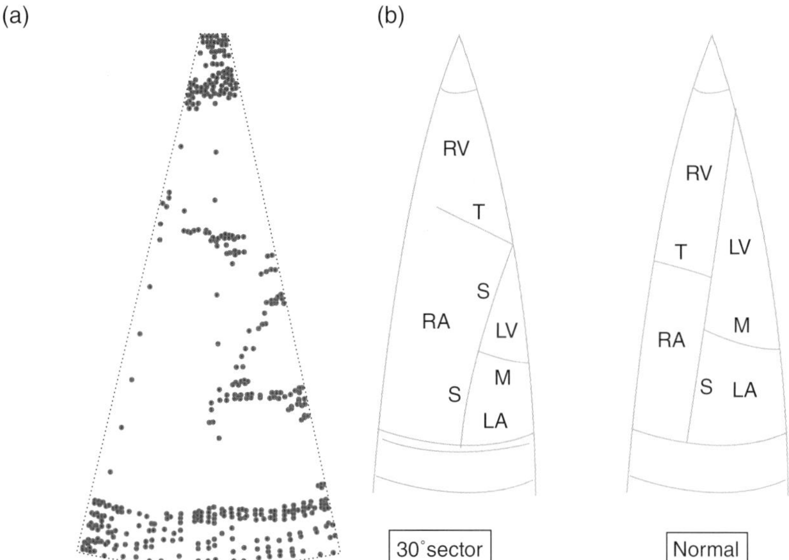

Figure 13.6 30° sector cardiography. M, mitral valve; S, septum; T, tricuspid valve.

8 Angiogram

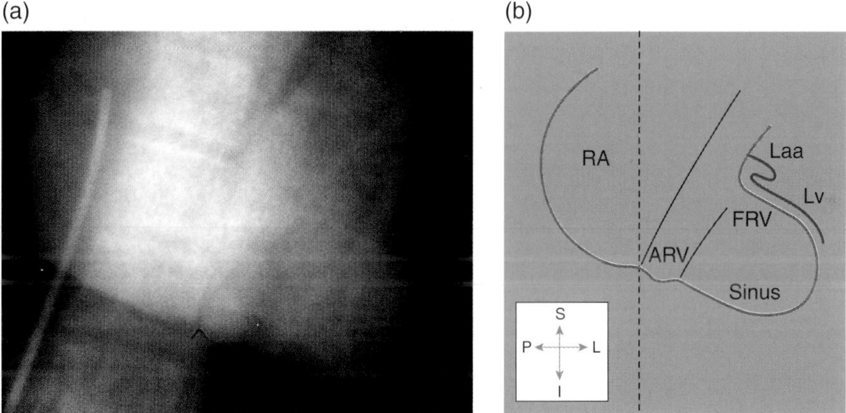

Figure 13.7 (a) RA angiogram AP view. The red arrow shows the position of the RA-atrialized RV junction. (b) RA angiogram in AP view. ARV, atrialized RV; FRV, functional RV; Laa, LA appendage.

9 Diagnosis

What is the diagnosis?

Answers and commentary

1 History and physical examination

History

Fatigue is a nonspecific symptom.

Physical findings

The presence of clubbing and cyanosis is indicative of a right to left shunt at atrial, ventricular, or great vessel level.

No description was available of the jugular venous waveform or the timing of the parasternal lift.

The systolic murmur recorded in this patient is probably a flow murmur across the pulmonic valve rather than that of tricuspid regurgitation. The murmur of tricuspid regurgitation is usually pansystolic and heard best at LLSB.

2 ECG

The rhythm is sinus with first-degree AV block (PR 0.24 s, QRS 0.10 s, rate 100 /min, QRS axis +120°.

Peaked P in 2, 3, F suggestive of RA enlargement.

Slurring of QRS complex seen in V1–2 and lead 2 suggests an intraventricular conduction disturbance. The right-axis deviation may in part be due to the age and habitus of the patient.

3 Chest X ray

The heart has a globular shape with some prominence of the right heart in PA view. The lung fields appear unremarkable. Physical examination showed cardiomegaly, which is not borne out by the normal C/T ratio.

In the lateral view the barium swallow study fails to show any posterior indentation of the esophagus, thus excluding LA enlargement.

4 Cardiac pressures

Right and left heart pressures were normal. The LA was entered via an atrial septal defect.

Normal pulmonary vasculature and normal PA pressures in the presence of cyanosis and clubbing point to Ebstein's anomaly.

5 Oxygen sample run

There is no significant step up in oxygen saturation on entering the RA from the vena cavae. The slight step up in oxygen saturation on entering RV from RA could be due to streaming of blood from the IVC to the RA or due to a small left to right shunt at atrial level. Additional blood samples from the right heart would have clarified the most likely diagnosis.

There is arterial oxygen desaturation, which could be due to a right to left shunt or lung disease (alveolar hypoventilation, diffusion defect, or abnormal ventilation/blood flow ratios). In the absence of known lung disease a right to left shunt is most likely present.

Calculation of pulmonary/systemic ratio (Q_p/Q_s)

In the absence of lung disease we assume that the pulmonary venous saturation is 95%.

Step 1: Calculate the total oxyhemoglobin content

As Hb is 18.3 g % we have total content = 1.34 × 18.3 = 24.5 vol%.

Step 2: Convert the corresponding saturations to oxygen content

$$C_{pv} = 23.3\text{ vol\%}$$
$$C_{pa} = 18.6\text{ vol\%}$$
$$C_{ao} = 21.9\text{ vol\%}$$

Step 3: Knowing the oxygen consumption is 185 cc/min. calculate the pulmonary (Q_p) and systemic (Q_s) blood flow

$$Q_p = \frac{185}{10(23.3-18.6)} = 3.93\text{ L/min}$$

$$Q_s = \frac{185}{10(21.9-18.6)} = 5.60\text{ L/min}$$

$$Q_p/Q_s = 0.7$$

Thus the right to left shunt is 5.6 – 3.93 L/min = 1.67 L/min.

6 Pressures and intracardiac ECG

The left panel of Figure 13.5a shows a large P wave in the intracardiac ECG when the catheter is in the RA. The P wave becomes much smaller when the recording is in the RV in the right panel. However, a pull back from RV to low RA shows an area where the intracardiac ECG is ventricular but the pressure contour is atrial. This atrialized RV implies the displacement of the tricuspid valve inferiorly into the RV.

7 Echocardiogram

The RA is enlarged and the tricuspid valve leaflet (usually the septal leaflet) is displaced much deeper into the RV. Normally the tricuspid leaflet is about level with the mitral valve leaflet in the four-chamber view. In M mode (not shown) the tricuspid valve closure was delayed and occurred 70 ms after the closure of the mitral valve.

8 Angiogram

The RA is enlarged. A small notch (see arrow on Figure 13.7a) separates the RA proper with the atrialized RV. There is filling of the LA and LV via an ASD.

9 Diagnosis

Ebstein's anomaly, with a right to left shunt at atrial level.

14 PATIENT STUDY 14

Sequence of data presentation

1 Phonocardiogram
↓
2 History
↓
3 Physical examination
↓
4 Chest X ray
↓
5 ECG
↓
6 Intracardiac pressures
↓
7 Oxygen sample run
↓
8 Diagnosis

1 Phonocardiogram

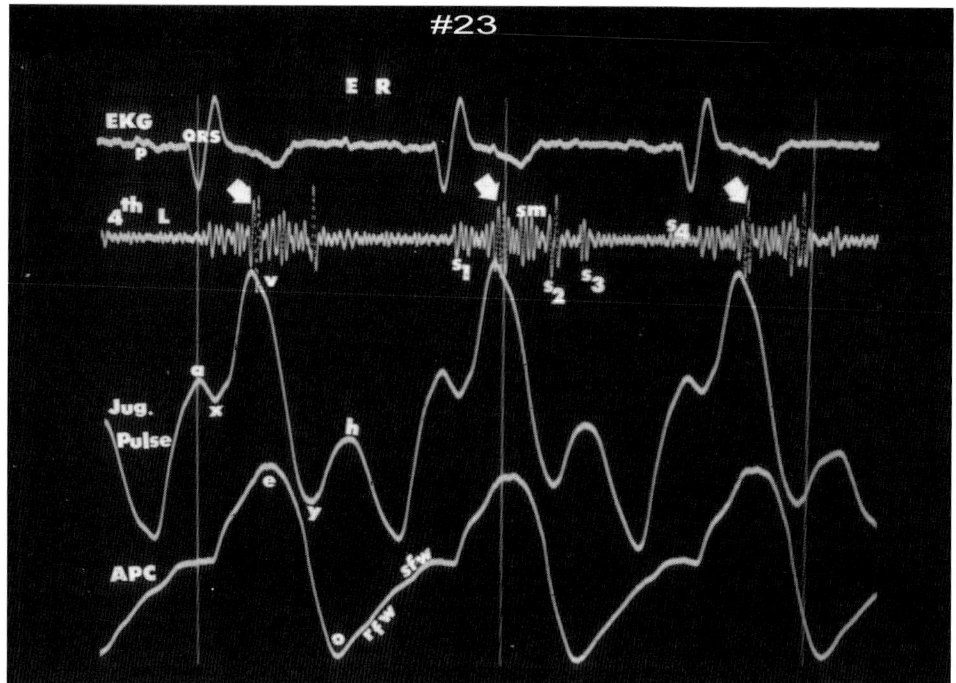

Figure 14.1 Phonocardiogram. From above downwards: ECG, phonocardiogram at the 4th left interspace parasternally, jugular venous pulse, apexcardiogram (apc) showing the rapid filling wave (rfw) and the slow filling wave (sfw).

What are the arrows pointing to?

2 History

29-year-old man admitted to hospital with progressive exertional dyspnea on walking one block over the last few months.

As a child he had easy fatigue on playing sports.

At age 17 he was told he had a heart murmur with cyanosis and clubbing.

At age 25 he had some exertional dyspnea, which did not improve with digoxin.

Patient Studies in Valvular, Congenital, and Rarer Forms of Cardiovascular Disease: An Integrative Approach, First Edition. Franklin B. Saksena.

Companion Website: www.wiley.com/go/saksena/patientstudies

No history of rheumatic fever, chest pain, edema, or palpitations.
Patient does not drink alcohol or smoke.

3 Physical examination

67 inches tall, 124 lb male with possible clubbing but no definite cyanosis.
No elevation of jugular venous pressure.
No cardiomegaly. No visible precordial pulsations.
S1 normal. S2 normal with physiological splitting. S3 noted at LLSB.
Grade 2/6 hololsystolic murmur heard at LLSB, increasing on inspiration.
No hepatosplenomegaly.
No edema. Good peripheral pulses.
Lungs were clear.

4 ECG

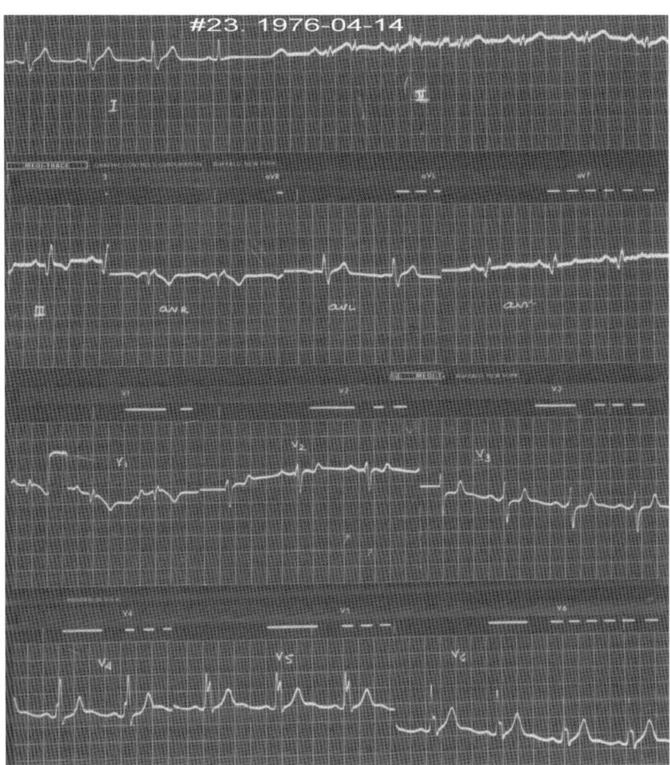

Figure 14.2 ECG.

5 Chest X ray

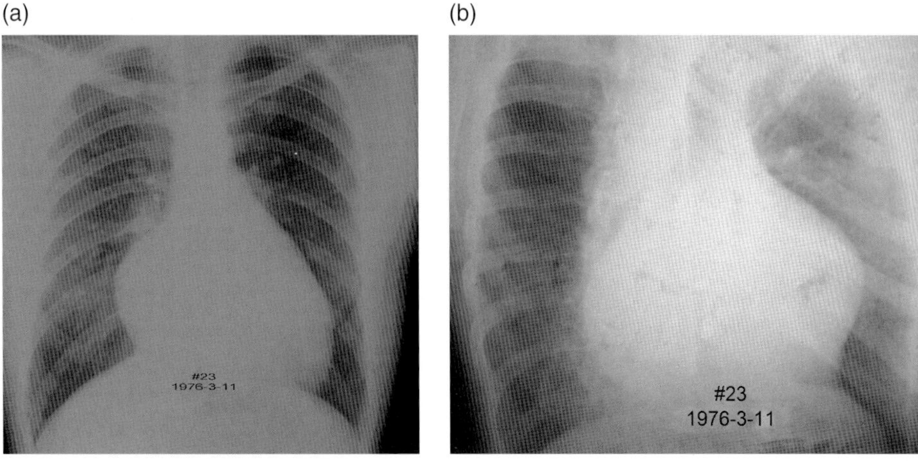

Figure 14.3 (a) Chest X ray PA view. (b) Chest X ray RAO view.

6 Intracardiac pressures

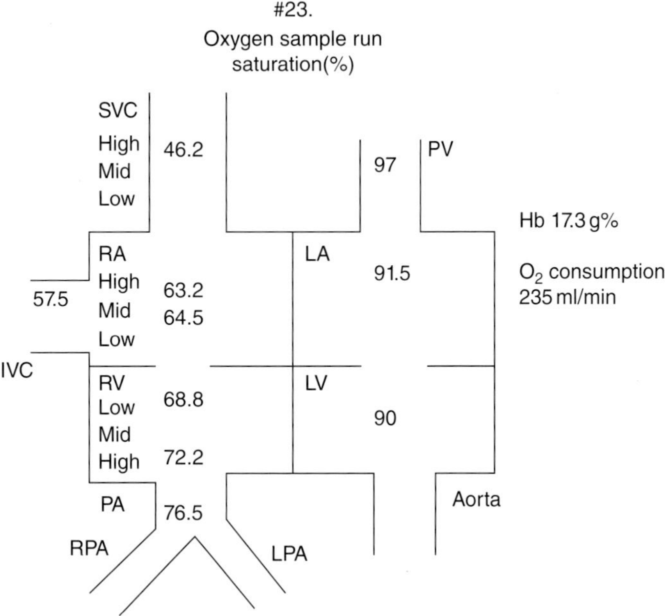

Figure 14.5 Oxygen sample run.

What is the pulmonary and systemic blood flow?

7 Oxygen sample run

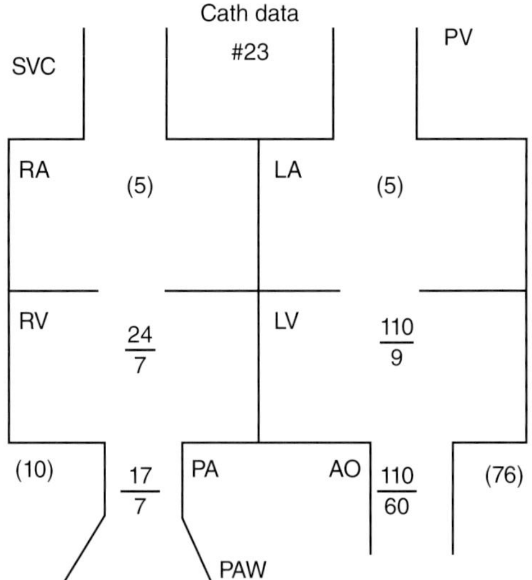

Figure 14.4 Pressures.

8 Diagnosis

What is the diagnosis?

Answers and commentary

1 Phonocardiogram

The arrows point to a high amplitude T1 ('sail sound'), which occurs about 0.10s later than the low amplitude M1 (labeled S1) component of the first sound. There is a late systolic murmur occurring after T1. No obvious splitting of S2 is seen at the 4th interspace parasternally. S3 is also seen.

There is a large 'v' wave seen in the jugular venous pulse, indicating tricuspid regurgitation.

2 and 3 History and physical examination

The history of a murmur, cyanosis, and clubbing suggest a right to left shunt. The systolic murmur is due to tricuspid regurgitation as corroborated by the phonocardiogram. The first sound was described as normal but the phonocardiogram showed a high-amplitude T1 component. The S3 is probably of physiological origin in a young man.

The absence of a loud P2 or an RV lift is against the diagnosis of pulmonary hypertension.

4 ECG

Rhythm sinus. Rate 75/min. PR 0.19s. QRS 0.08s. QRS axis indeterminate.

Impression: incomplete RBBB, low QRS voltage.

Despite the large RA on the chest X ray the P wave morphology does not show RA enlargement.

5 Chest X ray

In Figure 14.3a the right heart is enlarged. Lung fields appear unremarkable. In the RAO view (Figure 14.3b) there is a bulge in the upper part of the right heart compatible with superior displacement of the RV by an enlarged RA.

6 Intracardiac pressures

Right and left heart pressures are normal.

7 Oxygen sample run

There is a step up in oxygen saturation on entering the RA from the SVC, indicative of a left to right shunt at atrial level. There is arterial oxygen desaturation, indicative of a right to left shunt assuming no lung disease.

The calculation of the bidirectional shunt is shown in stepwise fashion.

Step 1: Find the total oxyhemoglobin content

Hemoglobin = 17.3 g/mL × 1.34 = 23.2 vol%, assuming 1 m of hemoglobin combines with 1.34 mL of oxygen

Step 2: Find the oxygen content of the PV, aorta (AO), PA, SVC, and IVC.

Oxygen content = oxygen saturation × total oxyhemoglobin content

$$\begin{aligned} PV &= 0.97 \times 23.2 = 22.5\,\text{vol\%} \\ AO &= 0.90 \times 23.2 = 20.8\,\text{vol\%} \\ PA &= 0.765 \times 23.2 = 17.7\,\text{vol\%} \\ SVC &= 0.462 \times 23.2 = 10.7\,\text{vol\%} \\ IVC &= 0.575 \times 23.2 = 13.3\,\text{vol\%} \end{aligned}$$

Step 3: Calculate the pulmonary (Q_p), systemic (Q_s), and effective (Q_{ep}) pulmonary blood flow

$$\text{Flow equals } \frac{\text{oxygen.consumption}}{\text{AVO}_2\text{ difference}}\ \frac{\text{mL/min}}{\text{mL/L}}$$

$$Q_p = \frac{235}{10(22.5-17.7)} = 4.9\,\text{L/min}$$

$$Q_s = \frac{235}{10(20.8-10.7)} = 2.32\,\text{L/min}$$

$$Q_{ep} = \frac{235}{10(22.5-10.7)} = 2.0\,\text{L/min}$$

$$Q_{L\text{-}R} = Q_p - Q_{ep} = 2.9\,\text{L/min}$$

$$Q_{R\text{-}L} = Q_s - Q_{ep} = 0.32\,\text{L/min}$$

Net left to right shunt is 2.9 – 0.32 = 2.58 L/min.

Note: (i) There is little difference in the results if 1.36 is used instead of 1.34 as the amount of oxygen combining with 1 g of hemoglobin. (ii) Using a weighted average of mixed vena cava blood, namely $\frac{2\,SVC + IVC}{3}$ yields an oxygen content of 11.6 vol% and a calculated Q_s of 2.6 L/min, so the net left to right shunt becomes 2.3 L/min.

8 Diagnosis

Ebstein's anomaly.
ASD with small right to left shunt.

Discussion

In Ebstein's anomaly there is apical displacement of the tricuspid valve annulus associated with abnormalities of the tricuspid valve and the RV structure [1, 2]. The posterior and septal leaflets are displaced apically whereas the anterior leaflet is still attached to the tricuspid valve annulus [2]. The anterior leaflet is enlarged and opens in a sail-like fashion [1, 3]. This downward or apical displacement of the tricuspid leaflet leads to tricuspid regurgitation, resulting in RA enlargement. Furthermore, the RV is divided into an atrialized portion and a functional portion (Figures 14.6 and 14.7).

In about 80–94% of cases there is a right to left shunt across the atrial septum [4], which can help to decompress the RA when there is severe tricuspid regurgitation.

Ebstein's anomaly occurs in about 1:20,000 of the general population [5]. Patients with cyanosis, clubbing and no apparent pulmonary hypertension may be suspected of having an Ebstein's anomaly.

Sometimes the bedside diagnosis can be difficult as there is usually no elevation of jugular venous pressure (because of the markedly enlarged RA) so the murmur of tricuspid regurgitation may not be apparent [4].

The ECG may be of some help as there are large P waves (Himalayan waves) in 2, 3, F in 60–90% of cases [1, 5, 6]. At least 25% of patients with Ebstein's anomaly have WPW syndrome type B – a feature not found in other forms of cyanotic heart disease [5] – and so are subject to atrial arrhythmias [7].

The chest X ray may suggest Ebstein's anomaly if there is right heart enlargement and relatively normal pulmonary vasculature in a patient with known cyanosis and clubbing.

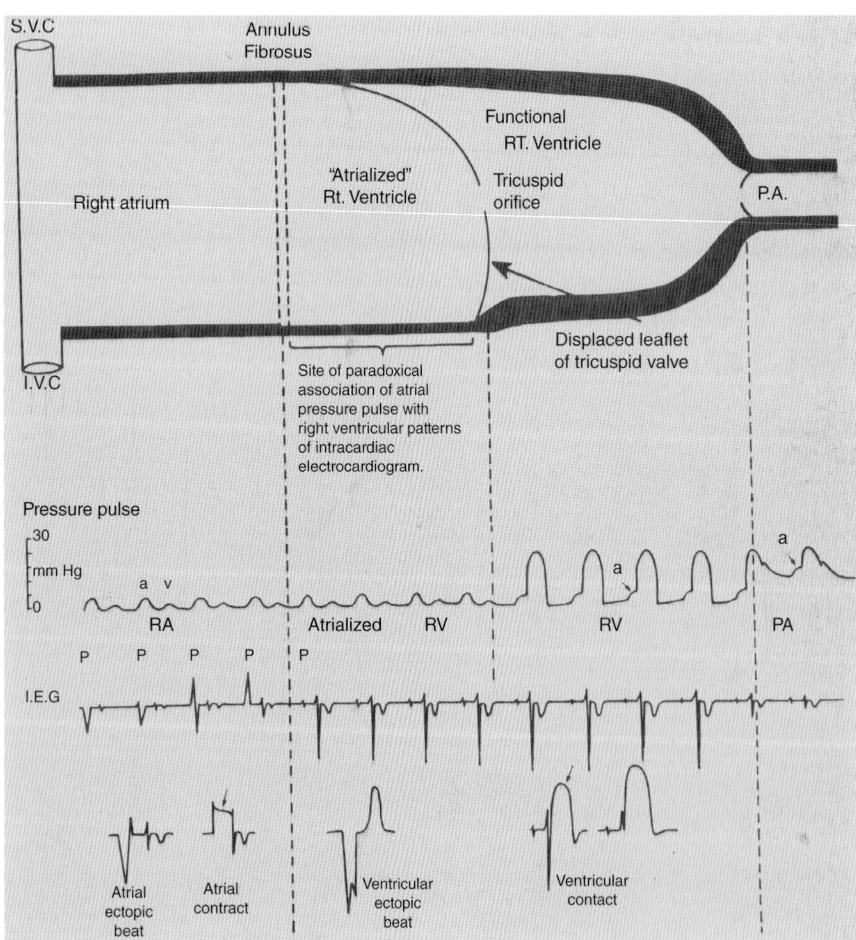

Figure 14.6 The relationship of surface ECG and intracardiac ECG to RA, atrialized RV, and functional RV. Source: Watson H. (1974). Reproduced with permission of BMJ Publishing Group.

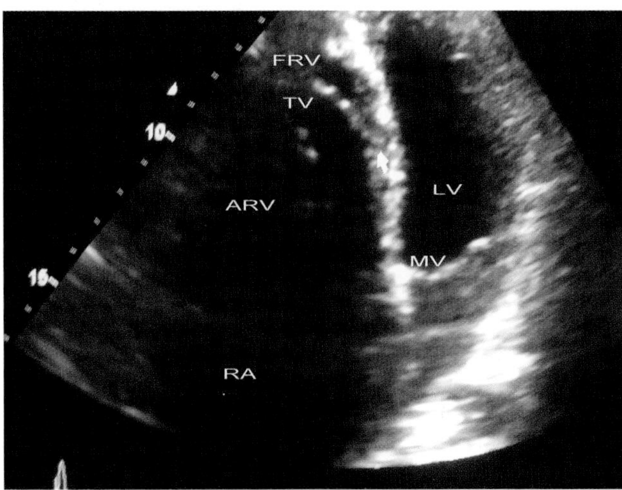

Figure 14.7 Ebstein's anomaly in a 52-year-old man. Four-chamber view showing apical displacement of tricuspid septal leaflet (tricuspid valve, TV). ARV, atrialized right ventricule; FRV, functional right ventricle; MV, mitral valve.

Conditions associated with Ebstein's anomaly are pulmonary stenosis, pulmonary atresia, VSD, PDA [2, 4, 8], tetralogy of Fallot, and corrected transposition of the great vessels [2, 4]. Left-sided lesions such as LV nonimpaction [9] and mitral valve disease have also been reported [9, 10].

Nowadays cardiac catheterization is seldom required to diagnose Ebsteins's anomaly unless coronary artery disease is suspected or it becomes necessary to measure the PA pressure [4, 11].

Two-dimensional or transesophageal echocardiography were not available at the time of these two studies (Patients 13 and 14). Two-dimensional echocardiography is now the preferred method of diagnosis [4, 11]. The apical displacement of the septal leaflet by at least 8 mm/m^2 body surface area from the insertion of the anterior mitral valve leaflet, best seen in the four-chamber view, is diagnostic of Ebstein's anomaly [4] (Figure 14.7).

Both these patients were followed medically as they were in Class 1–2. Surgical treatment is recommended in Class 3–4 patients, especially if there is right heart failure or a cardiothoracic ratio over 65% [7]. Paradoxical embolism, progressive cyanosis, or atrial arrhythmias refractory to medical treatment and percutanerous radiofrequency ablation are additional surgical indications [7, 12, 13].

Surgical treatment consists of repair or replacement of the tricuspid valve and closure of the atrial septal defect [12, 13]. If there is severe tricuspid regurgitation and poor RV function then a caval–PA shunt may be required [13]. Accessory pathways may be surgically ablated [4, 14] in Ebstein patients who also require surgery.

Key points

1. The presence of a loud T1 ('sail sign'), tricuspid regurgitation, and the absence of pulmonary hypertension may suggest Ebstein's anomaly.
2. A patient with cyanosis and clubbing along with normal or near-normal pulmonary vasculature on chest X ray points towards Ebstein's anomaly.
3. Ebstein's anomaly is probably the only cyanotic heart disease associated with WPW Type B.
4. Two-dimensional echocardiography readily demonstrates one of the cardinal features of Ebstein's anomaly, namely the apical displacement of the tricuspid valve.
5. Ebstein's anomaly is most commonly associated with an atrial septal defect. Other anomalies, such as pulmonary atresia, pulmonary stenosis, VSD, PDA, or tetralogy of Fallot, may also be present.
6. Patient 13 illustrates the relationship of the intracardiac ECG to the right heart pressures and Patient 14 shows a phonocardiogram that demonstrates some of the physical findings in Ebstein's anomaly.

References

[1] Anderson KR, Zuberbuhler JR, Anderson RH et al. Morphologic spectrum of Ebstein's anomaly of the heart. *A review. Mayo Clin Proc* 1979; 54: 174–180.

[2] Daliento L, Angelini A, Ho SY et al. Angiographic and morphologic features of the left ventricle in Ebstein's malformation. *Am J. Cardiol* 1997; 80: 1051–1059.

[3] Sondergaard L, Cullen S. *Ebstein anomaly*. In: Diagnosis and management of adult congenital heart disease, Gatzoulis MA, Webb GD, Daubeney PEF (eds), Churchill Livingston, Edinburgh, 2003, pp 283–287.

[4] Lev M, Liberthson RR, Joseph RH et al. The pathologic anatomy of Ebstein's disease. *Arch Path* 1970; 90: 334–343.

[5] Danielson GK, Driscoll DJ, Nair DD et al. Operative treatment of Ebstein's anomaly. *J Thorac Cardiovasc Surg* 1992; 104: 1195–1202.

[6] Giuliani ER, Fuster V, Brandenburg RO et al. Ebstein's anomaly. The clinical features and natural history of Ebstein's anomaly of the tricuspid valve. *Mayo Clin Proc* 1979; 54: 163–173.

[7] Dearani JA, Danelson GK. Tricuspid valve repair for Ebstein's anomaly. *Oper Tech Thorac Cardiovasc Surg* 2003; 8: 188–192.

[8] Khositseth A, Danielson GK, Dearani JA, et al. Supraventricular tachyarrhythmias in Ebsteins anomaly. *Management and outcome. J Thorac Cardiovasc Surg* 2004; 128: 826–833.

[9] Deutsch V, Wexler L, Blieden LC et al. Ebstein's anomaly of tricuspid valve: Critical review of roentgenological features and additional angiographic signs. *Am J Roentgenol Ther Nucl Med* 1975; 125: 395–411.

[10] Attenhofer CH, Connolly HM, Dearani JA et al. Ebstein's anomaly. *Circulation* 2007; 115: 227–285.

[11] Watson H. Natural history of Ebstein's anomaly of the tricuspid valve in childhood and adolescence. An international co-operative study of 505 cases. *Br Heart J* 1974; 36: 417–427.

[12] Perloff JK. *Ebstein's anomaly of the tricuspid valve*. In: The clinical recognition of congenital heart disease. WB Saunders, Philadelphia, 2003, pp 194–215.

[13] Lowe KG, Emslie-Smith D, Roberson PG, Watson H. Scalar, vector, and intracardiac electrocardiograms in Ebstein's anomaly. *Br Heart J* 1968; 30: 617–629.

[14] Attenhofer CH, Connolly HM, O'Leary PW et al. Left heart lesions in patients with Ebstein anomaly. *Mayo Clin Proc* 2005; 80: 361–368.

15 PATIENT STUDY 15

Sequence of data presentation

Phase 1 1966–1979

1 Chest X ray 1966
↓
2 ECG 1967
↓
3 Cardiac catheterization 1967
↓
4 History and physical examination 1967
↓
5 Cardiac catheterization 1968 (post operation)
↓
6 Course 1968–1974
↓
7 Exercise stress test 1974
↓
8 Course 1977
↓
9 M-mode echocardiography 1977
↓
10 Exercise stress test 1977
↓
11 Right heart catheterization 1977
↓
12 Course 1977–1979
↓
13 ECG 1978
↓
14 Exercise stress test 1978
↓
15 Chest X ray 1978
↓
16 Cardiac catheterization 1977 & 1978
↓
17 Pressure curves 1978
↓
18 Additional hemodynamic data 1978
↓
19 Surgical results 1979

Phase 2 1979–1994

20 Outpatient follow-up
↓
21 Repeat surgery 1994

Phase 3 1994–2005

22 Outpatient follow-up
↓
23 Chest X rays 2004–2005

Phase 1 1996–1979

1 Chest X ray 1966

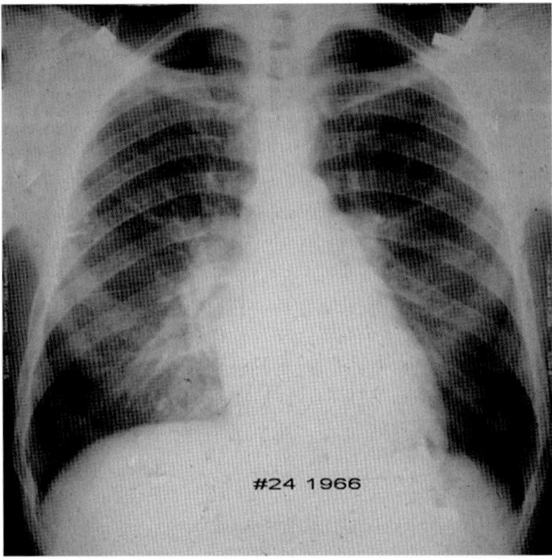

Figure 15.1 PA chest X ray 1966.

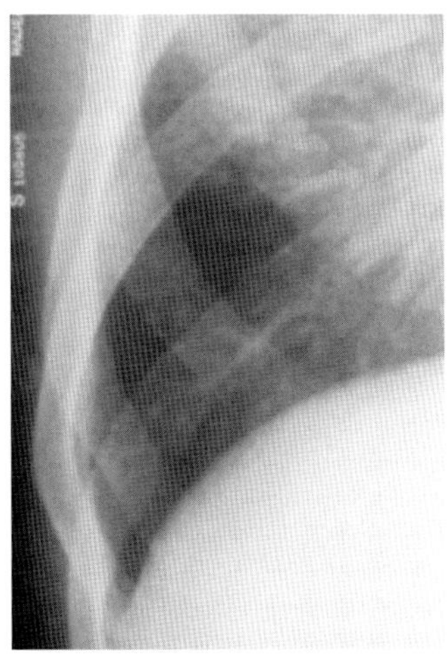

Figure 15.2 Right lower zone of chest X ray 1966.

Patient Studies in Valvular, Congenital, and Rarer Forms of Cardiovascular Disease: An Integrative Approach, First Edition. Franklin B. Saksena.

Companion Website: www.wiley.com/go/saksena/patientstudies

2 ECG 1967

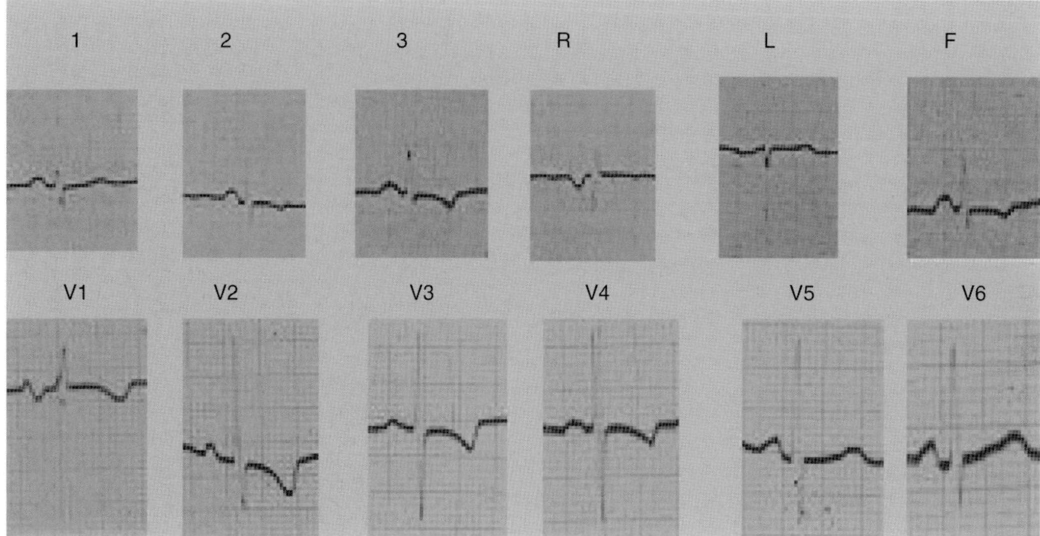

Figure 15.3 V1–V6 ECG 1967.

3 Cardiac catheterization 1967

(a)

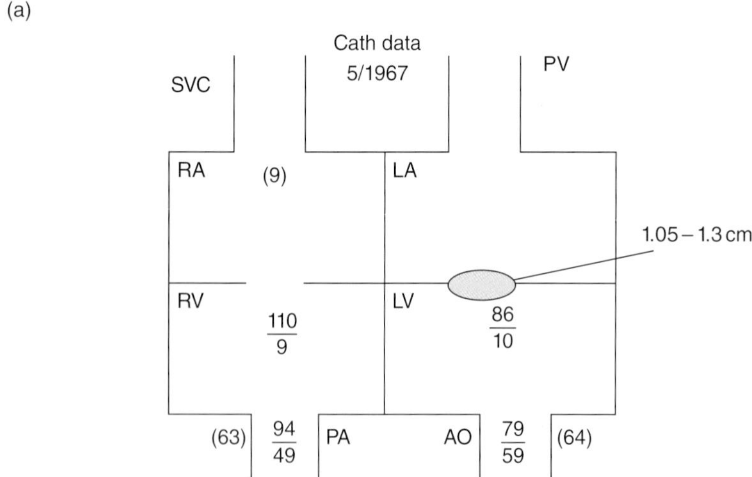

Figure 15.4a Intracardiac pressures (a) 1967 and (b) 1968. The mean mitral diastolic gradient was 17 mmHg in 1967 and 7 mmHg in 1968. Numbers in brackets are mean pressures (mmHg). Numerators in RV and LV are systolic pressures. Denominators in the ventricles are end-diastolic pressures, whereas denominators in the aortic and pulmonary arteries are diastolic pressures (mmHg).

4 History and physical examination 1967

History

32-year-old foundry worker with a possible history of rheumatic fever as a child.

Between 1963 and 1966 he had intermittent hemopytsis, atypical chest pain, and progressive exertional dyspnea.

No history of diabetes, hypertension, or alcoholism.

Physical examination 1967

72 inches tall, 162 lb male. BP 112/80. Pulse 72/min regular.

The apex beat was in the 5th interspace, 10 cm from the mid-sternal line.

There was a 2/4 left lower sternal lift.
S1 was increased in intensity. S2 was narrowly split.
There was an opening snap (OS) at the LLSB.
The S2–OS interval was 0.08 s.
There was a grade 3/6 diastolic apical rumble with presystolic accentuation.
Lungs were clear.

5 Cardiac catheterization 1968 (post operation)

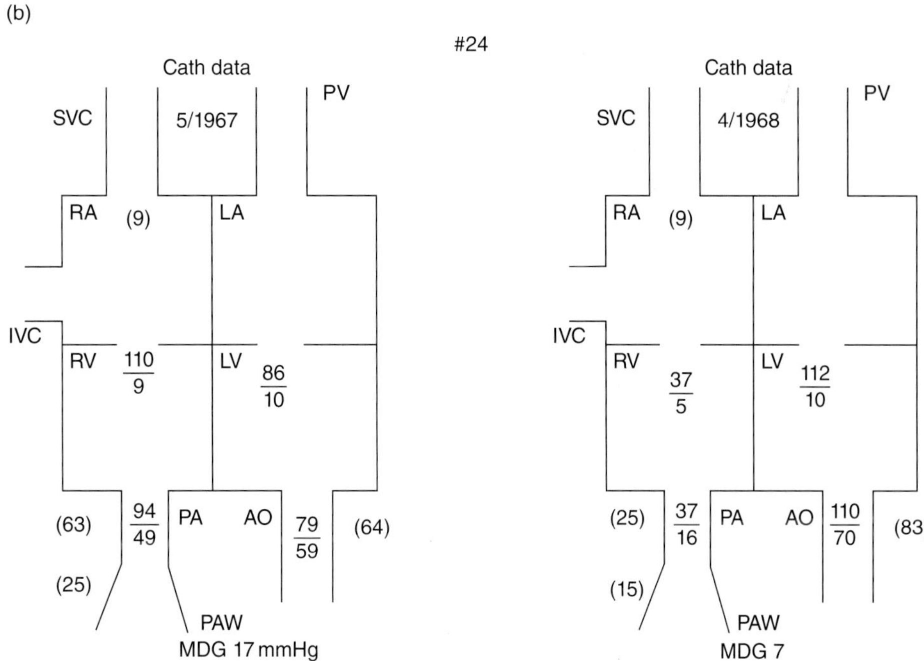

Figure 15.4b

6 Course 1968–1974

The patient was diagnosed with severe mitral stenosis in 1967 and underwent successful mitral valve commissurotomy in 1968.

He did well after the operation, as confirmed by his asymptomatic status and improved hemodynamics (April 1968).

7 Exercise stress test 1974

Table 15.1 Exercise test 1974.

Naughton-Balke protocol		
	Rest	**Exercise**
Heart rate	85 /min	140/min*
Rhythm	sinus	rare PVC
Blood pressure	110/70	160/80
Estimated mets		8
Reason for stopping		dyspnea
Level of ex achieved		3mph, 12.5% grade

*Max target HR for pts age 186/min.

8 Course 1977

In 1977 the patient entered hospital in pulmonary edema and atrial flutter.

Comment on the noninvasive workup (Figures 15.5 and 15.6) and right heart catheterization (Figure 15.6).

9 M-mode echocardiography 1977

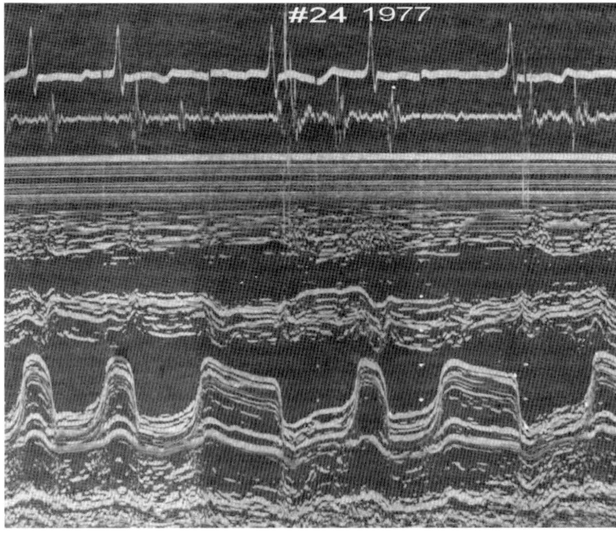

Figure 15.5 M-mode echocardiogram 1977.

10 Exercise stress test 1977

Table 15.2 Exercise test 1977.

Naughton-Balke protocol		
	Rest	**exercise**
Heart rate	100/min	210/min
Blood pressure	120/80	200/80
Rhythm	Atrial fibrillation	Atrial fib, pvcs
O_2 consumption ml/kg/min	4.0	21.5
Mets	1.1	6.6
Speed		3 mph@15% grade

11 Right heart catheterization 1977

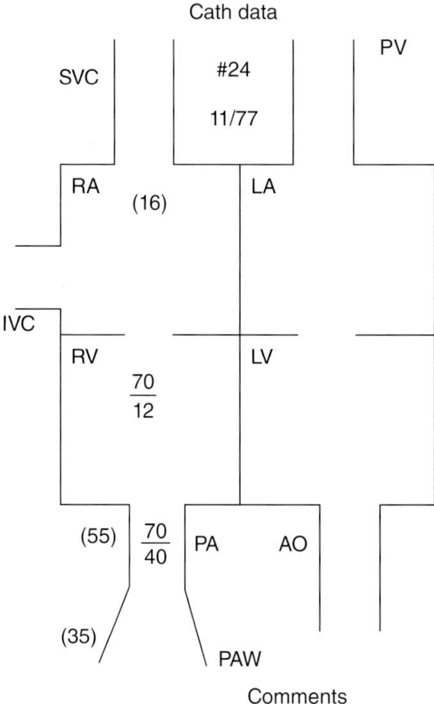

Figure 15.6 Right heart catheterization 1977.

12 Course 1977–1979

The patient improved medically on digoxin, diuretics, and warfarin, and was discharged home in November 1977. In March 1978 the patient returned to hospital with dyspnea and a syncopal episode.

Physical examination

72 inches tall, 172 lb male. BP 134/82. HR 60/min irregular.
No elevation of jugular venous pressure.
Apex beat was in the 5th interspace, 12 cm from the mid-sternal line.
S1 increased in intensity. S2 single. No opening snap heard.
Grade 2/6 diastolic apical rumble (it had disappeared after mitral valve surgery in 1968).
Diffuse expiratory wheezing heard bilaterally.
No leg edema or calf tenderness.

13 ECG 1978

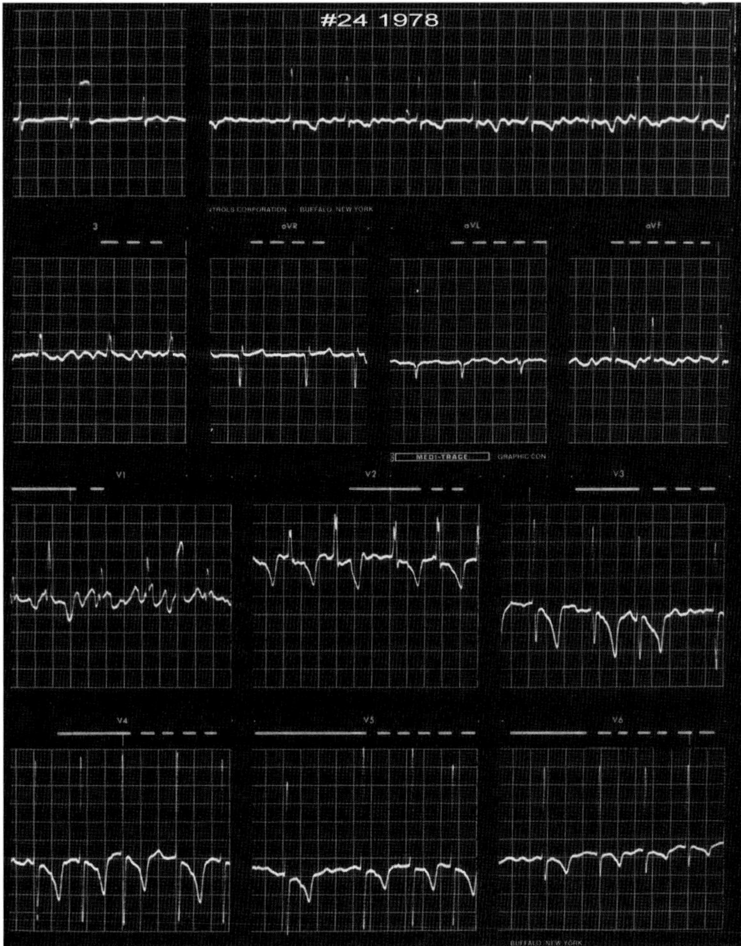

Figure 15.7 12-lead ECG 1978.

14 Exercise stress test 1978

Table 15.3 Exercise test 1978.

Protocol used: Naughton-Balke		
	Rest	**Exercise**
Heart rate	110	170
Blood pressure s/d mm Hg	130/80	140/90
EKG	atrial fibrillation	same, occasional PVC's
Oxygen consumption cc/kg/min	5.6	14.9
Mets	1.7	4.5
Reason for stopping test		dyspnea, fatigue
Level of exercise reached		3mph, 5% grade

15 Chest X ray 1978

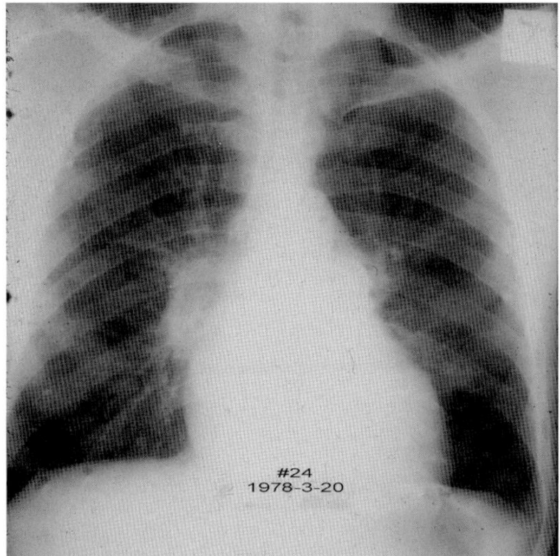

Figure 15.8 Chest X ray 1978.

16 Cardiac catheterization 1977 & 1978

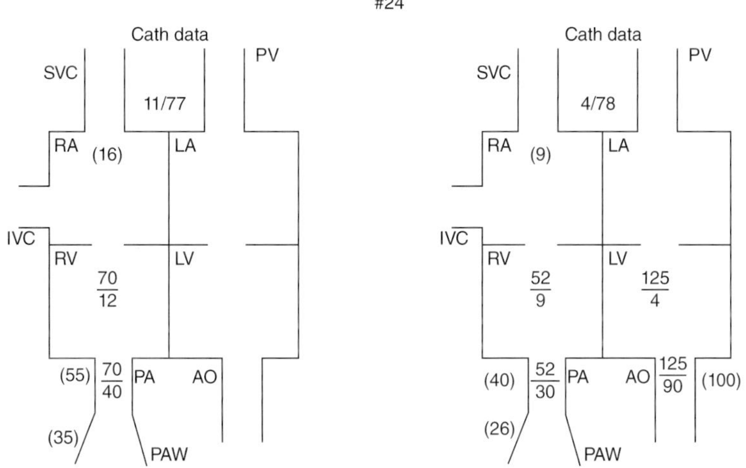

Figure 15.9 Cardiac catheterization 1977 & 1978.

17 Pressure curves 1978

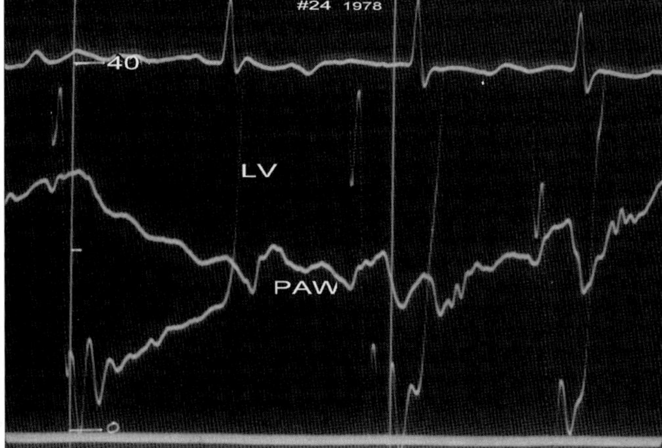

Figure 15.10 Simultaneous LV and wedge pressures. 0–40 mmHg scale.

18 Additional hemodynamic data 1978

Table 15.4 Additional data from 1978 cardiac catheterization.

1) Oxygen consumption	275 ml/min
Arterial oxygen saturation	96.4%
Mixed venous oxygen saturation	61.1%
Hemoglobin	12.4 gm%
2) Pressures see Figure 24–9	
3) Heart rate	116/min
Diastolic filling period	0.26 seconds
Mean mitral diastolic gradient	15.4 mmHg
4) Left ventricular end diastolic volume index	79ml/m^2
Left ventricular end systolic volume index	30 ml/m^2

Calculate (i) the cardiac output, (ii) the pulmonary and systemic resistance, (iii) the mitral valve area, and (iv) the LV ejection fraction.

19 Surgical results 1979

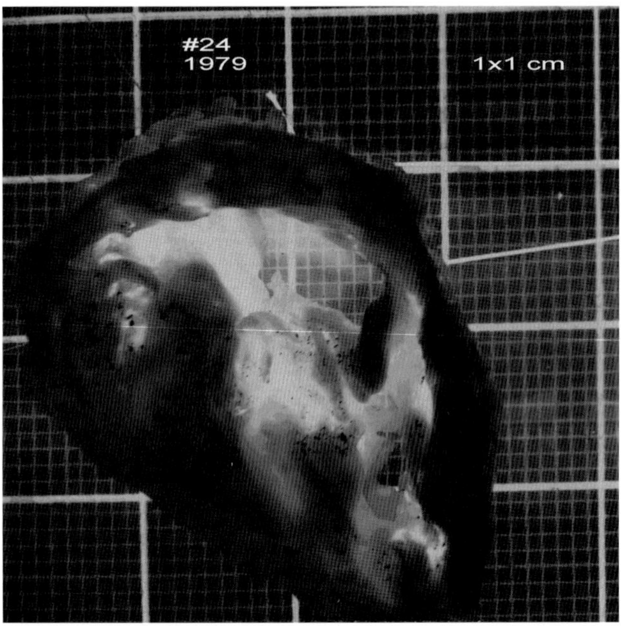

Figure 15.11 Mitral valve 1979. Each large square is 1 cm^2.

Comment on the physical examination, ECG, chest X ray, exercise test, and cardiac catheterization tests (Figures 15.7, Table 15.3, Figures 15.8, 15.9, and 15.10, and Table 15.4).
Comment on the surgical specimen (Figure 15.11).

Phase 2 1979–1994

20 Outpatient follow-up

The patient underwent successful mitral valve replacement in 1979 and did well until 1994, when the mitral valve was replaced with a St Jude mitral valve prosthesis.

21 Repeat surgery 1994

The mitral valve was replaced with a St Jude mitral valve prosthesis.

Phase 3 1994–2005

22 Outpatient follow-up

The patient was followed as an outpatient over the next 11 years on digoxin, diuretics, warfarin, and subsequently enalapril.

23 Chest X rays 2004–2005

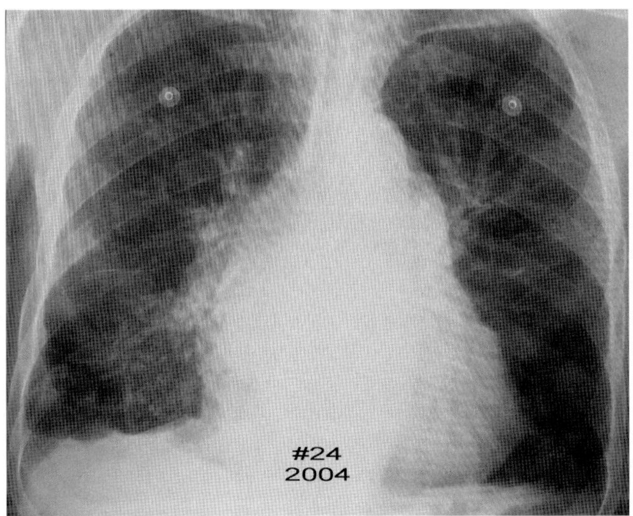

Figure 15.12 Chest X ray 2004.

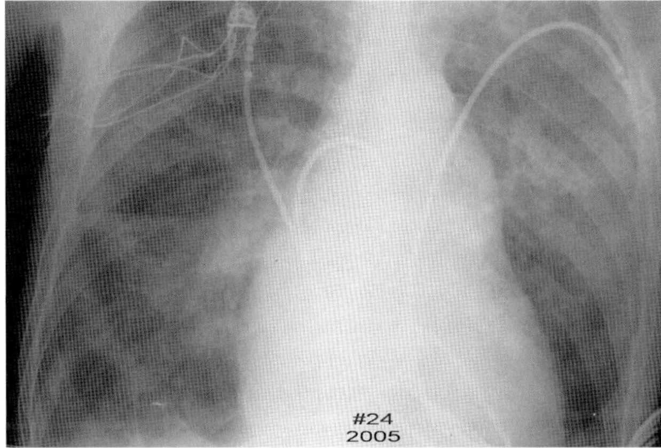

Figure 15.13 Chest X ray 2005.

Two-dimensional echocardiography (2001) showed moderate LA enlargement, a reduced LV ejection fraction of 41% (it had been 62% in 1978) and a functioning mitral valve prosthesis.

He was admitted to hospital with dyspnea and edema in 2004 and 2005.

Comment on the chest X rays taken in 2004 and 2005 (Figures 15.12 and 15.13).

Answers and commentary

1 Chest X ray 1966

There is straightening of the left heart border, implying LA appendage enlargement. The proximal PAs are enlarged and there is upper lobe hyperemia. Kerley B lines were seen on the original film but are not well seen in Figure 15.1. The cardiothoracic ratio is normal. Figure 15.2 shows the Kerley B lines better.

The impression is mitral stenosis with pulmonary hypertension. Kerley B lines are associated with a PA wedge pressure of 20–25 mmHg and often dyspnea at rest [1].

2 ECG 1967

The rhythm is sinus with a rate of 72/min. PR interval 0.16 s. QRS interval 0.06 s. QRS axis +90°.

P is biphasic in V1, suggestive of LA enlargement. There is RV hypertrophy based on rightward axis and a tall R wave in lead V1 (>7 mm). The inversion of T waves in V1–V4 is suggestive of RV overload [2, 3].

RVH and LA enlargement are often seen in mitral stenosis.

3 Cardiac catheterization 1967

The mean RA atrial and RVEDP are slightly elevated, possibly due to RV dysfunction. There is severe pulmonary hypertension and the wedge pressure is at pulmonary edema levels (hence the Kerley B lines). There is a large gradient in diastole across the mitral valve (17 mmHg). Mild systolic hypotension is noted.

The mitral valve area was reduced to 1.3 cm^2 using the original K of 31 in the Gorlin formula and 1.05 cm^2 using 37.8 for K.

Impression: severe mitral stenosis with severe pulmonary hypertension.

4 History and physical examination 1967

Patients with mitral stenosis give a history of rheumatic fever in about 60% of cases. Hemoptysis is seen in mitral stenosis if there is acute bronchitis, pulmonary embolism, pulmonary hypertension, or pulmonary edema [4].

A prominent RV impulse is indicative of RV hypertrophy. The presence of an opening snap implies that the anterior leaflet is pliable. A short 2–OS interval implies a significant gradient across the mitral valve in diastole (in the absence of AR or LV dysfunction).

Impression: moderate mitral stenosis with pulmonary hypertension.

5 Cardiac catheterization 1968 (post operation)

(This followed the patient's mitral commissurotomy in 1968.)

The PA mean pressure has fallen to near-normal values and the PA wedge pressure is only slightly elevated. There is now only a small gradient across the mitral valve in diastole (reduced from 17 to 7 mmHg). Left heart pressures are normal.

The striking reduction in the patient's mean PA pressure following operative relief of his mitral stenosis is consistent with the hypothesis that most of the pulmonary hypertension seen in mitral stenosis is of hypoxemic origin rather than due to obliterative vascular disease [5, 6].

6 and 7 Course 1968–1974 and exercise stress test 1974

The patient remained asymptomatic. He was in sinus rhythm. An exercise stress test in 1974 showed that the patient was in functional class 1 as he achieved >7 mets on the treadmill [7]. The resting oxygen consumption is normally 1 met or 3.5 mL oxygen consumed per kilogram per minute.

8 Course 1977

The patient did well for 9 years but his symptoms of dyspnea recurred. Atrial arrhythmias appeared in 1977.

9 M-mode echocardiogram 1977

The rhythm is atrial fibrillation. The anterior and posterior mitral leaflets are thickened and move concordantly.

Diagnosis: mitral stenosis.

10 Exercise stress test 1977

There was systolic hypertension on exercise, with only slightly reduced exercise tolerance (early functional class 2). The rhythm was atrial fibrillation.

11 Right heart catheterization 1977

The RA pressure is moderately elevated, possibly due to RV dysfunction and/or tricuspid regurgitation. There is severe pulmonary hypertension and the wedge pressure is at pulmonary edema levels.

12 Course 1977–1979

Physical examination in March 1978 revealed that the opening snap was no longer audible, implying loss of pliability of the anterior mitral leaflet from either fibrosis or calcification. The presence of a diastolic apical rumble points to a recurrence of mitral stenosis.

13 ECG 1978

The rhythm is atrial fibrillation. Ventricular rate 100/min. QRS interval 0.07 s. QRS axis +80°. Taller R waves in V1 and more deeply inverted T inV2–6 as compared to the 1967 ECG.

Impression: increase in RV strain pattern compared to 1966 ECG.

14 Exercise stress test 1978

This showed further deterioration in the patient's exercise tolerance to functional class 3 as he only achieved 4.5 mets on the treadmill [7].

15 Chest X ray 1978

The cardiothoracic ratio is 0.48. The proximal PAs are dilated, with some increase in pulmonary plethora since the 1966 X ray.

16 Cardiac catheterization 1978

There is mild RV dysfunction, moderately severe pulmonary hypertension, and evidence of mitral restenosis. See below for detailed calculations.

The incidence of mitral restenosis following commissurotomy in a 10-year period varies from 1% to 5% [8].

17 Pressure curves 1978

There is a gradient in diastole across the mitral valve. During a long diastolic period the end-diastolic gradient is at its least.

18 Additional hemodynamic data 1978

1 Find the cardiac output from the following data.
Oxygen consumption = 275 mL/min
Arterial oxygen saturation = 96.4%
Mixed venous oxygen saturation = 61.1%
Hemoglobin = 12.4 g%
Total oxyhemoglobin content = 1.34 × 12.4 g % = 16.6 vol%
Arterial O_2 content = 96.4 × 16.6 = 16 vol%
Mixed venous O_2 content = 61.1 × 16.6 = 10.1 vol%
Hence AV O_2 difference = 5.9 vol% or 59 vol/L
Cardiac output = oxygen consumption/AV O_2 difference = 275/59 = 4.7 L/min

2 Calculate the pulmonary vascular resistance (PVR) and systemic vascular resistance (SVR) from the following data.
RA mean pressure = 9
PA mean pressure = 40
PA wedge = 26
Aortic mean pressure = 100
Cardiac output from 1.
PVR = 80(PA mean – PAW mean)/cardiac output = 80(40–26)/4.7 = 238 dyn.sec.cm^{-5}
SVR = 80(Ao mean – RA mean)/cardiac output = 80(100–9)/4.7 = 1549 dyn.sec.cm^{-5}

3 Calculate the mitral valve area (MVA) from the following data.
Heart rate = 116/min
Diastolic filling period (dfp) = 0.26 s
Mean mitral diastolic gradient (mdg) = 15.4 mmHg
Cardiac output from 1.
The Gorlin formula for the MVA (cm^2) is:

$$\frac{CO}{HR \times dfp \times 38 \times \sqrt{mdg}} = \frac{4700}{116 \times 0.26 \times 38 \times 3.92} = 1.05\,cm^2$$

4 Calculate the LV ejection fraction from the following data.
LV end-diastolic volume index (LVEDVI) = 79 mL/m^2
LV end-systolic volume index (LVESVI) = 30 mL/m^2
Ejection fraction is equal to $\frac{LVEDVI - LVESVI}{LVEDVI}$ or (79–30)/79 or 62%
Impression: there is a reduced cardiac output, mild increase in PVR and SVR, and severe mitral stenosis.
The LV ejection fraction is normal.
Note that LV and aortic root angiography did not show any mitral or aortic regurgitation. Coronary angiography was normal.

19 Surgical results 1979

There is commisuural fusion, cuspal thickening, and marked narrowing of the mitral valve orifice. The valve area is at least 0.5 cm^2 (assuming the valve is seated squarely on the grid and all the tiny squares are visible).

20 and 21 Phase 2 1979–1994: Outpatient follow-up and repeat surgery 1994

The patient did well from 1979 until 1994, when he underwent a second mitral valve replacement, 15 years after his first one in 1979.

22 and 23 Phase 3 1994–2005: Outpatient follow-up and chest X rays 2004–2005

He was followed as an outpatient from 1994 to 2005 on digoxin, diuretics, and warfarin. There was an asymptomatic decline in his LV function in 2001(LV ejection fraction on echocardiography was 43%). Throughout this time the patient remained in atrial fibrillation.

In 2004 he was admitted to hospital in heart failure and enalapril was added to his regimen.

The 2004 chest X ray (Figure15.12) showed increased prominence of proximal PAs, an enlarged LA, pulmonary plethora, and probable RV enlargement.

The patient finally succumbed to pulmonary edema in 2005, as seen in his last chest X ray (Figure 15.13). Death was attributed to a combination of myocardial dysfunction from rheumatic heart disease, deterioration of prosthetic valve function, and possibly underlying coronary artery disease.

Discussion

Severity of mitral stenosis

The patient had moderately severe mitral stenosis on the basis of a short 2–OS interval of 0.08 s (range 0.6–0.13 s), a long diastolic apical rumble, and moderately severe pulmonary hypertension.

Two-dimensional echocardiography and Doppler studies in pure mitral stenosis may also be helpful in assessing the severity of mitral stenosis by calculating the mitral valve area, the mitral diastolic gradient, and the RV systolic pressure from the tricuspid regurgitant jet.

At cardiac catheterization if the cardiac output is normal then a mean mitral diastolic gradient of 5 mmHg suggests mild mitral stenosis, a gradient of 10 mmHg indicates moderate mitral stenosis, and a gradient of ≥15 mmHg is due to severe mitral stenosis.

A valve area of 1 cm^2 (normal 4–5 cm^2) suggests critical mitral stenosis.

Mitral re-stenosis

The patient had striking relief of symptoms for 10 years after surgical mitral valve commissurotomy. He is an example of mitral valve re-stenosis because he had clinical and hemodynamic improvement 1 year after commissurotomy followed by hemodynamic deterioration 9 years later. Mitral restenosis has been over-diagnosed in the past as it has been equated only with symptomatic deterioration. These patients lacked hemodynamic evidence that mitral stenosis had recurred [8].

The incidence of mitral restenosis following surgical commissurotomy is uncommon, occurring in about 1–5% of cases [8–10]. Restenosis may occur 6–12 years after an adequate commissurotomy has been performed [8–10].

Restenosis has been attributed to continued nonspecific valvular fibrosis and calcium deposits related to the effects of turbulent flow around a stenotic mitral valve rather than to an active rheumatic process [11]. Inadequate mitral valvotomy may [12] or may not [10] be another reason for mitral restenosis.

Percutaneous transatrial mitral commissurotomy has emerged as an effective nonsurgical technique for patients with symptomatic mitral stenosis, with a similar rate of re-stenosis as surgical mitral commissurotomy [13].

Atrial fibrillation

Patients with mitral stenosis usually develop atrial fibrillation in about their fourth decade [4], as was the case in this patient, who then went into acute pulmonary edema. Patients with atrial fibrillation and mitral stenosis have a lower cardiac output, a higher pulmonary resistance, a larger LA, and a higher risk of thromboembolism than in those patients in sinus rhythm [4].

Key points

1. Patients with at least moderate mitral stenosis have a loud S1 (in the absence of calcification), a short 2–OS interval (<0.08 s) a prolonged diastolic apical rumble, and evidence of pulmonary hypertension (loud P2, RV lift).
2. Patients with mitral stenosis may develop pulmonary hypertension, leading to RV failure.
3. Atrial fibrillation in mitral stenosis also occurs, resulting in pulmonary edema and systemic embolism.
4. This patient with mitral stenosis attained a near-normal life expectancy but required three open-heart surgeries over a 38-year period.
5. Following mitral commissurotomy there is a significant fall in PA pressures over several months. The rate of mitral restenosis is up to 5% over a 6–12 year period.

References

[1] Friedberg CK. *Diseases of the heart*, 3rd edn. WB Saunders, Philadelphia, 1966, p 1055.

[2] Fraser HRL, Turner R. Electrocardiography in mitral valvular disease. *Br Heart J* 1955; 17: 459–483.

[3] Murphy ML, Thenabada PN, de Soyza N et al. Re-evaluation of electrocardiographic criteria for left, right and combined cardiac ventricular hypertrophy. *Am J Cardiol* 1984; 53: 1140–1147.
[4] Wood P. An appreciation of mitral stenosis. Part 1 Clinical features. *Br Med J* 1954; 1: 1051–1063.
[5] Braunwald E, Braunwald NS, Ross J et al. Effects of mitral valve replacement on pulmonary vascular dynamics of patients with pulmonary hypertension. *New Engl J Med* 1965; 273: 509–514.
[6] Dalen JE, Matloff JM, Evans GL et al. Early reduction of pulmonary vascular resistance after mitral valve replacement. *New Engl J Med* 1967; 277: 387–394.
[7] Kattus AA, Bruce RA, Naughton J et al. *Exercise testing and training of apparently healthy individuals: A handbook for physicians*. American Heart Association, New York, 1972, p 13.
[8] Higgs LM, Glancy DL, O'Brien KP et al. Mitral stenosis: An uncommon cause of recurrent symptoms following mitral commissurotomy. *Am J Cardiol* 1970; 26: 34–37.
[9] Biswas B, Datta S, Dutta AL et al. Role of closed mitral commissurotomy for mitral stenosis. *J Indian Med Assoc* 1999; 97: 255–258.
[10] John S, Bashi VV, Jairaj PS et al. Closed mitral valvotomy: early results and long term follow-up of 3724 consecutive patients. *Circulation* 1983; 68: 891–896.
[11] Otto CM, Bonow RO. *Valvular heart disease*. In: Braunwald's Heart Disease, 8th edn. WB Saunders/Elsevier, Philadelphia, 2008, p 1656.
[12] Rahimtoola SH, Durairaj A, Mehra A. Current evaluation and management of patients with mitral stenosis. *Circulation* 2002; 106: 1183–1188.
[13] Kalra AR, Murty GS, Trehan V et al. Percutaneous transatrial mitral commissurotomy: Immediate and intermediate results. *J Am Coll Cardiol* 1994; 23: 1327–1332.

Further reading

Bruce CJ, Nishimura RA. Newer advances in the diagnosis and treatment of mitral stenosis. *Curr Probl Cardiol* 1998; 23: 125–196.

16 PATIENT STUDY 16

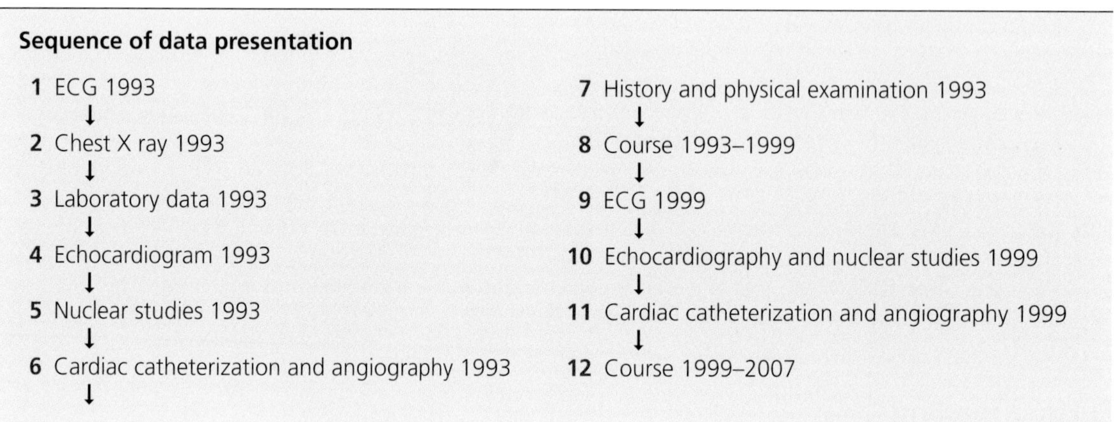

Sequence of data presentation

1 ECG 1993
↓
2 Chest X ray 1993
↓
3 Laboratory data 1993
↓
4 Echocardiogram 1993
↓
5 Nuclear studies 1993
↓
6 Cardiac catheterization and angiography 1993
↓
7 History and physical examination 1993
↓
8 Course 1993–1999
↓
9 ECG 1999
↓
10 Echocardiography and nuclear studies 1999
↓
11 Cardiac catheterization and angiography 1999
↓
12 Course 1999–2007

1 ECG 1993

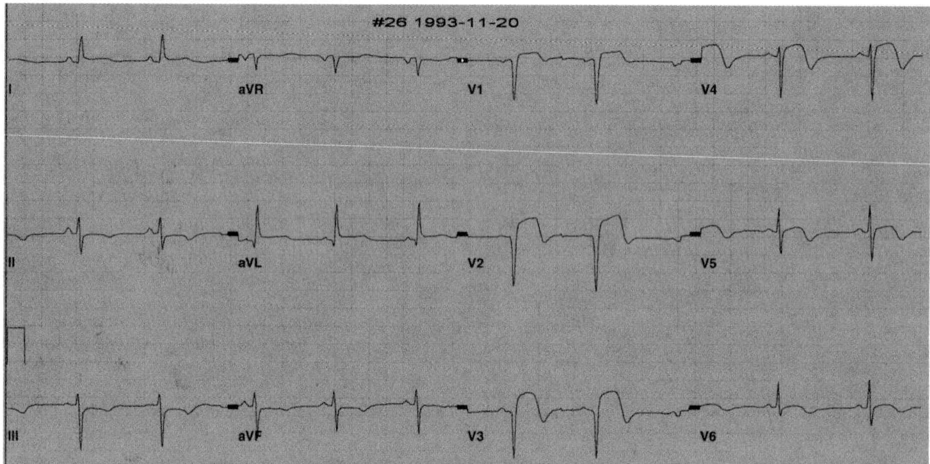

Figure 16.1 ECG 20 November 1993.

Patient Studies in Valvular, Congenital, and Rarer Forms of Cardiovascular Disease: An Integrative Approach, First Edition. Franklin B. Saksena.

Companion Website: www.wiley.com/go/saksena/patientstudies

2 Chest X ray 1993

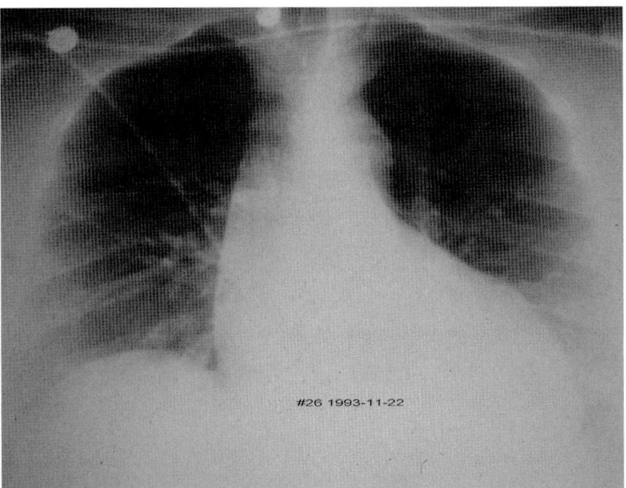

Figure 16.2 Chest X ray 1993.

3 Laboratory data 1993

Hb 16.0g %. WBC 16,400/mm^3.
Serial CPKs between 19 and 21 November were 2474, 1584, 824, and 310 U/L.
Serum glucose 125 mg%. Serum cholesterol 269 mg%.
Stool negative for occult blood.

4 and 5 Echocardiogram 1993 and nuclear studies 1993

LV apical and septal hypokinesia. LVH.
MUGA ejection fraction 24%.

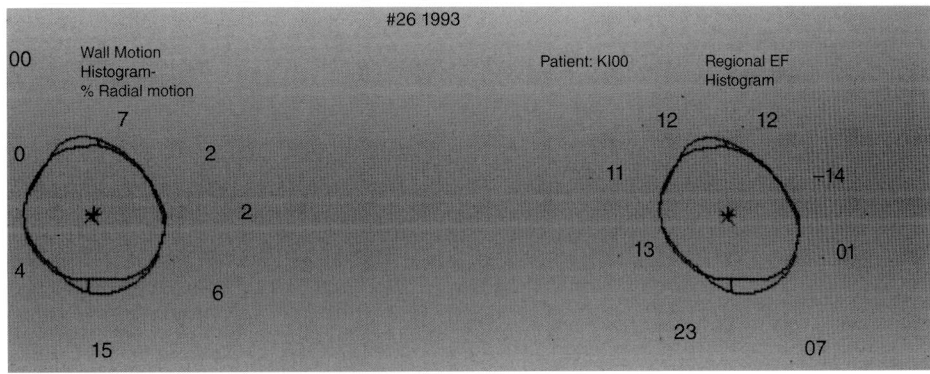

Figure 16.3 Nuclear scan of LV showing regional wall motion 1993.

6 Cardiac catheterization and angiography 1993

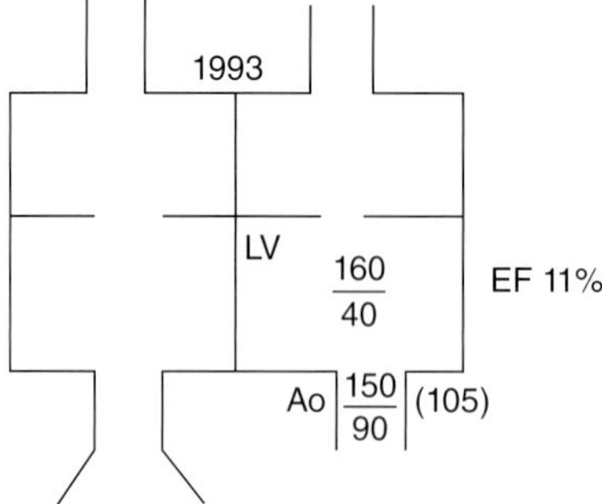

Figure 16.4 Cardiac catheterization and angiograms 1993.

7 History and physical examination 1993

History

55-year-old female mail carrier admitted to hospital on 19 November 1993 with exertional chest pain on and off for 3 days. This was associated with dyspnea and sweating.

One day prior to admission she had recurrent chest pain and vomiting of dark-red clotted blood. In the emergency room she had a BP of 160/112. HR 108/min. R 22. T 100 °F.

She was diagnosed as having an acute myocardial infarction and started on nitroglycerine IV, nifedipine, and IV heparin. She was not given t-PA because of her recent hematemesis.

She has had hypertension since the 1970s but stopped her antihypertensive medicine in 1981. No history of diabetes, peptic ulcer disease, or CVA. She has smoked for 19 pack years and drinks alcohol occasionally.

She has been a mail carrier for 12 years, works 45 h/week and lifts 40–50 lb of mail at a time.

Physical examination 1993

61 inches tall female weighing 185 lb. BP 127/65. HR 107/min regular (following treatment in the emergency room). Two microaneurysms noted in the fundus. The optic discs were normal.

There was a positive ear crease sign.

Inspiratory tracheal tug sign. Lungs clear.

No elevation of jugular venous pressure. Normal carotid upstroke.

Apex beat was in the 5th interspace 10 cm from the mid-sternal line.

S1 normal. S2 normal. S4 + 1 apex. No murmurs.

2+/4+ femoral pulses. No edema, cyanosis, or clubbing.

Abdomen showed only an old hysterectomy scar. No CNS findings.

8 Course 1993–1999

The patient was treated with beta blockers, amlodipine, ACE inhibitors, warfarin, and a statin, and was discharged as improved on 2 December 1993.

Between 1993 and 1999 the patient was followed as an outpatient on the above medicines plus furosemide.

A dobutamine–MUGA study showed that the LV ejection fraction improved from 11 to 27% on 40 mcg/kg/min of dobutamine in February 1994.

She resumed her 50 h/week work in March 1994.and was walking up to six blocks a day delivering mail.

In July 1999 she had an episode of dyspnea, wheezing, and weakness. Systolic BP was 90 mmHg, HR 150/min. She was admitted to hospital (see Figure 16.5). She had successful cardioversion, was started on amiodarone, and received anticongestive measures. She then underwent evaluation of her LV function (Table 16.1) and had a cardiac catheterization (Figure 16.6).

9 ECG 1999

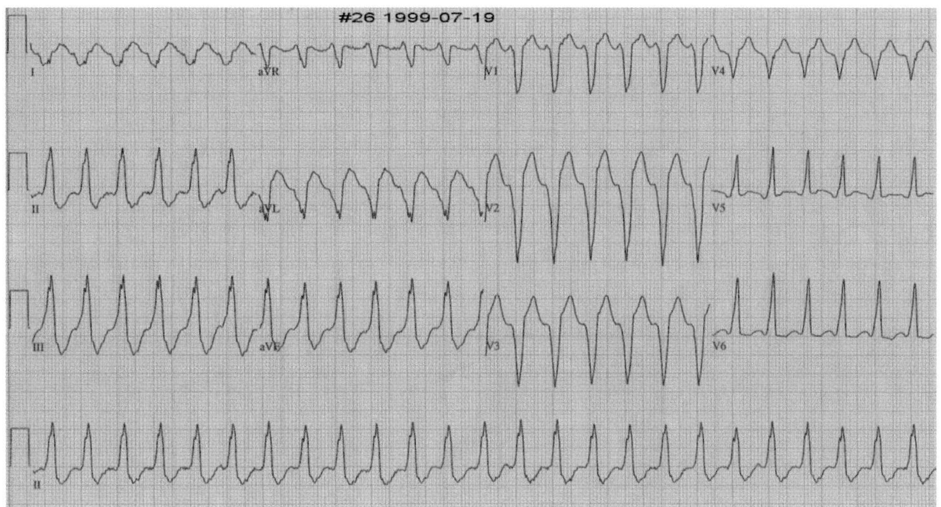

Figure 16.5 ECG 19 July 1999.

10 Echocardiography and nuclear studies 1999

Table 16.1 Echocardiogram and nuclear studies 1999

Echocardiogram	
LV severe diffuse hypokinesia	
LV apical thrombus	
LA end-diastolic diameter	5.6cm
LV end-diastolic diameter	7.4cm
LV ejection fraction	15–20%
MUGA ejection fraction was	14%

There was severe diffuse LV hypokinesia and a LV apical thrombus.

11 Cardiac catheterization and angiography 1999

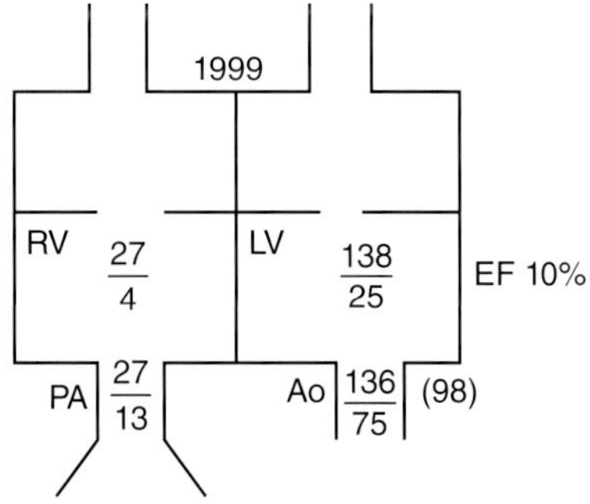

Figure 16.6 Cardiac catheterization and angiograms 1999.

12 Course 1999–2007

The patient retired from work in 2000. She was able to walk two to three blocks every other day but gained 20 lb over the next 6 years. She was continued on nifedipine XL, amiodarone, warfarin, ACE inhibitors, furosemide, and simvastatin. There were no further episodes of VT and she never had any systemic emboli. She died in 2007 from cancer of the colon.

Answers and commentary

1 ECG 1993

Sinus rhythm. Rate 62/min. PR 0.16 s. QRS 0.08 s. QRS axis −30°. QTc 0.48 s.
QS in V1–3. Elevated ST in V1–4. T inverted in 2, 3, F, V5–6.
Impression acute anterior wall infarction.

2 Chest X ray 1993

Cardiomegaly. Mild pulmonary congestion.

3 Laboratory data 1993

The white count is increased. Marked elevation of serum CPK levels to 2,474 U/L with subsequent fall to 310 U/L (normal 26–140 U/L in women) in a 2-day period suggestive of myocardial necrosis.
No evidence of subsequent GI bleeding. Serum cholesterol is moderately elevated.

4 and 5 Echocardiography and nuclear studies 1993

There is severe diffuse LV hypokinesia and a marked reduction in the LV ejection fraction to 11%.

6 Cardiac catheterization and angiography1993

There was severe LV hypokinesia and the LVEDP was three times the normal value. Both findings are due to severe LV dysfunction.
As the LAD was occluded at its origin the patient was not considered a suitable surgical candidate.

7 History and physical examination 1993

The patient was admitted to hospital with symptoms of an acute myocardial infarction over a 3-day period. She had risk factors for coronary artery disease, was post-menopausal, had untreated hypertension and hypercholesterolemia, and she was a smoker. If she had come to the hospital sooner and we had been able to give her t-PA she might not have had quite as much myocardial damage.
She had hypertensive retinopathy and an S4 probably due to LVH. A diagonal ear crease sign is a marker for coronary artery disease. An inspiratory tracheal tug sign indicates increased work of breathing, in this case to mild congestive heart failure.

8 Course ECG 1993-1999

The patient did well on medical therapy and resumed her job.

9 ECG 1999

Wide QRS complex tachycardia. Rate 150/min. QRS 0.17 s. QRS axis +100°.
QTc 0.56 s. QS in V1–4. There is now marked right-axis deviation.
Retrograde conduction of P waves were seen in lead 2. No AV dissociation seen.
Diagnosis: ventricular tachycardia is highly likely in view of the QS waves in V1–4 as well as the prolonged QRS duration compared to a previously normal QRS duration in 1994.

10 Echocardiogram and nuclear studies 1999 (Table 16.1)

The LA is moderately enlarged with marked enlargement of the LV.
The LV is severely hypokinetic. The LV ejection fraction is still very low and unchanged from 1993.

11 Cardiac catheterization and angiography 1999

Moderately elevated LVEDP (25 mmHg). LVEF unchanged from 1994 and still markedly reduced. The cardiac output was 3.6 L/min.

Severe diffuse LV hypokinesia with apical calcification.

Left anterior descending coronary artery was occluded at its origin, but filled retrogradely from the right coronary artery (RCA).

There was 50% stenosis of the circumflex coronary artery. RCA was essentially normal.

12 Course 1999–2007

The patient lived another 8 years on medical therapy without any further cardiovascular complications.

Key points

1. New onset of angina warrants prompt admission to hospital to minimize myocardial damage.
2. Patients with an LV aneurysm can be treated conservatively with warfarin and ACE inhibitors, diuretics, and, when indicated, antiarrhythmic agents.
3. Ventricular tachycardia and LV apical thrombi are common complications of an LV aneurysm.

17 PATIENT STUDY 17

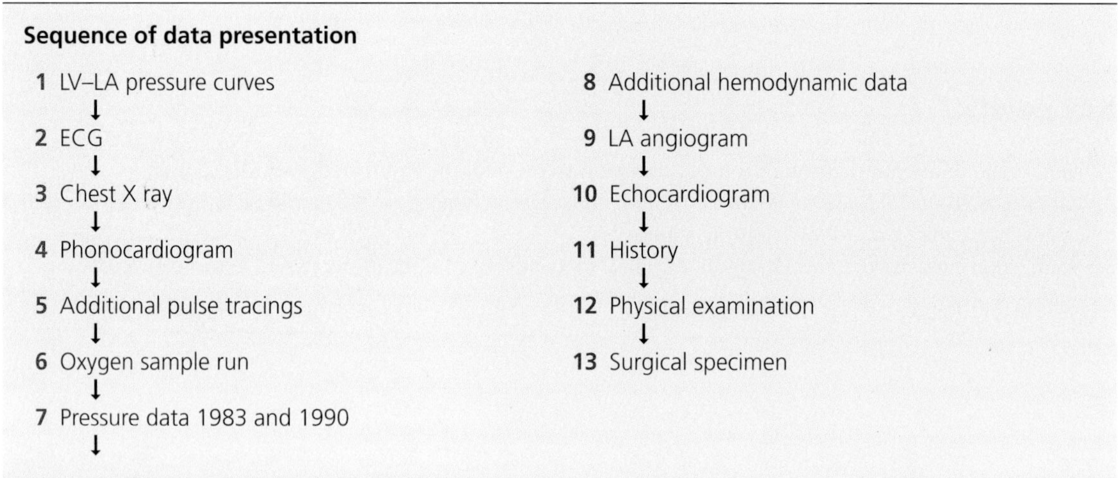

Sequence of data presentation

1 LV–LA pressure curves
↓
2 ECG
↓
3 Chest X ray
↓
4 Phonocardiogram
↓
5 Additional pulse tracings
↓
6 Oxygen sample run
↓
7 Pressure data 1983 and 1990
↓
8 Additional hemodynamic data
↓
9 LA angiogram
↓
10 Echocardiogram
↓
11 History
↓
12 Physical examination
↓
13 Surgical specimen

1 LV–LA pressure curves

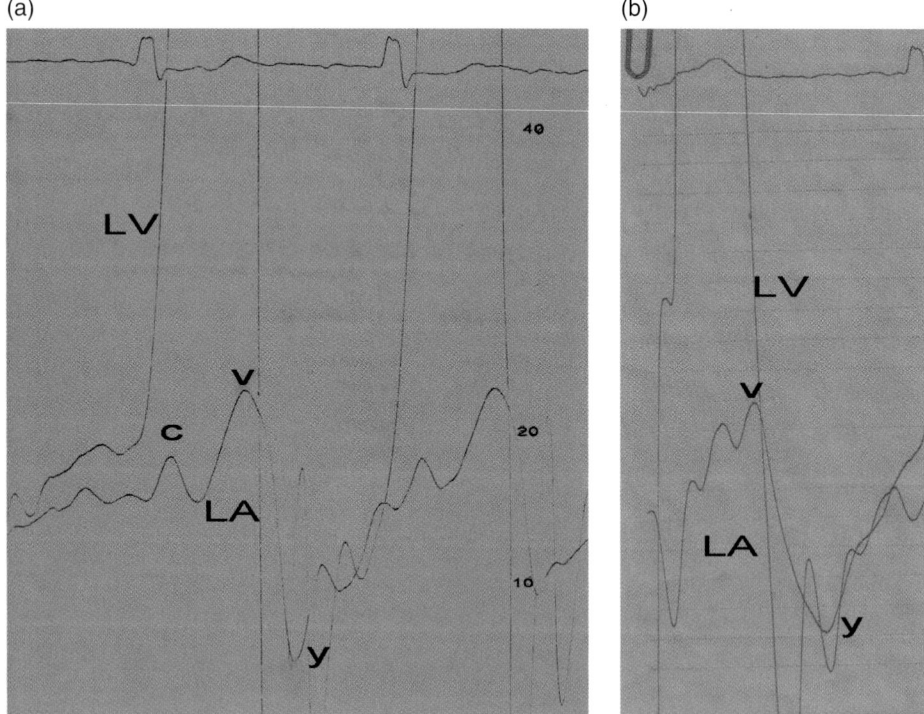

Figure 17.1 Simultaneous recording of LV and LA pressure tracings. 0–40 mmHg scale, taken at different times during the catheterization.

Patient Studies in Valvular, Congenital, and Rarer Forms of Cardiovascular Disease: An Integrative Approach, First Edition. Franklin B. Saksena.

Companion Website: www.wiley.com/go/saksena/patientstudies

2 ECG

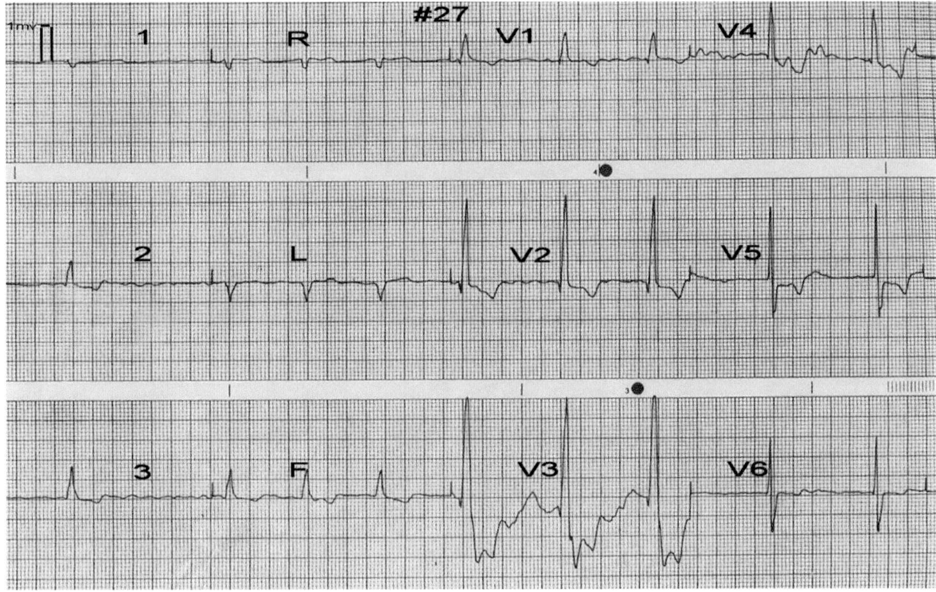

Figure 17.2 12-lead ECG 1990.

3 Chest X ray

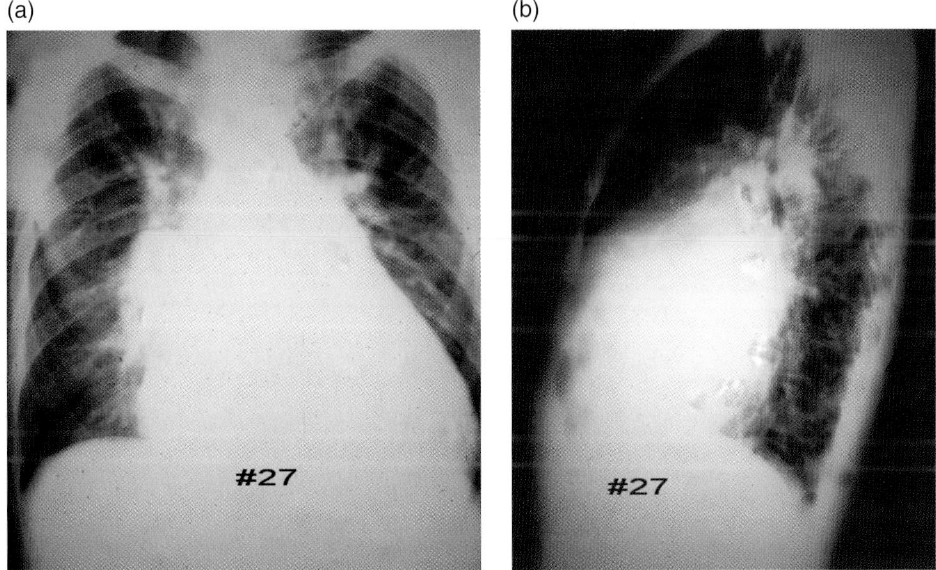

Figure 17.3 (a) PA chest X ray. (b) Lateral chest X ray.

4 Phonocardiogram

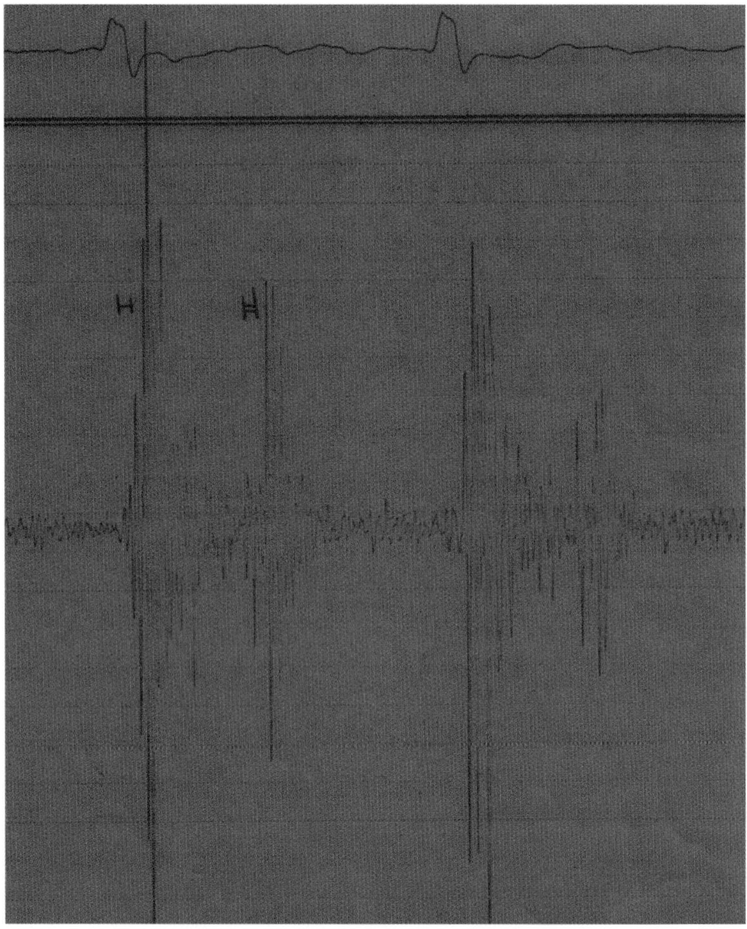

Figure 17.4 Phonocardiogram at left 3rd interspace parasternally.

5 Additional pulse tracings

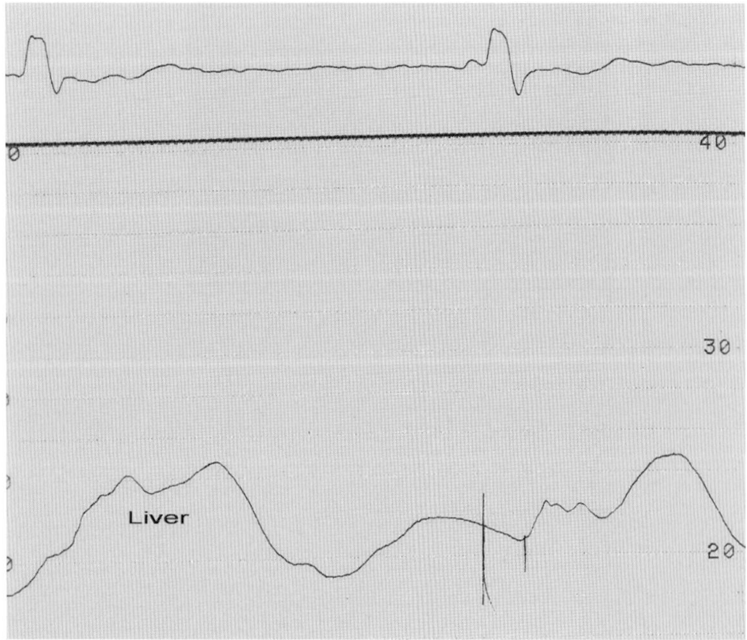

Figure 17.5 Pulsations recorded over liver.

6 Oxygen sample run

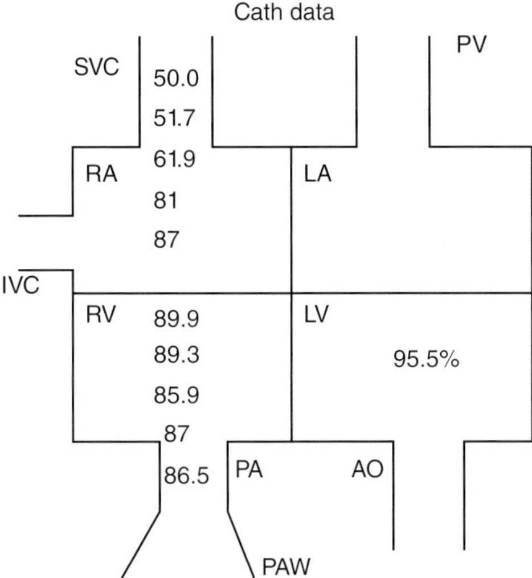

Figure 17.6 Oxygen sample run 1990.

7 Pressure data 1983 and 1990

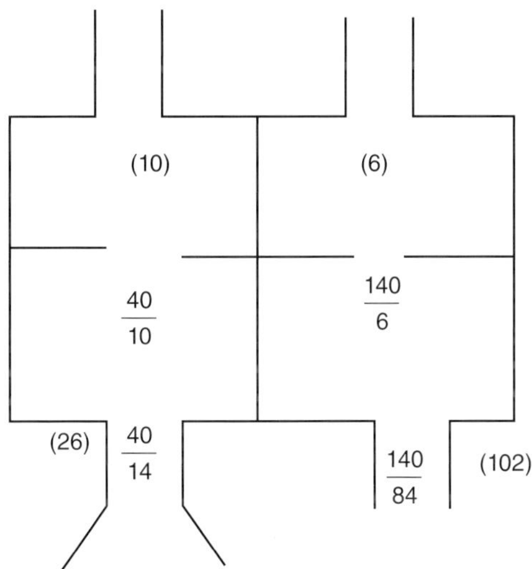

Figure 17.7 Intracardiac pressures 1983.

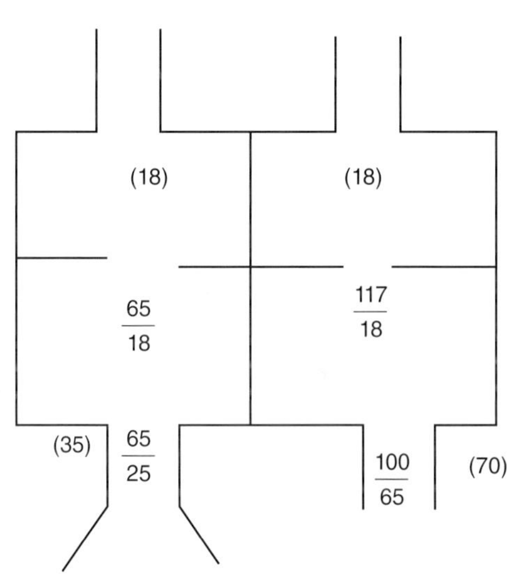

Figure 17.8 Intracardiac pressures 1990.

8 Additional hemodynamic data

Table 17.1 1990

Oxygen consumption	239 mL/min
Hemoglobin	15.1 g%
Average superior vena cava oxygen saturation	50.8%
Average pulmonary artery saturation	86.8%
Arterial oxygen saturation	95.5%
LV end-diastolic volume index	199 mL
LV end-systolic volume index	43 mL
Aortic regurgitation	2+
Mitral regurgitation	0
Normal coronary angiography	

Calculate the pulmonary blood flow, systemic blood flow, and the LV ejection fraction. Comment on the results.

9 LA angiogram

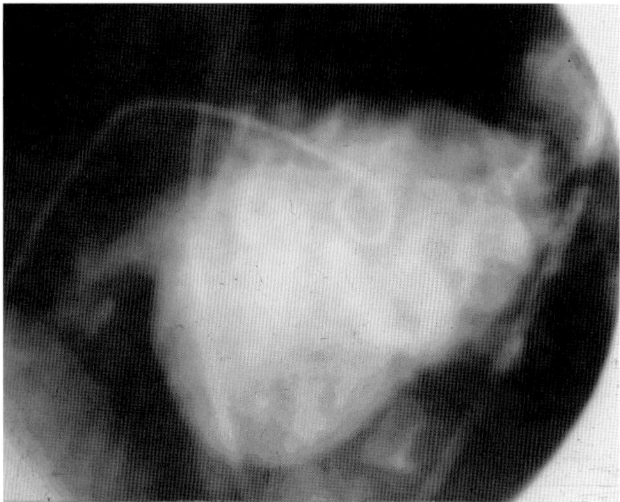

Figure 17.9 LA angiogram in LAO view 1990, about 3 s after contrast was injected.

10 Echocardiogram

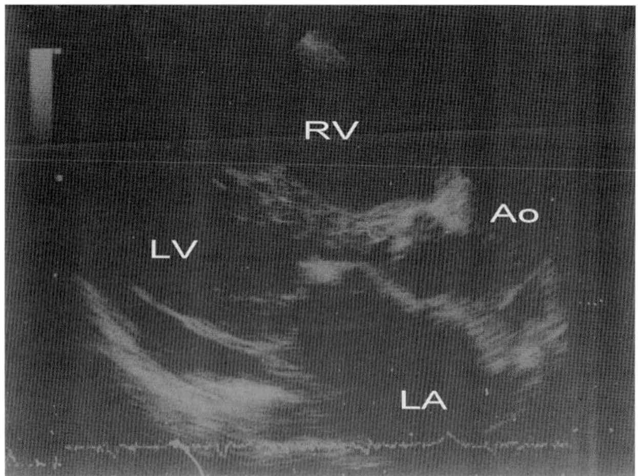

Figure 17.10 Two-dimensional echocardiogram long axis view.

11 History

33-year-old man with dyspnea and leg edema for 6 weeks (1990).

He was diagnosed as having an ASD with a pulmonary/systemic flow ratio of 4:1 in 1983. At that time he also had mild aortic regurgitation and mild pulmonary hypertension. He declined surgery and was followed up intermittently by his family doctor. He was taking digoxin, furosemide, isordil, potassium chloride, and hydralazine.

He was apparently well until 6 weeks prior to admission in 1990, when he developed easy fatigue, dyspnea on walking half a block and leg edema. No history of chest pain.

Past history: he had rheumatic fever at age 13, was an occasional drinker and had smoked for 10 pack years.

12 Physical examination

5 ft 11 inches tall male weighing 150 lb. BP 105/70. HR 56/min irregular. There was an extra digit on the 5th finger of the left hand (Figure 17.11).

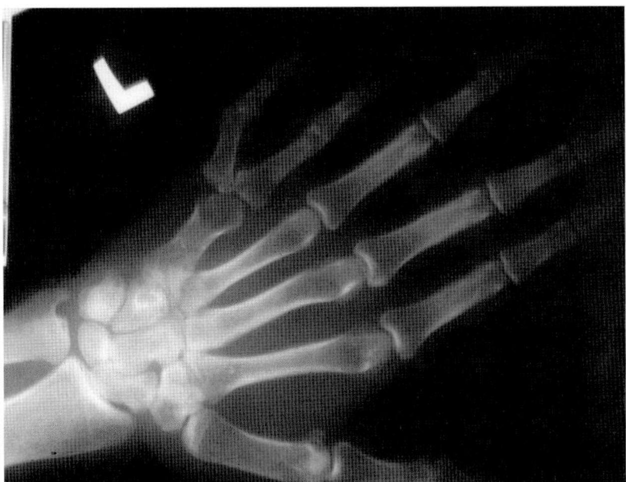

Figure 17.11 X ray of left hand showing extra digit attached to the 5th finger.

The jugular venous pressure was increased.
The apex beat was in the 6th and 7th interspace, 12 cm from the mid-sternal line.
There was a parasternal lift at left lower sternal area.
S1 was loud. S2 was narrowly split.
There was a grade 3/6 crescendo-decrescendo systolic murmur best heard at left 3rd interspace parasternally.
There was a grade 3/6 pansystolic murmur heard at the apex and increasing on inspiration.
The liver was enlarged and pulsatile (Figure 17.5).

13 Surgical specimen

Comment on the surgical specimen (Figure 17.12).

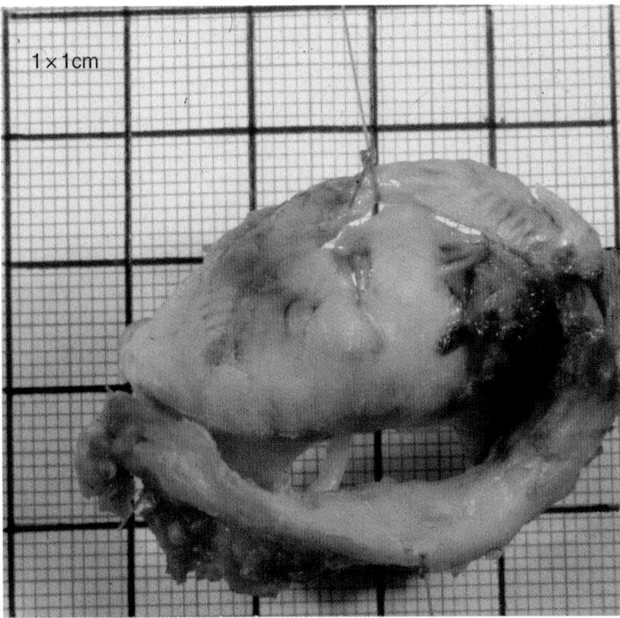

Figure 17.12 Mitral valve excised at operation. Each large square is 1 × 1 cm.

Answers and commentary

1 LV–LA pressure curves

The rhythm is atrial fibrillation. The LA pressure curve shows two positive waves, a 'c' wave and a 'v' wave. The y descent is rapid. There is no gradient in diastole across the mitral valve.

2 ECG

The rhythm is atrial fibrillation. Rate 60–70/min. PR–QRS 0.16s. QRS axis +100°.
qR pattern in V1. R in V1 = l mv. T inverted V1–4.
Impression: (i) atrial fibrillation, (ii) RBBB, (iii) RVH likely.
Patients with RBBB and atrial fibrillation can be seen in chronic lung disease or ASD.

3 Chest X ray

PA view

There is cardiomegaly with a cardio-thoracic ratio of ~0.7. There is straightening of the left heart border suggestive of LA enlargement. The pulmonary vessels are enlarged proximally and extend to its tertiary branches.

Lateral view

There is marked RV enlargement. The combination of RV and LA enlargement is a common feature of mitral stenosis.

4 Phonocardiogram

The amplitude of the first heart sound is much greater than the second sound. Its amplitude is variable because of the patient's atrial fibrillation.

A high amplitude first sound can be seen in high output states or mitral stenosis.

The systolic murmur at the left 3rd space is not well defined. It could represent a flow murmur across the pulmonic valve.

5 Additional pulse tracings

The presence of liver systolic pulsations is indicative of tricuspid regurgitation.
The most common cause of tricuspid regurgitation is pulmonary hypertension

6 Oxygen sample run

There is a significant step up in oxygen saturation in the mid to high RA indicative of a left to right shunt at atrial level. Other causes of such a step up in oxygen saturation in the RA include an anomalous pulmonary venous return, ruptured sinus of valsalva into the RA, a VSD with tricuspid regurgitation, or a coronary AV fistula.

The presence of a pulmonary flow murmur, pulmonary plethora, and a step up of oxygen saturation in the RA should suggest a secundum ASD.

7 Pressure data 1983 and 1990

In 1983 there is mild pulmonary hypertension (PA mean 26 mmHg). This increased to 35 mmHg 7 years later. There is RV dysfunction, which has become worse since 1983 (RVEDP has increased from 10 to 18 mmHg). LV dysfunction has also worsened, with an increase in LVEDP from 6 to 18 mmHg.

In 1990 the RA, LA and LVEDP are identical due to a significant ASD when all three chambers are in open communication in diastole.

8 Additional hemodynamic data

To find the pulmonary and systemic blood flows

Step 1: Find the total oxygen carrying capacity

Total oxygen carrying capacity $= 1.36 \times \text{Hgb (g\%)}$
$= 1.36 \times 15.1 = 20.54\,\text{mL\%}$

Step 2: Find the oxygen content of SVC, PA and aorta

Superior vena cava oxygen content (C_{svc}) = saturation × total oxygen carrying capacity

$$= 50.8 \times 20.54 = 10.4\,\text{mL\%}$$

Pulmonary oxygen content (C_{pa}) = $86.8 \times 20.54 = 17.8\,\text{mL\%}$

Arterial oxygen content (C_{ao}) = $95.5 \times 20.54 = 19.6\,\text{mL\%}$

Step 3: Find the pulmonary blood flow and systemic flow using Fick's principle

$$\text{Pulmonary blood flow} = \frac{V_{O_2}}{C_{ao} - C_{pa}} = \frac{239}{10(19.6 - 17.8)} = 13.3\,\text{L/min}$$

$$\text{Systemic blood flow} = \frac{V_{O_2}}{C_{ao} - C_{svc}} = \frac{239}{10(19.6 - 10.4)} = 2.6\,\text{L/min}$$

$$\text{Pulmonary/systemic flow ratio} = \frac{13.3}{2.6} = 5.12$$

This a large left to right shunt.

Calculate the LV ejection fraction

$$\text{LV ejection fraction} = \frac{\text{Stroke volume}}{\text{LV end diastolic volume}} = \frac{199 - 43}{199} = 0.78$$

The LV ejection fracton is above normal.

9 LA angiogram

The LA is enlarged. Contrast is seen entering the RA due to the ASD. Only a small amount of contrast enters the LV due to severe mitral valve obstruction.

10 Echocardiogram

The RV and LA are enlarged. LV is not enlarged. The anterior mitral valve leaflet is thickened and has a hockey stick appearance characteristic of mitral valve stenosis.

The RV and LA were also noted to be enlarged on chest X ray.

11 History

The patient had recurrence of dyspnea and edema, implying that there has been further progression of his right heart failure due to his known ASD.

12 Physical examination

There was evidence of pulmonary hypertension. The patient had tricuspid regurgitation on the basis of a pansystolic murmur at the apex, increasing on inspiration and liver pulsations (Figure 17.5). The pulmonary systolic murmur is related to increased pulmonary blood flow across the pulmonary valve, which in turn is related to his ASD.

There is an extra digit attached to his fifth finger (Figure 17.11). Digital abnormalities are not uncommon in an ASD. A fingerized thumb (Holt–Oram syndrome) is another digital abnormality seen in an ASD [1].

13 Surgical specimen

The commissures are fused and thickened. The mitral valve area is less than 1 cm^2, which is indicative of rheumatic mitral stenosis.

Discussion

The patient had a large secundum ASD and severe rheumatic mitral stenosis (valve area < 1 cm^2), indicative of Lutembacher's syndrome.

Attempts have been made to broaden the definition of Lutembacher's syndrome to include:

1. other congenital left to right shunts at atrial level along with rheumatic mitral stenosis [2]
2. patients who having undergone trans-septal mitral valvuloplasty develop a persistent ASD, and subsequently develop mitral valve restenosis [3].

Mitral stenosis is seen in about 4% of patients with a secundum ASD [4] and was overlooked in the first cardiac catheterization as there was no detectible gradient across the mitral valve in diastole.

In comparison to the 1983 data the patient's left to right shunt and PA pressures had further increased in 1990, probably as a result of silent mitral stenosis.

Mitral stenosis delays the emptying of the LA into the LV and thereby increases the left to right shunt at atrial level [5].

In this patient there was no detectible gradient in diastole across the mitral valve, but the delayed emptying of the LA, detected angiographically, as well as the calcified mitral valve pointed to the presence of mitral valvular disease. The M-mode echocardiogram also confirmed the presence of mitral valvular disease along with LA and RV enlargement.

Further information can be obtained with two-dimensional echocardiography and Doppler flow studies in patients with Lutembacher's syndrome.

Two-dimensional echocardiography and color Doppler studies can readily visualize the ASD and mitral stenosis [6]. As the AV half-time ($T_{1/2}$) does not reliably reflect the severity of mitral stenosis in the presence of an ASD, it should not be used in the calculation of the mitral valve area (mitral valve area = $230/T_{1/2}$) [7]. The mitral valve area is best calculated on two-dimensional echocardiography by direct planimetry [7] in the Lutembacher syndrome.

Key points

1. Lutenbacher's syndrome consists of a secundum ASD and rheumatic mitral stenosis.
2. The murmur of mitral stenosis can be silent as the left to right shunt decompresses the LA and thus abolishes the mitral diastolic gradient.
3. An extra digit or a fingerized thumb is seen in patients with a secundum ASD.

References

[1] Holt M, Oram S. Familial heart disease with skeletal malformations. *Br Heart J* 1960; 22: 236–242.

[2] Goldfarb B, Wang Y. Mitral stenosis and left to right shunt at the atrial level. A broadened concept of the Lutembacher syndrome. *Am J Cardiol* 1966; 17: 319–326.

[3] Sadaniantz A, Luttman C, Shulman RS, Block PC et al. Acquired Lutembacher syndrome or mitral stenosis and acquired atrial septal defect after transseptal mitral valvuloplasty. *Cathet Cardiovasc Diagn* 1990; 21: 7–9.

[4] Perloff JK, Marelli AJ. *Lutembacher's syndrome.* In: Perloff's Clinical recognition of congenital heart disease 2012, 6th edn. WB Saunders/Elsevier, Philadelphia.

[5] Perloff JK. Lutembachers's syndrome—A contemporary appraisal. *Med Ann District of Columbia* 1970; 39: 71–77.

[6] Ansari A, Maron BJ. Lutembacher's syndrome. *Tex Heart J* 1997; 24: 230–231.

[7] Vasan RS, Shrivastava S, Kumar MV. Value and limitations of Doppler echocardiographic determination of mitral valve area in Lutembacher syndrome. *J Am Coll Cardiol* 1992; 20: 1362–1370.

18 PATIENT STUDY 18

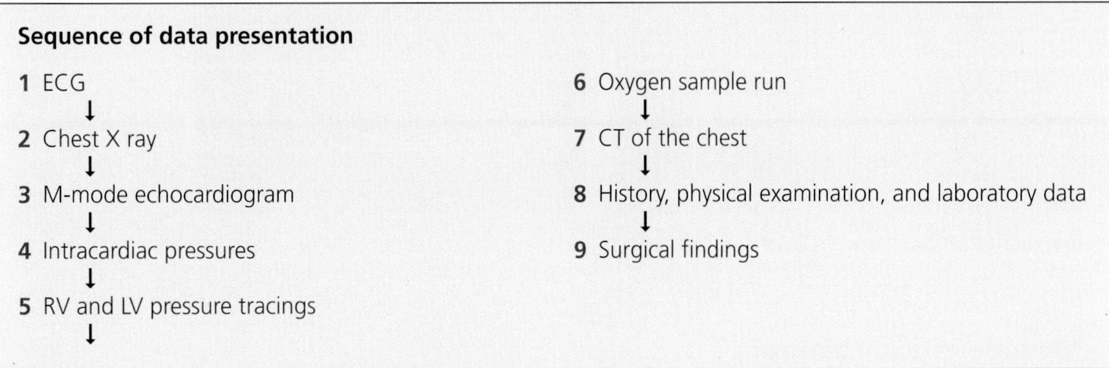

Sequence of data presentation

1 ECG
↓
2 Chest X ray
↓
3 M-mode echocardiogram
↓
4 Intracardiac pressures
↓
5 RV and LV pressure tracings
↓
6 Oxygen sample run
↓
7 CT of the chest
↓
8 History, physical examination, and laboratory data
↓
9 Surgical findings

1 ECG

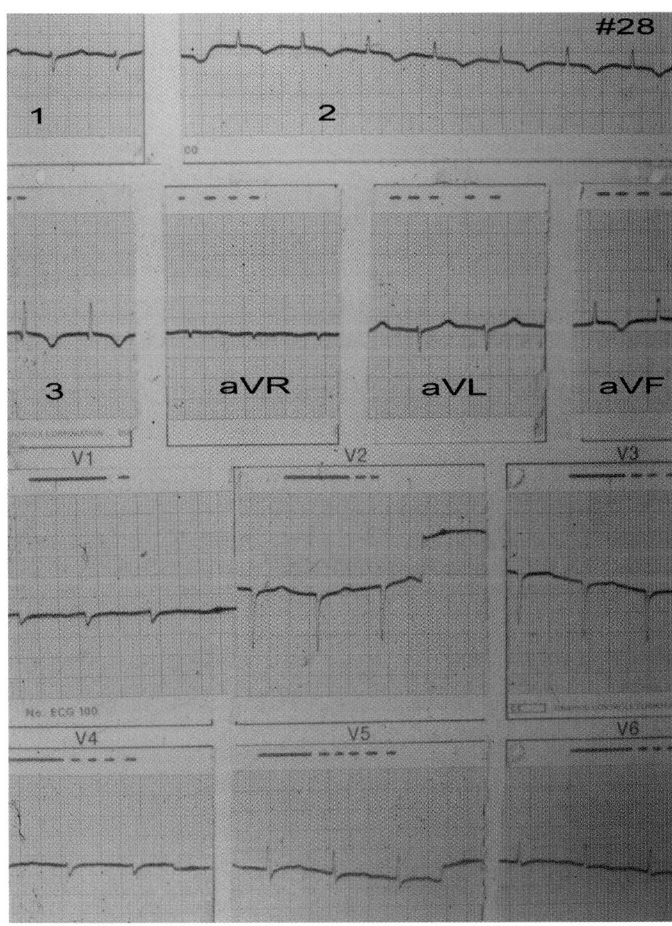

Figure 18.1 12-lead ECG. 10 mm = 1 mv standardization.

Patient Studies in Valvular, Congenital, and Rarer Forms of Cardiovascular Disease: An Integrative Approach, First Edition. Franklin B. Saksena.

Companion Website: www.wiley.com/go/saksena/patientstudies

2 Chest X ray

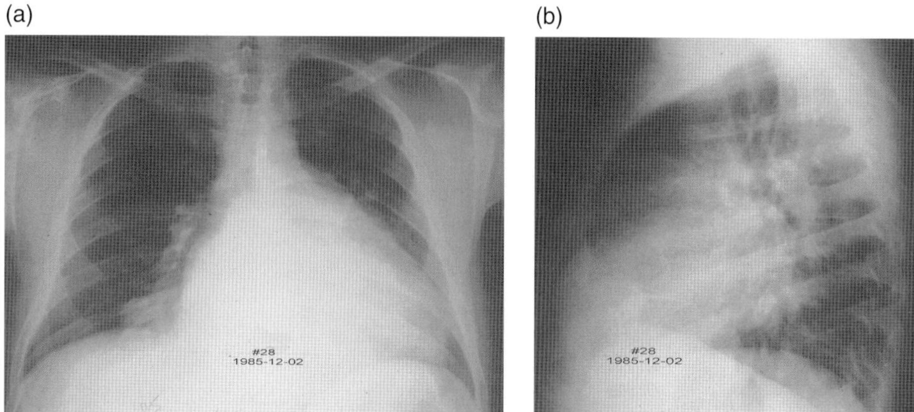

Figure 18.2 (a) PA chest X ray. (b) Lateral chest X ray.

3 M-mode echocardiogram

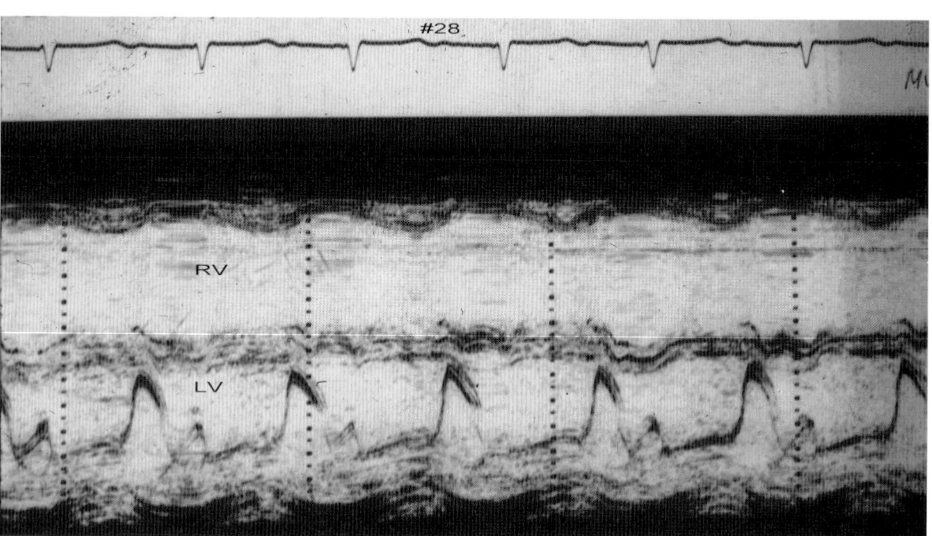

Figure 18.3 M-mode echocardiogram. The vertical dots are 1 cm apart.

4 Intracardiac pressures

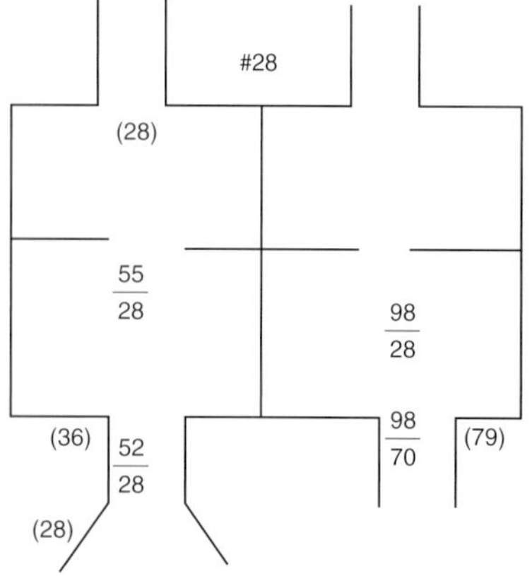

Figure 18.4 Intracardiac pressures.

5 RV and LV pressure tracings

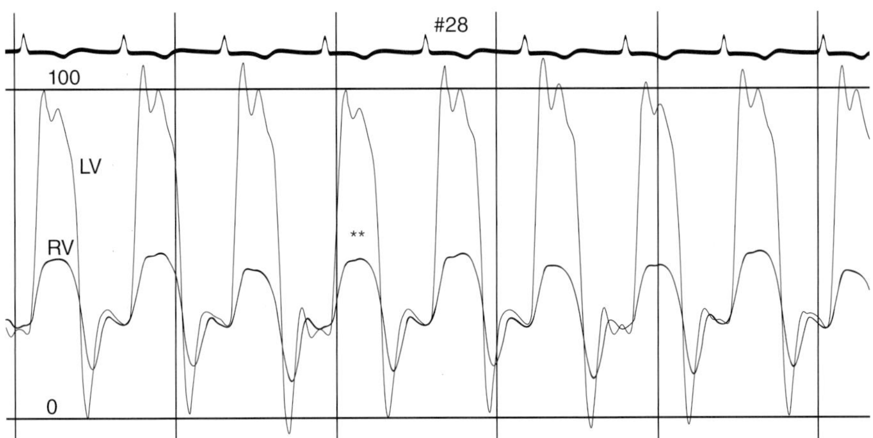

Figure 18.5 Simultaneous RV and LV pressure curves. 0–100 mmHg scale.
Comment on the 4th beat (**).

6 Oxygen sample run

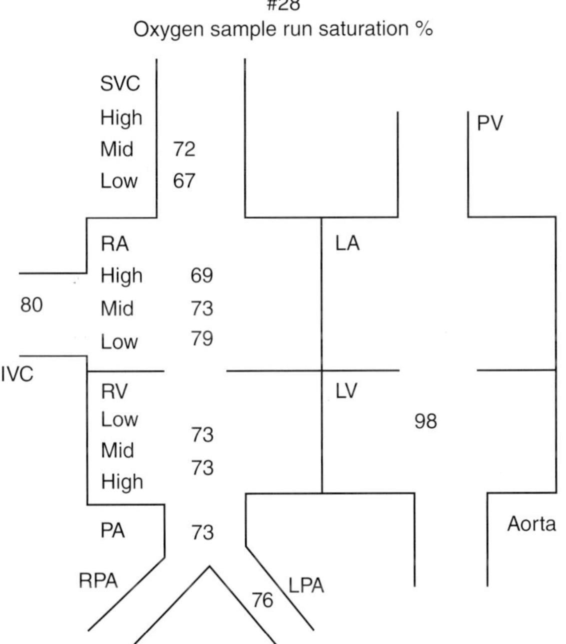

Figure 18.6 Oxygen saturation sample run.

7 CT of the chest

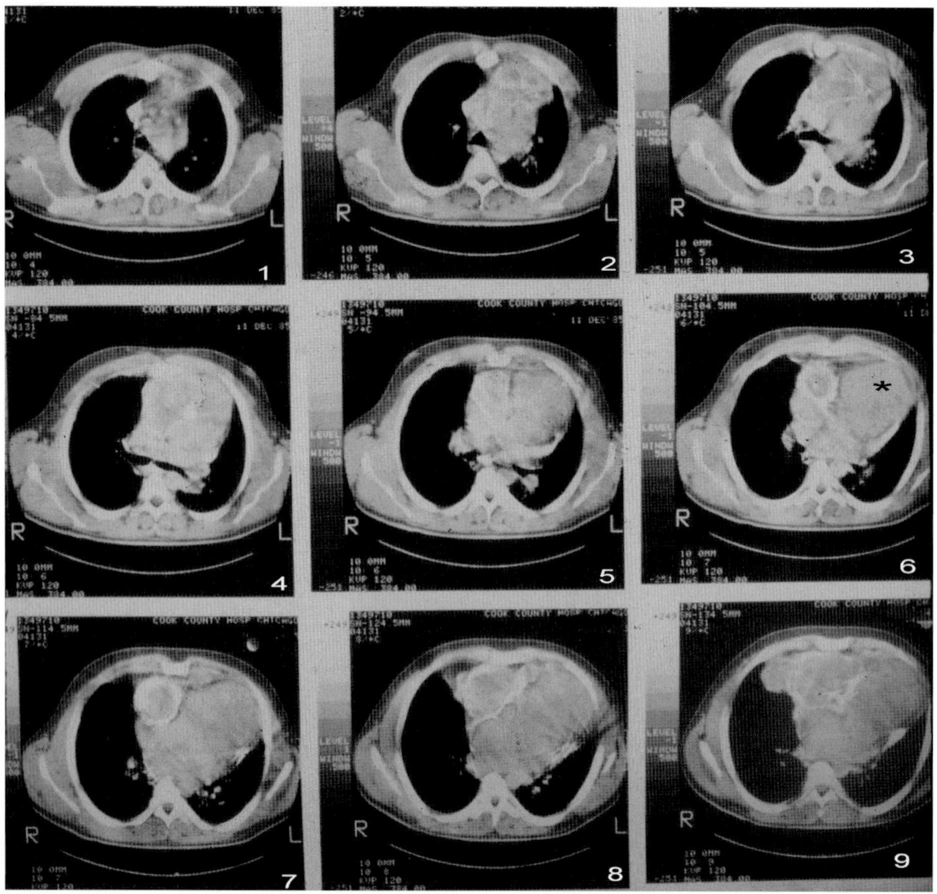

Figures 18.7 Nine successive CT slices of the chest from above downwards. * indicates the RV.

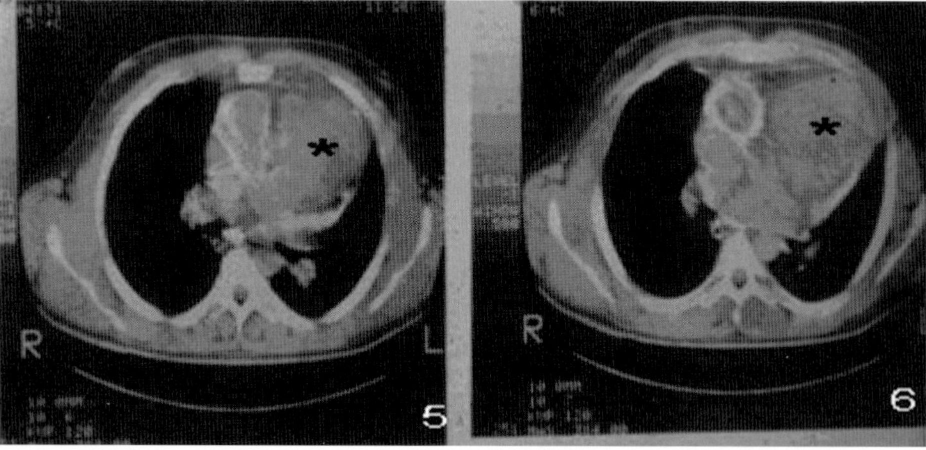

Figure 18.8 Enlargement of Panels 5 and 6 of the chest CT. * indicates the RV.

8 History, physical examination, and laboratory data

History

29-year-old black male admitted to hospital with bilateral pleuritic chest pain for the last 3 months (November 1985).

He has had progressive exertional dyspnea for the last 3 months. In the last week he has had one block dyspnea as well as leg edema. No paroxysmal nocturnal dyspnea, fever, or chills.

No history of rheumatic fever, hypertension, or liver disease. He does not smoke or use drugs. He has drunk three cans of beer a day over last 3 years.

Physical examination

BSA 2.05 m^2. BP 110/70. Pulse 94/min regular. RR 20/min. Temperature normal.
Borderline scleral icterus.
There was marked elevation of jugular venous pressure to the angle of the jaw.
There was hepatojugular reflux.
The apex beat was not palpable.
There was 1+ left lower sternal lift.
S1 decreased. S2 increased with loud P2. Apical S3.
Grade 1/6 systolic murmur heard at the 3rd left interspace parasternally.
2+ pitting edema of legs and ankles. No cyanosis or clubbing.
Lungs clear to percussion and auscultation.
Liver span is 18 cm. Smooth edge. Non tender.

Laboratory data

Hb 14.4 g%. WBC 5910/mm^3. Bilirubin 2.6 mg%.
PPD negative. VDRL test negative.
Liver biopsy: cardiac cirrhosis.
V/Q scan of lung: low probability of pulmonary embolism.

9 Surgical findings

At surgery a large anterior necrotic mediastinal abscess was found, which was displacing the heart leftwards. Viral, TB and bacterial studies of this abscess were negative.

Answers and commentary

1 ECG

P waves are not well seen. QRS duration 0.05 s. QRS axis +110°. QS in V1–4. Low QRS voltage. T inversion 2, 3, F.
Impression: (i) the low QRS voltage could account for the inapparent P waves so rhythm is either sinus or junctional, (ii) right-axis deviation could be due to RVH or cardiac rotation and distortion [1], (iii) the QS waves in V1–4 could be due to an anteroseptal myocardial infarction, but in this young patient is mostly likely a pseudoinfaction pattern that is occasionally seen in CCP [2].

2 Chest X ray

In the PA view there is cardiomegaly. If the apex is displaced laterally and inferiorly then LV enlargement is more likely, but in this case the apex beat is displaced laterally and horizontally, suggestive of RV enlargement. The lateral view tends to confirm that the RV is enlarged in that the anterior cardiac shadow occupies at least two interspaces. The lung fields show some prominence of the proximal pulmonary arteries.

3 M-mode echocardiogram

The RV end-diastolic diameter is increased to 3 cm (normal < 2.3 cm). The LV size is normal. A DE amplitude of 3 cm is at the upper limits of normal (normal 1.7–3 cm). The EF slope is normal, thus making mitral stenosis unlikely.
Impression: (i) RV enlargement, (ii) restrictive filling of LV.

4 Intracardiac pressures

The RA pressure is markedly elevated, possibly due to tricuspid regurgitation, left to right shunt or right heart failure.
RA mean = RVEDP = PA diastolic pressure = PAW mean = LVEDP = 28 mmHg.
This equalization of diastolic pressures may be due to a restrictive cardiomyopathy (RCM) or CCP.

5 RV and LV pressure tracings

This confirms the equalization of RVEDP and LVEDP. These pressure contours show a rapid y descent followed by a plateau for the rest of diastole (a square root sign) and indicate restrictive or constrictive pathology. The 4th beat (**) shows a slight rise in RV systolic pressure with a slight fall in LV systolic pressure, presumably during inspiration (as a nasal respirometer was not used). This discordance of ventricular pressures is more in favor of a chronic constrictive pattern. In RCM the LV and RV pressures move concordantly on inspiration [3].

6 Oxygen sample run

The sample run is normal, thus excluding a significant left to right shunt.

7 CT of the chest

Panel 6 in Figure 18.7 shows calcification around an enlarged RV (*) and part of the LV. The RV is displaced to the left by a large calcified mass surrounding the RA. Panels 7–9 show calcification around the RA. An anterior calcified mediastinal mass is pushing the heart leftwards. The RV is enlarged.

Enlargement of panels 5 and 6 to better show the calcification around the RA and RV (*) is given in Figure 18.8.

These findings confirm the diagnosis of CCP.

8 History, physical examination, and laboratory data

The patient had chest pain aggravated by deep breathing, which could have been of pleural/ pericardial origin. He had moderately severe pulmonary hypertension and RV failure along with tricuspid regurgitation but no evidence of left heart failure.

9 Surgical findings

The patient had CCP and moderately severe pulmonary hypertension.

The treatment is to carry out pericardial stripping.

The cause of the patient's pulmonary hypertension is uncertain. It could be due to pulmonary fibrosis, obstructive sleep apnea, or a cardiomyopathy. The patient underwent successful pericardial stripping and was doing well 1 year later.

Discussion

The patient presented in RV failure due to CCP. The diagnosis of CCP was based on the following findings: (i) a diastolic plateau in the right heart pressures, (ii) possible discordant motion of the RV and LV pressures during inspiration, (iii) extensive calcification and fibrosis around the heart on CT, (iv) resolution of symptoms following pericardial stripping.

Unexplained is the pulmonary hypertension in this patient, which is higher than expected in CCP [4]. Underlying lung disease such as fibrosis, obstructive sleep apnea, or cardiomyopathy are possible considerations. There was no evidence of obstructive lung disease.

The differentiation between CCP and RCM has continued to be refined since 1985, when this patient was first seen.

In 1989 Doppler echocardiography differentiated these two entities by noting the effects of inspiration on the RV and LV pressures [3]. In CCP the thickened pericardium fixes the total ventricular volume and prevents the complete transmission of intrathoracic pressure to the cardiac chambers. On inspiration there is a fall in the intrathoracic pressure, which is transmitted to the pulmonary vessels but not to the cardiac chambers. This leads to a fall in the pulmonary venous return and a reduction in LV filling and LV size. This decrease in LV size results in the LV septum bulging into the LV, which allows an increase in RV filling. This sequence of events is reversed in expiration. Thus, in CCP on inspiration the LV systolic pressure falls and the simultaneous RV pressure rises – a discordant reaction [4–6]. This distinguishes CCP from RCM, in which the LV and RV pressures respond concordantly during inspiration [5].

The systolic area index (SAI) is a useful way of quantifying ventricular discordance.

The areas under the RV and LV systolic pressure curves are measured on inspiration (I) and expiration (e), represented by RV_I and RV_e LV_I and LV_e respectively, and the SAI is calculated as below:

$$\mathrm{SAI} = \frac{\mathrm{RVarea_I \backslash LVarea_I}}{\mathrm{RVarea_e \backslash LVarea_e}}$$

An SAI ratio > 1.1 has a 97% sensitivity and 100% predictive accuracy of diagnosing CCP [6].

Additional ways of distinguishing CCP from RCM are summarized in Table 18.1.

Table 18.1 A comparison of CCP and RCM

Measurement	CCP	RCM	Reference
Autonomic dysfunction	Severe	Mild	7
Doppler E′	≥8 cm/s	≤6 cm/s	8, 9
Myocardial velocity gradient of LV posterior wall	$4.4 \pm 1.0\,s^{-1}$	$2.8 \pm 1.2\,s^{-1}$	10
Longitudinal strain	Normal	Reduced	5

The tissue Doppler of early diastolic velocity = E′ reflects early diastolic relaxation.

Key points

1. Patients with CCP show equalization of the end-diastolic pressures: $\overline{RA}$ = RVEDP = PADP = $\overline{PAW}$ = LVEDP, similar to RCM.
2. There is discordant motion of LV and RV pressures on inspiration in CCP but not in RCM.
3. The presence of calcification and fibrosis around the heart favors CCP over RCM.
4. Tissue Doppler studies and strain measurements are additional ways of distinguishing CCP from RCM.

References

[1] Chesler E, Mitha AS, Matisonn RE. The ECG of constrictive pericarditis – pattern resembling right ventricular hypertrophy. *Am Heart J* 1976; 91: 420–424.

[2] Levine HD. Myocardial fibrosis in constrictive pericarditis. Electrocardiographic and pathologic observations. *Circulation* 1973; 48: 1268–1281.

[3] Hatle LK, Appleton CP, Popp RL. Differentiation of constrictive pericarditis and restrictive cardiomyopathy by Doppler echocardiography. *Circulation* 1989; 79: 357–370.

[4] Goldstein JA. Cardiac tamponade, constrictive pericarditis and restrictive cardiomyopathy. *Curr Probl Cardiol* 2004; 29: 503–567.

[5] Dal-Bianco JP, Sengupta PP, Mookadam F et al. Role of echocardiography in the diagnosis of constrictive pericarditis. *J Am Soc Echocardiogr* 2009; 22: 24–33.

[6] Sorajja P. Invasive hemodynamics of constrictive pericarditis, restrictive cardiomyopathy, and cardiac tamponade. In: Lim MJ (ed.), Catheterization Hemodynamics. *Cardiol Clin Saunders* 2011; 29: 191–199.

[7] Singh M, Juneja R, Bali HK et al. Autonomic functions in restrictive cardiomyopathy and constrictive pericarditis: a comparison. *Am Heart J* 1998; 136: 443–448.

[8] Choi E-Y, Ha J-W, Kim J-M et al. Incremental value of combining systolic mitral annular velocity and time difference between mitral inflow and diastolic mitral annular velocity for differentiating constrictive pericarditis from restrictive cardiomyopathy. *J Am Soc Echocardiogr* 2007; 20: 738–743.

[9] McCall R, Stoodley PW, Richards DAB et al. Restrictive cardiomyopathy versus constrictive pericarditis: making the distinction using tissue Doppler imaging. *Eur J Echocardiogr* 2008; 9: 591–594.

[10] Palka P, Lange A, Donnelly JE et al. Differentiation between restrictive cardiomyopathy and constrictive pericarditis by early diastolic Doppler myocardial velocity gradient at the posterior wall. *Circulation* 2000; 102: 655–662.

19 PATIENT STUDY 19

Sequence of data presentation

1 Chest X ray 27 October 1988
↓
2 12-lead ECG 27 October 1988
↓
3 Laboratory data
↓
4 Lung scan 27 October 1988
↓
5 Follow-up chest X rays 27 October 1988 and 1 November 1988
↓
6 Angiogram 5 November 1988
↓
7 Lung scans 27 October 1988 and 8 November 1988
↓
8 History
↓
9 Physical examination
↓
10 Diagnosis and treatment
↓
11 Follow-up chest X rays 27 October, 1 November, and 15 November 1988

1 Chest X ray 27 October 1988

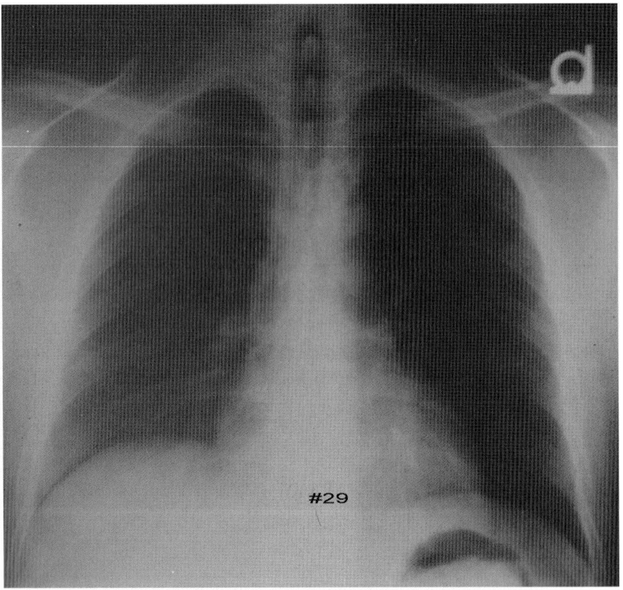

Figure 19.1 Chest X ray PA view 27 October 1988.

Patient Studies in Valvular, Congenital, and Rarer Forms of Cardiovascular Disease: An Integrative Approach, First Edition. Franklin B. Saksena.

Companion Website: www.wiley.com/go/saksena/patientstudies

2 12-lead ECG 27 October 1988

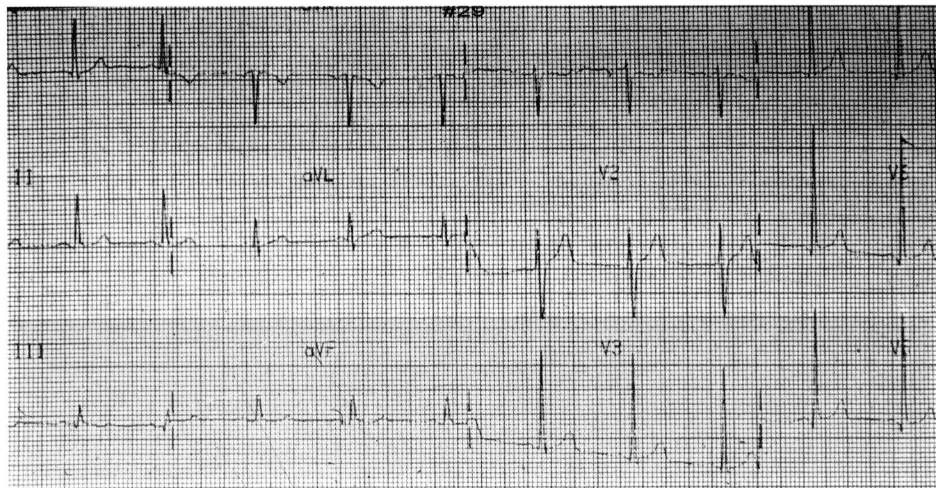

Figure 19.2 12-lead ECG 27 October 1988.

3 Laboratory data

Hemoglobin 16.1 g%. WBC 4670/mm^3. Platelet count 274,000/mm^3.
TB skin test negative.
Normal echocardiogram and ECG.

4 Lung scan 27 October 1988

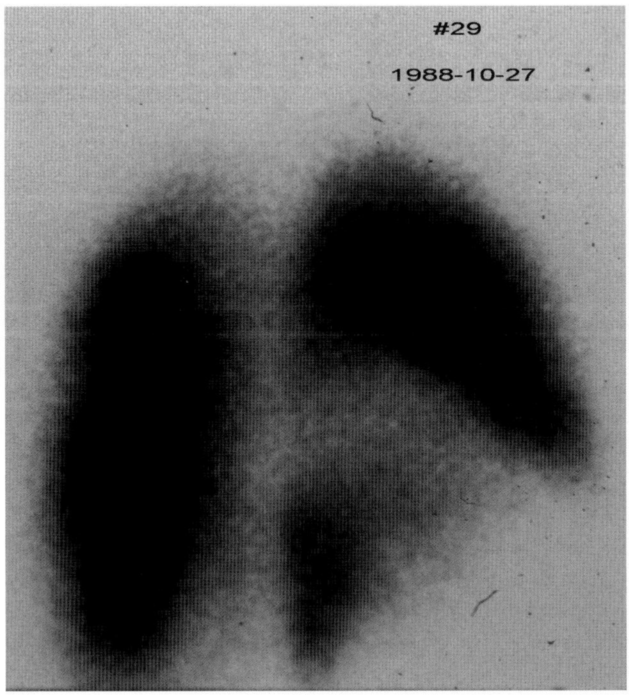

Figure 19.3 Lung scan, right posterior oblique view 27 October 1988.

5 Follow-up chest X rays 27 October 1988 and 1 November 1988

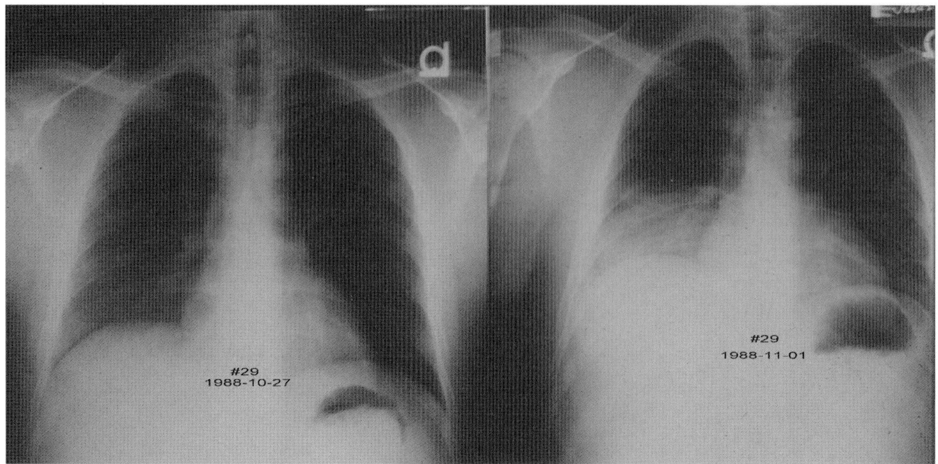

Figure 19.4 Chest X rays 27 October and 1 November 1988.

6 Angiogram 5 November 1988

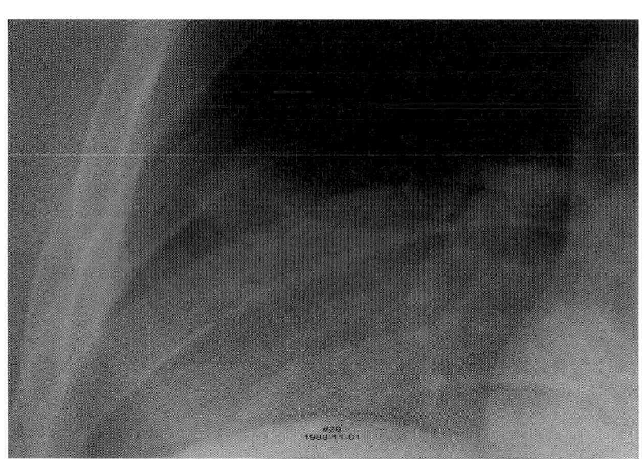

Figure 19.5 RLL chest X ray area 1 November 1988. PA view.

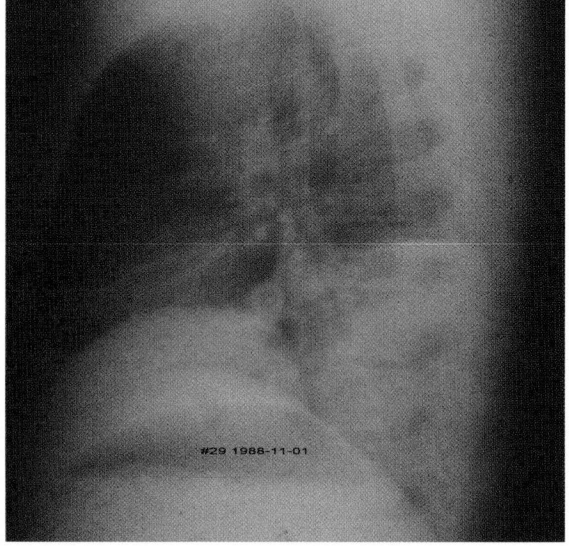

Figure 19.6 Lateral view of chest X ray 1 November 1988.

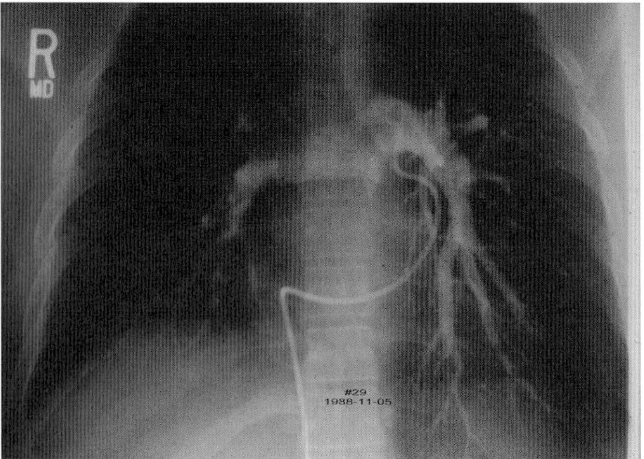

Figure 19.7 PA angiogram AP view 5 November 1988. Tip of catheter is in left PA.

7 Lung scans 27 October 1988 and 8 November 1988

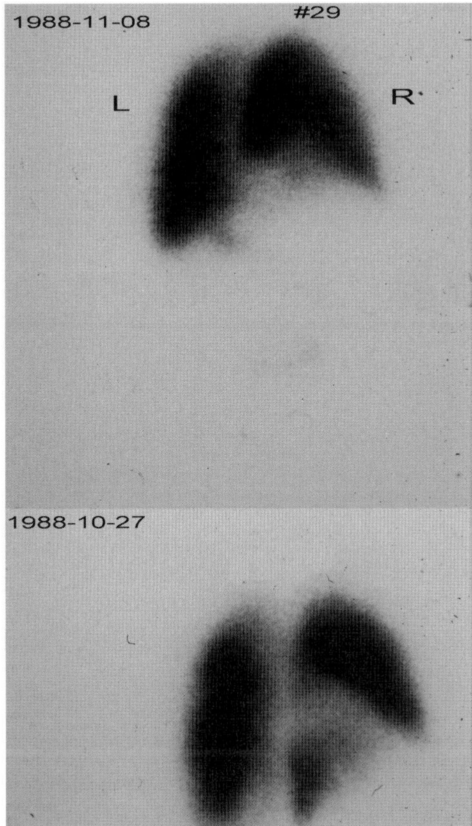

Figure 19.8 Lungs scans 27 October and 8 November 1988.

8 History

25-year-old man admitted to hospital with hemoptysis for one day (~500 mL in 24 h).
No history of chest or leg pain.
He had traveled recently from Pakistan on a 16-h flight under cramped conditions.
One year ago a chest X ray was normal.

9 Physical examination

5 foot 7 inches tall, 160 lb male. BP 110/70. HR 90/min regular. RR 28/min. Temperature normal.
No elevation of jugular venous pressure. Normal carotid upstroke.
Apex beat 5th interspace, 7 cm from mid-sternal line.
S1 normal. S2 normal. No murmurs.
Lungs clear to percussion and auscultation.
No edema, cyanosis, or clubbing.

10 Diagnosis and treatment

On 4 November he developed RLL consolidation and fever.

What is your diagnosis and proposed treatment?

11 Follow-up chest X rays 27 October, 1 November, and 15 November 1988

Comment on the serial chest X rays shown in Figure 19.9.

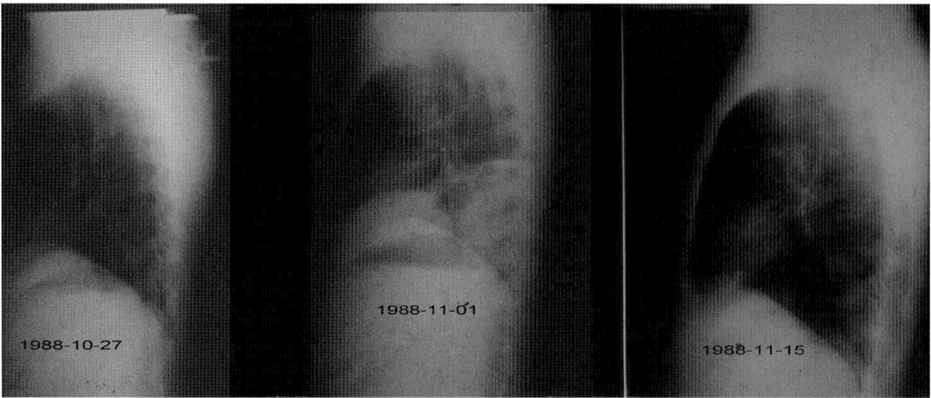

Figure 19.9 Sequential lateral chest X rays taken on 27 October, 1 November, and 15 November.

Answers and commentary

1 Chest X ray 27 October 1988

The heart size is normal. Right diaphragm is slightly elevated. Lung fields are clear.

2 12-lead ECG 27 October 1988

The rhythm is sinus. Rate 77/min. PR interval 0.16 s. QRS 0.05 s. QRS axis +40°.
Impression: normal ECG.

3 Laboratory data

A normal echocardiogram also rules out any RVH. The negative TB skin test makes TB an unlikely cause of hemoptysis in an otherwise healthy man.

4 Lung scan 27 October 1988

There is a segmental perfusion defect in right lower zone of lung field. This is suggestive of a pulmonary embolism as the corresponding chest X ray showed no abnormalities.

5 Follow-up chest X rays 27 October 1988 and 1 November 1988

1 November 1988

The right lower lung zone shows consolidation best seen in Figures 19.4 and 19.5. The absence of an air bronchogram within the area of consolidation makes it less likely that this is a pneumonia [1].

1 November 1988

Figures 19.4 and 19.5 show a consolidated area with a rounded upper edge that is often seen in pulmonary infarction and is referred to as Hampton's hump [2].

6 Angiogram 5 November 1988

The tip of the PA catheter is in the left PA, which could account for underfilling of the right lung. There may be some filling defects in the RLL artery due to clots. No PA pressures were measured prior to angiography.

7 Lung scans 27 October 1988 and 8 November 1988

The scan for 8 November shows a more extensive perfusion defect area in RLL as compared to the scan for 27 October, corresponding to the consolidation seen on 8 November.

8 History

The patient was admitted to hospital with hemoptysis. He had developed a leg clot and subsequent pulmonary embolism whilst travelling for 16 h by air in cramped quarters (economy class syndrome) [3].

9 Physical examination

Initially he had only a tachypnea without evidence of RV dysfunction. Four days after admission he developed RLL consolidation due to an extensive pulmonary infarct.

10 Diagnosis and treatment

Pulmonary embolism.
Pulmonary infarction.
He received intravenous heparin and oxygen.

11 Follow-up chest X rays 27 October, 1 November, and 15 November 1988

There has been a regression of RLL consolidation with better lung perfusion seen on 15 November as compared to 1 November.

He initially improved on heparin and oxygen, but on 4 November he developed hemoptysis and fever. He was continued on IV heparin and showed gradual clinical and radiographic improvement. He was discharged on warfarin. He was lost to follow-up.

Discussion

The patient had economy class syndrome or traveler's thrombosis [3–5]. Passengers traveling on long air flights have an increased tendency to develop blood clots in the legs, with subsequent pulmonary embolism [4].

Table 19.1 Economy class syndrome showing incidence of pulmonary embolism to the number of air miles travelled [4]

Economy Class syndrome	
Miles travelled	**Incidence of pulmonary embolism/ million**
<3100	0.01
>3100	1.5
>6200	4.8

Ref. Lapostolle et al. New.Eng J. Med 2001;345:779–783

Prolonged immobilization, dehydration, and excessive use of alcohol may be factors that contribute to venous stasis in the legs. In addition air travel may decrease fibrinolytic activity because of low air pressure and relative hypoxemia [5].

Patients who are obese, have had a prior venous thromboembolism, or a recent history of surgery or lower extremity fracture are at an additional risk of developing traveler's thrombosis [5].

This patient had a right lower lobe consolidation without an air bronchogram, which is in favor of a pulmonary infarction, as an air bronchogram is rarely seen in a pulmonary infarction [1].

A pulmonary infarction may be shaped like a truncated cone but has a wide variety of shapes when viewed in the PA and lateral chest X rays [2]. Usually one or more sides are pleural based with a convex or hump-shaped cardiac margin. The long axis of the infarct is always parallel to the longest pleural surface involved [2]. In our patient the long axis of the infarct paralleled the diaphragmatic surface.

As the infarct resolved within a few days there probably was little or no alveolar wall destruction (incomplete pulmonary infarction) [2].

Alveolar wall destruction is seen in a complete pulmonary infarct, which may take 2–5 weeks to resolve [2,6]. A resolving pulmonary infarct tends to retain its shape as it shrinks in size (melting sign) [7], in contrast to a pneumonic area, which is apt to clear in small patches. A pleural effusion is seen in 40% of patients with a pulmonary infarction [2] but was not seen in this patient.

A spiral CT of the chest would now be the preferred method of diagnosing a pulmonary embolism [8,9].

Key points

1. The patient developed a pulmonary embolism and infarction after a prolonged air flight in cramped quarters (economy class syndrome).

2. Economy class syndrome is more likely to develop in flights over 6000 miles long, but the incidence of pulmonary embolism is quite low.
3. The chest X ray in a patient with a pulmonary infarct may show an area of consolidation without an air bronchogram. Hampton's hump is also a feature suggesting a pulmonary infarction.
4. Spiral CT of the chest is now the method of choice (but was not available in 1988) to diagnose a pulmonary embolism.

References

[1] Bachynski JE. Absence of the air bronchogram sign. A reliable finding in pulmonary embolism with infarction or hemorrhage. *Radiology* 1971; 100: 547–552.
[2] Hampton AO, Castleman B. Correlation of postmortem chest teleroentgenograms with autopsy findings. With special reference to pulmonary embolism and infarction. *Am J Roentgenol* 1940; 43: 305–326 (400 cases studied, 21 figures).
[3] Cruickshank JM, Gorlin R, Jennett B. Air travel and thrombotic episodes: the economy class syndrome. *Lancet* 1988; 2: 497–498.
[4] Lapostolle F, Surget V, Borron SW et al. Severe pulmonary embolism associated with air travel. *N Engl J Med* 2001; 345: 779–783.
[5] O'Keefe DJ, Baglin TP. Traveller's thrombosis and economy class syndrome: incidence, aetiology and prevention. *Clin Lab Haem* 2003; 25: 277–281.
[6] Wolfe MW, Skibo LK, Goldhaber SZ. Pulmonary embolic disease: diagnosis, pathophysiologic aspects, and treatment with thrombolytic therapy. *Curr Probl Cardiol* 1993; 18: 585–636.
[7] Woesner ME, Sanders I, White GW. The melting sign in resolving transient pulmonary infarction. *Am J Roentgenol* 1971; 111: 782–790.
[8] Schoepf UJ, Golhaber SZ, Costello P. Spiral computed tomography for acute pulmonary embolism. *Circulation* 2004; 109: 2160–2167.
[9] Stein PD, Matta F. Acute pulmonary embolism. *Curr Probl Cardiol* 2010; 35: 312–376 (207 references).

20 PATIENT STUDY 20

Sequence of data presentation

1 Chest X ray 31 August 1998
↓
2 12-lead ECG 31 August 1998
↓
3 Echocardiogram 31 August 1998
↓
4 Lung scan 31 August 1998
↓
5 Lung scan 5 September 1998
↓
6 ECG follow-up 8 September 1998
↓
7 CT of chest 8 September 1998
↓
8 Admission history, physical examination, and laboratory data 31 August 1998
↓
9 Diagnosis and treatment
↓
10 Lung scan 14 September 1998
↓
11 CT of chest follow-up 19 September 1998
↓
12 Course 14 September 1998 to 9 December 1998

1 Chest X ray 31 August 1998

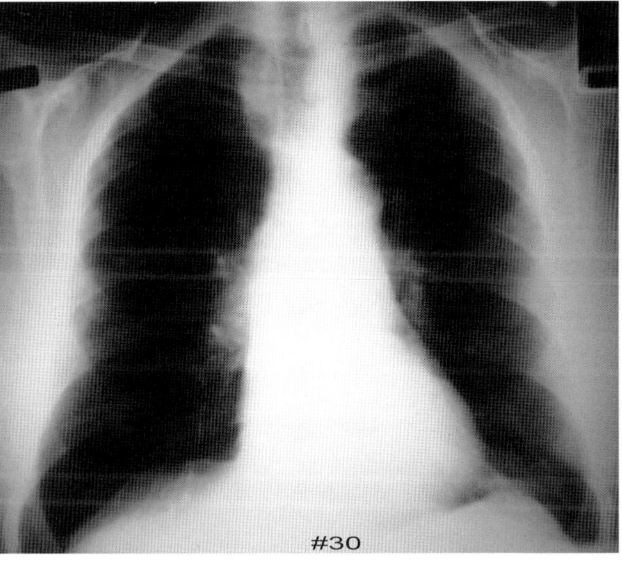

Figure 20.1 PA view of chest X ray 31 August 1998.

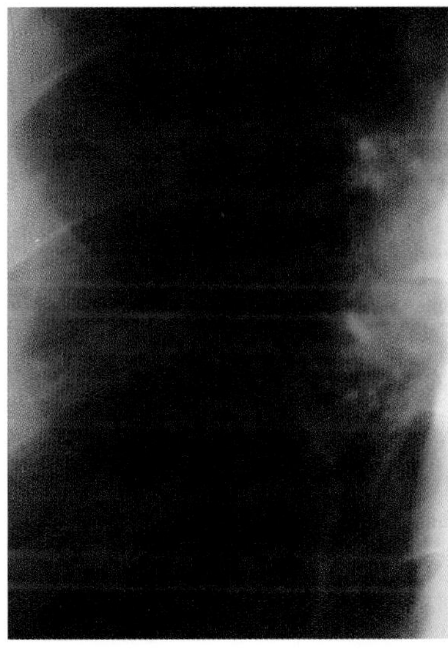

Figure 20.2 Right lung X ray 31 August 1998.

Patient Studies in Valvular, Congenital, and Rarer Forms of Cardiovascular Disease: An Integrative Approach, First Edition. Franklin B. Saksena.

Companion Website: www.wiley.com/go/saksena/patientstudies

2 12-lead ECG 31 August 1998

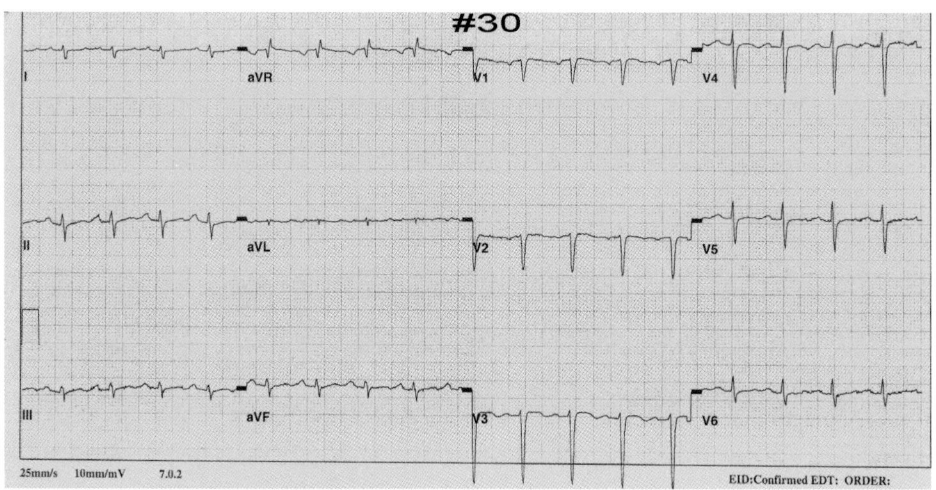

Figure 20.3 12-lead ECG 31 August 1998.

3 Echocardiogram 31 August 1998

Table 20.1 Two-dimensional echocardiographic dimensions 31 August 1998

Site	Measurement (cm)	Normal values (cm)
Aortic valve excursion	1.8	>1.6
Aortic root dimension	3.6	2.0–3.7
LA dimension	3.6	1.9–3.6
RV dimension	2.7	0.7–2.0
RA	>4.9	3.4–4.9
LV septal thickness	1.3	0.7–1.2
LV posterior wall thickness	1.0	0.8–1.1
LV end-diastolic dimension	4.5	3.5–5.8
LV end-systolic dimension	2.4	3.1–4.6
Tricuspid valve regurgitant velocity	3 m/s	

Calculate the RV systolic pressure.

4 Lung scan 31 August 1998

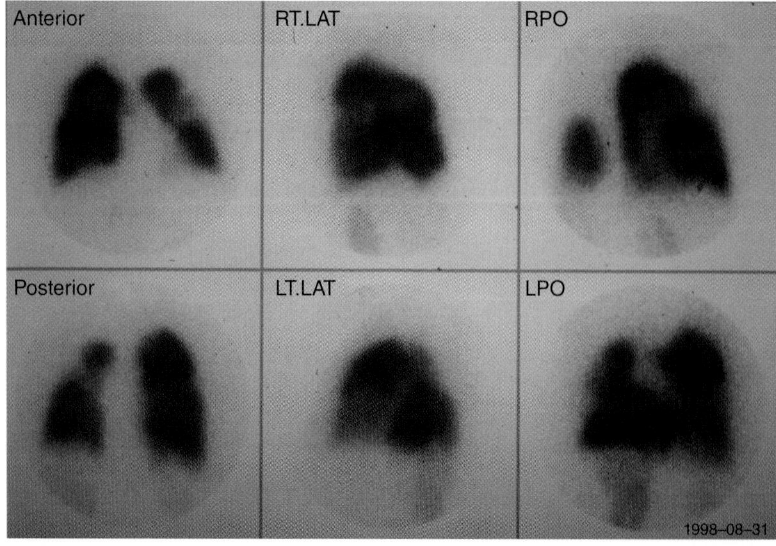

Figure 20.4 Perfusion lung scan (six views) 31 August 1998.

5 Lung scan 5 September 1998

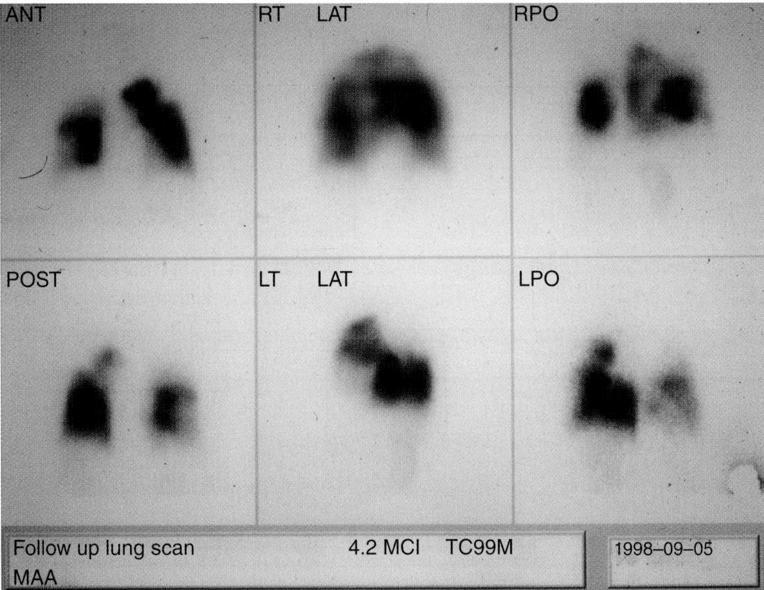

Figure 20.5 Follow-up perfusion lung scan 5 September 1998.

6 ECG follow-up 8 September 1998

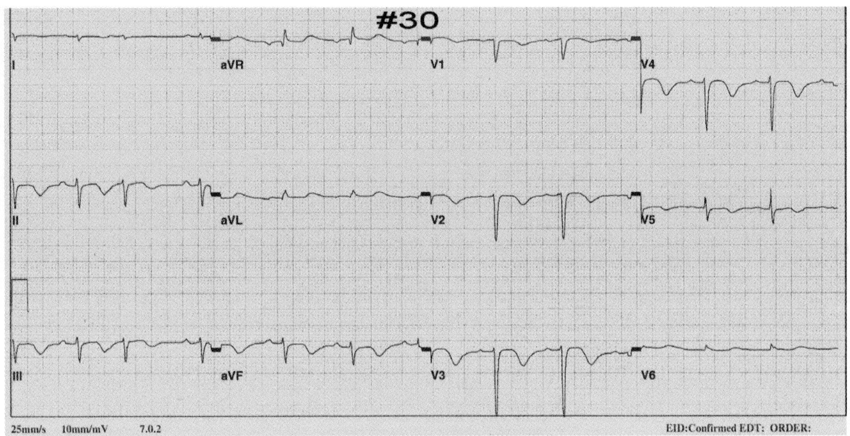

Figure 20.6 12-lead ECG 8 September 1998.

7 CT of chest 8 September 1998

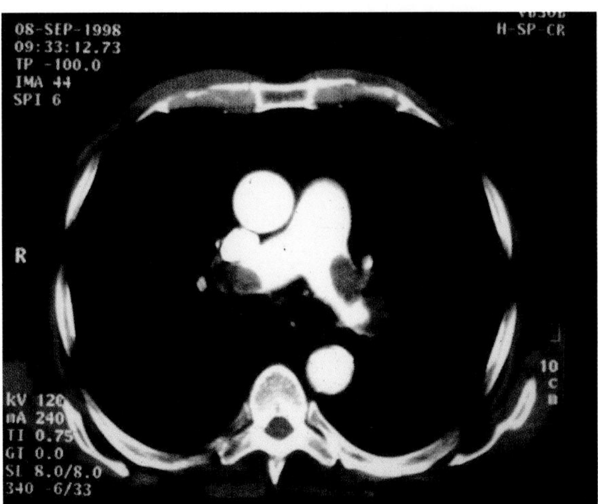

Figure 20.7 Spiral CT of chest at about T 7 level.

8 Admission history, physical examination, and laboratory data 31 August 1998

History

80 year old man admitted to hospital with dyspnea and hemoptysis. No chest pain.
He has a past history of smoking, hypertension, and a transient ischemic episode.

Physical examination

Patient is 70 inches tall and weighs 195 lb. BP 169/97. HR 103/min. Regular rhythm.
No elevation of jugular venous pressure.
No cardiomegaly. S1 normal. S2 normal. No murmurs or S3.
Lungs clear.
Normal peripheral pulses. No leg edema.

Laboratory data

Hemoglobin 13.3 g%. Platelet count 144,000/mm^3.
pO_2 was 94 mmHg on 28% oxygen via nasal cannula. Normal troponin levels.

9 Diagnosis and treatment

What is the diagnosis and treatment for this patient?

10 Lung scan 14 September 1998

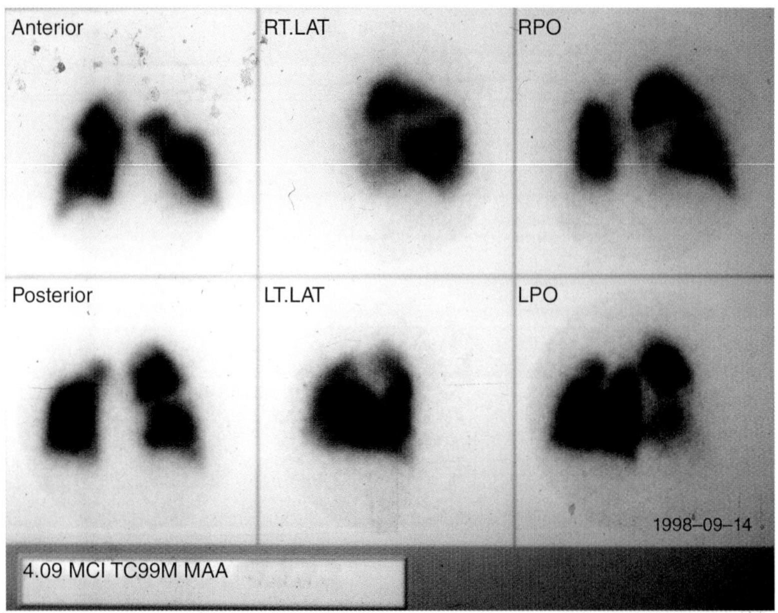

Figure 20.8 Follow-up perfusion lung scan 14 September 1998.

11 CT of chest follow-up 19 September 1998

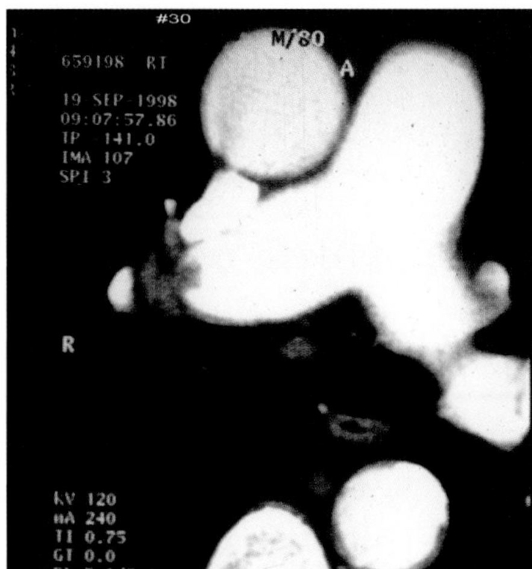

Figure 20.9 Spiral CT of chest 19 September 1998.

12 Course 14 September 1998 to 9 December 1998

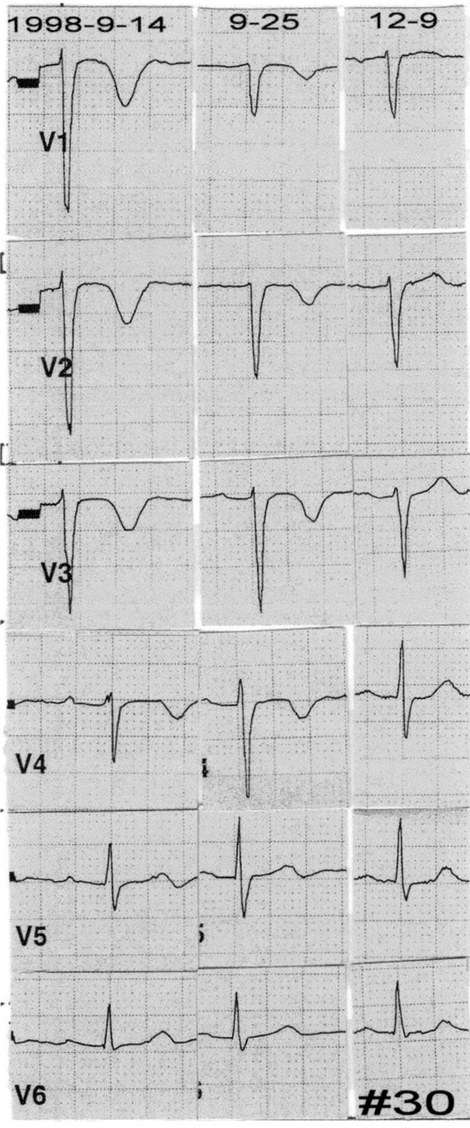

Figure 20.10 Serial ECGS (V1–6 leads) 14 September 1998, 25 September 1998, and 9 December 1998.

Answers and commentary

1 Chest X ray 31 August 1998

There is no cardiomegaly. There may be some pulmonary hypertension based on the prominence of the proximal pulmonary arteries and paucity of vessels in the lung fields, but the latter needs to be interpreted cautiously as the 'dark lung fields' may be simply due to an overexposed X ray.

The right upper mediastinal shadow confluent with the cardiac silhouette is probably due to an ectatic right subclavian artery.

In Figure 20.2 the right lung field is free of infiltrates, and shows a prominent right hilum and a paucity of peripheral blood vessels.

2 12-lead ECG 31 August 1998

The rhythm is sinus. Rate 103/min. PR 0.19 s. QRS 0.09 s. QRS axis +210°.

Poor R wave progression V1–3. Deep S wave in V5. Low or biphasic T wave abnormalities in 2,3,F and V1–6.

Impression: (i) sinus tachycardia, (ii) probable RVH on the basis of marked right-axis deviation and deep S in lateral leads, (iii) nonspecific T wave abnormalities, (iv) possible pseudo-infarction pattern in anterior precordial leads.

3 Echocardiogram 31 August 1998

The RV and RA are enlarged. Normal LV size. The calculated RV systolic pressure is 46 mmHg (RV systolic pressure $= 10 + 4v^2$, where 10 mmHg is the assumed RA mean pressure and v is the peak velocity across the tricuspid valve, which in this case is 3 m/s).

Thus there is evidence of pulmonary hypertension and RV dysfunction on the basis of all of the above findings.

4 Lung scan 31 August 1998

There are perfusion defects in the left upper lobe and possibly right upper lung.

5 Lung scan 5 September 1998

There is now absence of perfusion of upper half of the right lung with an increase in the left upper lobe defect. A new defect is seen in the right lower lobe.

These lung scans are diagnostic of extensive bilateral pulmonary emboli.

6 ECG follow-up 5 September 1998

1 The rhythm is sinus with a rare premature atrial contraction. Rate 70/min. PR 0.20 s. QRS 0.09 s. QRS axis +270°. T is now deeply inverted in V2–6 as well as 2, 3, F. Poor R wave progression V1–3.

Impression: (i) sinus rhythm with rare PAC, (ii) marked left-axis or right-axis deviation, (iii) anterior and inferior wall ischemia, (iv) possible pseudo-infarction pattern in anterior leads.

2 Compared to 31 August the rate has slowed from 103 to 70/min and the QRS axis has increased from 210 to 270°, with new evidence of anterior and inferior wall ischemia/necrosis.

7 CT of chest 8 September 1998

There are filling defects close to the origin of the right and left pulmonary branches of the main PA. The ascending aorta and the descending aorta are unremarkable. The paucity of the vessels in the peripheral lung fields suggests pulmonary emphysema.

Not shown in Figure 20.7 are additional filling defects in both lung fields close to the hilum and that there were no blood clots seen in the IVC.

Impression: (i) extensive bilateral pulmonary embolization, (ii) emphysema.

8 History, physical examination, and laboratory data 31 August 1998

The patient was admitted with dyspnea with no apparent evidence of left heart failure.

Hemoptysis would suggest some underlying lung disease. Laboratory data showed evidence of hypoxemia as the pO_2 should have risen to >300 mmHg on 28% oxygen via nasal cannula. The patient's hypoxemia may have been due to underlying lung disease such as emphysema or pulmonary embolism.

Thus far none of the above findings are diagnostic of pulmonary embolism.

9 Diagnosis and treatment

With the addition of ECG, echocardiogram, lung scans and CT of the chest the diagnosis of pulmonary embolism was established.

The patient was started on heparin and oxygen on 31 August. In addition, he received an infusion of t-PA from 8 to 11 September because he continued to have evidence of pulmonary emboli on lung scan while on warfarin. CT of the chest confirmed that he had very extensive peripheral and central pulmonary emboli.

10 Lungs scan 14 September 1998

There is marked improvement of the perfusion in the right upper lobe.

Some improvement in perfusion is also seen in the right lower lobe, left upper and left lower lobes. Bilateral segmental defects still persist.

Impression: resolving pulmonary emboli.

11 CT of chest follow-up 19 September 1998

There is almost complete resolution of pulmonary emboli in the left and right PAs.

12 Course 14 September 1998 to 9 December 1998

The patient was given warfarin and sent home symptomatically improved on 19 September 1998.

Serial ECGs showed gradual regression of the ischemic-like anterior T wave changes over the next 3 months. These ischemic-like T wave changes are often seen in patients with submassive pulmonary embolism and their slow disappearance rate is an adverse prognostic sign [1]. The mechanism of these T wave changes remains obscure as RV ischemia does not appear to be a factor [2].

Discussion

CT pulmonary angiography or spiral CT became available in the early 1990s. Spiral CT produces a two-dimensional image of the chest by rotating a detector around the chest in less than 30 s per imaging slice [3]. This single slice method was useful in detecting pulmonary embolism in the main PAs and its interlobar branches but less sensitive in detecting clots in the subsegmental vessels [5]. The multi-slice technique became available in the late 1990s and allowed better visualization of the clots in the subsegmental arteries [4].

Since 2006 multi-slice CT angiography has become the most commonly used imaging modality for diagnosing pulmonary embolism [2], so that there is now much less need to do lung scanning or catheter pulmonary angiography.

Pulmonary embolism is usually treated with heparin, reserving t-PA for patients with severe hypoxemia or shock [2,3,5] or who have thrombi in the right heart [6]. t-PA was used in this patient because he continued to have pulmonary emboli on warfarin and had a significant embolic load on chest CT.

Key points

1. Spiral CT angiography is the method of choice in diagnosing a pulmonary embolism and assessing the efficacy of therapy.
2. Fibrinolyic therapy for pulmonary embolism has a role if the patient continues to have pulmonary emboli on warfarin and has a large embolic load.
3. Persistent negative T wave abnormalities in the precordial leads following a submassive pulmonary embolism is an adverse prognostic sign.

References

[1] Ferrari E, Imbert A, Chevalier T et al. The ECG in pulmonary embolism. Predictive value of negative T waves in precordial leads – 80 case reports. *Chest* 1997; 111: 537–543.

[2] Stein PD, Matta F. Acute pulmonary embolism. *Curr Probl Cardiol* 2010; 35: 309–376.

[3] Rahimtoola A, Bergin JD. Acute pulmonary embolism: An update on diagnosis and management. *Curr Probl Cardiol* 2005; 30: 55–114.

[4] Remy-Jardin M, Remy J, Mayo JR et al. *CT angiography of the chest*. Lippincott Williams and Wilkins, Philadelphia, 2001, pp 51–66.

[5] Dalen JE. The uncertain role of thrombolytic therapy in the treatment of pulmonary embolism. *Arch Int Med* 2002; 162: 2521–2523.

[6] Fedullo PF. *Pulmonary embolism*. In: Hurst's The Heart, 13th edn. Fuster V, Walsh RA, Harrington R (eds). McGraw Hill, New York, 2011.

Further reading

Schoepf UJ, Goldhaber SZ, Costello P. Spiral computed tomography for acute pulmonary embolism. *Circulation* 2004; 109: 2160–2167.

21 PATIENT STUDY 21

Sequence of data presentation

1 ECG
↓
2 Chest X rays
↓
3 Hands
↓
4 Phonocardiogram
↓
5 Oxygen saturation sample run
↓
6 Pressures
↓
7 RV–PA pressures
↓
8 RV and aortic pressures
↓
9 Echocardiogram
↓
10 LV angiogram
↓
11 Pulmonary angiograms
↓
12 RV angiograms
↓
13 Diagnosis
↓
14 History
↓
15 Physical examination
↓
16 Laboratory data and additional angiographic data

1 ECG

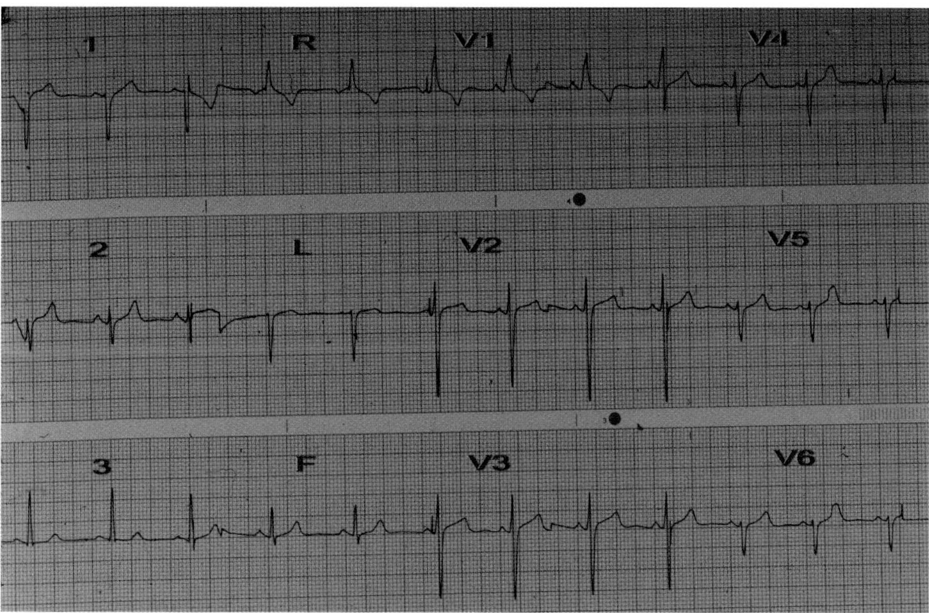

Figure 21.1 ECG 1989.

Patient Studies in Valvular, Congenital, and Rarer Forms of Cardiovascular Disease: An Integrative Approach, First Edition. Franklin B. Saksena.

Companion Website: www.wiley.com/go/saksena/patientstudies

2 Chest X rays

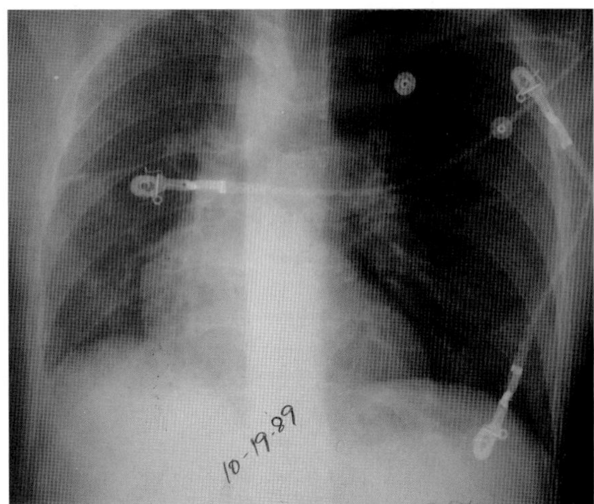

Figure 21.2 Chest X ray PA view 1989.

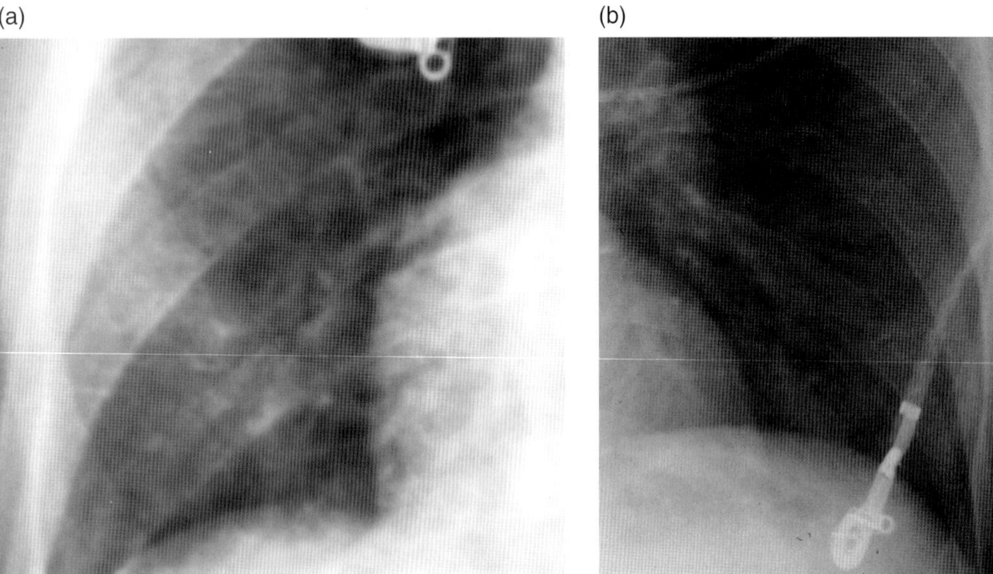

Figure 21.3 (a) Right lung field 1989. (b) Left lung field 1989.

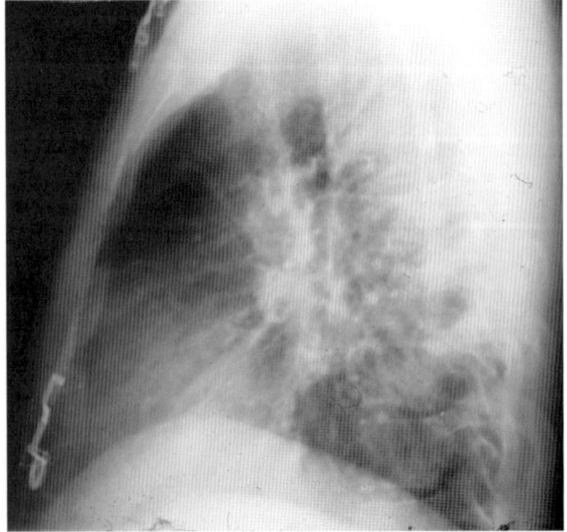

Figure 21.4 Lateral view of chest X ray 1989.

3 Hands

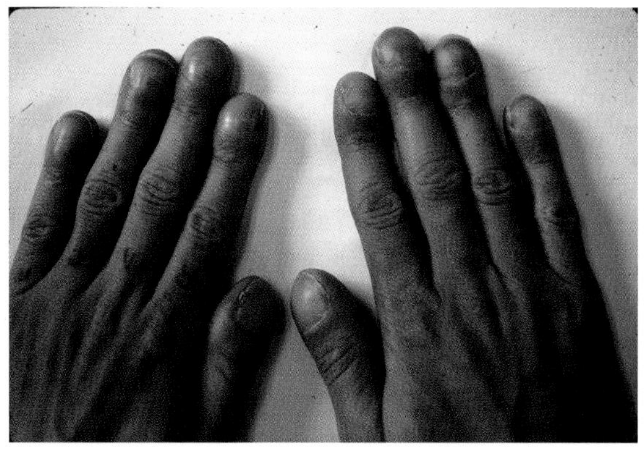

Figure 21.5 Hands.

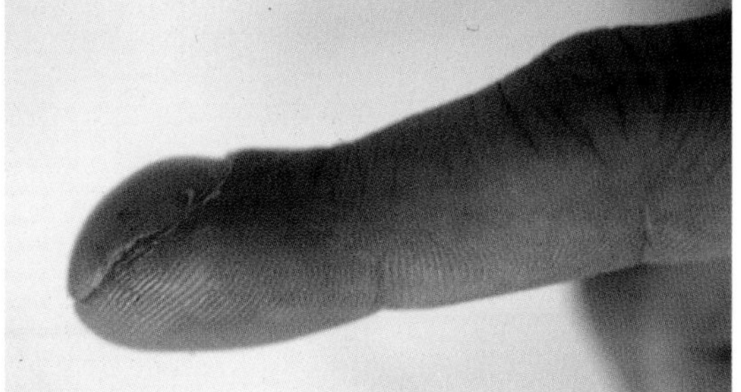

Figure 21.6 Lateral view of finger.

4 Phonocardiogram

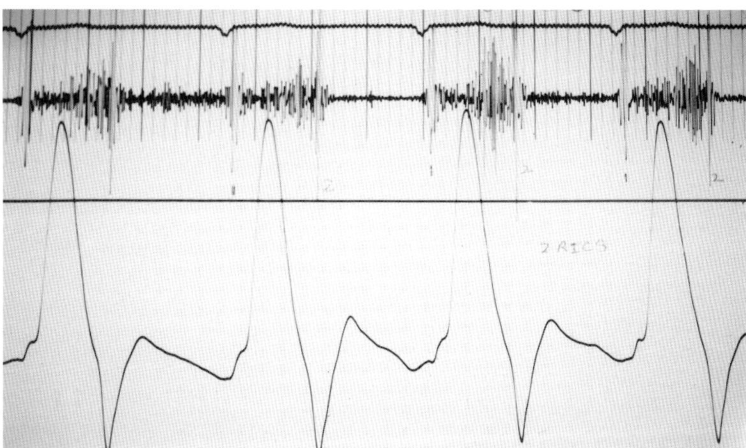

Figure 21.7 Phonocardiogram.

5 Oxygen saturation sample run

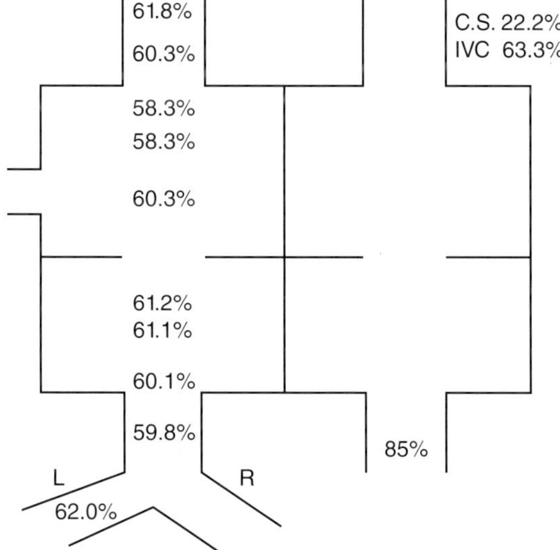

Figure 21.8 Oxygen saturation sample run.

Calculate the pulmonary and systemic blood flow given hemoglobin is 21.4 g% and oxygen consumption is 284 mL/min.

6 Pressures

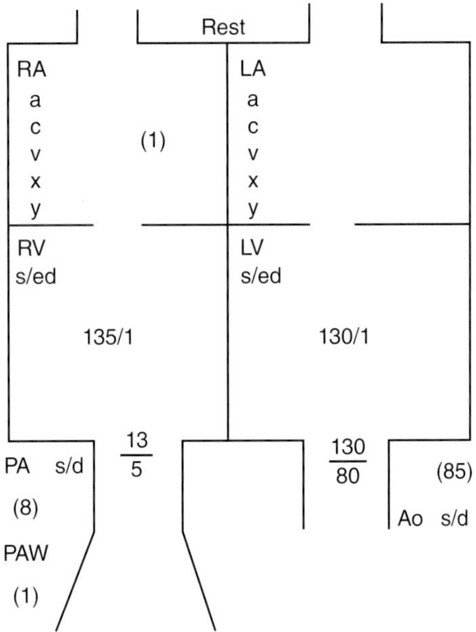

Figure 21.9 Intracardiac pressures.

7 RV–PA pressures

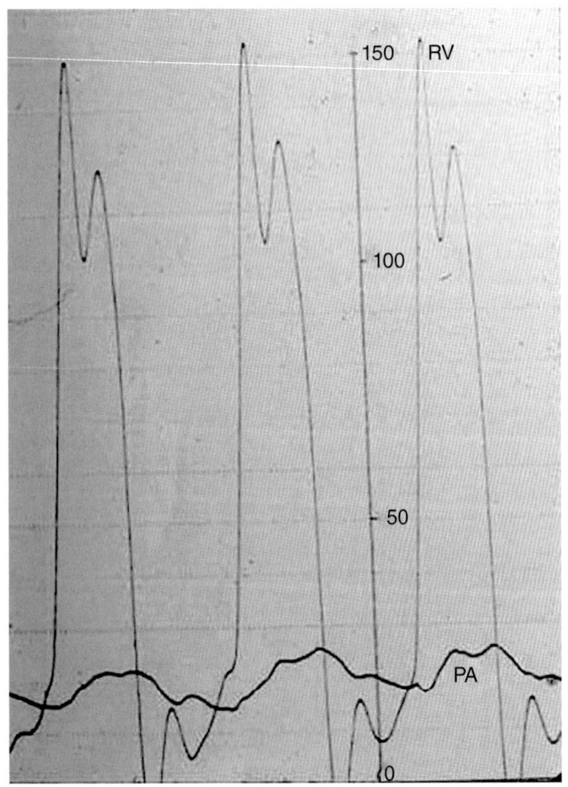

Figure 21.10 Simultaneous RV and PA pressures. 0–150 mmHg scale.

8 RV and aortic pressures

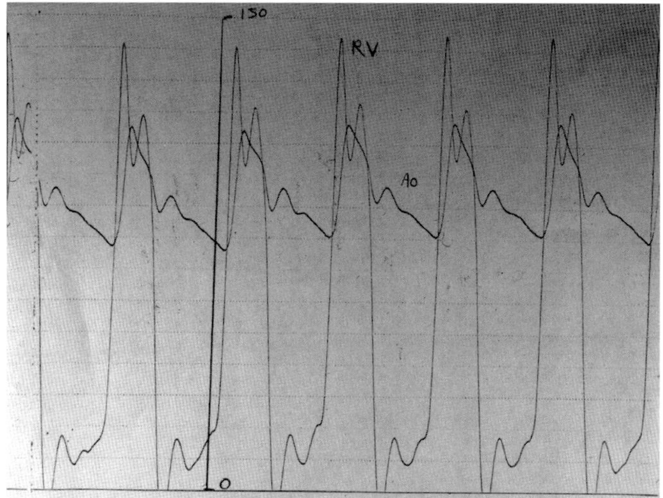

Figure 21.11 Simultaneous RV and aortic pressures. 0–150 mmHg scale.

9 Echocardiogram

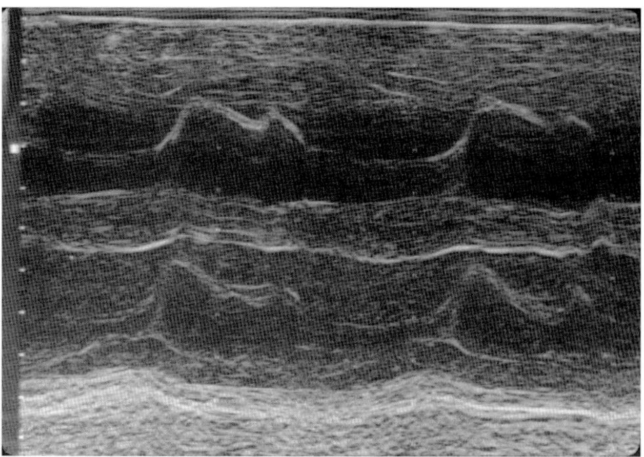

Figure 21.12 M-mode echocardiogram showing tricuspid and mitral valves. Two-dimensional echocardiogram (not shown) revealed a VSD with bidirectional flow.

10 LV angiography

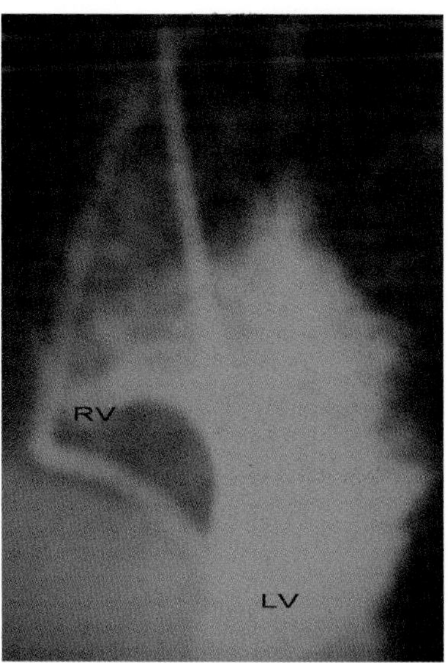

Figure 21.13 LV angiography in 60° LAO view.

11 Pulmonary angiograms

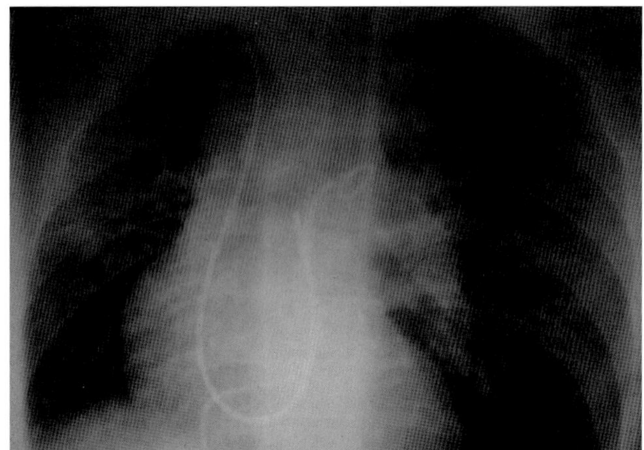

Figure 21.14 PA angiogram (pre-injection).

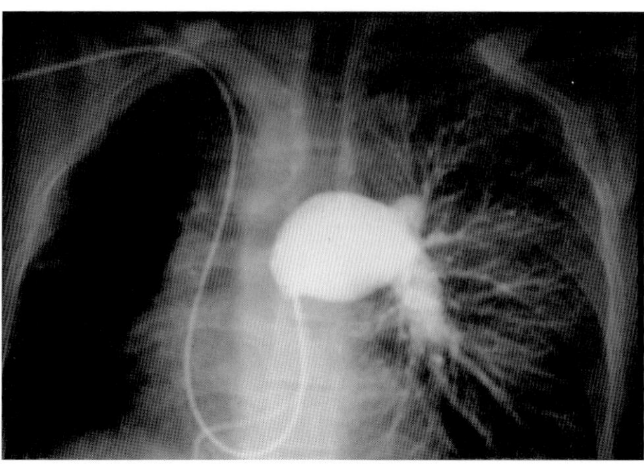

Figure 21.15 PA angiogram (arterial phase).

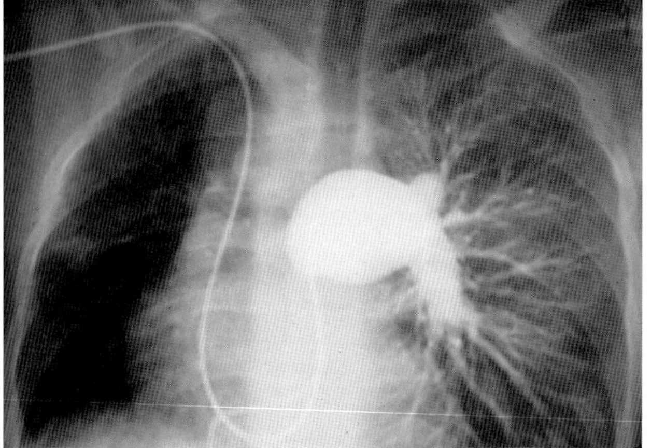

Figure 21.16 PA angiogram (late arterial phase).

12 RV angiograms

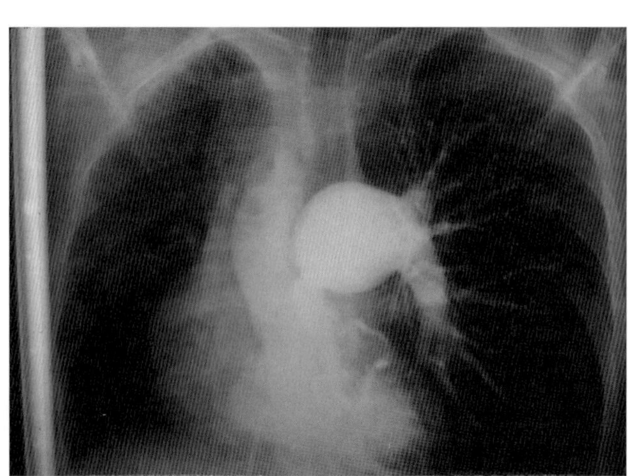

Figure 21.17 RV angiogram AP view.

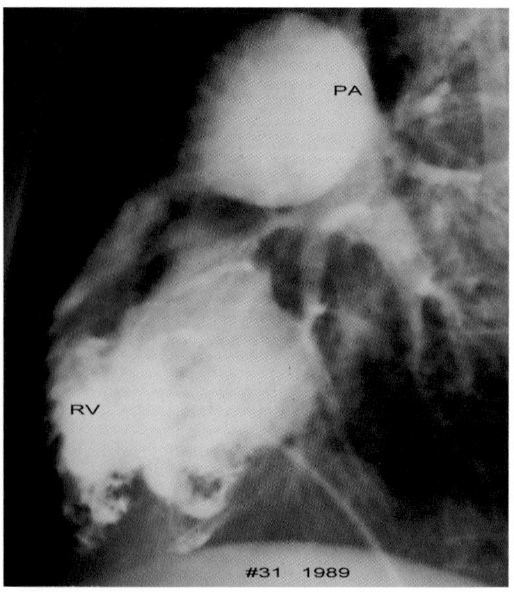

Figure 21.18 RV angiogram lateral view.

13 Diagnosis

What is the diagnosis?

14 History

21-year-old man admitted to hospital with hemoptysis for one day. He had had an upper respiratory tract infection for the last 4 weeks. He had mild impairment of exercise tolerance He was diagnosed with a heart murmur at age of 16.

Patient does not drink, smoke, or use drugs. No history of rheumatic fever.

15 Physical examination

66 inches tall, 130 lb. The patient had flushed cheeks and dark red conjunctiva.

Cardiovascular system: 4+ clubbing with cyanosis.

No elevation of jugular venous pressure. Normal carotid upstroke.

Apex beat was in the 5th intercostal space, 8 cm from the mid-sternal line. No left parasternal lift.

There was a systolic thrill at RUSB.

S1 normal. S2 normal. No S3 or S4.

Grade 3/6 diamond-shaped systolic murmur maximum at LLSB, radiating to left second interspace and right second interspace parasternally.

No leg edema.

Respiratory system.

Normal percussion note bilaterally.

The breath sounds were diminished on the right side compared to the left side.

Vocal fremitus equal bilaterally.

Abdominal exam and CNS exams were normal.

16 Laboratory data and additional angiographic data

Hemoglobin 21.4 g%. Hematocrit 63%. WBC 6800/mm^3. Platelets 229,000/cu mm.

PPD skin test positive. Sputum negative for acid fast bacillus on three successive occasions.

Oxygen consumption 284 mL/min.

Normal aortic and selective coronary angiography.

Normal LV volumes and LV ejection fraction.

Answers and commentary

1 ECG

The rhythm is sinus with a rate of 75/min. PR interval 0.16 s. QRS interval 0.08 s.

QRS axis +120° R in V1 is 10 mm. Deep S in V5–6.

Impression: severe RVH.

2 Chest X rays

In Figure 21.2 the PA view of the chest shows shrinkage of the right lung volume. The heart is shifted to the right. There is a right-sided indentation of the trachea by a right-sided aorta. A right-sided aorta may be seen in **T**etralogy of Fallot in 13–34% of cases. It also occurs in persistent **T**runcus arteriosus, **T**ricuspid atresia and **T**ransposition of the great vessels in 36%, 8% and 5% of cases, respectively [1].

In Figure 21.3a and b the right lung field appears devoid of vasculature as compared to the left lung field.

Figure 21.4 shows possible RV enlargement in the lateral chest X ray.

3 Hands

There is advanced clubbing with cyanosis. The hyponychial angle is 180° and the subungal angle is 210°. There is subcuticular edema. While pulmonary disease is the most common cause of clubbing (80% of cases), cardiovascular causes comprise almost 20% of causes, usually right to left shunts [2].

4 Phonocardiogram

There is a crescendo systolic murmur recorded at the right 2nd interspace.

This murmur is due to pulmonic stenosis. The late peaking of the murmur indicates that the pulmonic stenosis is severe [3].

5 Oxygen saturation sample run

There is no step up in oxygen saturations in the right heart, making a left to right shunt less likely. There is arterial oxygen desaturation, which could be due to a right to left shunt assuming that there is no lung disease.

Calculation of the pulmonary blood flow (Q_p), systemic blood flow (Q_s), effective blood flow (Q_{ep}), right to left blood flow (Qr–l), and left to right blood flow (Ql–r).

Step 1 Calculate the total oxygen-carrying capacity of hemoglobin (Hb)

Total oxygen-carrying capacity of Hb = 1.34 × 21.4 g% = 28.67 mL/100 mL blood, i.e. 28.67 mL% ≡ 100% saturation.

Step 2 Convert the averaged oxygen saturations (%) to oxygen content (mL/100 mL blood)

RA content = (averaged saturations) × total Hb content = 0.59 × 28.67 = 16.91 mL%

PA content = (averaged saturations) × total Hb content = 0.61 × 28.67 = 17.5 mL%

Ao content = arterial saturation × total Hb content = 0.85 × 28.67 = 24.4 mL%

Pulmonary venous (PV) saturation in absence of lung disease is assumed to be 95%

∴PV content = 0.95 × 28.67 = 27.24 mL%

Step 3 Calculate Q_p, Q_s, and Q_{ep} using the Fick principle

$$\text{Blood flow (L/min)} = \frac{VO_2}{A - VO_2 \text{ difference}}$$

As the oxygen consumption is 284 mL/min we have:

$$Q_p = \frac{284}{10(27.24 - 17.5)} = 2.91 \text{ L/min}$$

$$Q_s = \frac{284}{10(24.4 - 16.91)} = 3.79 \text{ L/min}$$

$$Q_{ep} = \frac{284}{10(27.24 - 16.91)} = 2.75 \text{ L/min}$$

Step 4 Calculate the right to left shunt (Q_{r-l}) and the left to right shunt flow (Q_{l-r})

$$Q_{r-l} = Q_s - Q_{ep} = 3.79 - 2.75 = 1.04 \text{ L/min}$$
$$Q_{l-r} = Q_p - Q_{ep} = 2.91 - 2.75 = 0.16 \text{ L/min}$$

The net right to left shunt is 1.04 – 0.16 = 0.88 L/min

Alternatively, net right to left shunt = $Q_s - Q_p$, which also yields 0.88 L/min.

6 Pressures

There is a large peak-to-peak gradient of 122 mmHg across the pulmonic valve in systole, indicative of severe pulmonic stenosis. Using the Gorlin formula the pulmonary valve area is 0.25 cm^2.

Left heart pressures are normal.

7 RV–PA pressures

The PA pressure is damped and has a delayed upstroke compared to the RV pressure tracing.

There is a large pressure gradient between RV and PA. The RVEDP is within normal limits (1–5 mmHg).

8 RV and aortic pressures

These confirm that the RV systolic pressure exceeds the aortic pressure. The aortic pressure tracing is normal.

9 Echocardiogram

The RV is thickened. There is no dilatation of the RV or LV. The tricuspid and mitral valve echograms appear normal.

The two-dimensional echocardiography report showed a VSD with bidirectional flow.

10 LV angiography

LV angiography showed partial filling of the RV via a large subaortic VSD. The right to left shunt prevented complete filling of the RV despite the pressure injection of contrast material into the LV.

11 Pulmonary angiograms

The tip of the right heart catheter is centrally positioned in the PA prior to angiography (Figure 21.14).

The left PA is dilated (post stenotic dilatation) and its arterial branches are filling with contrast material. The right PA is absent (Figure 21.15).

Complete filling of only the left pulmonary arterial tree is now seen (Figure 21.16).

12 RV angiograms

In Figure 21.17 the RV is highly trabeculated. Contrast material is seen entering the huge left PA and the ascending aorta. The ascending aorta is indenting the right side of the trachea, as also noted on the plain chest X ray (Figure 21.1). The ascending aorta overrides the RV, which accounts for its prompt filling via RV angiography.

Figure 21.18 shows the lateral view of the RV with marked narrowing of the RV outflow tract and post-stenotic dilatation of the left PA.

13 Diagnosis

1. TOF with severe pulmonary stenosis, VSD, RVH, and overriding aorta.
2. Absent right PA.
3. Right-sided aortic arch.

14–16 History, physical examination, laboratory data, and additional angiographic data

The patient had polycythemia, cyanosis, and clubbing, suggesting a right to left shunt.

As indicated earlier the systolic murmur found on this patient is due to pulmonic stenosis rather than a VSD.

The reduced expansion of the right lung is because the right lung was hypoplastic. The absence of the right PA means that the blood supply of the right lung has to be obtained from aortopulmonary collaterals. In a subsequent study, a descending aortogram demonstrated such collaterals.

Coronary angiograms were normal and free of anomalies. The coronary arteries may rarely supply a hypoplastic right lung via collateral circulation [4] but this was not the case in this patient.

A normal aortogram excludes aortic regurgitation or a PDA.

Discussion

The patient had TOF on the basis of severe pulmonic stenosis, VSD, RV hypertrophy, and an overriding aorta.

An adult with advanced clubbing, cyanosis, and polycythemia has a high likelihood of having a TOF.

The severity of the pulmonic stenosis determines the degree of right to left shunting (see Figure 21.18).

As patients with pure pulmonic stenosis very rarely have a right-sided aortic arch, its presence should suggest a coexistent VSD [5].

Cardiac catheterization, and pulmonary and coronary angiography is required in TOF patients who are to undergo a complete repair as 10–15% will have associated findings such as an ASD, PA branch stenosis, or anomalous left anterior descending artery originating from the right coronary artery [6].

Untreated, 70–75% of patients with TOF die by the age of 10 [6, 7].

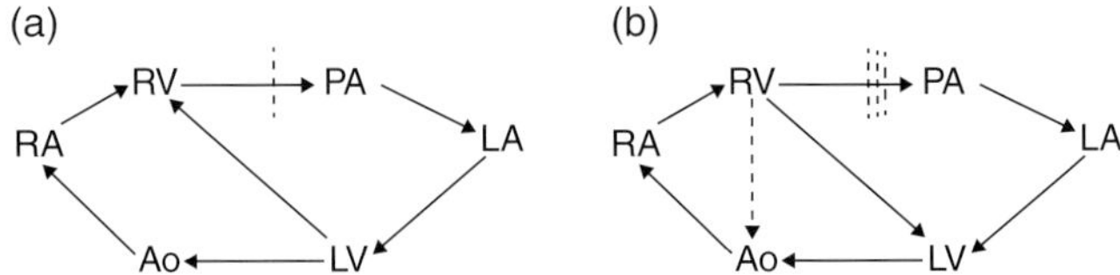

Figure 21.19 (a) Blood flow in a patient with mild pulmonic stenosis (denoted by a single line between RV and PA) and predominant left to right shunt at ventricular level (pink tetralogy). (b) Blood flow in a patient with severe pulmonic stenosis (denoted by a triple line between RV and PA) with predominant right to left shunt at ventricular level. Some blood will also flow from RV to the overriding aorta as in case study patient (blue tetralogy).

Surgical results of patients with TOF undergoing a complete repair have been good (86% survival in 36 years) [8]. A successful complete repair consists of complete closure of the VSD and relief of the RV outflow tract obstruction with minimal development of pulmonary regurgitation post operatively [7]. However, a palliative intervention has been recommended as a first step of surgical treatment in patients who have TOF with unilateral absence of the PA [9].

This patient was recommended for surgery but unfortunately was lost to follow-up.

An isolated absence of a PA is very rare (1 in 200,000) and may present with hemoptysis or pulmonary hypertension [10]. It is most often associated with TOF [11] and very rarely with an ASD [12] or an anomalous pulmonary venous return [13].

Key points

1. TOF consists of a VSD, pulmonic valvular or infundibular stenosis, overriding aorta, and RVH.
2. TOF is the most common form of cyanotic congenital heart disease.
3. The more severe the valvular or infundibular pulmonic stenosis in TOF the greater is the likelihood of a right to left shunt and the development of cyanosis (blue tetralogy).
4. A mild infundibular or valvular pulmonic stenosis in TOF may be associated with a left to right shunt without cyanosis (pink tetralogy).
5. Absence of the right PA is rare. It is often associated with TOF.
6. A right-sided aortic arch may be seen in TOF, truncus arteriosus, tricuspid atresia, or transposition of the great vessels.

References

[1] Hastreiter AR, D'Cruz IA, Cantez T et al. Right-sided aorta. I Occurrence of right aortic arch in various types of congenital heart disease. II Right descending aorta and associated anomalies. *Br Heart J* 1966; 28: 722–739.

[2] Coury C. Hippocratic fingers and hypertrophic osteoarthropathy. A study of 350 cases. *Br J Dis Chest* 1960; 54: 202–209.

[3] Zuberbuhler JR, Lenox CC, Neches WH et al. *Auscultatory spectrum of the Tetralogy of Fallot*. In: Physiologic principles of heart sounds and murmurs. American Heart Association Monograph No. 46, Leon DF, Shaver JA (eds). AHA, New York, 1975, pp 187–196.

[4] Gupta K, Livesay JJ, Lufschanowski R. Absent right pulmonary artery with coronary collaterals supplying the affected lung. *Circulation* 2001; 104: e12–e13.

[5] Wood P. *Right sided aorta*. In: Paul Wood's diseases of the heart and circulation, 3rd edn. Eyre and Spottiswoode, London, 1968, p 387.

[6] Foster E, Webb G, Human D et al. *The adult with Tetralogy of Fallot*. ACC Current Journal Review March/April 1998; 62–66 (contains a useful list of surgical procedures for tetralogy of Fallot).

[7] Gatzoulis MA. *Tetralogy of Fallot*. In: Diagnosis and Management of Adult Congenital Heart Disease, Gatzoulis MA, Webb GD, Daubney PEF (eds), Churchill Livingstone, Edinburgh, 2003, p 318.

[8] Nollert G, Fischlein T, Bouterwek S et al. Long term survival in patients with repair of Tetralogy of Fallot: 36 year follow-up of 490 survivors of the first year after surgical repair. *J Am Coll Cardiol* 1997; 30: 1374–1383.

[9] Bockeria LA, Podzolkov VP, Makhachev OA et al. Surgical correction of Tetralogy of Fallot with unilateral absence of pulmonary artery. *Ann Thorac Surg* 2007; 83: 613–618.

[10] Koga H, Hidaka T, Miyako K et al. Age related clinical characteristics of isolated congenital unilateral absence of a pulmonary artery. *Pediatr Cardiol* 2010; 8: 1186–1190.

[11] Reading DW, Oza U. Unilateral absence of a pulmonary artery: a rare disorder with variable presentation. *Proc* (Bayl Univ Med Cent) 2012; 25: 115–118.

[12] Orun UA, Yilmaz O, Bilici M et al. Congenital right pulmonary artery agenesis with atrial septal defect and pulmonary hypertension. *Congenit Heart Dis* 2012; 7: e6–e9.

[13] Binnetoglu K, Ayabakan C, Sarisoy O et al. Absence of the right pulmonary artery associated with a partial anomalous pulmonary venous connection. *Pediatr Cardiol* 2012; 33: 182–184.

22 PATIENT STUDY 22

Sequence of data presentation

1 History
↓
2 12-lead ECG 18 October 1992
↓
3 Angiograms
↓
4 Cardiac catheterization data
↓
5 Coronary angiography
↓
6 Physical examination
↓
7 Laboratory data
↓
8 Doppler pressure studies
↓
9 Diagnosis
↓
10 Course

1 History

23-year-old Hispanic female with 1 year history of exertional chest pain. She has also recently complained of dimming of vision and jaw claudication (1992). No history of hypertension, diabetes, or rheumatic fever.

2 ECG

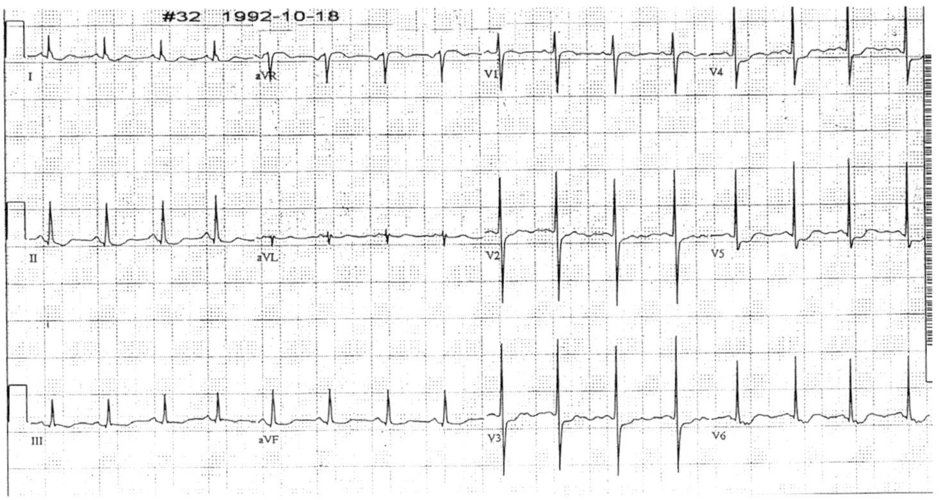

Figure 22.1 12-lead ECG 18 October 1992.

Patient Studies in Valvular, Congenital, and Rarer Forms of Cardiovascular Disease: An Integrative Approach, First Edition. Franklin B. Saksena.

Companion Website: www.wiley.com/go/saksena/patientstudies

3 Angiograms

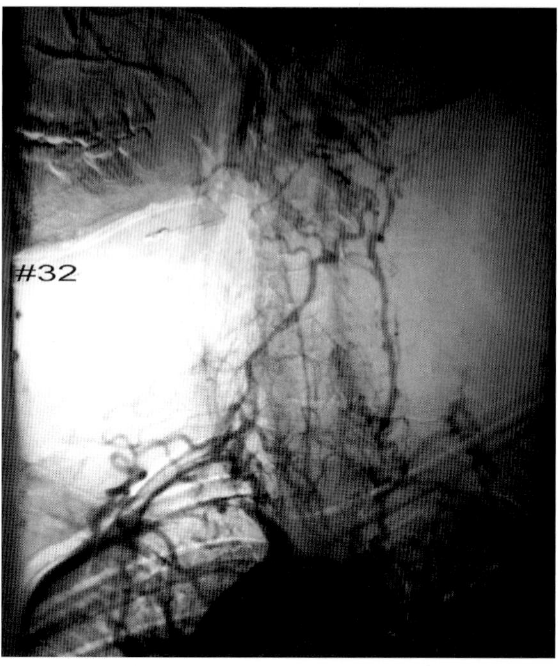

Figure 22.2 Aortic arch angiogram LAO view 18 October 1992.

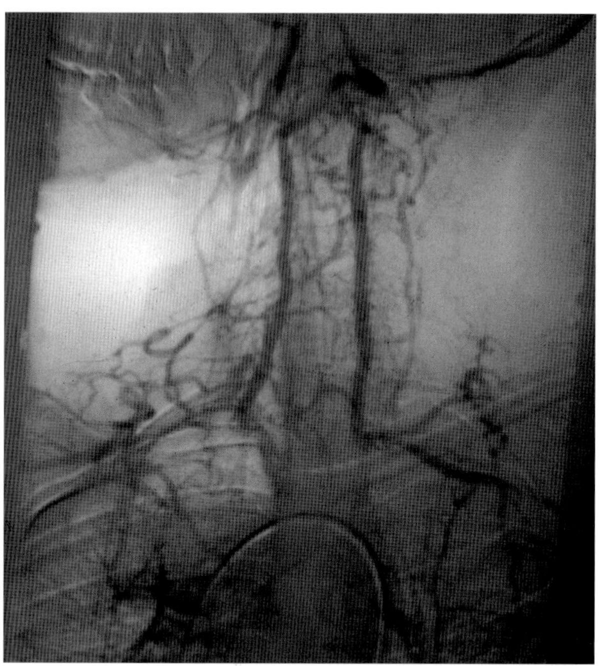

Figure 22.3 Aortic arch angiogram LAO view late phase 18 October 1992.

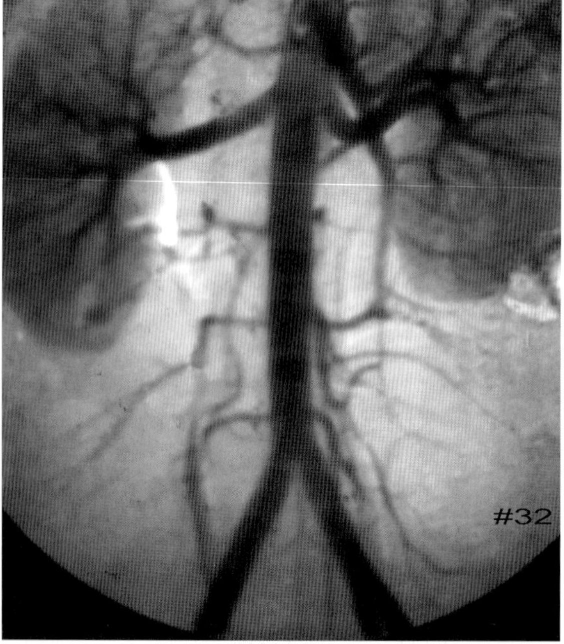

Figure 22.4 Abdominal aorta angiogram.

4 Cardiac catheterization data

Table 22.1 Cardiac catheterization data

Pulmonary artery wedge pressure	8 mmHg
Aortic pressure	140/80 mmHg
LV end-diastolic volume index	72 mL/m^2
LV ejection fraction	62%
Normal LV, pulmonary and abdominal angiograms	
Moderately severe aortic regurgitation	

5 Coronary angiography

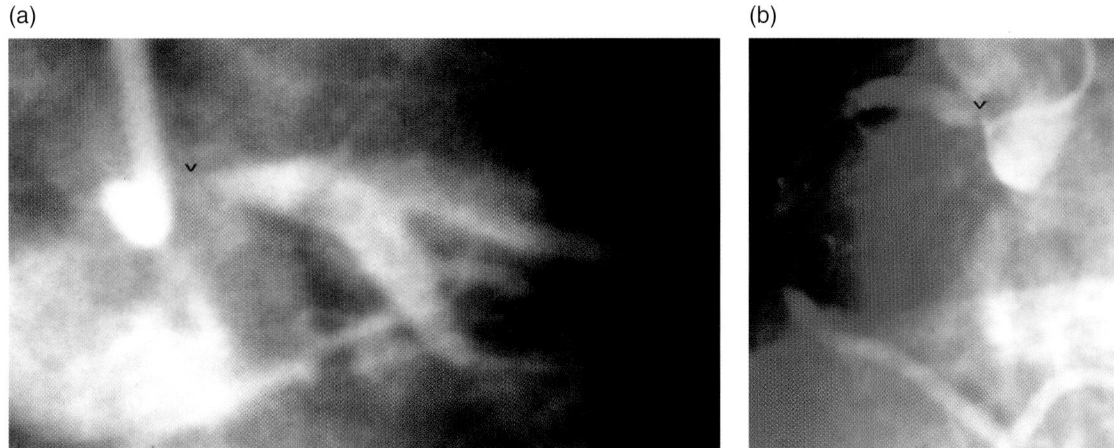

Figure 22.5 (a) Left coronary artery angiogram RAO view. (b) Right coronary artery angiogram LAO view.

What do the arrow heads point to?

6 Physical examination

The carotid pulses were impalpable. BP was not obtainable (right arm). HR 100/min.
No cardiomegaly or heart murmurs detected.

7 Laboratory data

Data on admission in October 1992: hemoglobin 11.9 gm%, normal WBC count, BUN 14 mg%, glucose 99 mg%.

8 Doppler pressure studies

Table 22.2 Doppler systolic pressure measurements in arms and legs (mmHg)

Arterial site	Right	Left
Brachial	50	47
Ulnar	42	52
Femoral	138	133
Posterior tibial	124	127
Toe	125	121

9 Diagnosis

What is the diagnosis?

10 Course

What is the course?

Answers and commentary

1 History

Anginal chest pain in a 23-year-old female is unlikely to be due to severe aortic stenosis or coronary artery disease. It may be seen if there is an anomalous coronary artery (e.g. arising from the PA), Kawasaki disease, or a vasculitis due to a collagen disease or involvement of the great vessels. In the absence of known diabetes the visual impairment and anginal chest pain could be caused by a vasculitis involving the heart and the eye.

Jaw claudication may be seen in occlusive arterial disease involving the temporal artery or the great vessels of the aorta.

2 12-lead ECG 18 October 1992

The rhythm is sinus with a rate of 100/min. PR interval 0.16 s. QRS 0.07 s. QRS axis +60°. There is ST depression in V3–6. Biphasic T in 2, 3, F. ST sagging in V6.

Impression: inferior and anterolateral ischemia.

On the basis of history and ECG there is evidence of myocardial ischemia. The absence of LVH or LAE makes valvular heart disease less likely. The other possibilities are listed in the history above.

3 Angiograms

The right innominate and left subclavian arteries are cut off close to their origin.

There is no filling of the right subclavian artery.

A few branches of these innominate and left subclavian arteries course to the head (Figure 22.2).

In Figure 22.3, as a result of bilateral subclavian occlusive disease, there is retrograde filling of the vertebral arteries into the distal arms (bilateral subclavian steal syndrome). In Figure 22.4 the abdominal aorta is normal with normal distal runoff.

4 Cardiac catheterization data

The PA wedge pressure is normal, implying a normal LVEDP. The aortic pressure shows borderline elevation in systolic pressure.

LV size and systolic function appear normal. Aortic regurgitation is probably of recent origin as there is no LVH or LV enlargement. The size of the aortic root was not mentioned. A normal pulmonary angiogram means that the PAs are not obviously affected by a vasculitis.

5 Coronary angiography

There is severe left main and proximal left coronary artery disease as well as a high-grade proximal right coronary artery stenosis (>90% narrowing). The red arrow heads point to the sites of the stenosis.

6 Physical examination

The visual impairment, the absence of the carotid pulses, and the unobtainable BP in the right arm are because the innominate artery and its main branches (right subclavian and right common carotid artery) were occluded. It is unclear why the murmur of aortic regurgitation was not detected.

7 Laboratory data

Initial hemoglobin and WBC count were within normal limits. No ESR measurement mentioned.

8 Doppler pressure studies

The systolic pressures in both arms are markedly reduced, thus corroborating the inability to obtain arm BPs. The systolic pressures in the lower extremities are within normal limits, which correlates well with the normal appearing femoral vessels as seen on the abdominal aortogram.

9 Diagnosis

1. Takayasu's arteritis (TA) involving aortic arch and its branches.
2. Severe proximal right and left coronary artery disease.
3. Aortic regurgitation.

10 Course

The patient was diagnosed as having a non-Q-wave infarction in October 1992 and treated with nitrates, metoprolol, and aspirin. She underwent right femoral to axillary bypass surgery on 19 November 1992. On

21 November 1992 the ECG (Figure 22.6) showed partial regression of ST–T wave abnormalities as compared to 18 October 1992.

Laboratory data in November 1992 was essentially unchanged from October 1992 except for a rise in WBC count (hemoglobin 11.5 g%, WBC 16,300/mm^3, glucose 61 mg%, BUN 16 mg%).

A left femoral to axillary bypass was planned in the near future.

Unfortunately she developed chest pain, hypotension, and ventricular fibrillation on 21 November 1992 and died.

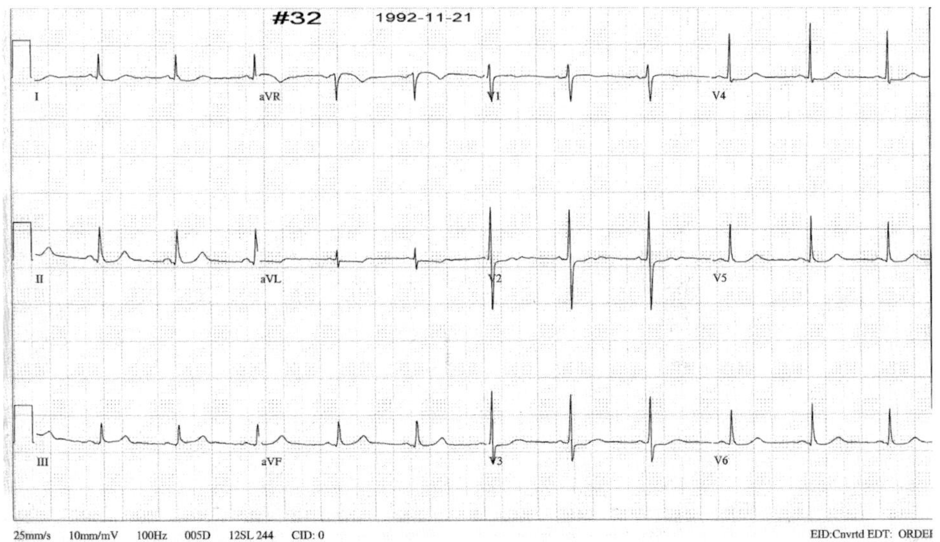

Figure 22.6 12-lead ECG 21 November 1992.

Discussion

TA (pulseless disease) is a chronic vasculitis of unknown cause involving the aorta and its branches. It is most common in Japan, where 150 new cases occur a year, predominantly in women [1]. TA occurs in other Asian countries as well as in Latin America (as in this patient) [2]. It is uncommon in the white population. In the USA there are one to three new patients with TA/year/million population [1].

The patients are usually between the ages of 10 and 40 [1], and usually present with nonspecific constitutional symptoms of fever, malaise, arthralgias, fatigue, and weight loss. These findings were not mentioned in this 23-year-old patient.

The presence of visual symptoms in this patient represents a late manifestation of the disease and may be attributed to extensive carotid artery occlusive disease [3,4].

This patient fulfilled the criteria for TA in that she was <40 years old, had bilateral subclavian artery involvement, and absence of arm and carotid pulses [5].

Aortic regurgitation occurred in this patient and may have been due to aortic root dilatation [2].

The diagnosis is often established with contrast aortic angiography, but newer techniques such as high-resolution Doppler ultrasound [5,6], MRI [5,7], and PET scanning [5] show considerable promise in diagnosing TA at an earlier stage.

Ten per cent of patients with TA have coronary artery disease [2], usually involving the ostia [8]. This patient had severe proximal coronary artery disease, which probably accounts for her sudden death. She might have benefited from coronary artery stenting but this was not available to us in 1992.

Prognosis in TA is worse if there are complications (hypertension TA retinopathy, aortic regurgitation, aneurysm) or if the course is progressive [9].

The mortality rate in TA may be up to 35% in 5 years [5] and 57% in 15 years if there are complications and a progressive course [9].

Medical treatment consists mostly of the use of steroids or possibly chemotherapeutic agents such as methotrexate or azathioprine. Surgical intervention in selected cases would include coronary artery angioplasty or stenting [10], bypass grafting or aortic valve replacement [2].

Key points

1. Patients with TA may present symptoms from occlusion of the great vessels or the coronary arteries. TA occurs most commonly in young women of Asian descent.
2. Complications of TA include aortic regurgitation, aortic aneurysms, and myocardial infarction.
3. Treatment is with steroids and chemotherapeutic agents.
4. TA has a high mortality rate and patients can die suddenly.

References

[1] Hunder GG. Clinical features and diagnosis of Takayasu arteritis. Uptodate www.uptodate.com,4 February 2010.
[2] Ogino H, Matsuda H, Minatoya K et al. Overview of late outcome of medical and surgical treatment for Takayasu Arteritis. *Circulation* 2008; 118: 2738–2747.
[3] Lewis JR, Glaser JS, Schatz NJ et al. Pulseless (Takayasu) disease with ophthalmic manifestations. *J Clin Neuro-Ophthalm* 193; 13: 242–249.
[4] Rodriguez-Pia A, de Miguel G, Lopez-Contreras J et al. Bilateral blindness in Takayasu's disease. *Scand J Rheumatol* 1996; 25: 394–395.
[5] Andrews J, Mason JC. Takayasu's arteritis – recent advances in imaging offer promise. *Rheumatology* 2007; 46: 6–15.
[6] Matsumura Y, Morimoto K, Ishikawa M et al. Ultrasonographic images of Takayasu's arteritis. *Circulation* 1998; 98: 1585–1586.
[7] Zimmer S, Nickenig G. Pulselessness in the upper extremities. *J Am Coll Cardiol* 2009; 54: 660.
[8] Soto ME, Melendez-Ramirez G, Kimura-Hayama E et al. Coronary CT angiography in Takayasu Arteritis. *J Am Coll Cardiol Img* 2011; 4: 958–966.
[9] Ishikawa K, Maetani S. Long term outcome for 120 Japanese patients with Takayasu's disease. Clinical and statistical analyses of related prognostic factors. *Circulation* 1994; 90: 1855–1860.
[10] Punamiya K, Bates ER, Shea MJ et al. Endoluminal stenting for unprotected left main stenosis in Takayasu's Arteritis. *Cathet Cardiovasc. Diagn* 1997; 40: 272–275.

23 PATIENT STUDY 23

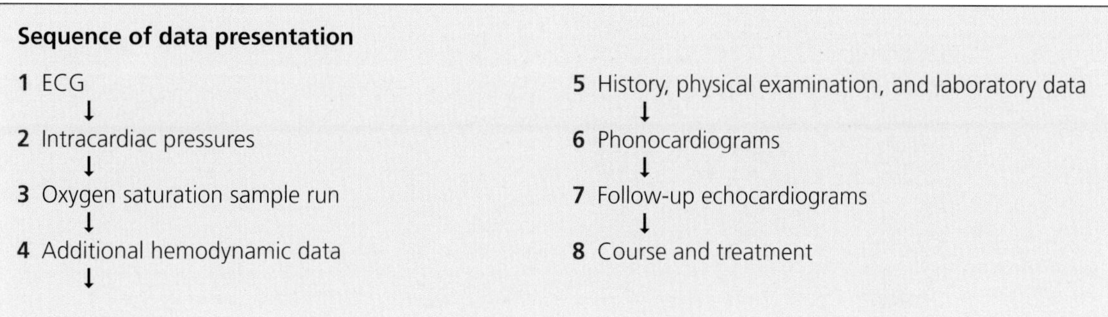

Sequence of data presentation

1 ECG
↓
2 Intracardiac pressures
↓
3 Oxygen saturation sample run
↓
4 Additional hemodynamic data
↓
5 History, physical examination, and laboratory data
↓
6 Phonocardiograms
↓
7 Follow-up echocardiograms
↓
8 Course and treatment

1 ECG

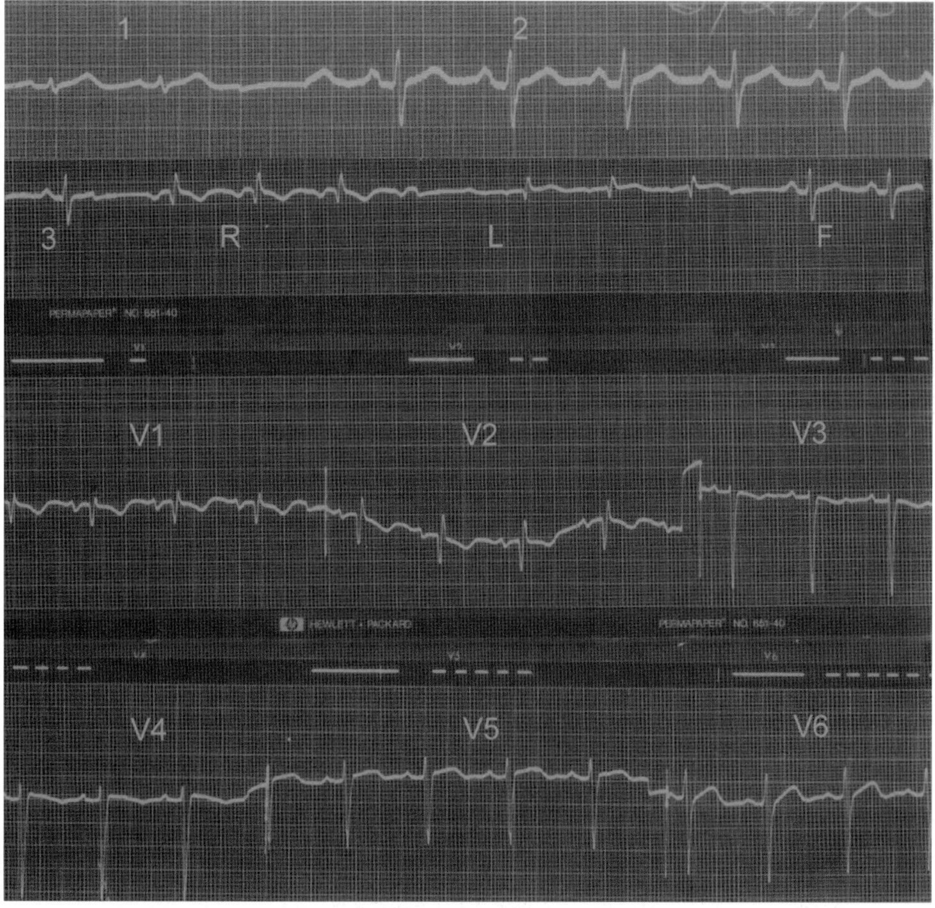

Figure 23.1 12-lead ECG 1975.

Patient Studies in Valvular, Congenital, and Rarer Forms of Cardiovascular Disease: An Integrative Approach, First Edition. Franklin B. Saksena.

Companion Website: www.wiley.com/go/saksena/patientstudies

2 Intracardiac pressures

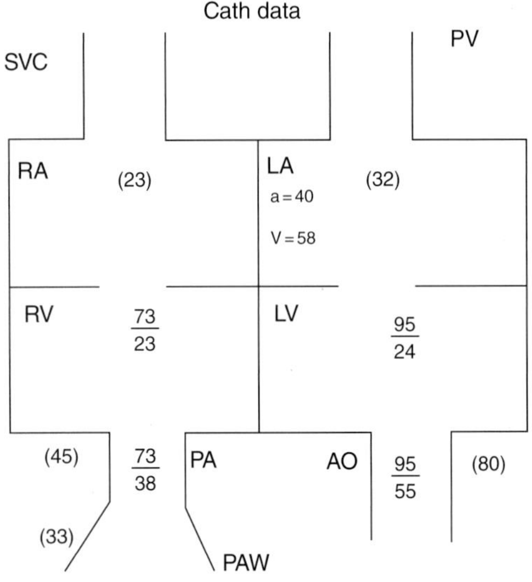

Figure 23.2 Intracardiac pressures 1975.

3 Oxygen saturation sample run

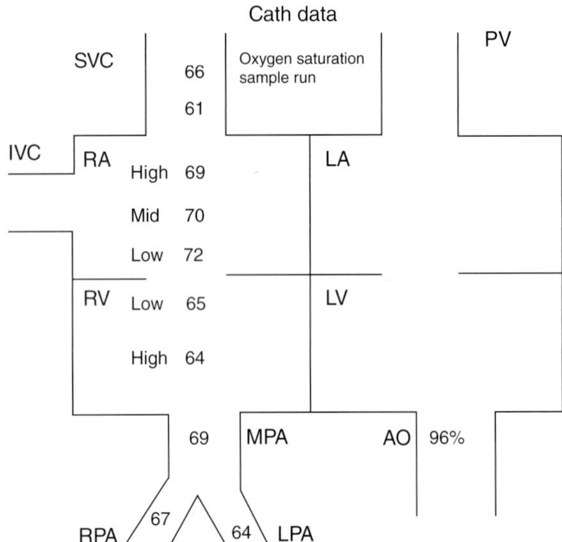

Figure 23.3 Oxygen sample run 1975.

Table 23.1 Additional hemodynamic data 1975

Additional data
Hemoglobin 14.7 gm%. BSA 1.94 m^2
Cardiac index 2.12 L/min/m^2
Mitral regurgitation 4+
Aortic regurgitation 0
LV end diastolic volume index 127 ml/m^2
LV end systolic volume index 48 ml/m^2
LV ejection fraction 0.62

4 Additional hemodynamic data

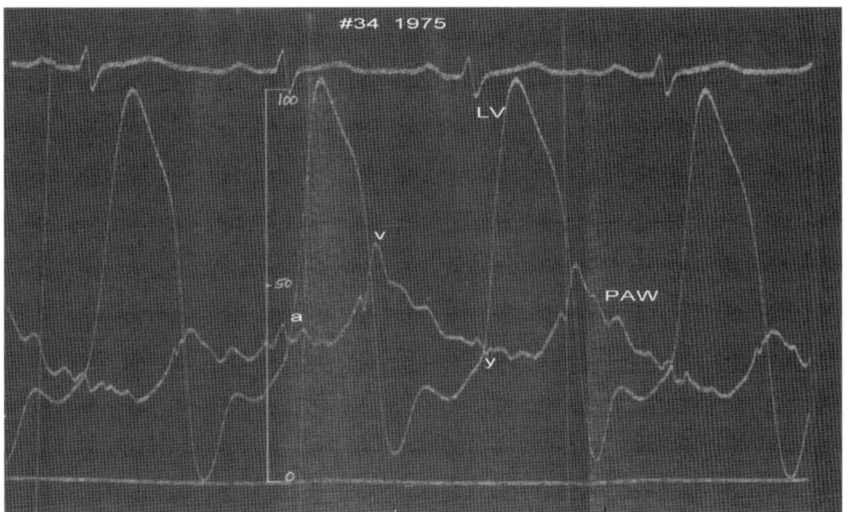

Figure 23.4 LV and pulmonary artery wedge pressures 1975. 0–100 mmHg scale.

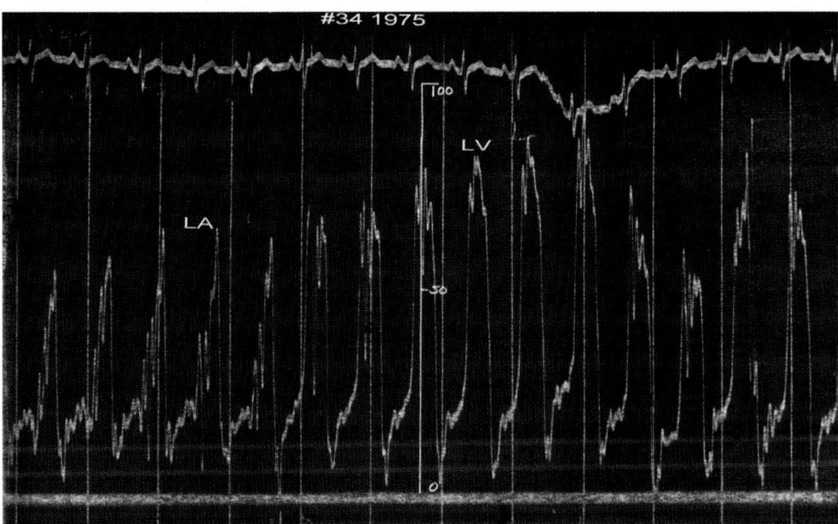

Figure 23.5 LV and LA pressures 1975. 0–100 mmHg scale.

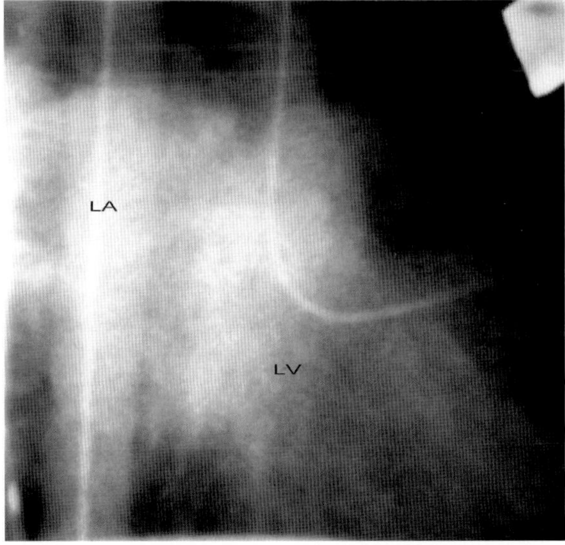

Figure 23.6 LV angiogram showing mainly LA in RAO view 1975.

5 History, physical examination, and laboratory data

History

40-year-old man admitted to hospital in 1975 with a history of dyspnea and edema for 3 months. He had been in hospital in 1974 for chronic alcoholism and peripheral neuropathy.

He has smoked for 40 pack years. He was told he had a heart murmur in 1961.

No history of hypertension, rheumatic fever, or TB.

Physical examination

6 ft, 3inches tall male weighing 152 lb. BP 110/80. HR 86/min regular.

Neck veins were distended to the angle of the jaw at 45°.

Apex beat was in the 5th interspace in the anterior axillary line.

There was a palpable systolic thrill at the apex.

S1 decreased. S2 showed normal splitting. P2 was louder than A2. Apical S3.

Grade 4/6 harsh holosystolic murmur was best heard at the apex and radiating to the axilla and interscapular area.

Grade 1/6 short diastolic blowing murmur heard down LLSB.

Normal breath sounds. No crackles or rhonchi. No clubbing.

2+ leg edema.

He had a sensory and motor neuropathy.

Laboratory data

Chest X ray showed cardiomegaly due to biventricular and LA enlargement. The hilar vessels were prominent and the peripheral lung fields oligemic.

6 Phonocardiograms

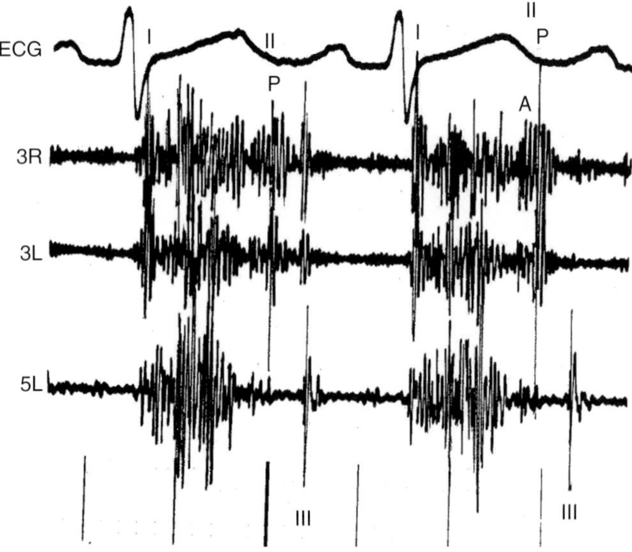

Figure 23.7 Phonocardiogram 1977 or1978.

7 Follow-up echocardiograms

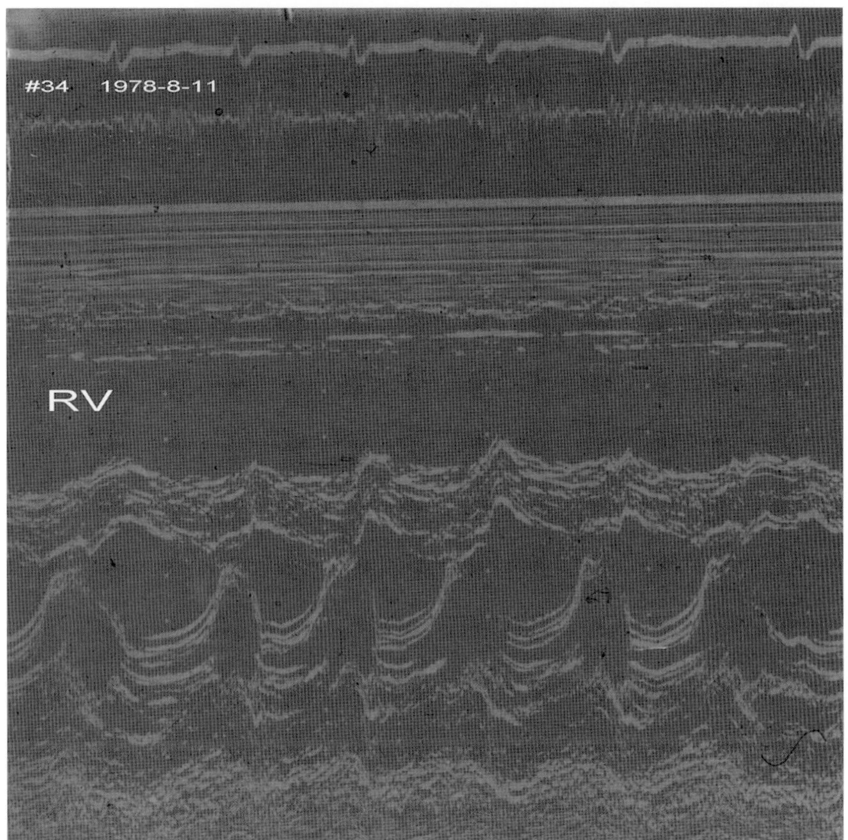

Figure 23.8 M-mode echocardiogram of mitral valve 1978.

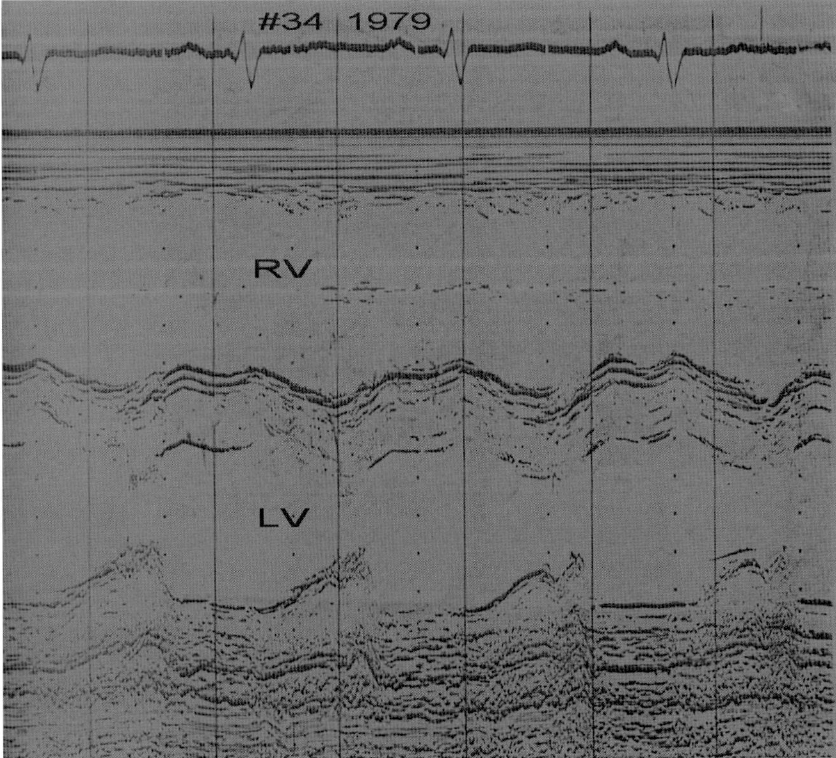

Figure 23.9 M-mode echocardiogram of LV and RV 1979.

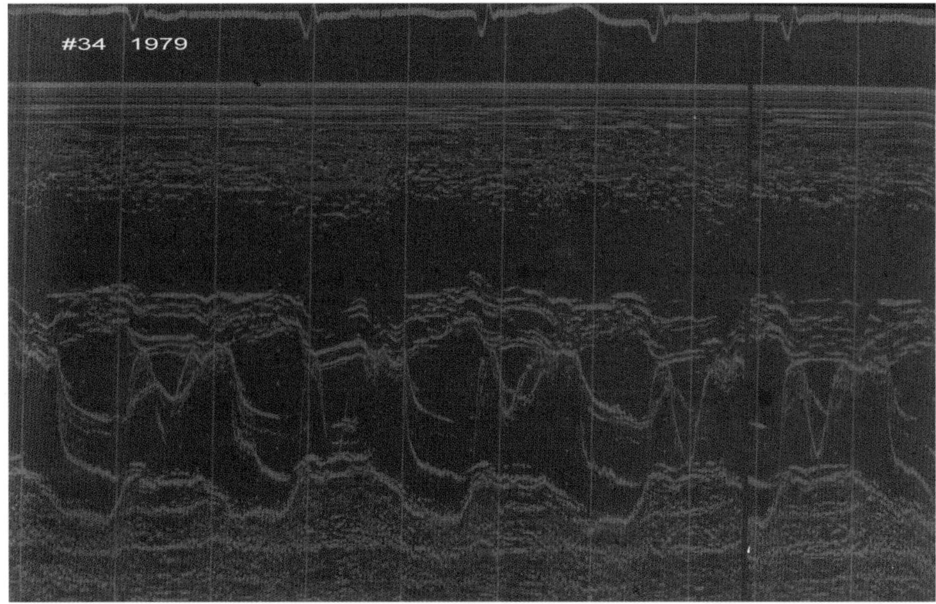

Figure 23.10 M-mode echocardiogram of mitral valve 1979.

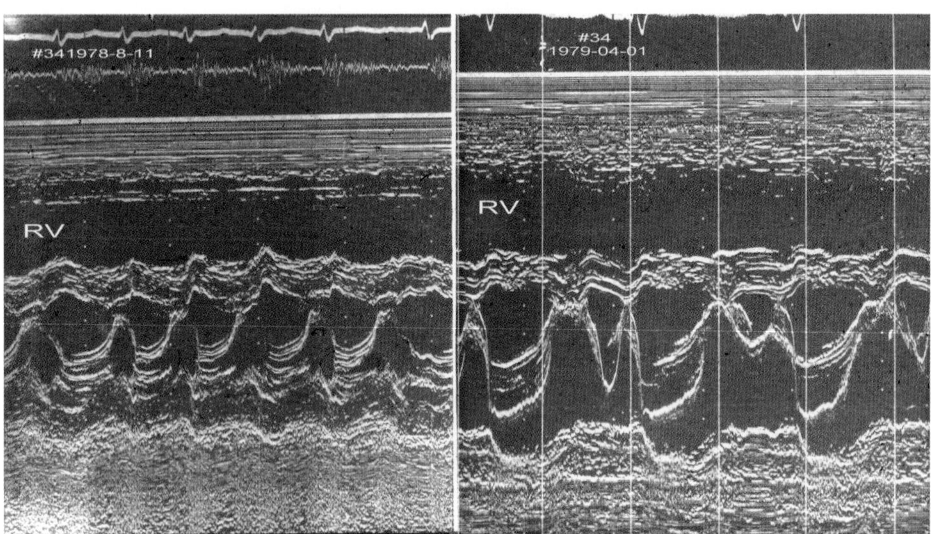

Figure 23.11 Comparison of 1978 and 1979 mitral echograms.

8 Course and treatment

The patient refused surgery in 1975. His heart failure did improve somewhat on medical therapy. He was readmitted in 1979 with recurrent heart failure.

How would you treat this patient?

Answers and commentary

1 ECG

The rhythm is sinus with a rate of 82/min. PR interval 0.16 s. QRS 0.08 s. QRS axis indeterminate. P biphasic in V1. Poor R wave progression V1–3. Deep S in V6.

Impression: (i) LA enlargement, (ii) possible RVH.

2 Intracardiac pressures

The RA pressure is very high, probably because of tricuspid regurgitation and/or RV failure. There is RV dysfunction (RVEDP is 23 mmHg) and moderately severe pulmonary hypertension.

The elevated LA pressure is due to LV failure. The 'v' wave is very high and almost double the LA mean pressure – a common finding in severe mitral regurgitation.

3 Oxygen saturation sample run

The oxygen saturation sample run is normal .thus ruling out a significant cardiac shunt.

4 Additional hemodynamic data

The cardiac index is reduced and there is severe mitral regurgitation. The LV end-diastolic volume of 127 mL/m^2 is moderately increased (normal 70 ± 20 mL/m^2). In mitral regurgitation the LV is unloaded and the LV ejection fraction should be supernormal. Thus an ejection fraction of 0.62 in the setting of mitral regurgitation is indicative of LV dysfunction.

LV and wedge pressures

The 'v' wave is dominant and much higher than the 'a' wave. The y descent is slower than usual but there is no significant end-diastolic gradient across the mitral valve.

LV and LA pressures

The 'v' wave in the LA pressure tracing is much higher than the 'v' wave seen in the wedge and the y descent is probably not delayed. The delay in the y descent in the wedge pressure is most likely due to an artifact. The catheter is going in and out of the LV probably because of the mitral regurgitant jet.

LV angiogram

The LA was completely filled with contrast material one beat after the LV injection. The mitral valve is not well seen. As contrast material refluxed into the pulmonary veins the patient had 4+ mitral regurgitation.

5 History, physical examination, and laboratory data

The patient had mitral regurgitation that could have been of rheumatic origin or due to mitral valve prolapse. Radiation of the systolic murmur to the scapular region is often seen when there is dysfunction of the anterior mitral valve leaflet. The short diastolic murmur is compatible with pulmonary regurgitation in keeping with the patient's pulmonary hypertension.

Biventricular enlargement and LA enlargement are seen on the chest X ray in mitral regurgitation and VSD. The latter is unlikely as the oxygen sample run was normal.

6 Phonocardiogram

There is an increase in the P2 closure sound in the 3rd right and 3rd left interspace. There is a mixed crescendo decrescendo and holosystolic murmur recorded at all three sites (3rd right and left interspaces as well as 5th left interspace parasternally). These findings are due to pulmonary hypertension, mitral regurgitation, and tricuspid regurgitation, respectively.

An S4 of low amplitude is seen at 5 L and a high amplitude S3 is noted at 5 L.

These findings are seen in severe mitral regurgitation with LV failure. VSD may have similar findings (pansystolic murmur at LLSB and biventricular failure) but this has been excluded by the normal sample run.

7 Follow-up echocardiograms

In 1978 the M-mode echocardiogram showed a thickened mitral valve and bowing of the posterior mitral leaflets suggestive of mitral valve prolapse.

In 1979 the M-mode echocardiogram showed large excursions and fluttering of the anterior mitral valve leaflet indicative of a flail anterior mitral valve. The posterior mitral valve leaflet is not well seen. A two-dimensional echocardiogram (not shown) also confirmed the diagnosis of a flail anterior mitral valve leaflet.

The RV is dilated and there is LVH.

8 Course and treatment

The patient finally agreed to have surgery in 1979. At surgery, three of the chordae of the anterior mitral valve leaflet were ruptured. He underwent mitral valve replacement using a 33 mm Porcine Hancock valve. He was doing well 3 months later and denied any dyspnea or chest pain. He was judged to be in functional class 2.

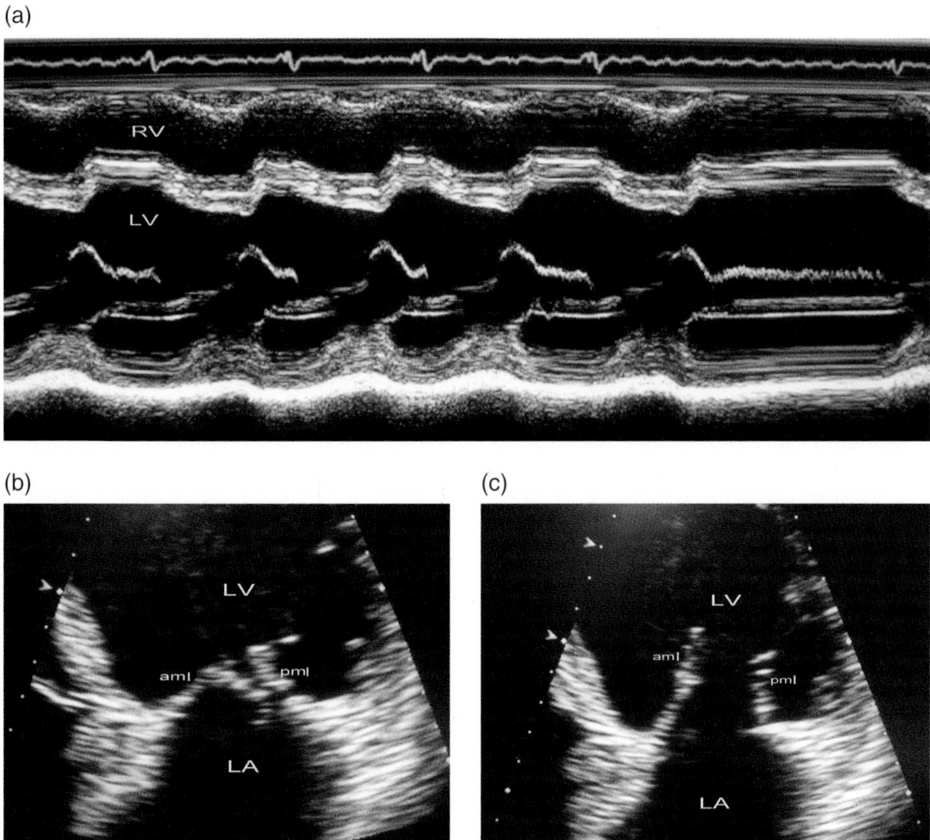

Figure 23.12 66-year-old man admitted to hospital in 2013 with atrial fibrillation and severe mitral regurgitation due to chordal rupture of the anterior mitral leaflet. (a) M-mode echocardiogram showing fluttering of anterior mitral valve leaflet and rounding of the E point, suggesting a flail mitral leaflet and mitral regurgitation. Atrial fibrillation may have also contributed to the mitral valve fluttering. (b) Two-dimensional echocardiography in four chamber view showing that the anterior leaflet fails to coapt with the posterior leaflet in systole. (c) Two-dimensional echocardiography in four-chamber view showing the leaflets opened in diastole. AML, anterior mitral leaflet; PML, posterior mitral leaflet.

Discussion

The patient had severe mitral regurgitation, presumably due to degenerative myxomatous mitral valve disease in 1975. The LV angiogram showed 4+ mitral regurgitation. The large amount of contrast material entering the LA can obscure the presence of mitral valve prolapse or a flail mitral valve [1]. In 1978 the M-mode echocardiogram did show possible mitral valve prolapse of the posterior leaflet. In 1979 the M-mode echocardiogram showed that the anterior mitral leaflet was flail on the basis of diastolic fluttering of the anterior leaflet [1]. Protrusion of the anterior leaflet into the LA in systole is another sign of a flail leaflet [1], but was not seen in this patient. At surgery only the chordae to the anterior mitral valve leaflet were torn. However, M-mode echocardiography has a much lower sensitivity and specificity than two-dimensional echocardiography in the diagnosis of a flail mitral valve [2]. Thus the preferred method of diagnosing a flail mitral valve is by either two-dimensional echocardiography [3] or TEE [4]. Two-dimensional echocardiography of a flail mitral valve shows (i) failure of the leaflets to coapt (see Figure 23.12), (ii) systolic fluttering of a leaflet as it protrudes into the LA, and (iii) chaotic diastolic motion of the leaflets [3, 5].

Rupture of the chordae to the anterior leaflets leads to a posteriorly directed systolic jet into the LA, which accounts for the radiation of the systolic murmur to the mid back. The presumed cause of the flail leaflet is often unknown [6], as in this patient, as there was no evidence of endocarditis or trauma.

Usually the posterior leaflet is flail (80% of cases) with 15% of cases involving the anterior leaflet and 5% involving both leaflets [6].

Valve replacement was carried out in this patient because of his severe heart failure. In later years a mitral valve repair might have been attempted. The surgical mortality is up to 4% for mitral valve repair [6].

Key points

1. Mitral valve prolapse is one of the most common causes of mitral regurgitation.
2. A flail anterior mitral valve leaflet usually results in acute LV failure. On physical examination the murmur of a flail anterior mitral valve leaflet may radiate from the apex to the interscapular area.
3. M-mode echocardiography and two-dimensional echocardiography can readily detect a flail mitral valve leaflet and its hemodynamic effects.
4. A flail mitral valve leaflet may be managed surgically by valve repair or replacement.

References

[1] Humphries WC, Hammer WJ, McDonough MT et al. Echocardiographic equivalents of a flail mitral leaflet. *Am J Cardiol* 1977; 40: 802–807.

[2] Mintz GS, Kotle MN, Parry WR et al. Statistical comparison of M mode and two dimensional echocardiographic diagnosis of flail mitral leaflets. *Am J Cardiol* 1980; 45: 253–259.

[3] Ballester M, Foale R, Presbitero P et al. Cross-section echocardiographic features of ruptured chordae tendineae. *Eur Heat J* 1983; 4: 795–802.

[4] Nanda NC, Domanski MJ. *Atlas of transesophageal echocardiography*. Williams and Wilkens, Baltimore, 1998, pp 83–85.

[5] Child JS, Skorton DJ, Taylor RD et al. M-mode and cross-sectional echocardiographic features of flail posterior mitral leaflets. *Am J Cardiol* 1979; 44: 1383–1390.

[6] Ling LH, Enriquez-Sarano M, Seward JB et al. Clinical outcome of mitral regurgitation due to flail leaflet. *New Engl J Med* 1996; 335: 1417–1423 (86 patients were treated medically and 143 were operated on).

24 PATIENT STUDY 24

Sequence of data presentation

1 Chest X ray
↓
2 ECG
↓
3 Echocardiogram
↓
4 Follow-up chest X ray
↓
5 Follow-up ECG
↓
6 Pressure tracings
↓
7 History, physical examination, and laboratory data
↓
8 Follow-up

1 Chest X ray

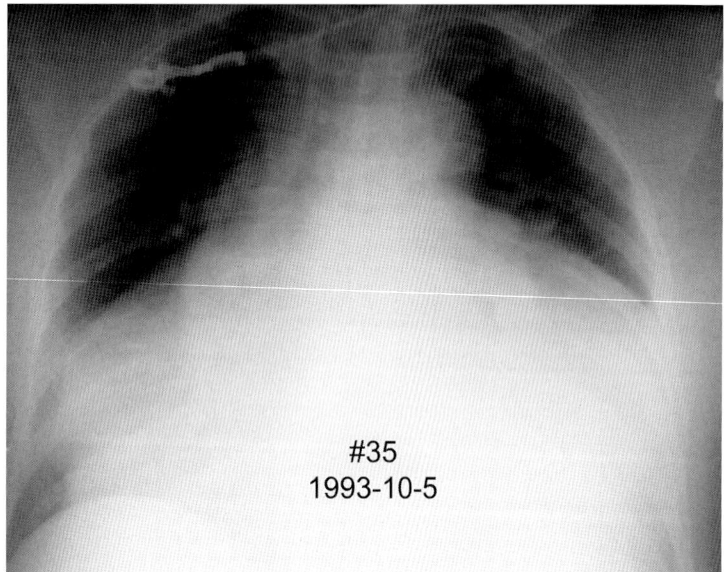

Figure 24.1 Chest X ray 5 October 1993.

Patient Studies in Valvular, Congenital, and Rarer Forms of Cardiovascular Disease: An Integrative Approach, First Edition. Franklin B. Saksena.

Companion Website: www.wiley.com/go/saksena/patientstudies

2 ECG

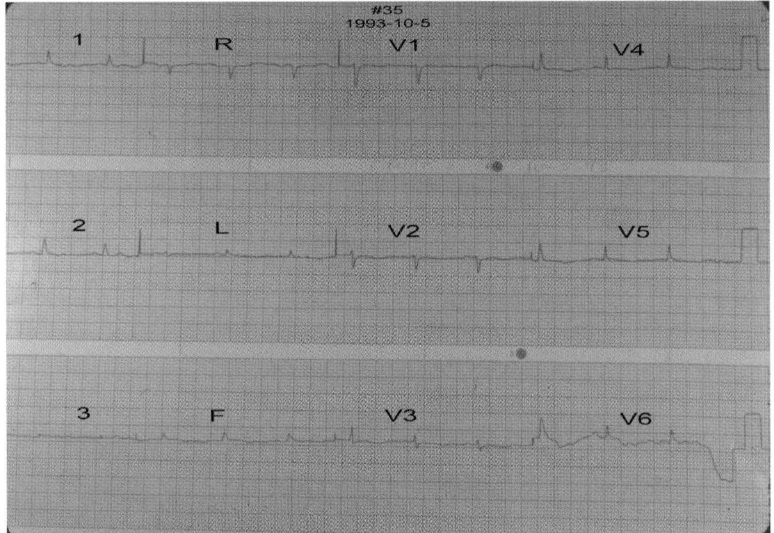

Figure 24.2 12-lead ECG 5 October 1993.

3 Echocardiogram

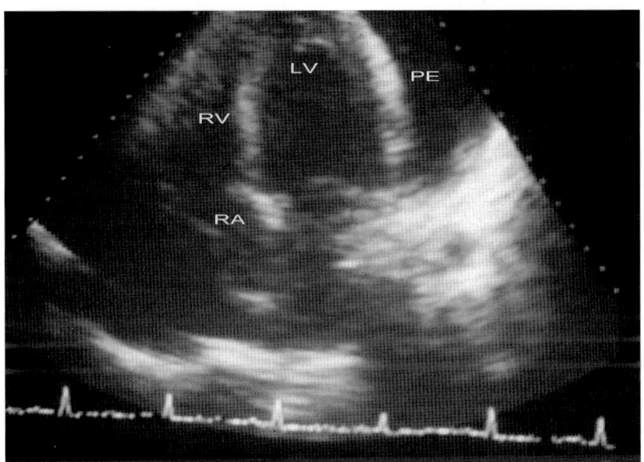

Figure 24.3 Two-dimensional echocardiography (four-chamber view) 5 October 1993.

4 Follow-up chest X ray

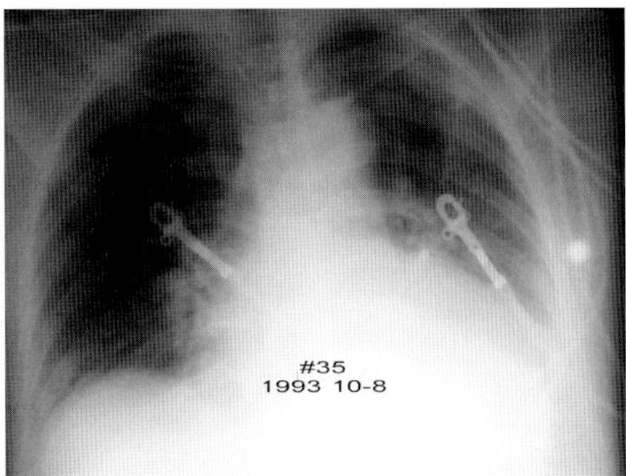

Figure 24.4 Chest X ray 8 October 1993.

5 Follow-up ECG

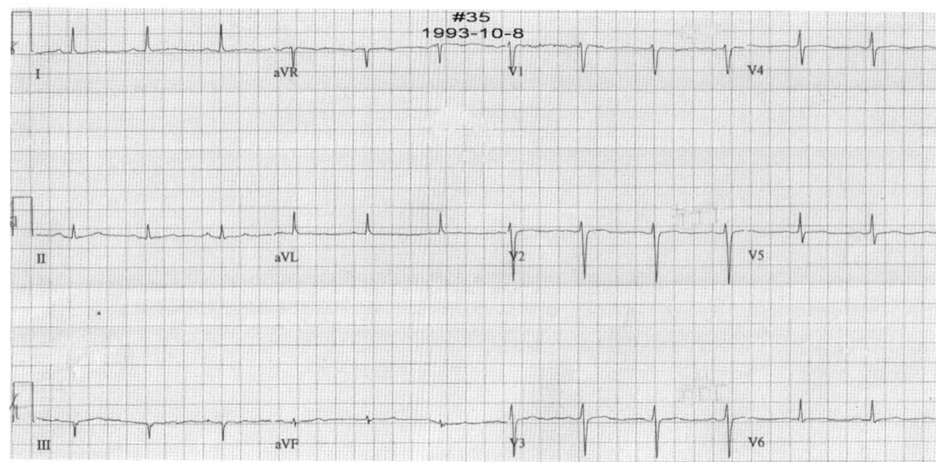

Figure 24.5 12-lead ECG 8 October 1993.

6 Pressure tracings

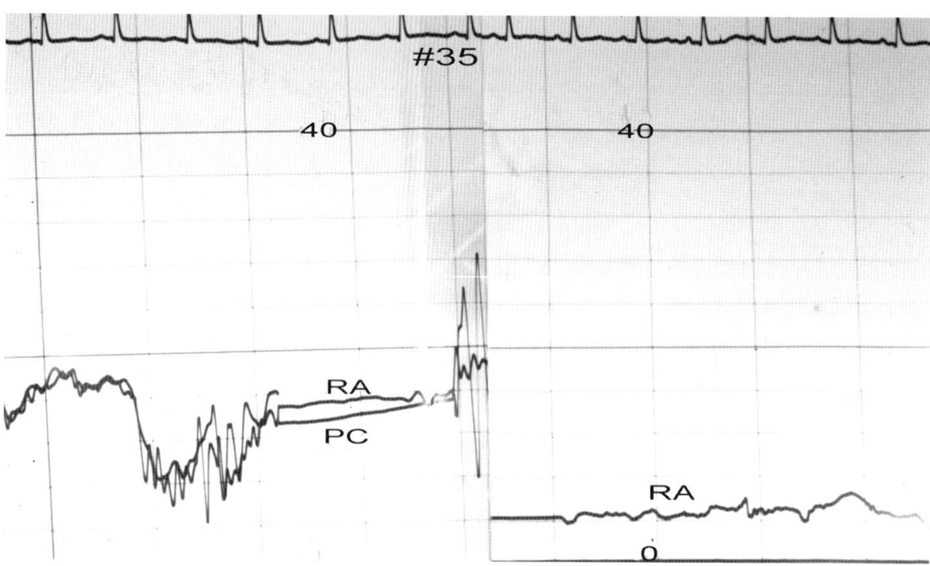

Figure 24.6 Pressure tracings. Left hand panel: initial recording of RA and intrapericardial pressures (PC); right hand panel: RA pressure after treatment. 0-40 mm Hg scale in both panels.

7 History, physical examination, and laboratory data

History

54-year-old female admitted to hospital with dyspnea and altered mental status for 3 days.
She had had Graves disease 30 years ago, treated with radioactive iodine without further follow-up.

Physical examination

HR 75/min. Reduced body temperature.
Height 65 inches, 140 lb.
She had periorbital puffiness with dry skin. Her voice was hoarse.
Cardiomegaly.
Leg edema.

Delayed relaxation of heel reflexes.

Laboratory data

Hemoglobin 11 g%. WBC 5500/mm^3.

Na 106 meq/L, Cl 76 meq/L, BUN 4 mg%, creatinine 0.6 mg%, blood glucose 126 mg%, cholesterol 318 mg%.

Creatine phosphokinase 5240 units/L (normal female 26–140 U/L).

Urine osmolality 280 mOsm/kg (normal 300–900 mOsm/kg).

Serum osmolality 222 mOsm/kg (normal 280–303 mOsm/kg).

Urine/serum osmolality 1.25 (normal 3/1).

TSH 9.9 mIU/L (normal 0.4–4.2 mIU/L) on 5 October 1993 and 17.5 on 14 October 1993.

C/T head normal.

8 Follow-up

Comment on the diagnosis and likely course.

Answers and commentary

1 Chest X ray

There is marked cardiomegaly (C/T ratio 0.9) without pulmonary congestion. The contour of the heart shadow resembles a water bottle due to either a pericardial effusion or a cardiomyopathy.

2 ECG

Sinus rhythm. Rate 75/min. Low-voltage PR 0.16. QRS 0.04. QRS axis +30 degrees. Low T waves in V1–6.

Impression: low QRS voltage may be seen in obesity, myocardiopathy, or pericardial effusion.

The latter is the most likely diagnosis when the X ray findings are taken into account.

3 Echocardiogram

There is a large echo free space (>2 cm) surrounding the heart, indicative of a large pericardial effusion. There is late diastolic collapse of the RA, suggestive of cardiac tamponade.

4 Follow-up chest X ray

The C/T ratio decreased from 0.9 to 0.73 in a 3-day period. The lungs remain clear. The implication is that fluid has been removed from the pericardium.

5 Follow-up ECG

The rhythm remains sinus, the QRS voltage has increased. The PR and QRS intervals and QRS axes remain unchanged.

6 Pressures

The RA and intra-pericardial pressures are nearly equal (~15 mmHg). Following pericardiocentesis the RA pressure (and by implication the intra-pericardial pressure) has fallen to 5 mmHg.

7 History, physical examination, and laboratory data

The patient had clinical and laboratory evidence of decompensated hypothyroidism (myxedema coma). The cardiomegaly was attributed to a massive pericardial effusion.

There was no mention as to whether there was a paradoxical pulse or an absent y descent in the RA pressure tracing.

8 Follow-up

The patient's dyspnea improved following a pericardial tap in which 2200 mL of straw-colored pericardial fluid were removed. The fluid was a transudate. She also received IV thyroxine and steroids for her myxedema coma as well as hypertonic saline for her hyponatremia. She was discharged in a satisfactory condition on her ninth hospital day on thyroxine and short-term steroids.

On 5 November 1993 serum sodium was 141 meq/L and CPK was 49 units/L.

She did well over the next 7 years, free of endocrine and CVS symptoms on a regimen of synthroid and pravastatin. Serum TSH was 0.53 mIU/L on 22 March 2000.

Discussion

The patient had an altered mental status, hypothermia periorbital puffiness, hoarseness, and delayed relaxation of heel jerks indicative of decompensated hypothyroidism or myxedema coma [1, 2].

The diagnosis of hypothyroidism is supported by the elevated serum TSH and associated findings of a very high CPK, an elevated serum cholesterol as well as hyponatremia [1, 2]. The initial TSH level was only slightly elevated, attributable to the effect of an intercurrent nonthyroidal illness [2], i.e. cardiac tamponade in this case.

A pericardial effusion is seen in myxedema in up to 80% of cases [3]. As fluid accumulates slowly cardiac tamponade is rarely seen [4].

When tamponade in myxedema does occur the heart rate is usually normal (as in this patient) rather than increased [3].

This patient had a marked elevation of the pericardial pressure (>15 mmHg), signifying that the tamponade is severe [5]. Supportive evidence is obtained from the echocardiogram, which showed a large pericardial effusion (>2 cm thick) with diastolic collapse of the RA [3].

Other features of cardiac tamponade include a shallow or absent y descent in the RA pressure contour, pulsus paradoxus (>15 mmHg fall in systolic pressure on inspiration = severe tamponade) [5], RV collapse [5], and abnormalities on Doppler echocardiography, consisting of a marked increase in flow velocities across the right heart valves on inspiration and an inspiratory decrease in flow velocities across the left-sided valves [5–7].

Key points

1. Patients with decompensated hypothyroidism have an altered mental status, hypothermia, hoarseness, delayed relaxation of the heel jerks, and high TSH and CPK levels.
2. Myxedema commonly produces a pericardial effusion, which rarely leads to cardiac tamponade. HR is normal in myxedema-induced tamponade.
3. Patients with cardiac tamponade may have an absent y descent, elevated intrapericardial and venous pressures, and pulsus paradoxus.
4. Echocardiography and Doppler studies also provide diagnostic information in cardiac tamponade.

References

[1] Jordan RM. Myxedema coma. Pathophysiology, therapy and factors affecting prognosis. *Med Clin North Am* 1995; 79: 185–194.

[2] Wiersinga WM. Hypothyroidism and myxedema coma. In: DeGroot LJ, Jameson JL (eds), *Endocrinology*, 4th edn, volume 2. WB Saunders, Philadelphia, 2001, p. 1502.

[3] Wang J-L, Hsieh M-J, Lee C-H et al. Hypothyroid cardiac tamponade: Clinical features, electrocardiography, pericardial fluid and management. *Am J Med Sci* 2010; 340: 276–281.

[4] Hsu Y-F, Huang Y-K, Lu M-S et al. Recurrent post traumatic cardiac tamponade as a presentation of hypothyroidism: A forgotten disease. *J Trauma* 2007; 63: E124–E126.

[5] Hoit BD. Pericardial heart disease. *Curr Probl Cardiol* 1997; 22: 355–400.

[6] Materazzo C, Piotti P, Meazza R et al. Respiratory changes in transvalvular flow velocities versus two-dimensional echocardiographic findings in the diagnosis of cardiac tamponade. *Ital Heart J* 2003; 4: 186–192.

[7] Merce J, Sagrista-Sauleda J, Permanyer-Miralda G et al. Correlation between clinical and Doppler echocardiographic findings in patients with moderate and large pericardial effusion: Implications for the diagnosis of cardiac tamponade. *Am Heart J* 1999; 138: 759–764.

25 PATIENT STUDY 25

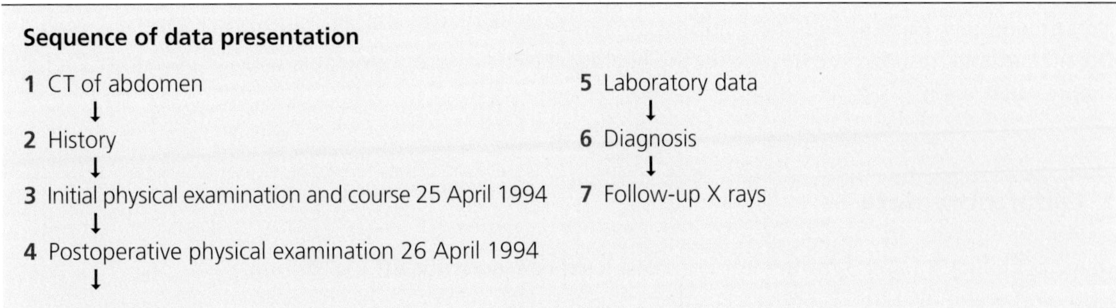

Sequence of data presentation

1 CT of abdomen
↓
2 History
↓
3 Initial physical examination and course 25 April 1994
↓
4 Postoperative physical examination 26 April 1994
↓
5 Laboratory data
↓
6 Diagnosis
↓
7 Follow-up X rays

1 CT of abdomen

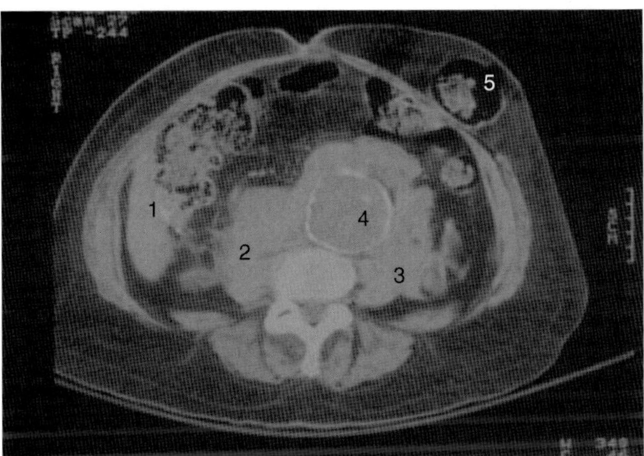

Figure 25.1 CT of abdomen without contrast at L2 level 1994.
Insert the names of the anatomic structures labeled 1–5.

2 History

74-year-old female admitted to hospital in 1994 with severe abdominal pain for 2 hours.

In 1993 she had undergone a colostomy following bowel resection for rectal cancer at another hospital. She also had coronary artery bypass surgery in 1993. Two weeks ago she was told she had an AAA that would need to be operated on.

3 Initial physical examination and course 25 April 1994

5 foot tall female weighing 140 lb. Initial BP 122/80. HR 96/min. RR 20/min.

The patient was unable to move her legs. Pulses in the legs were diminished.

The patient became stuporous with respiratory distress, sweating, and pallor. Her BP fell to 33/24. She was started on dopamine and sent to the operating room once the CT of the abdomen had confirmed the rupture of an AAA.

Patient Studies in Valvular, Congenital, and Rarer Forms of Cardiovascular Disease: An Integrative Approach, First Edition. Franklin B. Saksena.

Companion Website: www.wiley.com/go/saksena/patientstudies

At surgery a ruptured AAA, just distal to the renal arteries and measuring 6 cm in diameter, was resected and replaced with an aorto-iliac Dacron graft. There was about 3000 mL of blood in the abdominal cavity. She received 2 units of blood.

4 Postoperative physical examination 26 April 1994

The patient was alert and on the ventilator. BP 130/90. HR 114/min. PA pressure 25/15.
Lungs were clear.
No cardiomegaly. Heart sounds were normal. No murmurs.
Doppler arterial sounds were heard over the popliteal arteries but not over the feet. The feet were cool and dusky in color.

5 Laboratory data

Hematocrit 36.5% (after 3 further units of blood had been given). WBC 15,790/mm.
BUN 57. Creatinine 4.6 mg%. Normal cardiac enzymes.
Chest X ray and ECG were normal.
Venous Doppler of legs was normal.

6 Diagnosis

What is the diagnosis?

7 Follow-up X rays

She had follow-up abdominal CTs in 2000 and 2007 (Figure 25.2).

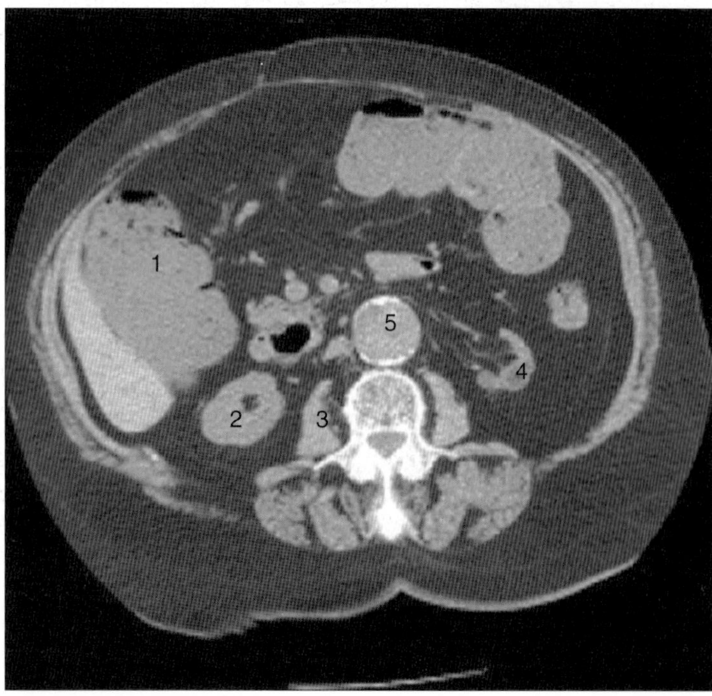

Figure 25.2 CT of abdomen without contrast material at ~ L2 level 2007.
Insert the names of the anatomic structures labeled 1–5.

Answers and commentary

1 Abdominal CT of abdomen

The abdominal CT (24 April 1994) was taken without contrast material ~ L2 level. There is a 6 cm diameter AAA (label 4) extending from below the renal arteries to the bifurcation of the aorta. The wall of the aorta is calcified. There is an irregular shaped mass (label 3) with the same opacity as the aortic lumen and psoas muscle (label 2) and involving the anterior and posterior pararenal space, attributable to blood leaking from a ruptured aortic aneurysm. Other frames show a normal right kidney and an atrophic left kidney.

Part of the liver (label 1) is seen in the right quadrant and a colostomy is seen in the left quadrant (label 5).

2 History

The sudden onset of abdominal pain and shock in a patient with a known abdominal aneurysm usually indicates that the aneurysm has ruptured [1].

3 Initial physical examination and course 25 April 1994

Details of the initial abdominal examination were not available. Often the physical signs of a pulsatile expansile aorta in the epigastric are either overlooked or difficult to detect in an obese patient [2].

The inability to move the legs with diminished leg pulses implies that thrombi from the aneurysm had embolized to the legs [1].

4 Postoperative physical examination 25 April 1994

The patient made a remarkable recovery following aortic graft surgery despite losing 3000 mL of blood from the aortic rupture. There was still evidence of some impairment of her peripheral circulation.

5 Laboratory data

The hematocrit stabilized after receiving a total of 5 units of blood. She had some azotemia, which later resolved.

6 Diagnosis

Ruptured AAA. Successfully repaired.

Hemorrhagic shock.

Residual peripheral vascular impairment.

Renal insufficiency.

Atrophic left kidney probably due to atherosclerosis.

7 Follow-up X rays

There is a 3.6 cm infrarenal abdominal aneurysm (label 5). An intact aortobifemoral graft is seen in other frames. The liver (label 1), right kidney (label 2), and right psoas muscle (label 3) are normal. The left kidney (label 4) is atrophic.

No change from a similar film taken in 2000.

Patient died of congestive heart failure in 2012.

Discussion

The normal abdominal aorta extends from T12 to L4, where it bifurcates into the common iliac arteries. It is normally 1.5–2.5 cm in diameter [3]. The renal arteries originate from the aorta opposite the second lumbar vertebra (L2).

An abdominal aneurysm is most commonly due to atherosclerosis and usually originates below the renal arteries. The aneurysmal wall may be calcified and its lumen often contains thrombus. An AAA occurs in up to 8% of men over the age of 65 [2]. The male/female ratio is 5/1 [2]. About 1 million new patients with AAAs are diagnosed each year, of which only about 70,000 are operated on [4]. Risk factors include smoking, dyslipidemia, hypertension, and a family history of AAA. Co-morbidities include coronary artery disease and diabetes [2].

Physical examination of the abdomen is a relatively insensitive way of detecting an AAA either because the aneurysm is small or because the patient is obese [2]. Abdominal ultrasound is a useful way of screening for a possible AAA in the high-risk group (typically a person over 65 who smokes, has hypertension, and especially if there is a family history of AAA) [2].

For aneurysms less than 6 cm in diameter the expansion rate is about 0.2–0.4 cm/year [5]. The chances of rupture are <1% per year if the aneurysm is <5 cm and 10% per year if it is >6 cm in diameter [2].

Elective surgery is recommended once the aneurysm has reached 5.5 cm in diameter for men and 5 cm for women [4]. The 30-day operative mortality for electively operated patients is 4–5% [4, 3, 6–8]. Once the aneurysm has ruptured, the operative mortality is 40–50%, with a 30-day survival rate of 11% [4]. This patient had a ruptured aortic aneurysm but had no further abdominal symptoms following successful grafting of her abdominal aneurysm and lived another 18 years.

Key points

1. Patients with an AAA are usually males over the age of 65. Risk factors are smoking, hypertension, hyperlipidemia, and a family history of AAA.
2. Elective repair of an AAA is recommended in women when the aortic diameter is 5 cm and for men 5.5 cm, with a 30-day surgical mortality rate of 5%.
3. Rupture of an AAA is heralded by sudden abdominal pain and shock, and carries a surgical mortality rate of 40–50% and 11% survival rate in 30 days.

References

[1] Isselbacher EM. *Abdominal aortic aneurysms*. In: Braunwald's Heart Disease, 8th edn, Libby P, Bonow RO, Mann DL, Zipes DP (eds). WB Saunders, Philadelphia, 2008, pp 1458–1459.

[2] Moxon JV, Parr A, Emeto TI et al. Diagnosis and monitoring of abdominal aortic aneurysm: current status and future prospects. *Curr Probl Cardiol* 2010; 35: 505–548.

[3] Bajwa TK, Shalev YA, Gupta A et al. Peripheral vascular disease part 1. *Curr Probl Cardiol* 1998; 23: 245–304.

[4] Allaqaband S, Kirvatis R, Jan MF et al. Endovascular treatment of peripheral vascular disease. *Curr Probl Cardiol* 2009; 34: 359–476.

[5] Bernstein EF, Chan EL. Abdominal aortic aneurysm in high-risk patients. *Ann Surg* 1984; 200: 255–262.

[6] Lovegrove RE, Javid M, Magee TR et al. A meta-analysis of 21,178 patients undergoing open or endovascular repair of abdominal aortic aneurysm. *Br J Surg* 2008; 95: 677–684.

[7] Schermerhorn ML, O'Malley AJ, Jhaveri A et al. Endovascular vs open repair of abdominal aortic aneurysms in the Medicare population. *New Engl J Med* 2008; 358: 464–474.

[8] de Vries SO, Hunink MGM. Results of aortic bifurcation grafts for aortoilicac occlusive disease. A meta-analysis. *J Vasc Surg* 1997; 26: 558–569.

26 PATIENT STUDY 26

Sequence of data presentation

1 ECG 26 February 2001
↓
2 CT of abdomen 2 March 2001
↓
3 History
↓
4 Physical examination 26 February 2001
↓
5 Laboratory data and course 26 February to 9 March 2001
↓
6 Coronary angiography 13 March 2001
↓
7 Diagnosis
↓
8 Management and immediate postoperative course 14–21 March 2001
↓
9 Postoperative course 21 March to 8 April 2001

1 ECG 26 February 2001

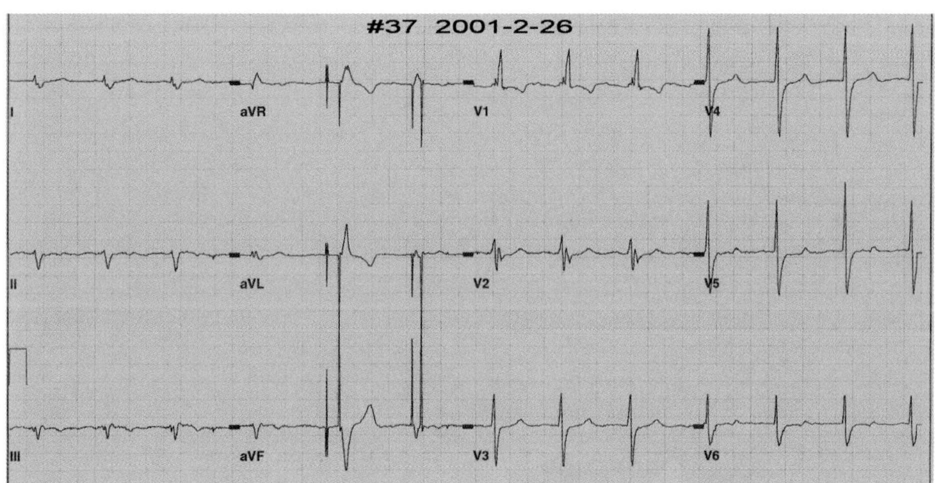

Figure 26.1 12-lead ECG 26 February 2001.

Patient Studies in Valvular, Congenital, and Rarer Forms of Cardiovascular Disease: An Integrative Approach, First Edition. Franklin B. Saksena.

Companion Website: www.wiley.com/go/saksena/patientstudies

2 CT of abdomen 2 March 2001

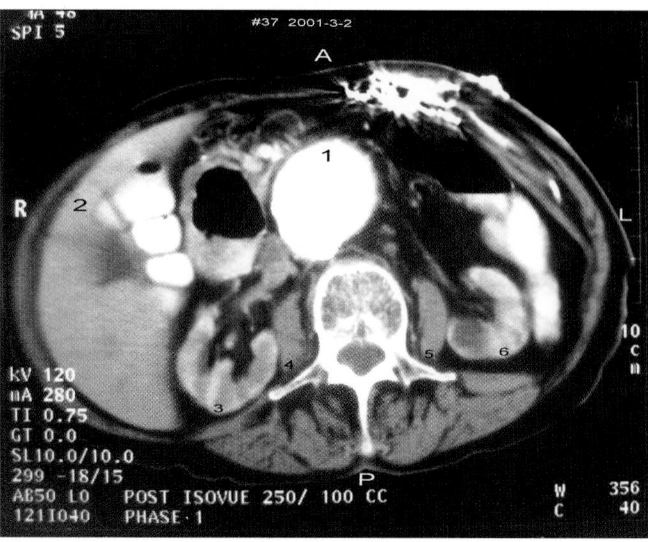

Figure 26.2 CT of abdomen with contrast material L2 level 2 March 2001.
Name the structures labeled 1–6.

3 History

82-year-old female admitted to hospital with recurrent lower GI bleeding due to angiodysplasia of the colon (26 February 2001). GI studies confirmed this diagnosis. She received blood and once she was considered stable she had follow-up X rays for a known AAA on 2 March 2001.

The patient had aortic valve replacement with a Starr–Edwards prosthesis in 1979 and a permanent pacemaker inserted via epicardial leads in 1975. She had undergone two-vessel CABG in 1993 and had had hypertension for many years. Patient does not drink alcohol, smoke, or use recreational drugs.

In 1993 she was first seen at our hospital with angina of effort. Coronary angiography via the femoral approach was unsuccessful because of severe atherosclerosis of the descending aorta and its iliac branches. At that time she was found to have a 3.2 cm AAA Follow-up studies between 1993 and 1998 showed that the aneurysm size had remained about the same (3.5 cm in 1998).

A follow-up U/S of the abdomen was recommended in 2000 but not carried out.

She was readmitted in February 2001 with melena.

4 Physical examination 26 February 2001

65 inches tall, 110 lb female. BP 170/90. HR 92/min irregular. Diagonal ear crease sign.

CVS: apex beat was in the 5th interspace, 9 cm from the mid-sternal line. There was a loud opening and closing click with an early grade 1/6 aortic systolic murmur.

Femoral pulses were normal but the foot pulses were decreased. No edema, cyanosis, or clubbing.

Respiratory system: lungs clear. No inspiratory tracheal tug sign. Well-healed median sternotomy scar.

Abdomen: pacemaker generator is implanted subcutaneously in the left upper quadrant, no abdominal tenderness.

5 Laboratory data and course 26 February to 9 March 2001

Chest X ray: cardiomegaly and mild pulmonary congestion.

Echocardiogram: mild LV hypokinesia; the mean gradient across the Starr–Edwards aortic valve in systole was only 17 mmHg.

Troponin levels on admission were normal.

GI work-up showed only a gastritis. Small bowel studies and colonoscopy were normal.

She was placed on a low dose of IV heparin (300 units/h) throughout her hospital course, having had warfarin stopped when she was first admitted.

She was transferred to another hospital on 9 March 2001 for insertion of an endovascular aortic graft for an AAA.

6 Coronary angiography 13 March 2001

Severe three-vessel disease. One saphenous graft to the circumflex artery was occluded but the second saphenous graft to the left anterior descending was open. No LV angiography was carried out.

7 Diagnosis

What is the diagnosis?

8 Management and immediate postoperative course 14–21 March 2001

The patient underwent successful endovascular graft stenting of the AAA on 14 March 2001 at another hospital.

Following surgery she required additional surgery on the right iliac artery to correct for ischemic changes in the right leg. She continued to experience abdominal pain and tenderness. At that time no definite endovascular leak was found, but she did have bilateral groin hematomas. Low-dose heparin was resumed because of her aortic valve Starr–Edwards prosthesis.

She returned to our hospital on 21 March 2001.

9 Postoperative course 21 March to 8 April 2001

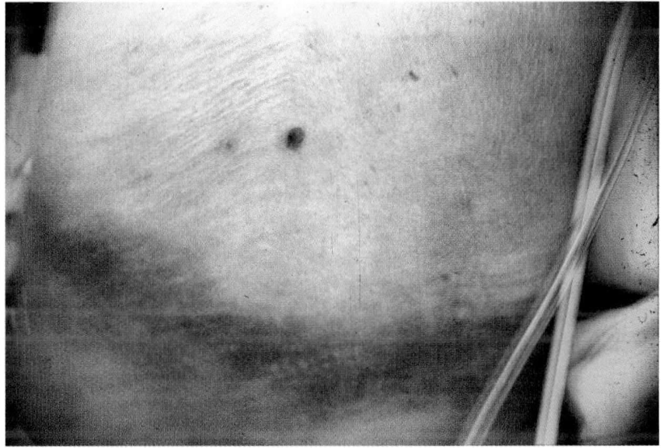

Figure 26.3 The patient's lumbosacral area 21 March 2001 (sitting position).

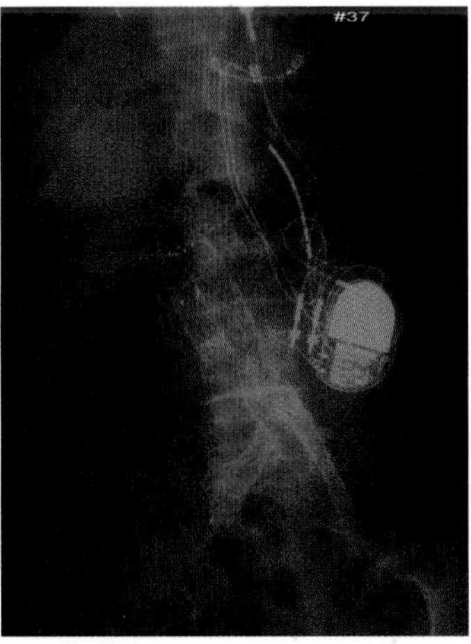

Figure 26.4 Plain abdominal film of aneurx graft in place.

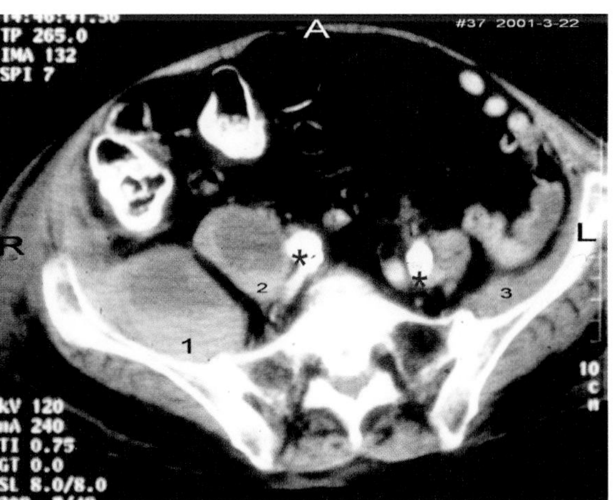

Figure 26.5 CT of abdomen with contrast material at L4 level 22 March 2001. *Name the structures labeled 1–3 and *.*

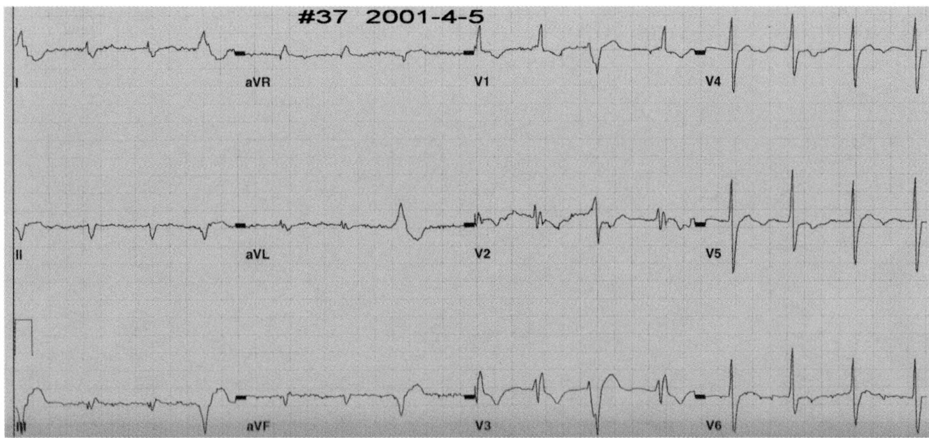

Figure 26.6 12-lead ECG 5 April 2001. Serum troponin levels (ng/mL): 58 (2 April 2001), 37 (3 April 2001), and 4 (7 April 2001). Normal troponin level < 0.03 ng/mL.

History and physical examination 21 March 2001

The patient was complaining of diffuse abdominal pain and melena. She had ecchymoses over the arms and back.

BP 120/70. HR 120/min. Atrial fibrillation.

CVS examination was essentially unchanged from 26 February 2001. There was a 10 × 5 cm hematoma over the left groin. The feet were cool but foot pulses were still present.

Respiratory system: bilateral basal crackles were noted.

Abdomen: there was abdominal tenderness and some distention, an extensive area of ecchymosis was seen over the lumbar area (Figure 26.3), compatible with the Grey–Turner sign.

Laboratory data

MUGA LV ejection fraction (24 March 2001) 23%.

Hemoglobin was 12 g% on 1 April 2001 and 8.5 g% on 6 April 2001.

Echocardiogram showed an estimated RV systolic pressure of 53 mmHg 4 April 2001.

The troponin levels (2–7 April 2001) were elevated. See legend for Figure 26.6.

Comment on the X rays (Figures 26.4 and 26.5) and ECG (Figure 26.6).

The patient received blood transfusions and anticongestive measures.

She had progressive heart failure (probably due to a silent myocardial infarction) despite diuretics and ACE inhibitor, and arrested on 8 April 2001.

Answers and commentary

1 ECG 26 February 2001

Dual chamber paced rhythm seen in AVR, AVL and AVF. HR 70/min. P waves not well seen. QRS 0.13 s. QRS axis +240°. RBBB pattern is seen in V1 (rather than LBBB) because epicardial pacing leads were placed over LV.

2 CT of abdomen 2 March 2001

There is an AAA measuring 6.2 cm in diameter (label 1).

Some suggestion of a clot in the distal portion of the aneurysm. The liver (label 2), kidneys (labels 3 and 6) and psoas muscles (labels 4 and 5) are normal.

The descending aorta was dilated to 4 cm in diameter in the same study.

3 History

The patient had a gradual increase in size of her AAA. Her course between 1993 and 2001 was complicated by the need to continually adjust her dose of anticoagulants (required because of her Starr–Edward aortic valve) in the face of several episodes of GI bleeding.

4 and 5 Physical examination, laboratory data, and course 26 February to 9 March 2001

The patient's aortic valve prosthesis was functioning well based on the physical examination and two-dimensional echocardiography. She probably was in functional class 2 and had only mild LV hypokinesia on echocardiography.

6 Coronary angiography 13 March 2001

Coronary angiography showed that the patient had three-vessel coronary artery disease and that one of her two saphenous bypass grafts had closed off. The LV ejection fraction was not measured at this time.

7 Diagnosis

1. AAA, 6.2 cm in diameter with thrombus.
2. Severe atherosclerosis of coronary arteries and its common iliac branches.
3. Functioning Starr–Edwards aortic valve prosthesis.
4. Functioning dual-chamber pacemaker.
5. Hypertension controlled.
6. History of angiodysplasia of right colon. Acute gastritis.

8 Management and immediate postoperative course 14–21 March 2001

Endovascular stent repair of AAA was indicated because of the large aneurysm (6.2 cm in diameter).

9 Postoperative course 21 March to 8 April 2001

History and physical examination

The presence of abdominal pain along with a Grey–Turner sign are compatible with retroperitoneal bleeding. The hematoma in the left groin suggests iliac artery injury.

Laboratory data

The patient is anemic from blood loss. The elevated troponin levels indicate myocardial necrosis. The LV function has declined significantly and there is moderately severe pulmonary hypertension.

Abdominal X rays

In Figure 26.4 the aortic stent graft is seen, extending from the infrarenal area to the common iliac arteries. The right limb of the bifurcating graft twists and enters the left common iliac artery.

CT of the abdomen at L4 level is seen in Figure 26.5 (22 March 2001). The iliac arteries are seen (*) just inferior to the bifurcation of the abdominal aorta. There is a large hematoma (label 1) in the right posterior zone showing layering of blood (heme level) and possibly a small (label 3) hematoma in the left abdominal area. The right psoas muscle (label 2) is enlarged and contains a layering of blood.

ECG 5 April 2001

Sinus rhythm with PVCs. Rate 80/min. PR 0.16 s. QRS 0.14 s. QRS axis +220°.

RBBB, as on 26 February 2001. Lateral T wave abnormalities have appeared since 26 February 2001.

Discussion

Patients with a significant AAA have been successfully treated with EVR with a lower mortality and early morbidity than open abdominal surgery [1]. Details of the complications of EVR are discussed elsewhere [1–3].

This patient had a large AAA 6.2 cm in diameter, which was a definite indication for surgical repair. Her risk factors were her age (82 years old), hypertension, and severe generalized atherosclerosis. She underwent successful EVR but succumbed in the postoperative period for the following reasons:

1. Iliac arterial injury, leading to retroperitoneal bleeding. The iliac vessels are smaller in women than in men and hence are more likely to be injured when inserting 16–24 French sized endovascular devices [2–4]. This retroperitoneal bleeding was aggravated by the need to resume her anticoagulants to prevent her aortic valve prosthesis from clotting. Retroperitoneal bleeding may be clinically detected by the Grey–Turner sign and confirmed by CT of the abdomen (as in this patient). The Grey–Turner sign usually appears about 24 h after the onset of bleeding [5] and is due to blood diffusing from the pararenal space to the subcutaneous tissue in the lumbosacral area.

2. Silent myocardial infarction leading to intractable heart failure. Females undergoing EVR have a worse prognosis than males and are 1.45 times as likely to die compared to males [6]. This may be because females have more advanced atherosclerosis than men as they present with AAA on average 5 years later than males [4] and also are more likely to have an unfavorable AAA anatomy, namely a short, wide, tortuous infrarenal aortic aneurysm neck [6]. Supra renal aortic dilatation was present in this patient and may [4] or may not [7] have been an adverse factor.

Key points

1. Patients with AAA usually have a lower morbidity and mortality with EVR than open abdominal repair.
2. Women who undergo EVR have a higher complication rate than men. This is because women are operated on at an older age than men (and thus have more advanced atherosclerosis) and their vessels are smaller and more easily injured.
3. Retroperitoneal bleeding following EVR may be due to an endovascular leak or damage to the aorta or its branches. It is readily detected by the Grey–Turner sign.

References

[1] Liaw JVP, Clark M, Gibbs R et al. Update: Complications and management of infrarenal EVAR. *Eur J Radiol* 2009; 71: 541–551.
[2] Desai M, Eaton-Evans J, Hillery C et al. AAA stent-grafts: Past problems and future prospects. *Ann Biomed Eng* 2010; 38: 1259–1275.
[3] Maleux G, Koolen M, Heye S. Complications after endovascular aneurysm repair. *Semin Interven Radiol* 2009; 26: 3–9.
[4] Norman PE, Powell JT. Abdominal aortic aneurysm: The prognosis in women is worse than in men. *Circulation* 2007; 115: 2865–2869.
[5] Dalal D, Mace SE. The clinical picture. A 60 year old man with abdominal bruising. *Cleveland Clin J Med* 2012; 79: 688–689.
[6] Velazquez OC, Larson RA, Baum RA et al. Gender related differences in infrarenal. Aortic aneurysm morphologic features: Issues relevant to Ancure and Talent endografts. *J Vasc Surg* 2001; 33: S77–S84.
[7] Lederle F, Johnson GR, Wilson SE et al. Abdominal aortic aneurysm in women. *J Vasc Surg* 2001; 34: 122–126.

27 PATIENT STUDY 27

Sequence of data display

1 12-lead ECG
↓
2 History and laboratory data
↓
3 Catheterization data
↓
4 Physical examination
↓
5 Course and diagnosis
↓
6 Surgical results

1 12 lead ECG

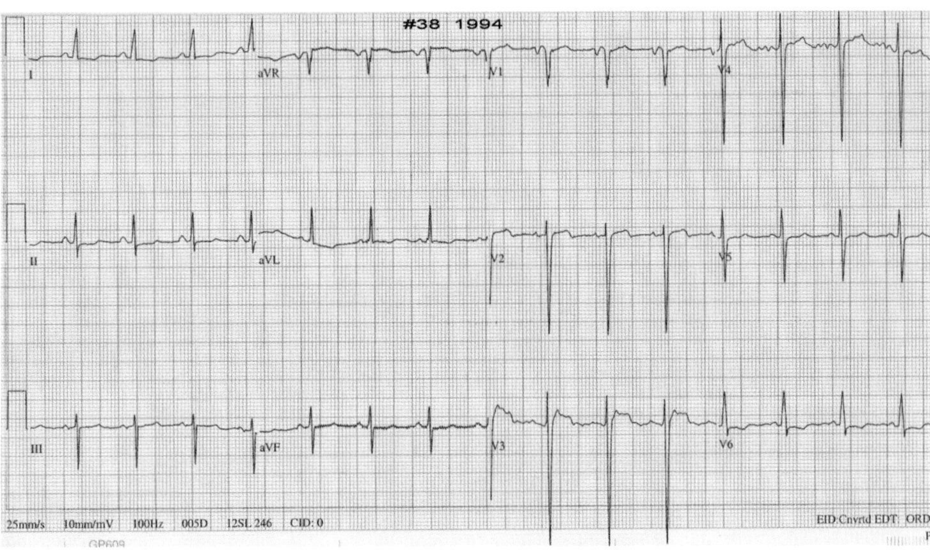

Figure 27.1 12-lead ECG.

2 History and laboratory data

History

41-year-old Asian Indian female admitted to hospital with exertional chest pain and dyspnea for 2 months. No history of rheumatic fever or myocardial infarction. Patient is a nonsmoker and does not drink alcohol.

Laboratory data

Chest X ray report: cardiomegaly and clear lung fields.
Hemoglobin 11 g%.

Patient Studies in Valvular, Congenital, and Rarer Forms of Cardiovascular Disease: An Integrative Approach, First Edition. Franklin B. Saksena.

Companion Website: www.wiley.com/go/saksena/patientstudies

3 Catheterization data

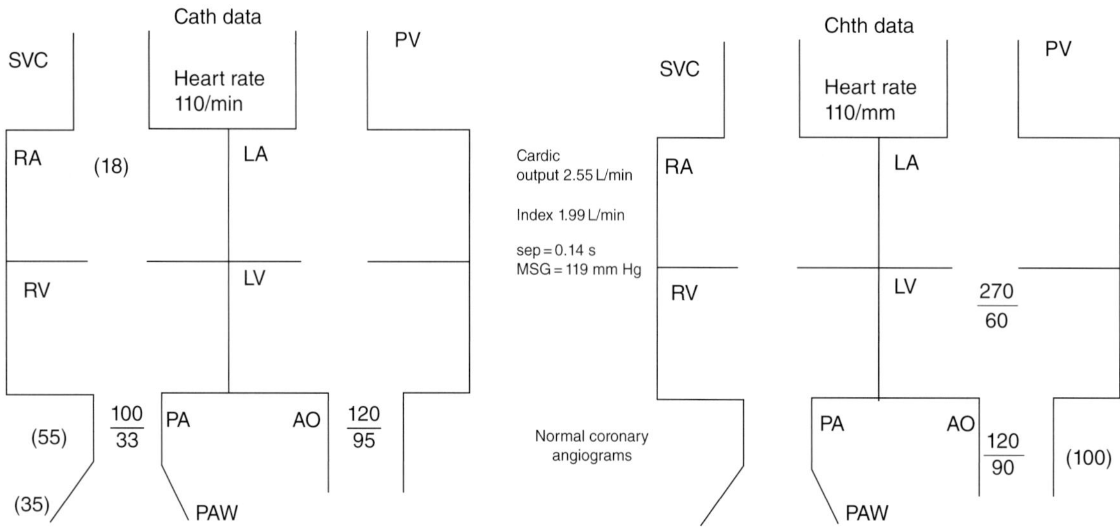

Figure 27.2 Right and left heart pressures before entry in LV. HR 110/min.

Figure 27.3 Left heart pressures after entering the LV. HR 150/min. MSG, mean systolic gradient (mmHg); sep, systolic ejection period (s).

Find the aortic valve area (cm²).

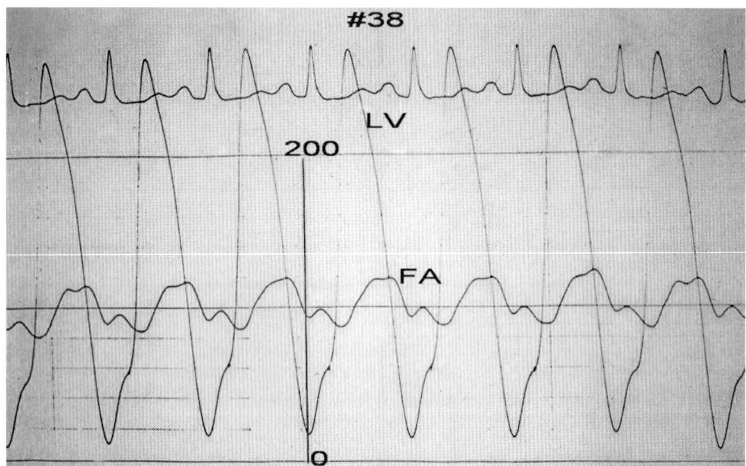

Figure 27.4 Simultaneous LV and femoral artery (FA) pressures. 0–200 mmHg scale.

4 Physical examination

An anxious female 55 inches tall and weighing 96 lb. BP 120/80. HR 100/min. Regular rhythm.
Carotid artery amplitude was diminished.
Apex beat was in the 6th interspace in the anterior axillary line, 11 cm from the mid-sternal line.
S1 normal. S2 –1 decreased. S4 at apex.
Grade 2/6 aortic systolic murmur.
Lungs were clear.
Foot pulses were 1+/4+.

5 Course and diagnosis

The patient developed sinus tachycardia and angina when the LV was entered. The catheter was quickly withdrawn from the LV and her symptoms subsided.

What is the diagnosis and treatment?

6 Surgical results

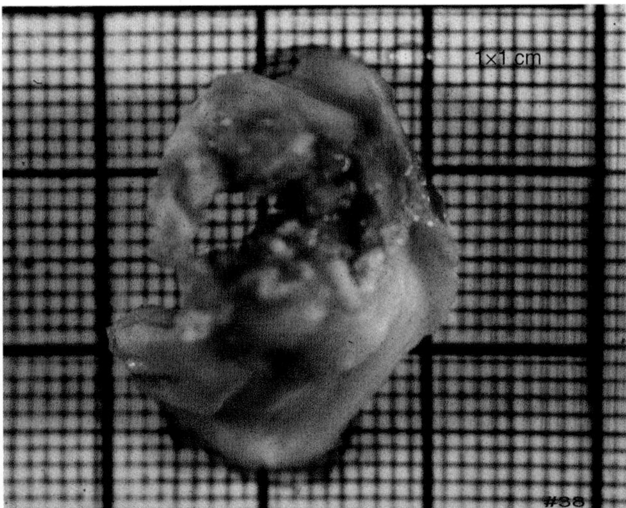

Figure 27.5 Aortic valve removed at surgery. The area of the large square is 1 cm^2.

Answers and commentary

1 ECG

The rhythm was sinus. Rate 93/min. PR 0.15 s. QRS 0.084 s. QRS axis −15°. QT_c 0.4 s. R in AVL + S in V3 > 20 mm. Impression: (i) LA enlargement, (ii) LVH by Cornell's criteria, (iii) nonspecific lateral T wave abnormalities.

2 History and laboratory data

The history and laboratory data suggest the presence of myocardial ischemia/necrosis.

3 Cardiac catheterization data

There is severe pulmonary hypertension (PA mean 55 mmHg) with an elevated wedge pressure of 35 mmHg (Figure 27.2). The wedge pressure may be elevated because of either mitral stenosis or severe LV dysfunction. There is mild diastolic hypertension (95 mmHg).

The LV systolic pressure is very high (270 mmHg), yielding a peak-to-peak gradient of 150 mmHg across the aortic valve (Figure 27.3). The LVEDP was also very high, indicating severe LV dysfunction.

Passing the catheter (cross-sectional area 0.045 cm^2) across the aortic valve was poorly tolerated by the patient, who developed angina and a rise in HR to 150/min. These symptoms subsided when the catheter was quickly withdrawn from the LV.

The calculated AVA using the Gorlin formula was 0.25 cm^2, as shown below.

Data

Cardiac output (CO) 2550 mL/min. HR 150/min.
Mean aortic systolic gradient 119 mmHg.
Systolic ejection period (sep) 0.14 s.

Answer

$$\text{AVA} = \frac{\frac{\text{CO}}{\text{HR} \times \text{sep}}}{44.4 \times \sqrt{\text{msg}}} = \frac{\frac{2550}{150 \times 0.14}}{44.4 \times \sqrt{119}} = 0.25\ \text{cm}^2$$

4 Physical examination

The patient had significant aortic stenosis on the basis of a delayed carotid upstroke, a soft S2, and an apical S4. The systolic murmur was only a grade 2 out of 6, probably because of a low output state. The presence of cardiomegaly is usually only seen in patients with advanced aortic stenosis. The cause of the aortic stenosis in this Indian lady is most likely due to rheumatic fever, which can occur at an earlier age in Asian patients than western ones.

5 Course and diagnosis

Severe aortic stenosis with low output state and severe pulmonary hypertension.

Ischemic chest pain probably due to inadequate blood supply to a hypertrophic LV as her coronary angiograms were normal.

6 Surgical results

The patient underwent successful aortic valve replacement.

The aortic valve commissures were fused, thickened, and calcified. The actual valve area was only 0.16 cm^2 (normal 4–5 cm^2) (Figure 27.5).

Discussion

The patient had severe aortic stenosis on the basis of physical examination, echocardiography (not shown), and hemodynamics.

When the aortic valve was crossed, the catheter (cross-sectional area 0.045 cm^2) further narrowed the valve area from 0.16 cm^2 to 0.115 cm^2, leading to a further fall in cardiac output, and producing symptoms of angina and marked sinus tachycardia.

Physicians need to be aware that crossing the aortic valve in patients with very severe aortic stenosis may be hazardous.

Key points

1. Aortic valve stenosis is often due to rheumatic heart disease in Asian patients.
2. Ischemic chest pain in patients with aortic stenosis can be due to coronary artery disease and/or from the greatly increased demands for oxygen from severe LVH.
3. Crossing the aortic valve orifice with a catheter in very severe aortic stenosis may narrow the valve area enough to lower the cardiac output and induce angina.

28 PATIENT STUDY 28

Sequence of data presentation

1 Aortograms 1994
↓
2 History 1994
↓
3 Doppler arterial studies
↓
4 Physical examination 1994
↓
5 Laboratory data 1994
↓
6 Treatment 28 September 1994
↓
7 Follow-up 1994–2009

1 Aortograms 1994

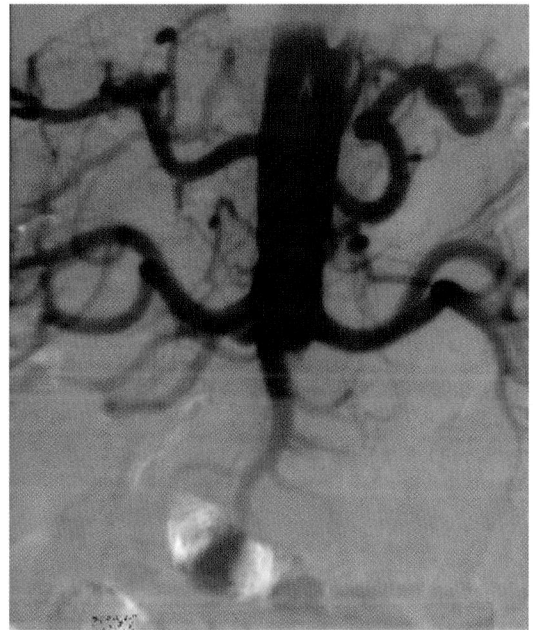

Figure 28.1 Abdominal aortogram 1994.

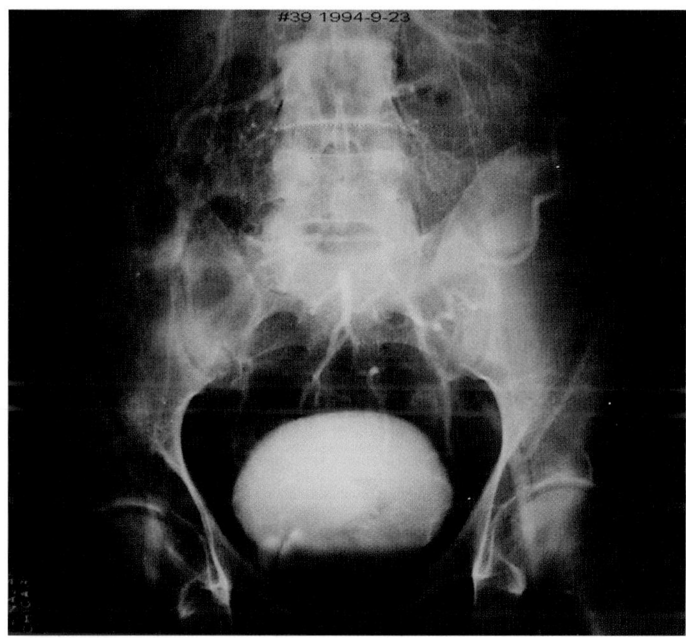

Figure 28.2 Delayed phase of aortogram.

What are the likely symptoms in this patient?

Patient Studies in Valvular, Congenital, and Rarer Forms of Cardiovascular Disease: An Integrative Approach, First Edition. Franklin B. Saksena.

Companion Website: www.wiley.com/go/saksena/patientstudies

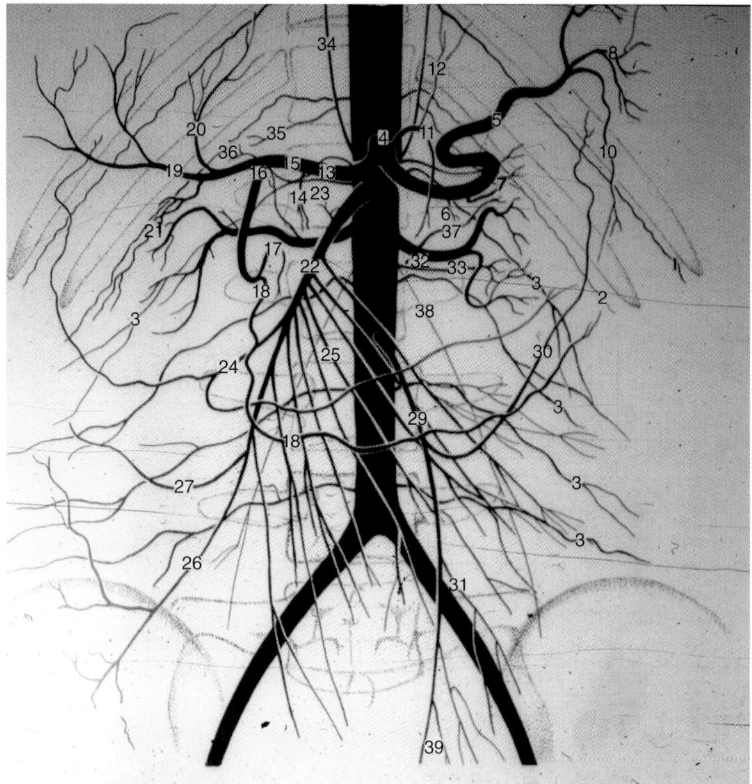

Figure 28.3 Normal abdominal arteriogram. 3, lumbar artery; 4, celiac axis; 22, superior mesenteric artery; 32, renal artery. Source: Muller RF, Figley MM. (1957). Reproduced with permission of the American Roentgen Ray Society.

2 History 1994

48-year-old male with history of right leg numbness for 3 months.
Pain in buttocks on walking half a block for 2 months.
Weakness of legs, unable to stand for 1 day.
Social history: Smoked for 25 pack years. Untreated hypertension for many years.
Daily beer drinker.

3 Doppler arterial studies

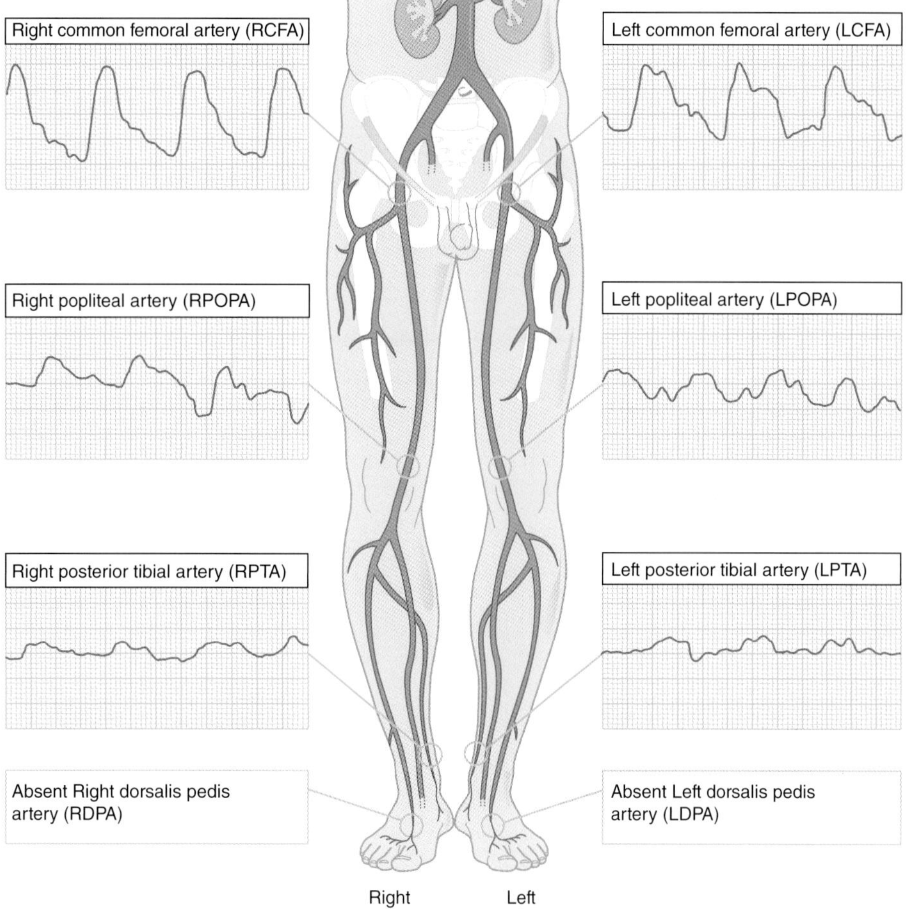

Figure 28.4 Doppler arterial study of lower extremity 22 September 1994.

Table 28.1 Doppler arterial pressures 22 September 1994

Systolic pressure mmHg	Right	left
Brachial	170	164
High thigh	54	52
Low thigh	62	58
Calf	56	46
Ankle	52	36

What is the ankle/brachial ratio?

4 Physical examination 1994

66 inches tall, 135 lb male. BP 180/100 right arm. HR 104/min.
Weak hip flexors, marked dorsiflexor weakness bilaterally.
He can stand up but not walk. Decreased sensation left leg.
No cardiomegaly or murmurs. Carotid a pulses are normal.
Femoral artery: bruits and 2+/4+ pulses bilaterally.
Feet: cool and pulseless.

5 Laboratory data 1994

ECG and chest X ray were normal.

6 Treatment 28 September 1994

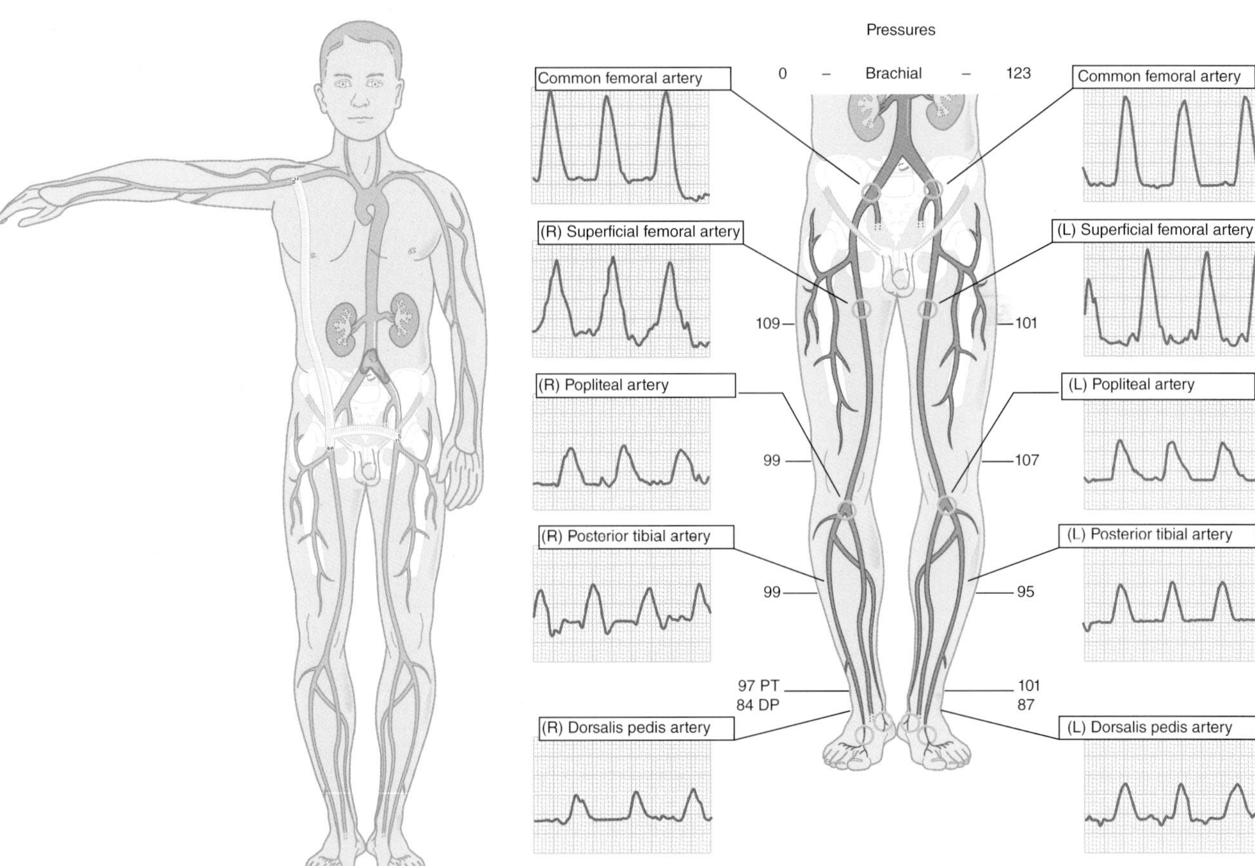

Figure 28.5 Surgical procedure 28 September 1994.

Figure 28.6 Doppler arterial study following surgery 4 October 1994.

7 Follow-up 1994–2009

Table 28.2 Doppler arterial studies 6 January 2006

Systolic pressure (mmHg)	Right	Left
Brachial	158	
High thigh	94	94
Low thigh	89	92
Calf	84	81
Ankle (post tibial)	76	77
Foot (dorsalis pedis)	59	64

Comment on the findings. What is the ankle/brachial ratio?

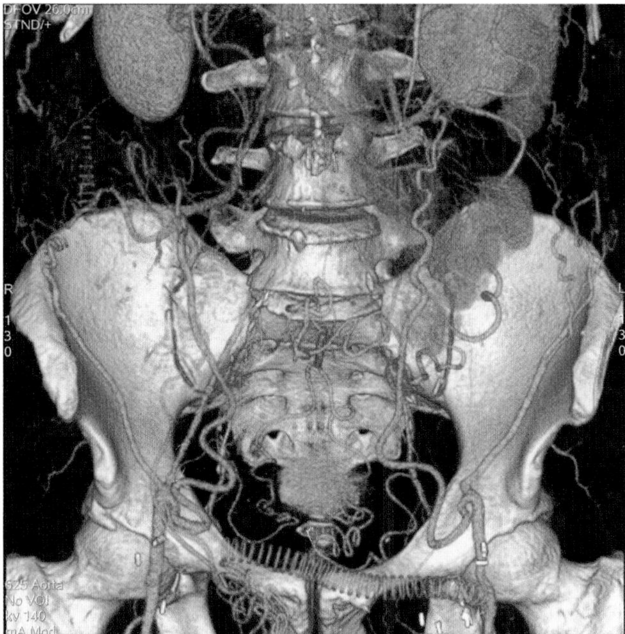
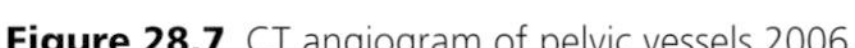

Figure 28.7 CT angiogram of pelvic vessels 2006.

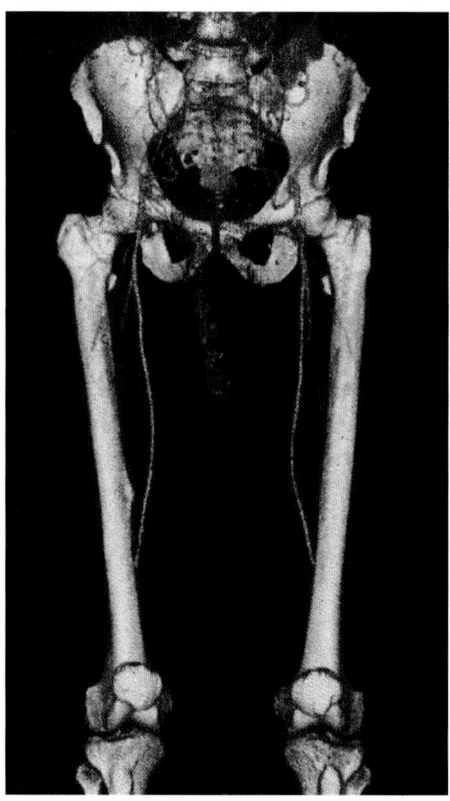

Figure 28.8 CT angiogram of femoral vessels 2006.

Answers and commentary

1 Aortograms 1994

In Figure 28.1 there is complete obstruction of the descending aorta just below the renal arteries. An enlarged lumbar artery issues from the distal aorta.

In Figure 28.2 there is delayed filling of the femoral arteries via an extensive collateral circulation.

These findings are diagnostic of Leriche syndrome.

Figure 28.3 shows the normal aortogram with its branches [1].

2 History 1994

The patient had buttock claudication which is a common symptom in Leriche syndrome. The weakness in the legs is probably due to lack of oxygen to the muscles but could easily be misinterpreted for motor weakness from a spinal cord lesion.

Some patients with Leriche syndrome may have impotence but this did not seem to be the case here.

3 Doppler arterial studies

Normally the systolic pressure in the thighs is about the same or slightly higher than that in the arm, with less than 30 mmHg difference at each level as one progresses from the thigh to the foot [2]. The waveform is normally triphasic, consisting of a large systolic forward flow, a brief reversal of flow in early diastole, and a smaller forward flow in mid diastole with no flow in late diastole [3].

In this patient the wave form is monophasic throughout the lower extremity with further fall in amplitude in the lower leg areas. These finding confirm the presence of severe peripheral vascular disease.

Right ankle/brachial artery ratio = 52/170 = 0.30

Left ankle/brachial artery ratio = 36/164 = 0.22

The normal ankle/brachial ratio is 1, assuming normal compressibility of the vessels. Erroneously high ankle/brachial artery ratios will occur if the vessels are stiff and difficult to compress, as in Monckeberg's disease.

Ankle/brachial ratios less than 0.5 indicate severe limb ischemia, as in this patient.

4 Physical examination 1994

The patient had evidence of severe ischemia of the buttocks and lower extremities.

The rest of the cardiac examination was normal except for hypertension (BP 180/100).

5 Laboratory data 1994

Normal chest X ray and ECG, implying that the hypertension was either of recent origin or only mildly elevated in the past.

6 Treatment 28 September 1994

The patient underwent a right axillary to femoral artery bypass as well as a femoral to femoral artery bypass to improve his lower extremity circulation. This approach poses a lower risk than entering the abdomen to perform an aortofemoral bypass, especially in view of the extensive collateral circulation seen on angiography. In more recent times an EVR repair would have been an alternative [4, 5] but this was not available to us in 1994.

7 Follow-up 1994–2009

1994–1999

Postoperatively, the pressures in the legs improved but the pressure wave form remained monophasic (4 October 1994).

The right brachial/ankle ratio was 97/123 (= 0.78) and the left brachial/ankle ratio was 101/123 (= 0.82) (Figure 28.6).

The patient was discharged on anticoagulants. His grafts were judged to be open in 1999.

January 2006

In January 2006 the patient returned to hospital with left leg pain for 2 weeks.

Doppler studies (Table 28.2) showed a fall in the ankle/brachial artery ratios.

Right ankle/brachial artery ratio = 59/158 = 0.37

Left ankle/brachial artery ratio = 64/158 = 0.40

CT of the pelvis area 13 January 2006

The abdominal aorta below the renal arteries is occluded and unchanged from 1994. The ilio-femoral arteries are receiving blood from inferior epigastric and iliolumbar collaterals.

The right axillary–femoral artery graft and the femoral–femoral grafts appear as long coils of wire. Both grafts are occluded.

CT of the thigh area 13 January 2006

The right femoral artery is patent down to the popliteal area. Subsequent views (not shown) reveal a patent popliteal artery and its three branches down to the ankle.

The left femoral artery is patent down to the popliteal artery. Subsequent views (not shown) show a patent popliteal artery. Only its anterior tibial artery branch is open. There are large collaterals extending into a hernial sac within the scrotum.

The patient's right axillary–femoral graft was occluded. He underwent left axillary–femoral (8 mm)artery graft bypass with right femoral artery endarterectomy.

November 2006

In November 2006 the patient returned with leg pain. On physical examination his blood pressure was 144/73, HR 75/min, RR 20/min, T 97.4 °F. He had decreased pulses in the feet.

CT of the abdomen showed that the left axillary–femoral artery graft was occluded. The patient elected to be followed medically. He was last seen in 2009.

Discussion

The patient had Leriche syndrome on the basis of buttock claudication, motor weakness of the legs, and decreased pulses in the lower extremities. He underwent right axillary–femoral and femoral–femoral bypasses, which remained patent for 12 years. Unfortunately his second axillary–femoral bypass done on the left side only remained open for 7 months.

Leriche syndrome or aortoiliac occlusive disease usually occurs in men between 30 and 40 years of age. It is characterized by claudication of the buttocks, absent femoral pulses, weakness of the lower extremity muscles, and impotence [6]. The risk factors are smoking and hyperlipidemia [6].

As the aortoiliac atherosclerosis progresses slowly, a rich collateral circulation has time to develop, thus averting the loss of a limb by ischemia [6].

Surgical treatment consists of aorto–iliac endarterectomy and aorto–bifemoral bypass or axillary–femoral bypass along with a graft connecting the right and left femoral arteries [7]. The disadvantage of the axillary–femoral bypass graft is its tendency to thrombose, as happened in this patient.

Newer approaches are an endovascular repair to the distal aorta providing the anatomy is suitable [4, 5].

Key points

1. Leriche syndrome often occurs in young men in their 30s who present with buttock claudication, weakness in the legs, and impotence.
2. It occurs when there is atherosclerotic occlusion of the aorto–iliac vessels.
3. Surgical treatment is to perform either an aortic endarterectomy and bypass grafting or an EVR.
4. Axillary–femoral bypass grafts can on occasion provide long-term symptomatic improvement.

References

[1] Muller RF, Figley MM. The arteries of the abdomen, pelvis and thigh. I Normal roentgenographic anatomy. II Collateral circulation in obstructive arterial disease. *Am J Roentgenol* 1957; 77: 296–311.

[2] Yao JST, Flinn WR, Bergan JJ. Noninvasive vascular diagnostic testing: techniques and clinical applications. *Prog Cardiovasc Dis* 1984; 26: 459–494.

[3] Blackshear Jr WM. Surgical indications for lower extremity arterial occlusive disease part 1. *Curr Probl Cardiol* 1981; 6: 7–48.

[4] Allaqaband S, Kirvaitis R, Jan MF, Bajwa T. Endovascular treatment of peripheral vascular disease. *Curr Probl Cardiol* 2009; 24: 351–476.

[5] Setacci C, Galzerano G, Setacci F et al. Endovascular approach to Leriche syndrome. *J Cardiovasc Surg (Torino)* 2012; 53: 301–306.

[6] Mcintyre KE. *Aortoiliac occlusive disease.* http://emedicine.medscape.com/article/471285 overview August 19, 2011.

[7] Marrocco-Trischitta MM, Bertoglio L, Tshomba Y et al. The best treatment of juxtarenal aortic occlusion is and will be open surgery. *J Cardiovasc Surg (Torino)* 2012; 53: 307–312.

29 PATIENT STUDY 29

Sequence of data presentation

1 History and physical examination 3 October 1995
↓
2 ECG 3 October 1995
↓
3 Intracardiac pressures 3 October 1995
↓
4 Course
↓
5 Phonocardiogram
↓
6 Oxygen saturation sample run 9 October 1995
↓
7 Right heart catheterization 9 October 1995
↓
8 Echocardiogram with Doppler study
↓
9 Diagnosis
↓
10 Treatment and course

1 History and physical examination 3 October 1995

67-year-old female admitted to hospital with chest pain on 3 October 1995. BP 70/0. HR 110/min.
No elevation of jugular venous pressure.
Apex beat 5th interspace 9 cm from the mid-sternal line.
No heart murmurs.
Bilateral basal crepitations.

2 ECG 3 October 1995

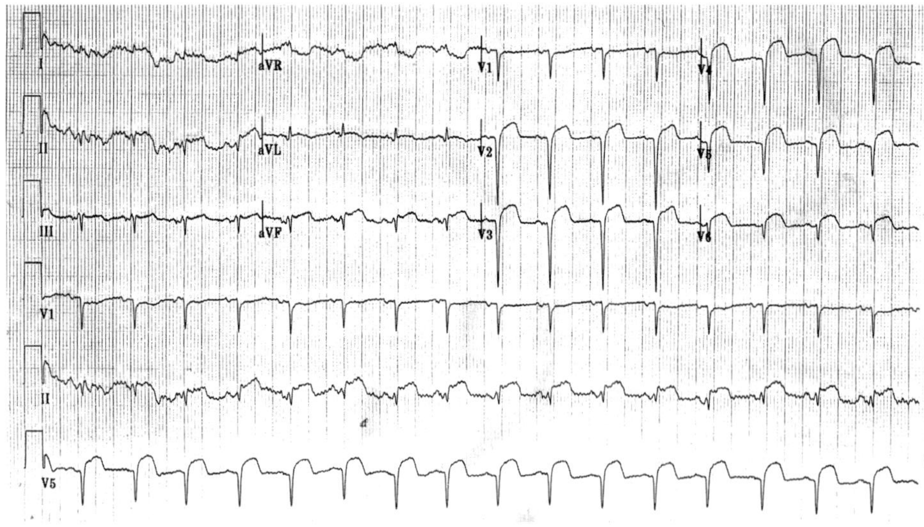

Figure 29.1 12-lead ECG 3 October 1995.

Patient Studies in Valvular, Congenital, and Rarer Forms of Cardiovascular Disease: An Integrative Approach, First Edition. Franklin B. Saksena.

Companion Website: www.wiley.com/go/saksena/patientstudies

3 Intracardiac pressures 3 October 1995

Table 29.1 Right heart pressures (mmHg) 3 October 1995

RV pressure	24/–
PA pressure	24/10, mean 14
PA wedge pressure	mean 8

4 Course

The patient underwent PTCA of the left anterior descending artery with partial reopening of the vessel. The patient was on the intra-aortic balloon pump for the next 2 days to stabilize BP.

On 9 October 1995 the patient went into acute LV failure and developed a systolic apical murmur. It was not stated whether the murmur was heard best just medial or just lateral to the apex beat (Figure 29.2).

5 Phonocardiogram

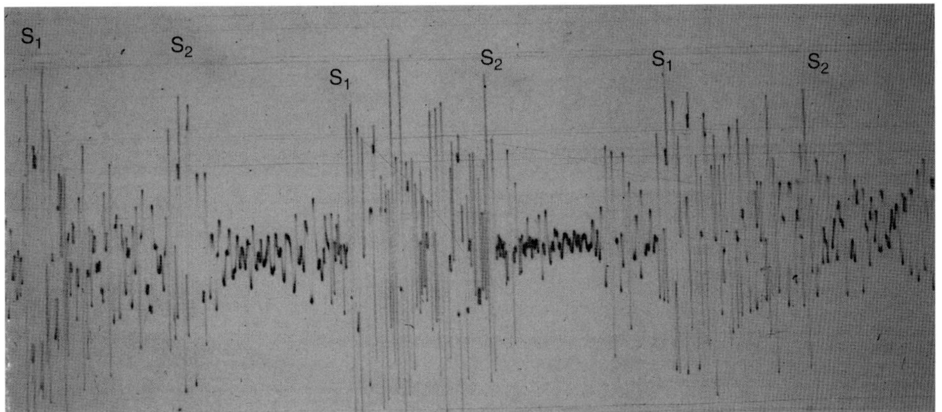

Figure 29.2 Phonocardiogram recorded at LV apex 8 October 1995. Medium frequency.

6 Oxygen saturation sample run 9 October 1995

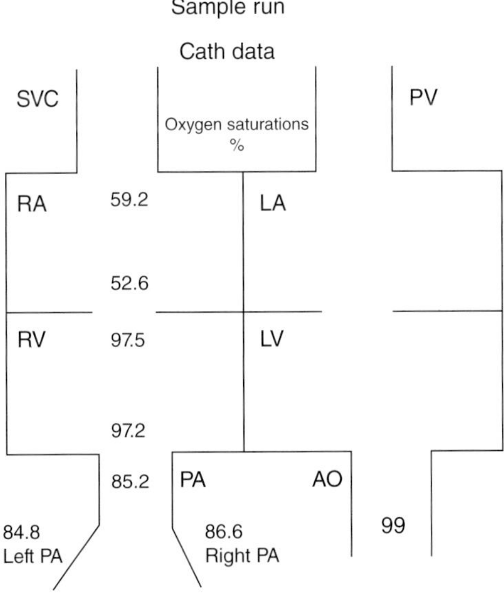

Figure 29.3 Oxygen sample run 9 October 1995.

What is the pulmonary/systemic flow ratio?

7 Right heart catheterization 9 October 1995

Table 29.2 Right heart catheterization 9 October 1995

PA pressure	70/30 (mean 50 mmHg)
PA wedge pressure	mean 30 mmHg
Cardiac index	1.99 L/min/m^2

What is the pulmonary vascular resistance index?

8 Echocardiogram with Doppler study

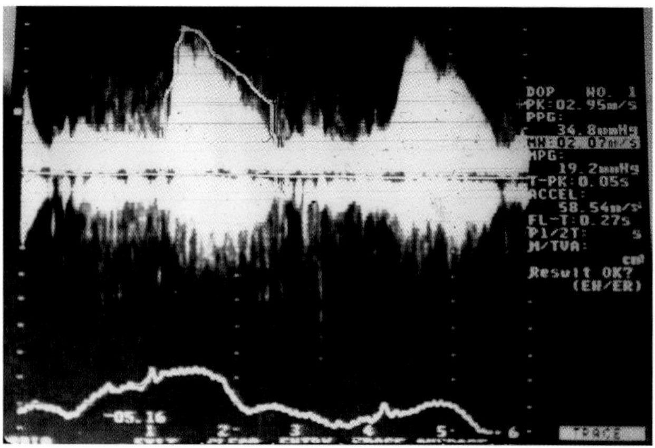

Figure 29.4 Doppler flow velocity across the VSD. VSD jet = 2.5 m/s.

Calculate the RV systolic pressure if the aortic systolic pressure is 100 mmHg.

9 Diagnosis

What is the diagnosis?

10 Treatment and course

She underwent VSD closure. Figure 29.5 shows the postoperative ECG.

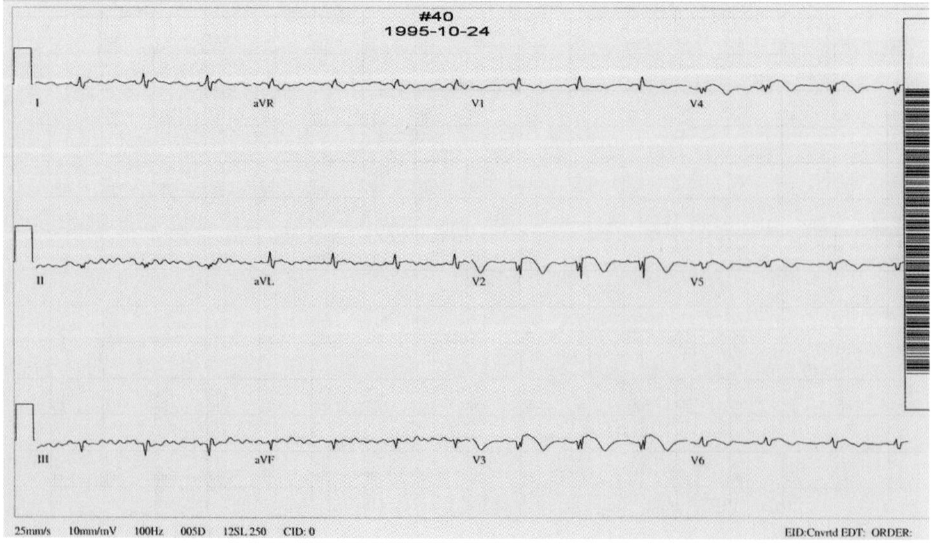

Figure 29.5 12-lead ECG postoperatively 24 October 1995.

Answers and commentary

1 History and physical examination 3 October 1995

This 65-year-old female had chest pain, hypotension, and tachycardia, which could be due to coronary artery disease, pericardial tamponade, or even aortic dissection.

2 ECG 3 October 1995

Rhythm: sinus tachycardia. Rate 110/min. PR interval 0.16 s. QRS 0.07 s. QRS axis –60°. Artifacts in leads 1 and 2. ST elevation and QS waves in V2–6.

Impression: acute anterior wall myocardial infarction.

3 Intracardiac pressures 3 October 1995

Intracardiac pressures were normal.

4 and 5 Course and phonocardiogram

A pansystolic murmur occurring 5 days after an acute myocardial infarction associated with LV failure could be due to acute mitral regurgitation (papillary muscle or chordal rupture) or less commonly a ruptured VSD. If the pansystolic murmur is loudest just medial to the apex beat this is in favor of a VSD, whereas if the murmur is best heard lateral to the apex beat then mitral regurgitation is more likely [1].

6 Oxygen saturation sample run 9 October 1995

There is a step up in oxygen saturation from the RA to the RV compatible with a left to right shunt at ventricular level. The arterial saturation is normal.

Calculation of pulmonary/systemic flow ratio (Q_p/Q_s)

Mean RA saturation 59.9%. Mean PA saturation 85.3%. Arterial saturation 99%.

$Q_p/Q_s = \dfrac{99-59.9}{99-85.3} = \dfrac{2.84}{1}$. This is a significant left to right shunt.

7 Right heart catheterization 9 October 1995

There is now severe pulmonary hypertension with a low cardiac index.

Calculate the pulmonary vascular resistance index

Pulmonary artery (PA) mean = 50 mmHg.
Pulmonary artery wedge (PAW) = 30 mmHg
Cardiac index (CI) = 1.99 L/min/m^2.
Pulmonary vascular resistance index (PVRI) = $\dfrac{\text{PA}-\text{PAW}}{\text{CI}} = \dfrac{50-30}{1.99} \times 80 = 800$ dyn.s/cm^{-5}/m^2
This is a moderately elevated PVRI.

8 Echocardiogram with Doppler study

To calculate the RV systolic pressure

Data

The velocity jet across the ventricular septum (V_s) = 2.5 m/s
Arterial systolic pressure = 100 mmHg

Method 1

The gradient in systole across the VSD = $4 \times (V_s)^2$ = 25 mmHg
The RVSP can then be calculated:
RVSP = arterial systolic pressure – gradient in systole across VSD = 100 – 25 = 75 mmHg
This is similar to the directly measured PA systolic pressure of 70 mmHg.

Method 2

The RVSP can also be calculated if there is significant tricuspid regurgitation (TR):
RVSP = mean RA pressure + $4(V_{TR})^2$
where V_{TR} is the velocity jet across the tricuspid valve.

9 Diagnosis

Ruptured ventricular septal defect secondary to an acute anterior wall myocardial infarction.

10 Treatment and course

The patient underwent surgical closure of a VSD with a 4 cm patch. She did well postoperatively, with some improvement in her ECG on 24 October 1995 compared to 3 October 1995, as seen below.

Sinus rhythm. Rate 80/min. PR 0.13 s. QRS 0.09 s. QRS axis –60°. Low voltage. Smaller Q waves in V2–6. Less ST elevation V2–6. T waves are now inverted in V2–6.

Discussion

A ventricular septal rupture occurred in 1–3 % of myocardial infarctions in the era before fibrinolysis [2]. The incidence has declined since the introduction of myocardial reperfusion to 0.34% of cases [2]. Sixty per cent of VSDs occur in anterior wall myocardial infarctions and 40% following an inferior or posterior wall infarction [3].

The rupture may be simple or complex. A simple rupture involves a through and through rupture of the ventricular septum at the same level, whereas a complex rupture involves an irregular serpiginous tract [2].

Patients who develop a VSD following an anterior wall infarct have an occluded left anterior descending coronary artery with little or no collateral circulation, as in this patient [2].

The development of a VSD typically occurs 3–7 [2] days after an acute myocardial infarction, heralded by a pansystolic murmur and shock.

The Doppler echocardiogram is invaluable in diagnosing what an acute apical systolic murmur in the setting of an acute myocardial infarction is due to, as it can distinguish between a VSD and acute mitral regurgitation [4].

Early surgical intervention is currently recommended because a ventricular septal rupture carries a high mortality rate [5, 6]. This patient was hemodynamically stable so surgery was delayed for 2 weeks as was the custom at that time [6]. The advantage of waiting is that the septum is less friable and easier to repair than in the acute stage. Some surgeons nowadays prefer to operate sooner rather than later to avoid the risk of sudden death.

Repair consists of patching the septal defect, as in this patient. Some authors have used a double patch [7] and others have used an infarct exclusion technique [8] (Figure 29.6). The use of an appropriately sized occluder to close the VSD while the patient in on a ventricular assist device has also been recently reported (Figure 29.7) [9].

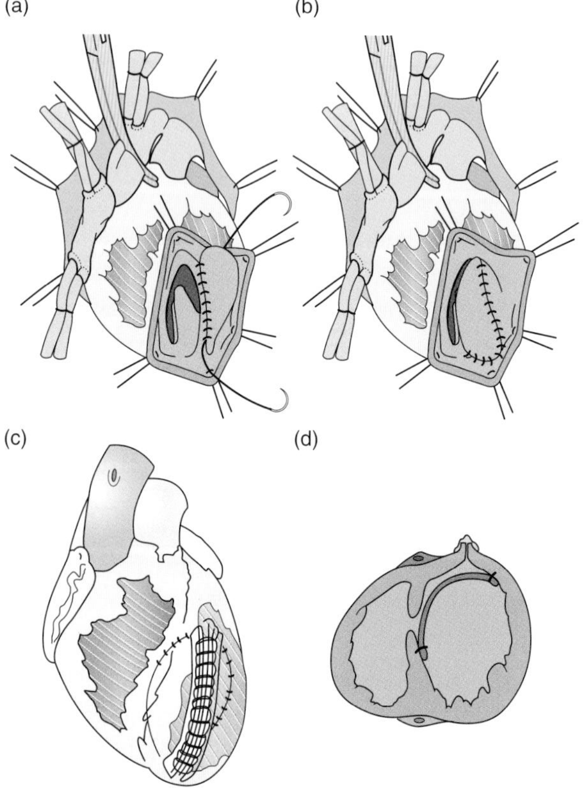

Figure 29.6 (a) 4x6 cm pericardial patch is attached to noninfarcted endocardium of the interventricular septum. (b) Patch is then sutured to noninfarcted endocardiium of anterolateral ventricular wall. (c) The ventriculotomy is then closed. (d) The LV cavity is now excluded from the infarcted myocardium. Source: David TE, Dale L, Sun Z. (1995). Reproduced by permission of Elsevier.

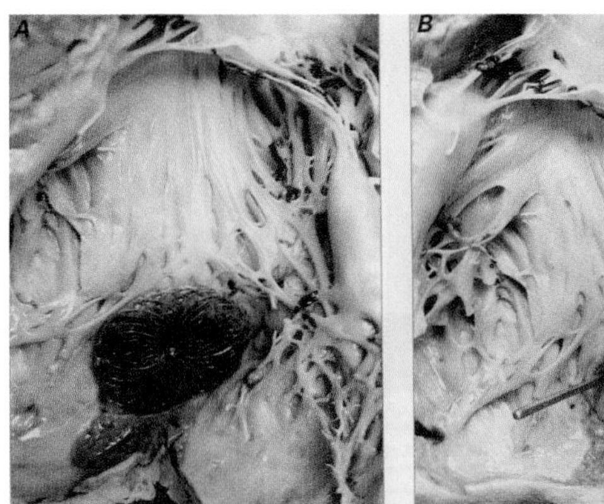

Figure 29.7 Closure of a VSD following a myocardial infarction using an occluder device while on a ventricular assist device. A, VSD occluder in place at autopsy. B, LV septum showing position of VSD after removal of occlude. The size of the occluder was determined beforehand by direct intracardiac echocardiography of the septum. Source: Loyalka P, Cevik C, Nathan S et al. (2012). Reproduced by permission of the Texas Heart Institute.

Key points

1. A pansystolic murmur occurring 3–7 days after an acute myocardial infarction could be due to acute mitral regurgitation or ventricular septal rupture.
2. The distinction between acute mitral regurgitation and a ventricular septal rupture may sometimes be made on physical examination, but right heart catheterization and/or Doppler echocardiography are most helpful in making the correct diagnosis.
3. Early surgical intervention of a ventricular septal rupture is now recommended, using a patch or an infarction exclusion technique.

References

[1] Constant J. *Bedside Cardiology*, 5th edn. Lippincott, Williams and Wilkins, Philadelphia, 1999, p. 267.

[2] Birnbaum Y, Fishbein MC, Blancha C et al. Ventricular septal rupture after acute myocardial infarction. *N Engl J Med* 2002; 347: 1426–1432.

[3] Bhijmi S. *Ventricular septal rupture following myocardial infarction*. Emedicine.medscape.com, 7 November 2008.

[4] Buda AJ. The role of echocardiography in the evaluation of mechanical complications of acute myocardial infarction. *Circulation* 1991; 84(suppl I): I–109–121.

[5] Lemery R, Smith HC, Giuliani ER et al. Prognosis in rupture of the ventricular septum after acute myocardial infarction and role of early surgical intervention. *Am J Cardiol* 1992; 70: 147–151.

[6] Morillon-Lutun S, Maucort-Boulch D, Mewton N et al. Therapeutic management changes and mortality rates over 30 years in ventricular septal rupture complicating acute myocardial infarction. *Am J Cardiol* 2013; 112: 1273–1278 (228 patients with ventricular septal rupture after myocardial infarction admitted from 1981 to 2010 of which 72% were operated on).

[7] Balkanay M, Eren E, Keles C et al. Double patch repair of postinfarction ventricular septal defect. *Tex Heart Inst.J* 2005; 32: 43–46.

[8] David TE, Dale L, Sun Z. Postinfarction ventricular septal rupture: Repair by endocardial patch with infarct exclusion. *J Thorac Cardiovasc Surg* 1995; 110: 1315–1322.

[9] Loyalka P, Cevik C, Nathan S et al. Closure of post-myocardial infarction ventricular septal defect with use of intracardiac echocardiographic imaging and percutaneous left ventricular assistance. *Tex Heart Inst J* 2012; 39: 454–456.

30 PATIENT STUDY 30

Sequence of data presentation

1 Chest X ray
↓
2 ECG
↓
3 Cardiac catheterization and aortography
↓
4 Echocardiogram
↓
5 History and physical examination
↓
6 Surgery

1 Chest X ray

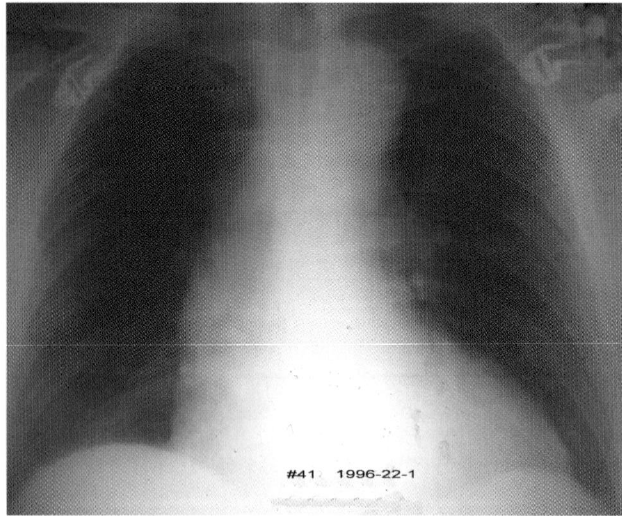

Figure 30.1 Chest X ray.

Patient Studies in Valvular, Congenital, and Rarer Forms of Cardiovascular Disease: An Integrative Approach, First Edition. Franklin B. Saksena.

Companion Website: www.wiley.com/go/saksena/patientstudies

2 ECG

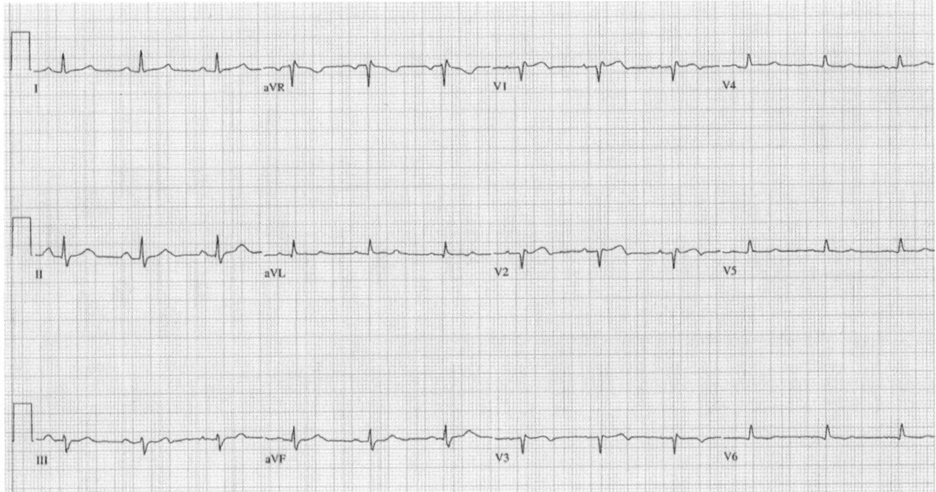

Figure 30.2 ECG. Sinus rhythm. Rate 72 /min.

3 Cardiac catheterization

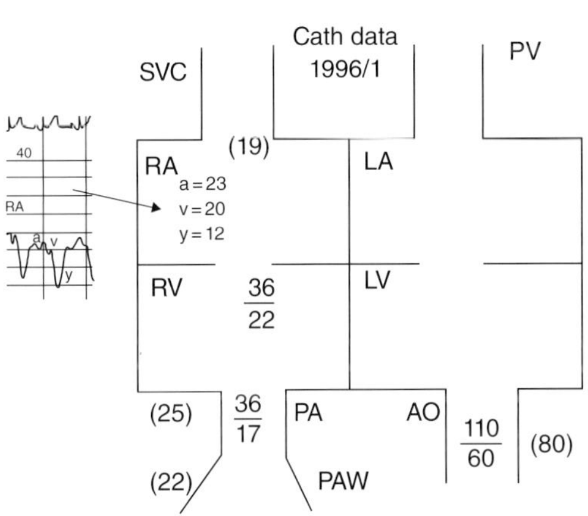

Figure 30.3 Cardiac catheterization.pressures. Inset showing the RA pressure tracing. 0–40 mmHg scale.

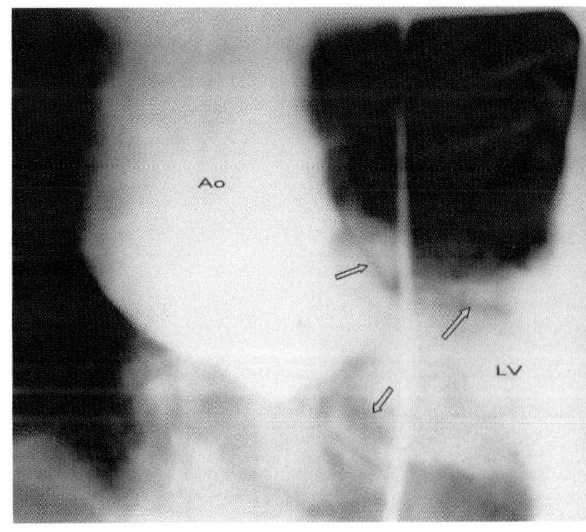

Figure 30.4 Aortogram 30°. RAO.

What are the arrows pointing to?

4 Echocardiogram

There were flickering echoes in the LVOT a pericardial effusion and aortic regurgitation.

5 History and physical examination

History

62-year-old man admitted to hospital with a 1-day history of severe retrosternal chest pain radiating to the jaw and dyspnea. He has a history of hypertension. Denies any myocardial infarction or diabetes.

Physical examination

68 inches tall, 185 lb male. BP 110/70. HR 70 R 22/min.

No jugular venous pressure elevation.

Apex beat 5th interspace, 11 cm from the mid-sternal line.

S1 normal. S2 normal. Loud S3 at apex.
Grade 2/6 diastolic blowing murmur at RLSB.
Lungs clear.
No edema.

6 Surgery

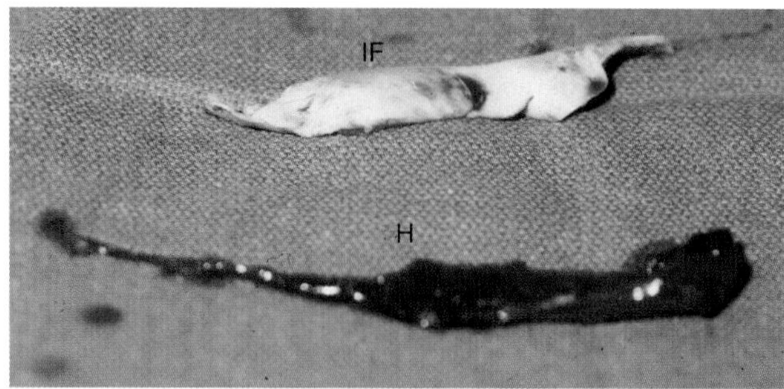

Figure 30.5 The intimal flap (IF) and dissecting hematoma (DH) removed at surgery.

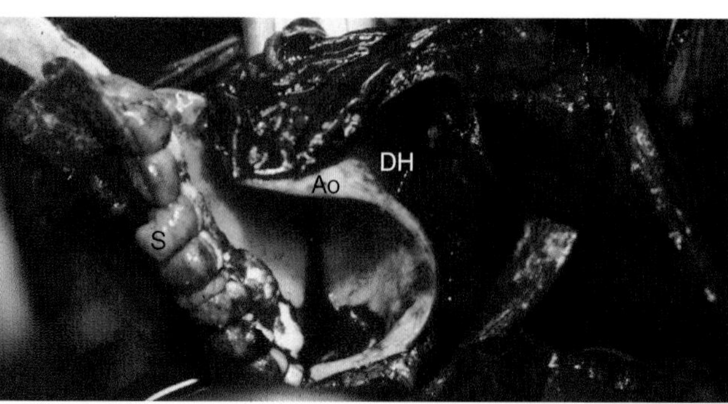

Figure 30.6 Surgical view of the proximal aorta (Ao) and dissecting hematoma (DH) within the false lumen, and the sandwich type (S) of closure of the aortic walls.

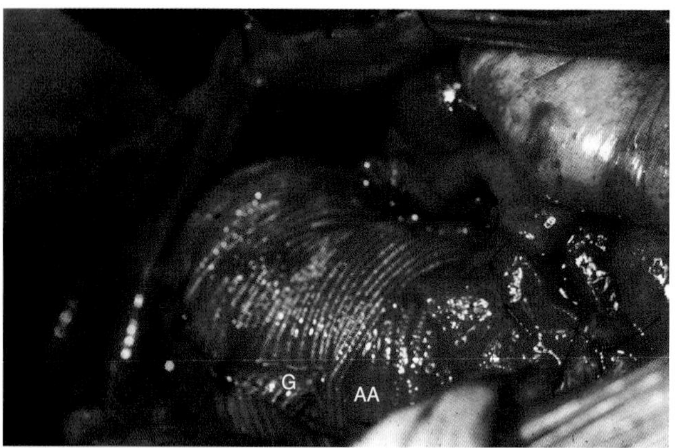

Figure 30.7 The Dacron tube graft (G) has been inserted between the proximal and distal ascending aorta. AA, proximal ascending aorta.

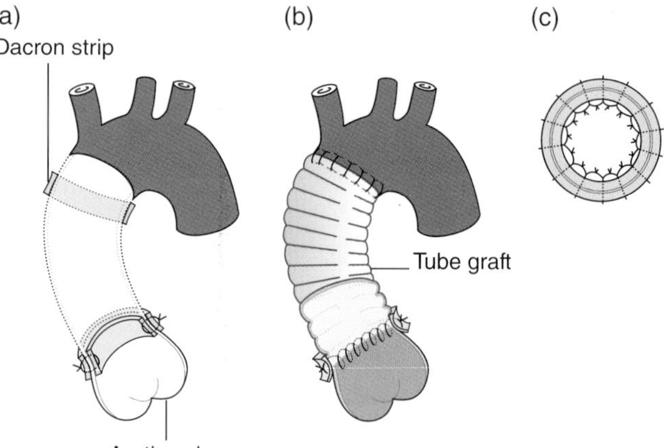

Figure 30.8 The repair of an aortic dissection involving the ascending aorta: (a) transection of ascending aorta (dotted lines), with ends of aorta oversewn to obliterate the false lumen. These sutures are reinforced by dacron strips to prevent them tearing through the fragile aortic walls. (b) Interposition of a Dacron tube graft between the proximal and distal ascending aorta. (c) Cross section of aorta showing obliteration of the false lumen after the aortic walls have been approximated.

Answers and commentary

1 Chest X ray

The chest X ray may be a portable one. Cardiomegaly, possible LVH. Ascending aorta and aortic knob are prominent. Lungs clear.

2 ECG

Sinus rhythm. Rate 72/min. PR 0.15 s. QRS 0.09 s. QRS axis +10°.
Low QRS voltage. Q waves in V1–3.
Impression: old anteroseptal wall myocardial infarction.
Low QRS voltage can be seen in obesity, pericardial effusion, emphysema, myocardial infiltrative disorders, or myocardial ischemia. As the patient is not obese and does not have emphysema then pericardial effusion or myocardial dysfunction remain as possibilities.

3 Cardiac catheterization

The rapid y descent indicates that there is rapid filling of the RA in end diastole (Figure 30.3), thus tending to exclude cardiac tamponade.

Mild pulmonary hypertension. Slightly widened pulse pressure.

The high RA mean, RVEDP, and PA wedge pressures are within 5 mm Hg of each other, suggesting a diastolic pressure plateau compatible with a restrictive filling pattern in at least early and mid diastole.

Aortogram

The ascending aorta is enlarged. Prolapsed intimal flaps (arrows) are seen entering the LV in diastole. There is also aortic regurgitation.

4 Echocardiogram

There was fluid in the pericardium. There were flickering echoes in the LVOT during diastole, which later proved to be a prolapsing intimal flap (cf also Figures 30.9 and 30.10 [1]). There was also aortic regurgitation.

5 History and physical examination

The initial presentation of chest pain was suggestive of an acute myocardial infarction. The patient had normal BP and aortic regurgitation. The diagnosis of an acute dissection was suggested by the widened mediastinum and the lack of enzyme evidence of myocardial necrosis [2]. The presence of aortic regurgitation and anterior chest pain may then suggest type A aortic dissection [2].

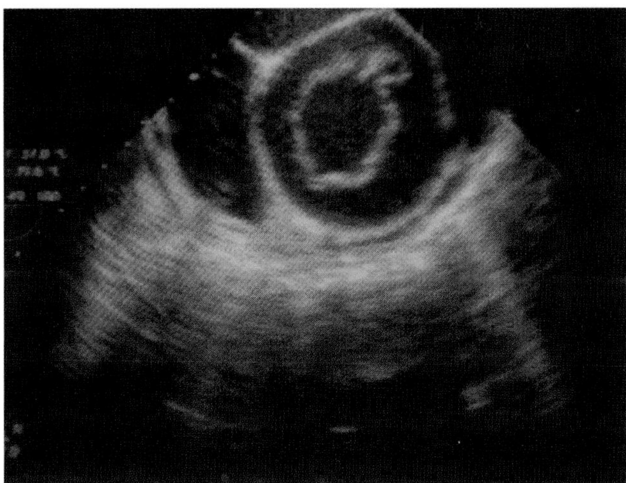

Figure 30.9 TEE appearance of the circumferentially free intimal flap in a 54-year-old man. Source: Oguz E, Apaydin AZ, Nalbantgil S et al. (2007). Reproduced with permission of the Texas Heart Institute.

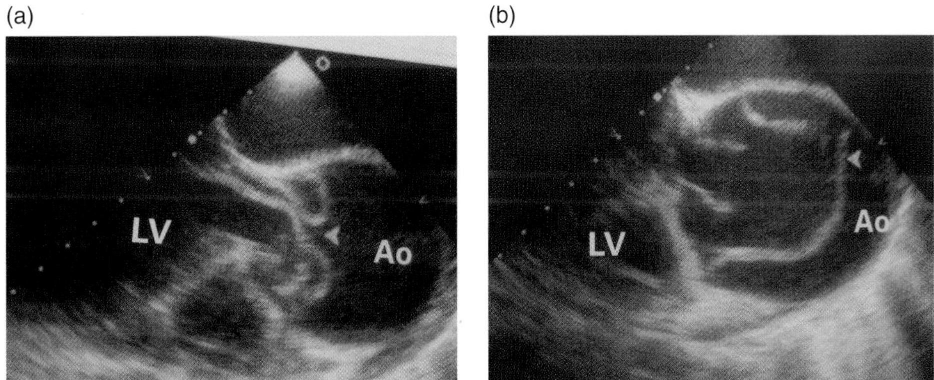

Figure 30.10 TEE shows the back and forth movement of the intimal flap in a 54-year-old man: (a), in diastole; (b), in systole. Source: Oguz E, Apaydin AZ, Nalbantgil S et al. (2007). Reproduced with permission of the Texas Heart Institute.

6 Surgery

The patient had a type A aortic dissection as well as a hemopericardium. A blood clot (DH) was removed from the pericardium and the false lumen of the ascending aorta (Figure 30.5). The distal ascending aorta containing the prolapsed intimal flap (IF) was resected (Figure 30.5).

The ascending aortic walls (Ao) were reapproximated (S) to eliminate the false lumen (Figures 30.6 and 30.8) and a tube graft (G) interposed between the proximal and distal parts of the ascending aorta (Figure 30.7). The aortic valve was spared.

Discussion

The patient had an aortic dissection beginning in the ascending aorta (type A). The dissection involved most of the circumference of the aorta, which resulted in an intimal flap. This intimal flap then crossed the aortic valve and entered the LV during each diastole. This movement of the intimal flap in and out of the LV would account for the patient's aortic regurgitation (see also Figures 30.9 and 30.10 in another patient).

Other mechanisms of aortic regurgitation in aortic dissection are (i) failure of leaflet coaptation due to aortic root dilatation, (ii) distortion of the valve leaflets by the dissection itself, and (iii) development of a flail aortic valve leaflet [1, 3].

The patient also had a hemopericardium, which probably accounts for the restrictive filling pattern of the right heart and the normalization of the BP in acute dissection. The rapid y descent in the RA pressure tracing would be against the presence of cardiac tamponade at the time of cardiac catheterization.

Key points

1. Hypertension, severe chest pain, aortic regurgitation, and mediastinal widening are findings that suggest aortic dissection.
2. A rare cause of aortic regurgitation in aortic dissection is prolapsing intimal flap into the LV in diastole.
3. Other causes of aortic regurgitation in aortic dissection are aortic root dilatation, distortion of the leaflets, or a flail leaflet.

References

[1] Oguz E, Apaydin AZ, Nalbantgil S et al. Circumferential intimal flap prolapsing into the left ventricle. *Tex Heart J* 2007; 34: 496–497. [Apaydin AZ, Almassi GH. Tex Heart J 2008; 35: 228 (letters).]

[2] Spittell PC, Spittell JA, Joyce JW et al. Clinical features and differential diagnosis of aortic dissection: Experience with 236 cases (1980 through 1990). *Mayo Clin Proc* 1993; 68: 642–651.

[3] Rosenzwieg BP, Goldstein S, Sherrid M et al. Aortic dissection with flap prolapse into the left ventricle. *Am J Cardiol* 1996; 77: 214–216.

31 PATIENT STUDY 31

Sequence of display data

1 12-lead ECG 17 October 1997
↓
2 Chest X rays
↓
3 Phonocardiogram
↓
4 Oxygen sample run
↓
5 Pressures and LV ejection fraction
↓
6 Echocardiograms
↓
7 History and physical examination
↓
8 Diagnosis

1 12- lead ECG 17 October 1997

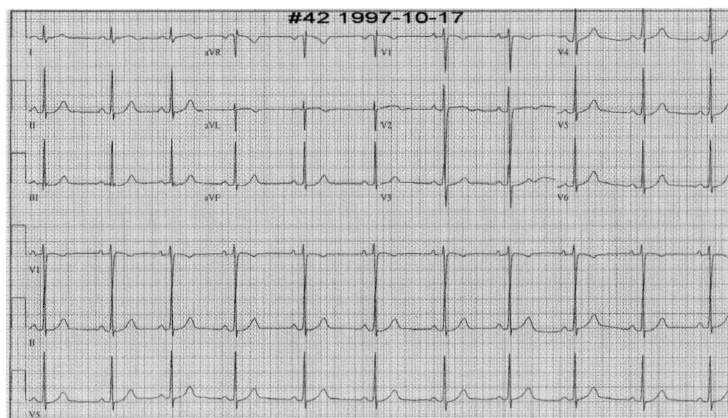

Figure 31.1 12-lead ECG.

2 Chest X rays

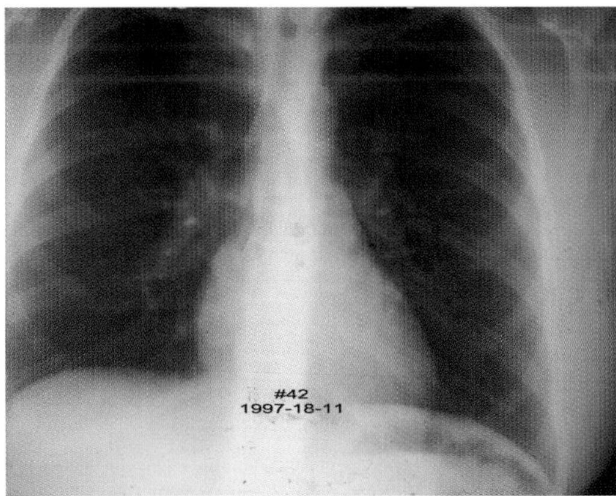

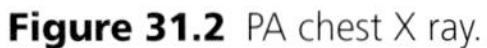

Figure 31.2 PA chest X ray.

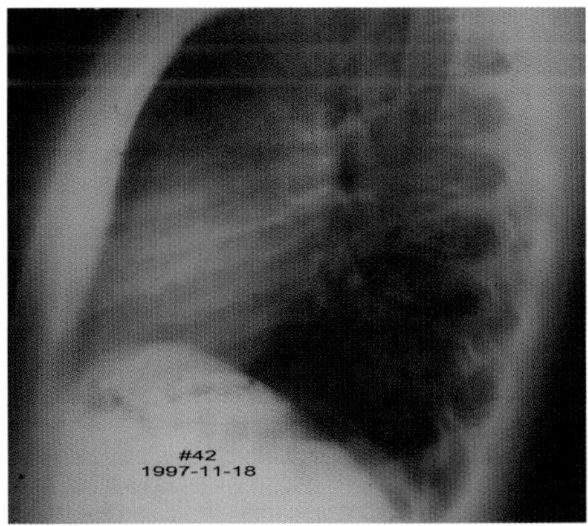

Figure 31.3 Lateral chest X ray.

Patient Studies in Valvular, Congenital, and Rarer Forms of Cardiovascular Disease: An Integrative Approach, First Edition. Franklin B. Saksena.

Companion Website: www.wiley.com/go/saksena/patientstudies

3 Phonocardiogram

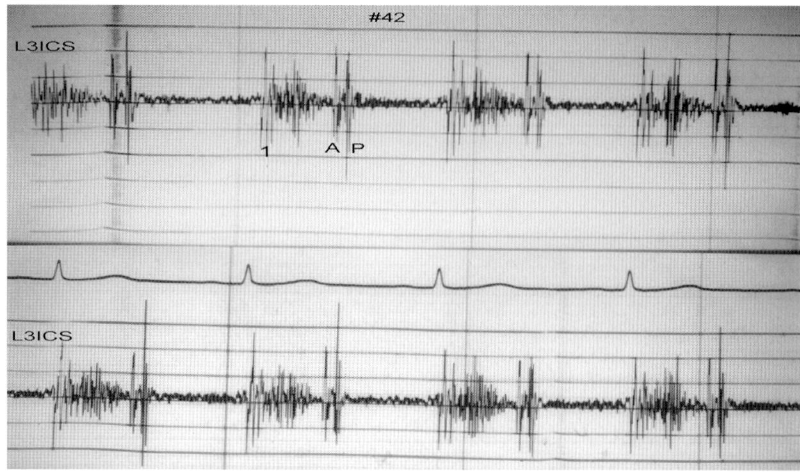

Figure 31.4 Phonocardiogram left 3rd interspace (8 beats in sequence).

4 Oxygen sample run

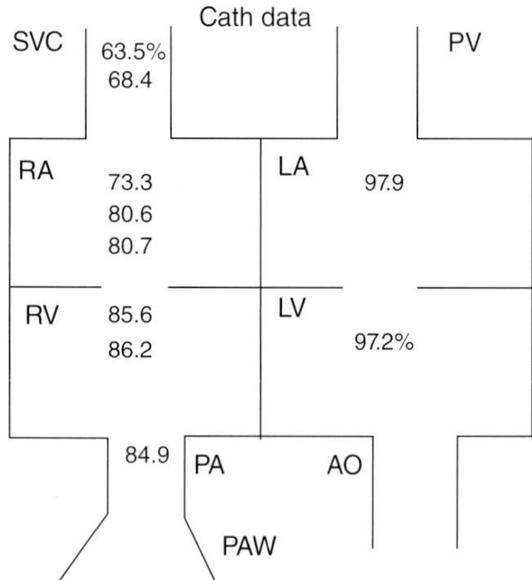

Figure 31.5 Oxygen saturation sample run.

Calculate the pulmonary/systemic flow ratio.

5 Pressures and LV ejection fraction

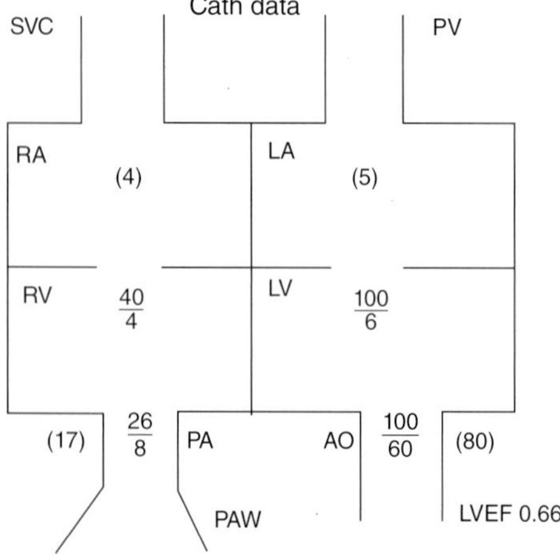

Figure 31.6 Pressures and LV ejection fraction.

6 Echocardiograms

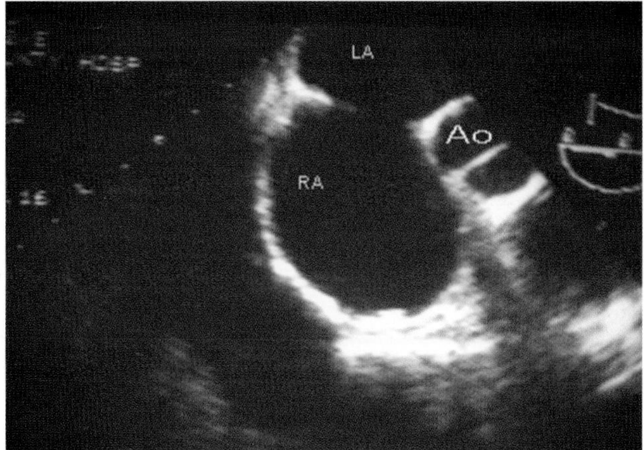

Figure 31.7 Short-axis view of the TEE at the mid-esophagus plane.

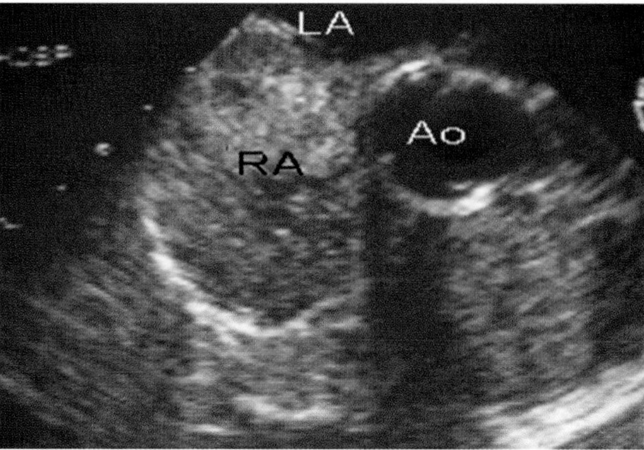

Figure 31.8 After an intravenous injection of saline, microbubbles are seen filling the RA using the same short-axis view of the TEE as Figure 31.7

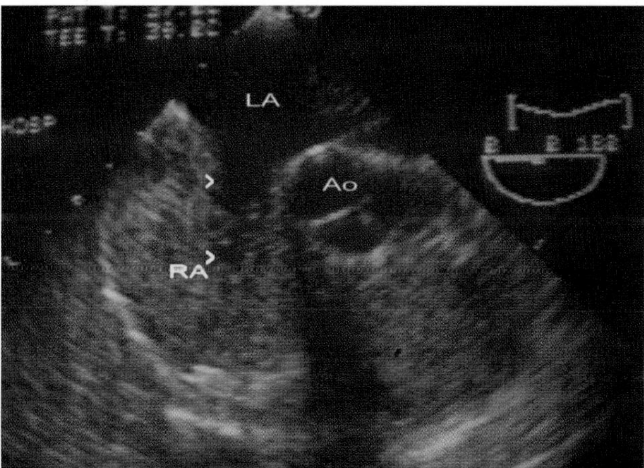

Figure 31.9 Short-axis view of the TEE showing microbubbles in the RA (late phase).
What are the arrowheads pointing to?

7 History and physical examination

History

17-year-old female admitted to hospital with a 6-month history of fatigue and dyspnea on walking two blocks. She was told she had had a heart murmur 6 months ago.

No history of rheumatic fever.

Physical examination

60 inches tall, 122 lb female. BP 108/57. HR 74/min.

No elevation of jugular venous pressure. Normal carotid upstroke.

Apex beat is in 5th interspace 11 cm from the mid-sternal line. No RV lift.

S1 normal. S2 wide fixed splitting (0.06 s).

Grade 2/6 systolic ejection murmur best heard at 3rd left interspace parasternally.

Lungs clear.

Normal peripheral pulses. No edema, cyanosis, or clubbing.

8 Diagnosis

What is the diagnosis?

Answers and commentary

1 12-lead ECG 17 October 1997

The rhythm is sinus. Rate 65/min. PR 0.16 s. QRS 0.08 s. QRS axis +80°.
Impression: normal ECG.

2 Chest X rays

In the PA view the cardiothoracic ratio (C/T) is 0.42 (normal). The proximal pulmonary arteries are enlarged. Based on the normal subcarinal angle (<70°) the LA is not enlarged.
In the lateral view about 50% of the retrocardiac space is occupied by the heart, indicative of RV enlargement.
The presence of RV enlargement and pulmonary plethora is suggestive of a left to right shunt.

3 Phonocardiogram

The wide fixed splitting of the second sound and the pulmonary ejection systolic murmur are indicative of an ASD. The absence of left-axis deviation on ECG suggests that this is a secundum rather than a primum defect.
Other causes of a fixed splitting of the second sound are idiopathic PA dilatation and acute massive pulmonary embolism [1], none of which are present in this patient.

4 Oxygen sample run

The arterial saturation is normal so that a right to left shunt is less likely.
There is a step up of oxygen saturation on entering the RA from the SVC, which is most often due to an ASD. Other causes of a step up in oxygen saturation from SVC to RA are a ruptured sinus of valsalva into RA, coronary AV fistula, VSD with tricuspid regurgitation, and anomalous pulmonary venous drainage.

Calculate the pulmonary/systemic (Q_p/Q_s) flow ratio

Given:
average SVC saturation = 65.5%
PA saturation = 84.9%
arterial saturation = 97.2% (LV)
PV saturation ≡ LA saturation = 97.9%

Step 1: Use Fick's principle
Q_p = oxygen consumption/($C_{pv} - C_{pa}$) where C is oxygen content
Q_s = oxygen consumption/($C_a - C_{svc}$)

Step 2: Find the Q_p/Q_s ratio using oxygen saturations
As oxygen content (C) = hemoglobin × 1.36 × saturation (S)
We have C is proportional to S

Hence $$\frac{Q_p}{Q_s} = \frac{C_a - C_{svc}}{C_{pv} - C_{pa}} = \frac{S_a - S_{svc}}{S_{pv} - S_{pa}} = \frac{97.2 - 65.5}{97.9 - 84.9} = \frac{2.4}{1}$$

This is a significant left to right shunt at atrial level.

5 Pressures and LV ejection fraction

The RV systolic pressure is mildly elevated. There is a small systolic gradient across the pulmonic valve due to increased flow across the valve. Left heart pressures are normal. There is no evidence of mitral stenosis as there is no gradient in diastole across the mitral valve. The LV ejection fraction is normal.

6 Echocardiograms

There is an ASD with a small inferior rim (Figure 31.7).
Saline injection showed microbubbles entering the RA (Figure 31.8) and a negative contrast jet seen in Figure 31.9, indicating a left to right shunt at atrial level.

7 History and physical examination

The patient was only mildly symptomatic but had the findings of ASD, i.e. wide fixed splitting of the second sound and a pulmonary flow murmur. However, the location of the apex beat did not correspond with the heart size on chest X ray.

8 Diagnosis

Secundum ASD with pulmonary/systemic flow ratio of 2.4/1.

Discussion

A secundum ASD involves the fossa ovalis and is mid-septum in location. It occurs in about 20% of all congenitial heart diseases [2]. The patient had the cardinal physical findings of an ASD, i.e. a wide fixed splitting of the second sound, a pulmonary flow murmur, and RV enlargement. Additional features include a loud first sound (attributed to the additive effect of the tricuspid closure sound to the mitral closure sound) and a diastolic murmur of relative tricuspid stenosis (due to increased flow across the tricuspid valve) [2–4].

Mitral stenosis can simulate some of the features of an ASD, in that a loud S1, a diastolic rumble, and RV enlargement are seen in both conditions. However, the wide fixed splitting of S2 and the absence of LA enlargement point to an ASD as being the correct diagnosis.

Cardiac catheterization is useful to establish the diagnosis of an ASD and exclude other congenital anomalies. After the age of 40, patients requiring closure of the ASD will require coronary angiography [4].

The pulmonary/systemic flow ratio (Q_p/Q_s) can be calculated at cardiac catheterization as well as by Doppler echocardiography, using the formula [5]:

flow across the RV or LV outflow tract = velocity × area, as follows

Q_p = time velocity integral across the RV outflow tract × area of pulmonic valve

Q_s = time velocity integral across the LV outflow tract × area of aortic valve

TEE is also useful in defining the size of the ASD and the direction of the shunt, determining rim adequacy, and excluding partial anomalous pulmonary venous drainage [4, 6].

In this patient, the rim of the defect was considered too small to recommend an Amplatzer septal occluder device [6] and so surgical closure with a pericardial patch was carried out. Closure of an ASD is recommended when the Q_p/Q_s ratio is over 1.5/1 as was the case in our patient [4, 6].

Closure is indicated to prevent long-term complications such as a reduced exercise tolerance, atrial arrhythmias, progression of tricuspid regurgitation, right to left shunting, overt congestive heart failure, embolism during pregnancy, and pulmonary vascular disease [7].

Operative mortality for ASD closure is about 1–2% at the present time [8, 9].

Key points

1. The physical findings of a secundum ASD are a loud S1, wide fixed splitting of S2, a pulmonary flow murmur, and RV enlargement.
2. The pulmonary/systemic flow ratio may be found from cardiac catheterization or Doppler echocardiography. A pulmonary/systemic flow ratio > 1.5/1 is an indication for closing the defect.
3. The ASD may be closed surgically or by using an Amplatzer septal occluder providing there is an adequate rim around the defect.

References

[1] Shaver JA, O'Toole JD, Curtiss EI et al. *Second heart sound: The role of altered greater and lesser circulation.* In: Physiologic Principles of Heart Sounds and Murmurs, Leon DF, Shaver JA (eds). American Heart Association Monograph Number 46, New York, 1975, pp 58–76 (discusses the hang out intervals for systemic and pulmonary circulation).

[2] Gerbode F, Carr I. Defects of the atrial septum. *Cardiovascular Clinics: Cardiac Surgery I* 1974; 3: 130–147.

[3] Leatham A, Gray I. Auscultatory and phonocardiographic signs of atrial septal defect. *Br Heart J* 1956; 18: 193–208.

[4] Webb G, Gatzoulis MA. Atrial septal defects in the adult. Recent progress and overview. *Circulation* 2006; 114: 1645–1653.

[5] Reynolds T. *The Echocardiographer's Pocket Reference*, 3rd edn. Heart Foundation, Phoenix, AZ, 2010, p. 355.

[6] Aboulhosn J, Levi DS, Child JS. Common congenital heart disorders in adults: Percutaneous therapeutic procedures. *Curr Probl Cardiol* 2011; 36: 261–284.

[7] Atrial septal defect. In: ACC/AHA 2008 Guidelines for the management of adults with congenital heart disease: Executive summary. *J Am Coll Cardiol* 2008; 52: 1905–1907.

[8] Horvath KA, Burke RP, Collins JJ et al. Surgical treatment of adult atrial septal defect: early and long term results. *J Am Coll Cardiol* 1992; 20: 1156–1159 (166 patients operated on, mean follow-up of 90 months).

[9] Zomer AC, Verheugt,CJ, Vaartjes I et al. Surgery in adults with congenital heart disease. *Circulation* 2011; 124: 2195–2201 (includes 1552 patients operated on for an ASD with a 15-year follow-up.)

32 PATIENT STUDY 32

Sequence of data presentation

1 History
↓
2 Echocardiogram 1991
↓
3 Cardiac catheterization 1991
↓
4 ECG 1997
↓
5 Chest X rays 1997
↓
6 Cardiac catheterization 1997
↓
7 Pressure tracings 1997
↓
8 Oxygen saturation sample run 1997
↓
9 Physical examination
↓
10 Laboratory data
↓
11 Follow-up studies 2001–2012

1 History

31-year-old female P2 G2 who was admitted to hospital in 1997 with a 1-month history of dizziness, fatigue, and a single episode of syncope. No history of dyspnea, chest pain, rheumatic fever, diabetes, or hypertension.

She had been seen at another hospital in 1991 and was placed on nifedipine following a cardiac catheterization in 1991 (Figure 32.2). She took nifedipine until 1993.

2 Echocardiogram 1991

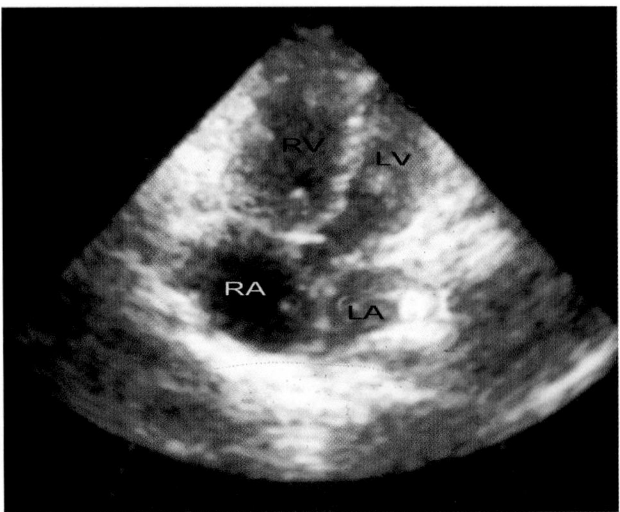

Figure 32.1 Two-dimensional echocardiogram showing four-chamber view 1991. The peak velocity across the tricuspid valve is 3.6 m/s. *What is the estimated RV systolic pressure?*

Patient Studies in Valvular, Congenital, and Rarer Forms of Cardiovascular Disease: An Integrative Approach, First Edition. Franklin B. Saksena.

Companion Website: www.wiley.com/go/saksena/patientstudies

3 Cardiac catheterization 1991

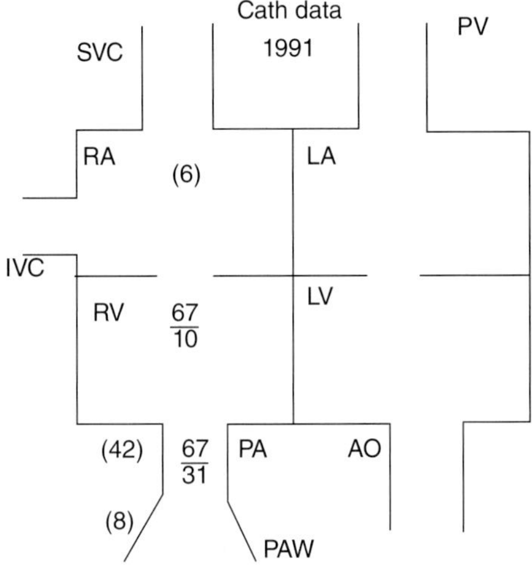

Figure 32.2 Right heart catheterization 1991.

4 ECG 1997

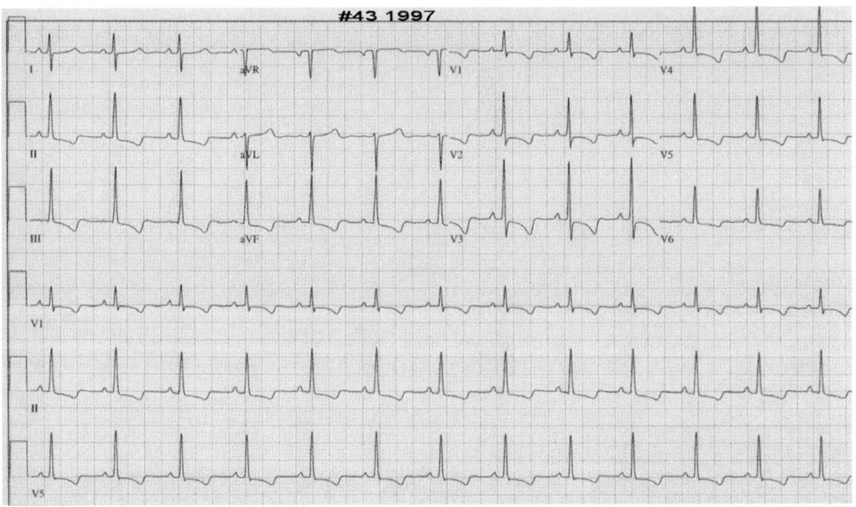

Figure 32.3 12-lead ECG 1997.

5 Chest X rays 1997

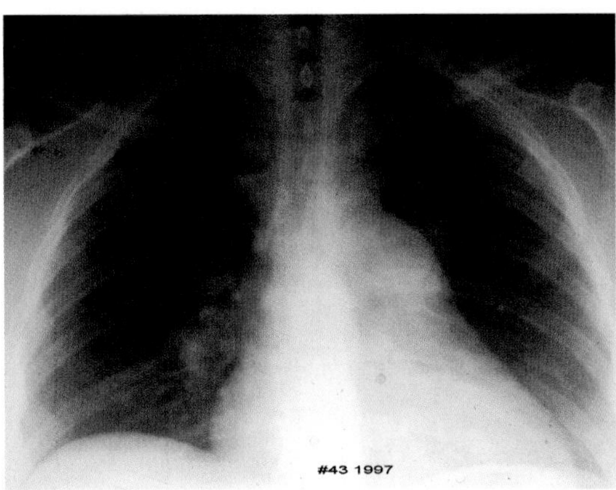

Figure 32.4 PA chest X ray 1997.

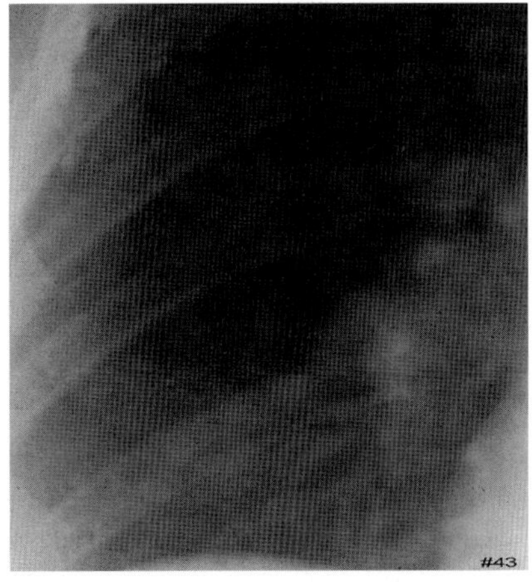

Figure 32.5 Right lung field. Same X ray as Figure 32.4.

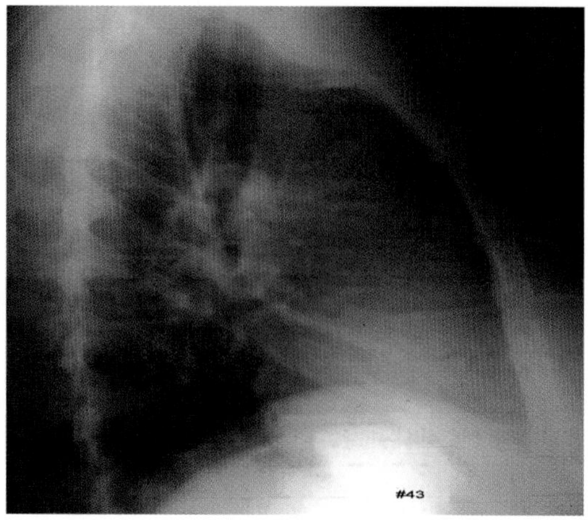

Figure 32.6 Lateral chest X ray 1997.

6 Cardiac catheterization 1997

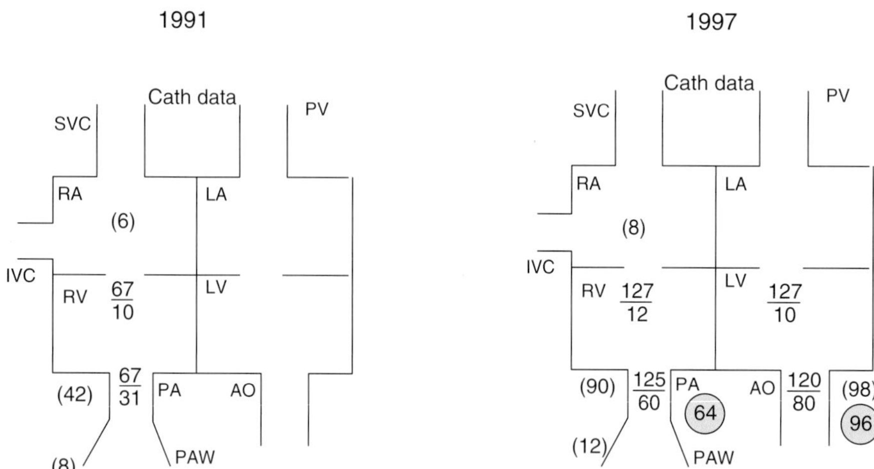

Figure 32.7 Right and left heart catheterization 1997, compared to 1991 study. Numbers in circles are oxygen saturations.

7 Pressure tracings 1997

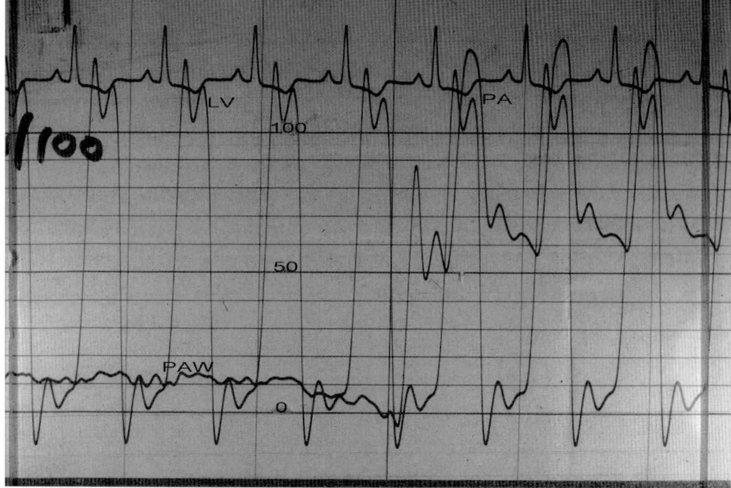

Figure 32.8 PA, PAW and LV pressure curves 1997. 0–100 mmHg scale.

8 Oxygen saturation sample run 1997

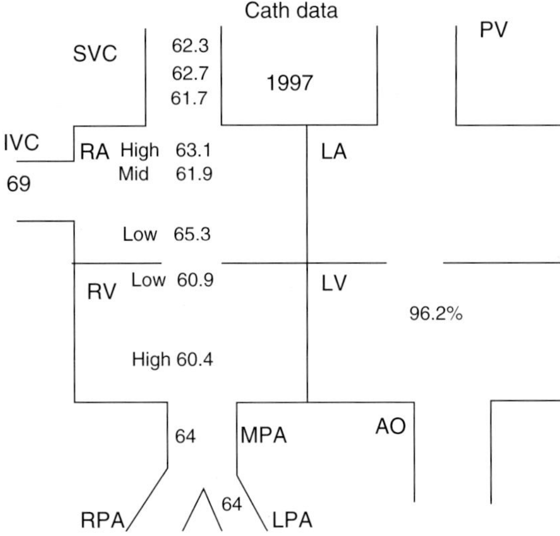

Figure 32.9 Oxygen saturation sample run 1997.

9 Physical examination 1997

65 inches tall female weighing 164 lb. BP 110/60. HR 90/min regular.
No elevation of jugular venous pressure.
Apex beat was in the 5th interspace, 9 cm from the mid-sternal line. RV lift 2+ out of 3+ (Figure 32.10).
S1 –l decreased. S2 is increased in intensity and widely split. S3 0.
Grade 3/6 pansystolic apical murmur.
Lungs clear.
Two out of 4+ femoral pulses. Trace leg edema.

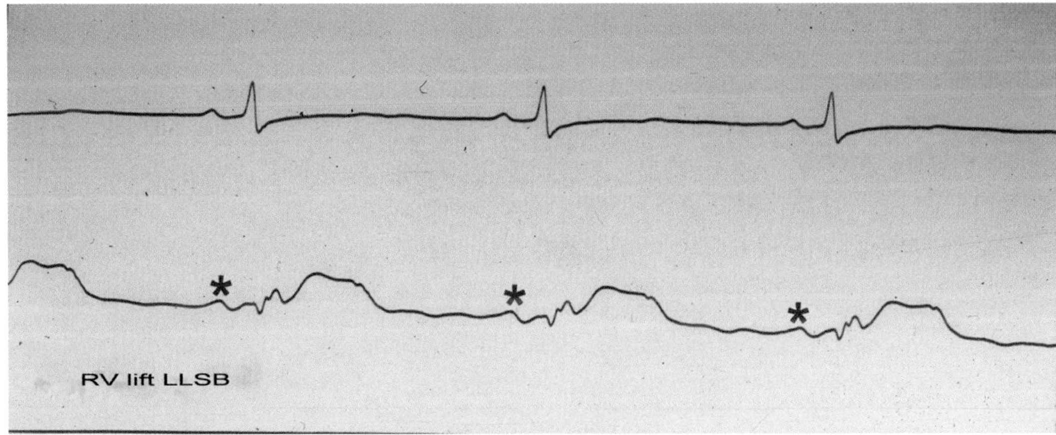

Figure 32.10 RV impulse at LLSB, 1997.
What do the red stars (*) refer to?

10 Laboratory data

Low probability of pulmonary embolism on lung scan.

11 Follow-up studies 2001–2012

The patient was referred to the pulmonary hypertension clinic for further treatment.

She was started on a continuous IV infusion of epoprostenol (synthetic prostacyclin, flolan). She also received warfarin and diuretics. In 2001 she was judged to be in functional class 2 on the basis of her exercise test.

In 2007 there was no appreciable change in the pulmonary pressure following an infusion of adenosine.

In 2008 she was doing well on epoprostenol and sildenafil, functional class 2.

In 2013 she was on epoprostenol and judged to be in functional class 1.

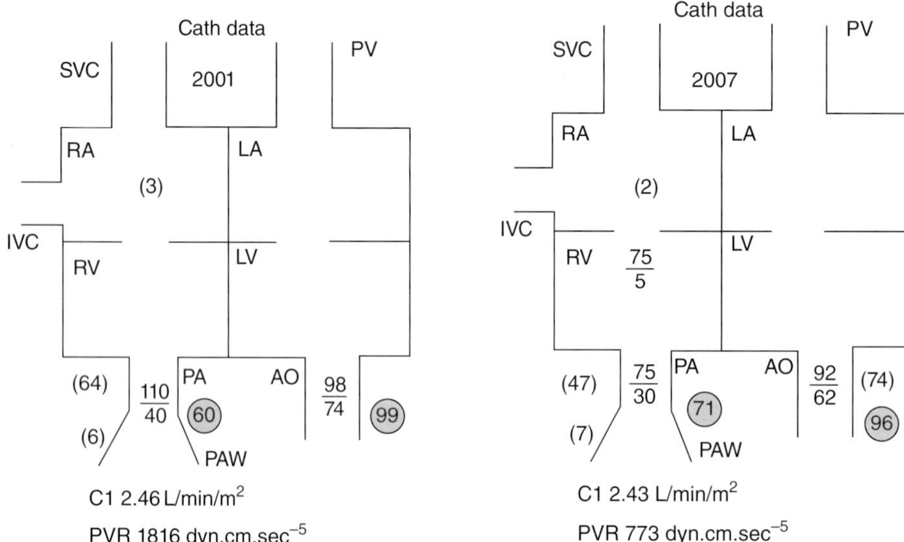

Figure 32.11 Right heart pressures in 2001 and 2007. Numbers in circles are oxygen saturations. (2001 and 2007 data courtesy of V. McLaughlin and M. Gomberg-Maitland, respectively).

12 Diagnosis

What is the diagnosis?

Answers and commentary

1 History

No specific diagnosis can be made on her initial symptoms of dizziness or dyspnea.

2 Echocardiogram 1991

The RV and RA are moderately enlarged. There was significant tricuspid regurgitation with an estimated RV systolic pressure of $4 \times (3.6)^2 + 10 = 62$ mmHg.

3 Cardiac catheterization 1991

There is moderately severe pulmonary hypertension (PA mean = 42 mmHg) with RV dysfunction (RVEDP = 10 mmHg). The wedge pressure is normal (8 mmHg), so mitral stenosis is unlikely to be present. These findings could represent pulmonary vascular disease or an intracardiac shunt.

The estimated RV systolic pressure on echocardiography is fairly similar to the actual pressure found at cardiac catheterization. Inaccuracies in the echocardiographic calculation of the RV systolic pressure often stem from the use of an estimated RA pressure.

4 ECG 1997

The rhythm is sinus with a rate of 75/min. PR 0.16 s. QRS 0.08 s. QRS axis +90°.

ST sagging/depression in 2, 3, F, V1–6. Tall R wave in V1.

Impression: RVH with ST-T wave abnormalities.

5 Chest X rays 1997

PA chest X ray showed an enlarged left PA and cardiomegaly (C/T ratio 0.52). The lung fields appear oligemic (best seen in Figure 32.5), implying significant pulmonary hypertension.

The lateral chest X ray shows some filling of the retrocardiac space suggestive of RV enlargement.

Impression: RV enlargement with significant pulmonary hypertension.

6 Cardiac catheterization 1997

The PA mean pressure has risen markedly from 42 mmHg in 1991 to 90 mmHg in 1997. There is RV dysfunction as the RVEDP is 12 mmHg. There is no significant gradient across the mitral valve in diastole. The PA saturation is slightly reduced, whereas the aortic saturation is normal.

7 Pressure tracings 1997

There is no gradient across the mitral valve in diastole. Withdrawal of the catheter from the PA wedge to the PA showed a PA systolic pressure that was higher than the LV pressure.

8 Oxygen saturation sample run 1997

There is no oxygen step up in the right heart study. The left-sided oxygen saturation is normal, thus there is no evidence of an intracardiac shunt.

9 Physical examination 1997

The pansystolic murmur is due to tricuspid regurgitation and there is evidence of RVH with a decreased RV compliance (based on the recordable impulse and presystolic impulse (see * in Figure 32.10) as well as pulmonary hypertension

10 Laboratory data

Pulmonary hypertension caused by a pulmonary embolism is mostly ruled out by the negative lung scan.

11 Follow-up studies 2001–2012

Cardiac catheterization data was collected in 2001 and 2007.

After treatment the PA mean fell from 90 mmHg in 1997 to 64 mmHg in 2001 and 47 mmHg in 2007. The pulmonary oxygen saturation also rose from 60% to 71%. There was a striking fall in pulmonary vascular resistance from 1816 to 773 dyn.sec.cm^{-5}.

12 Diagnosis

Idiopathic pulmonary hypertension, responsive to epoprostenol and sildenafil. A 21-year follow-up.

Discussion

The patient had idiopathic (primary) pulmonary hypertension [1] diagnosed in 1991. She was initially treated with nifedipine, which reduces pulmonary hypertension in only about 25% of patients [1, 2]. By 1997 her pulmonary hypertension had become severe. She did, however, do well from 1997 onwards with continuous infusion of epoprostenol [1, 3, 4] and subsequently sildenafil (approved for use in 2005) [5].

Idiopathic pulmonary hypertension is usually seen in young females in their 30s and was associated with a poor prognosis, many dying suddenly (Figure 32.12). The incidence in the general population is 2–5 per million/year [5]. A relative deficiency of prostacyclin may be a factor in the development of idiopathic pulmonary hypertension [3]. Patients usually present with dyspnea, angina, syncope, or right heart failure [5]. The median survival before the introduction of specific therapy is only 2.8 years. The 5-year survival rate is 34% [5].

Diagnosis of idiopathic pulmonary hypertension requires demonstrating a PA mean > 25 mmHg, PVR > 150 dyn.sec.cm^{-5} and PAW < 15 mmHg, in the absence of other causes [5].

Therapy consists of long-term use of a prostacyclin analogue (e.g. epoprostenol, treprostinil, iloprost) [3–6], an endothelin receptor antagonist (bosentan, sitaxsentan, ambrisentan) [5] or a phosphodiesterase inhibitor (sildenafil) [5]. The survival rate in patients treated with epoprostenol is 55% in 5 years [5].

Supportive measures include the use of anticoagulants, digoxin, diuretics, supplementary oxygen therapy, and exercise training [6].

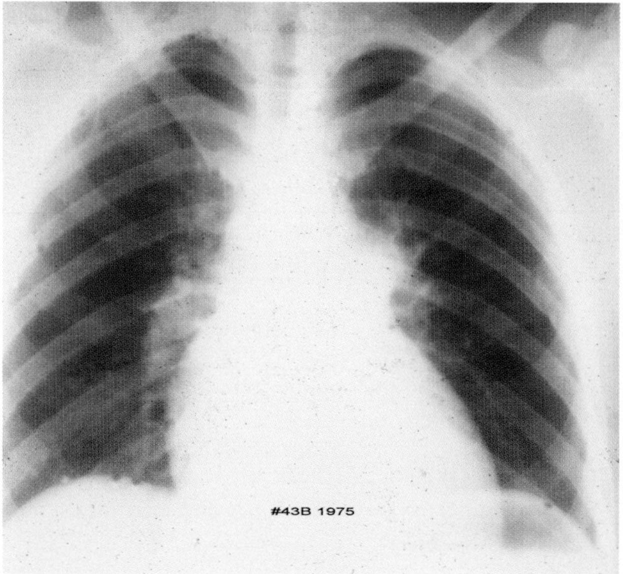

Figure 32.12 Chest X ray taken in 1975 of a 34-year-old female with idiopathic pulmonary hypertension. There is prominence of proximal pulmonary arteries and paucity of vessels in lung periphery. She had a normal sample run. PA pressures were 86/8 at rest and 134/21 when she became anxious .The respective aortic pressures were 110/6 and 140/100. She was in severe RV failure in 1976 despite treatment with digoxin, diuretics, and warfarin. She died suddenly in late 1976.

Key points

1. Idiopathic pulmonary hypertension is usually seen in women in their 30s. They may present with RV failure, chest pain, syncope, or sudden death.
2. Physical findings show evidence of pulmonary hypertension (loud P2, RVH, prominent 'a' wave in the neck veins, and secondary tricuspid regurgitation).
3. The diagnosis of idiopathic pulmonary hypertension can only be made if other causes (valvular heart disease, pulmonary disease, or cardiac shunts) have been excluded.
4. Treatment needs to be carried out in a clinic specializing in pulmonary hypertension as it requires the long-term use of prostacyclin, endothelial receptor antagonists, or a phosphodiesterase inhibitor. These medications are responsible for the marked improvement in survival in these patients.

References

[1] Shapiro SM, Oudiz RJ, Cao T et al. Primary pulmonary hypertension: improved long term effects and survival with continuous intravenous epoprostenol infusion. *J Am Coll Cardiol* 1997; 30: 343–349.

[2] Rich S, Brundage BH. High dose calcium channel blocking therapy for primary pulmonary hypertension: evidence for long term reduction in pulmonary arterial pressure and regression of right ventricular hypertrophy. *Circulation* 1987; 76: 135–141.

[3] Badesch DB, McLaughlin VV, Delcroix M et al. Prostanoid therapy for pulmonary arterial hypertension. *J Am Coll Cardiol* 2004; 43: 56S–61S (approved for use by FDA in 1995).

[4] Ventetuolo CE, Klinger JR. WHO group 1 pulmonary arterial hypertension: Current and investigative therapies. *Prog Cardiovasc Dis* 2012; 55: 89–103.

[5] McLaughlin VV, McGoon MD. Pulmonary arterial hypertension. *Circulation* 2006; 114: 1417–1431 (reviews pathogenesis, classification, and therapy).

[6] Judge EP, Gaine SP. Management of pulmonary arterial hypertension. *Curr Opin Crit Care* 2013; 19: 44–50.

General reference

Galie N, Simonneau G. (eds). Update in Pulmonary hypertension. Proceedings of the 5th world symposium on pulmonary hypertension. *J Am Coll Cardiol Suppl D.* 2013;62:D1–D126 (13 articles discussing etiology, classification, diagnosis and treatment of idiopathic and secondary pulmonary hypertension.

Simonneau G, Gatzoulis MA, Adatia I et al. Updated clinical classification of pulmonary hypertension. *J Am Coll Cardiol* 2013;62 Suppl:D34–41.

33 PATIENT STUDY 33

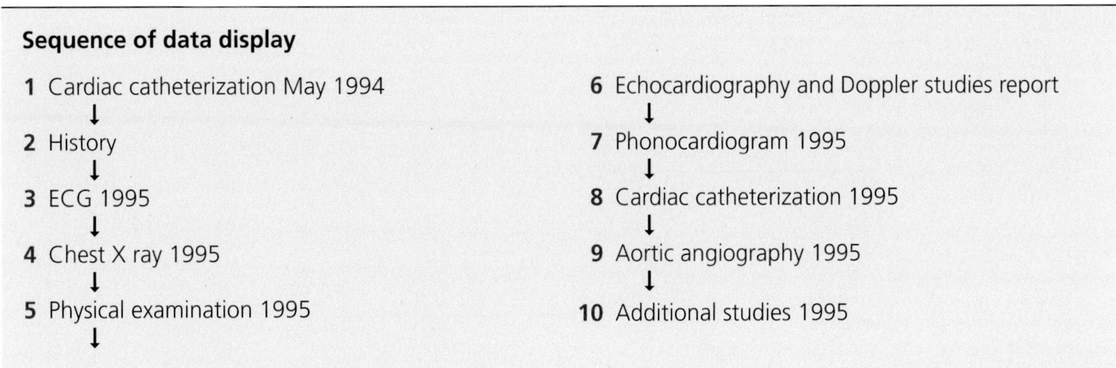

Sequence of data display

1 Cardiac catheterization May 1994
↓
2 History
↓
3 ECG 1995
↓
4 Chest X ray 1995
↓
5 Physical examination 1995
↓
6 Echocardiography and Doppler studies report
↓
7 Phonocardiogram 1995
↓
8 Cardiac catheterization 1995
↓
9 Aortic angiography 1995
↓
10 Additional studies 1995

1 Cardiac catheterization May 1994

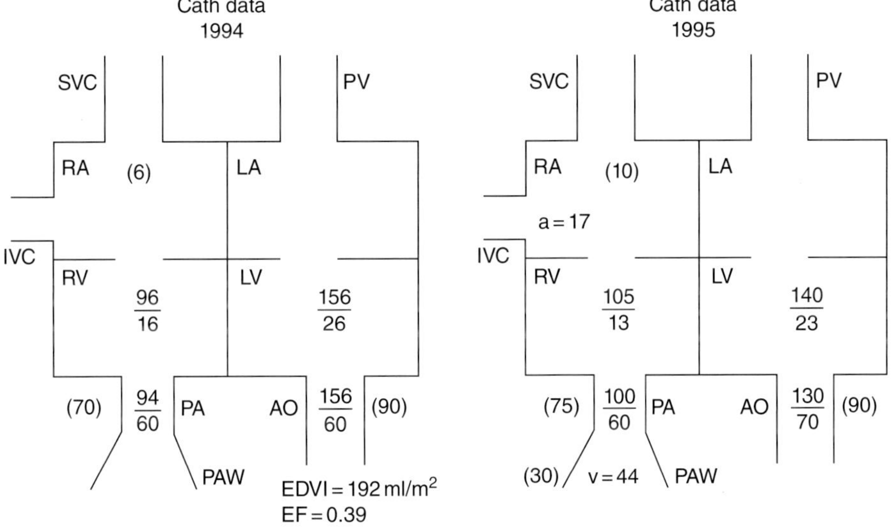

Figure 33.1 Cardiac catheterization data May 1994.

What is the pulmonary/systemic vascular resistance ratio?

Patient Studies in Valvular, Congenital, and Rarer Forms of Cardiovascular Disease: An Integrative Approach, First Edition. Franklin B. Saksena.

Companion Website: www.wiley.com/go/saksena/patientstudies

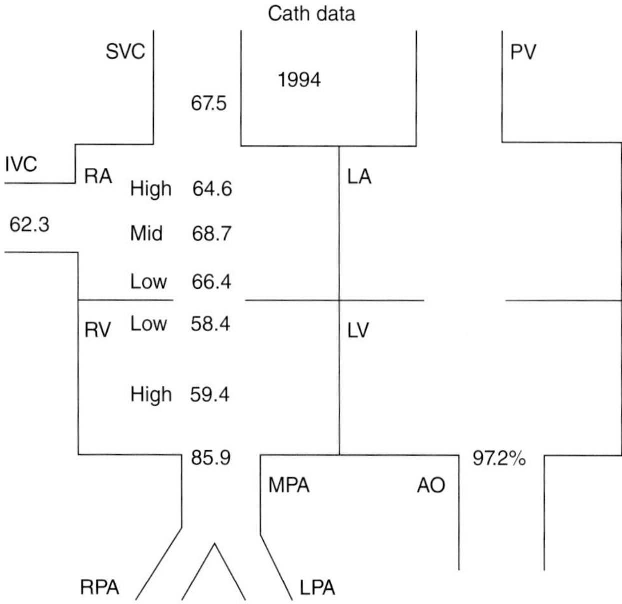

Figure 33.2 Oxygen saturation sample run 1994.

What is the pulmonary/systemic flow ratio?

Comment on the catheterization data. What is the recommended treatment?

2 History

33-year-old female P5 G5 admitted to hospital with dyspnea and leg edema in April 1994. She was told she had a heart problem in her last pregnancy. She underwent cardiac catheterization and surgery was recommended, which she refused. She returned a year later with the same symptoms and was then agreeable for surgery.

3 ECG 1995

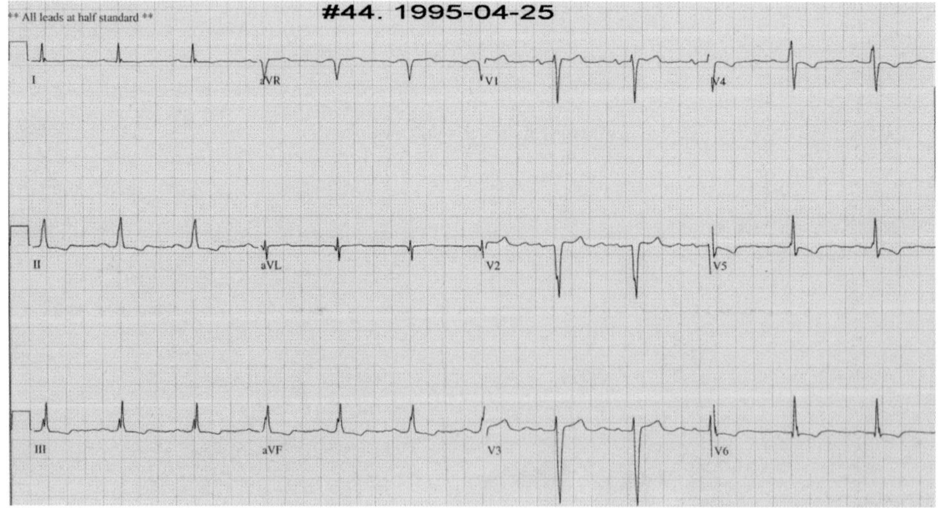

Figure 33.3 12-lead ECG 25 April 1995.

4 Chest X ray 1995

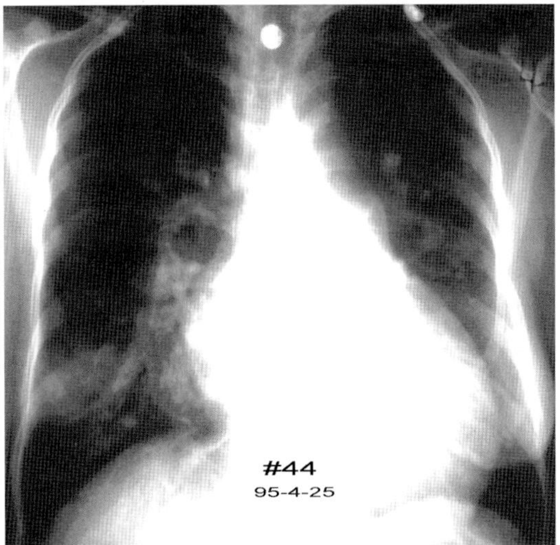

Figure 33.4 PA chest X ray 1995.

5 Physical examination 1995

The patient is 60 inches tall and weighs 82 lb. BP 110/50. P 88/min bounding.
BP in right leg 110 systolic.
Apex beat is in 5th and 6th interspaces, 14 cm from the mid-sternal line.
S1–1 decreased. S2+2 increased.
There was a 3/6 systolic ejection murmur heard at the 3rd LUSB, increasing after a PVC. There was a grade 2/6 diastolic blowing murmur heard best in 2nd and 3rd left interspace parasternally.
A continuous murmur was heard in the back.
Mildly enlarged liver.
No edema or clubbing. Peripheral pulses were all bounding.

6 Echocardiography and Doppler studies report

There was LV and LA enlargement as well as LV hypokinesia. Mild pulmonary and aortic regurgitation.

Comment on the 1995 and 1994 data.
What additional tests would you do to determine if surgery could be undertaken safely?

7 Phonocardiogram 1995

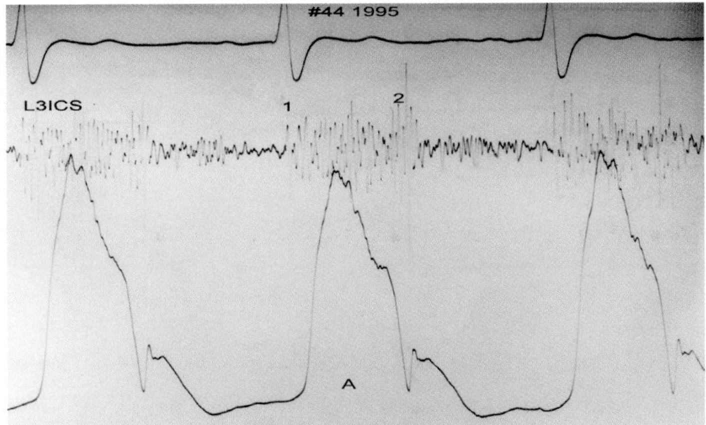

Figure 33.5 Phonocardiogram recorded at 3rd left sternal border with aortic pressure (A).

8 Cardiac catheterization 1995

See Figure 33.1 for 1995 data.

9 Aortic angiography 1995

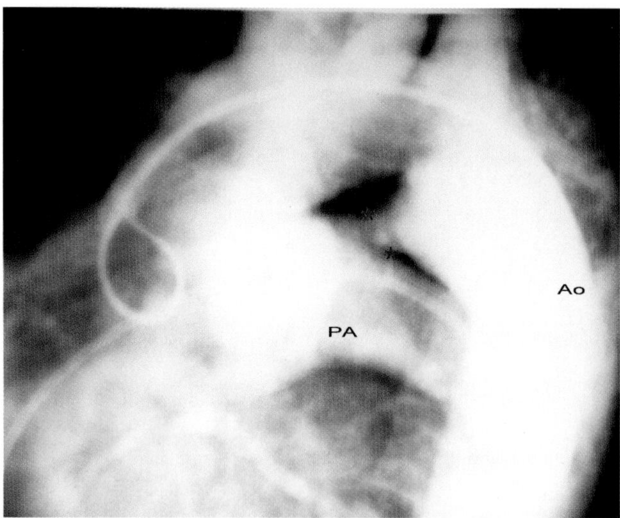

Figure 33.6 Aortic angiogram in 60° LAO cranial projection.

What is the structure between the 2 red stars?

10 Additional studies 1995

What additional tests would you do to determine if surgery could be undertaken safely?

Answers and commentary

1 Cardiac catheterization May 1994

Pressures

The RVEDP is moderately increased due to RV dysfunction.

There is severe pulmonary hypertension (PA mean = 70 mmHg). The LVEDP is markedly elevated due to LV dysfunction. There is a wide pulse pressure, which could be due to an AV fistula, high output failure, or aortic regurgitation.

The LV end-diastolic volume is almost three times normal size and the LV ejection fraction is reduced.

Oxygen sample run

This shows a step up at the pulmonic level, most likely due to a left to right shunt from a PDA.

In conclusion the patient has a PDA with severe pulmonary hypertension, aortic regurgitation, and biventricular dysfunction.

Treatment recommended: surgical closure of the PDA.

2 History

The patient agreed to have surgery in 1995.

3 ECG 1995

Sinus rhythm. Rate 72/min. PR 0.18 s. QRS 0.11 s. QRS axis +70°. T low in 1.L and inverted in V4–6. LVH by voltage criteria.

Impression: LVH with repolarization abnormality.

4 Chest X ray 1995

The C/T ratio is 14/24. The right heart is enlarged. The inferior displacement of the apex suggests LV enlargement and there is pulmonary plethora.

5 Physical examination 1995

The presence of a continuous murmur, a wide pulse pressure, and cardiomegaly may be explained on the basis of a PDA. It is unclear why a continuous murmur was heard in the back but not in the left 2nd interspace parasternally. The diastolic blowing murmur heard at the left 2nd and 3rd interspaces parasternally could be due to aortic regurgitation and/or pulmonary regurgitation.

6 Echocardiography and Doppler studies report

The findings on echocardiography corroborated the above findings on physical examination as to the presence of LV enlargement, and pulmonary and aortic regurgitation.

7 Phonocardiogram 1995

There is a diamond-shaped systolic murmur recorded at the 3rd left interspace parasternally, attributed to a PDA. Its diastolic component was not well recorded for either technical reasons or because the diastolic component of the PDA has become shorter as a result of severe pulmonary hypertension.

8 Cardiac catheterization 1995

There has been a further increase in pulmonary hypertension since 1994. Biventricualar dysfunction remains unchanged.

The pulmonary vascular resistance/systemic vascular resistance ratio is 0.56, as follows:

PA mean = 75, PAW mean = 30, Ao mean = 90, RA mean = 10 mmHg

$$\text{PVR} / \text{SVR} = \left(\overline{\text{PA}} - \overline{\text{PAW}}\right) / \left(\overline{\text{Ao}} - \overline{\text{RA}}\right) = (75-30)/(90-10) = 0.56$$

(lines over a variable indicate a mean value)

$$\text{Pulmonary/systemic flow ratio} = \frac{97.2-67.5}{97.2-85.9} = \frac{2{,}6}{1}$$

This pulmonary/systemic flow ratio is approximate at best in a PDA because ductus preferencial flow into the left PA and pulmonary regurgitation result in an unreliable mixed PA saturation.

9 Aortic angiography 1995

A large ductus without constriction (Krichenko type C) [1] is seen between the descending aorta and the left PA.

Aortic root angiography did show mild aortic regurgitation, unchanged from 1994 (between the 2 red stars in Figure 33.6).

10 Additional studies 1995

1. 100% oxygen was given for 10 minutes and the PA and aortic pressures were measured.
2. The ductus was occluded with a balloon catheter for 5 min, and PA and aortic pressures were measured.

There were no changes in the PA and aortic pressures in both instances (see Table 33.1).

The patient underwent successful ligation of the ductus in 1995. The aortic valve was not operated on. She was doing well as of 2003, with a reduction in heart size (Figures 33.7 and 33.8) seen on chest X ray.

Table 33.1 PA and aortic pressures before and after (a) breathing 100% oxygen and (b) occlusion of the PDA

	Aortic pressure mmHg S/D	Pulmonary artery pressure S/D
Baseline	140/76	100/76
100% O_2 × 10 min	140/76	98/76
Baseline	120/80	104/56
Ductus occlusion × 5 min	120/80	107/60

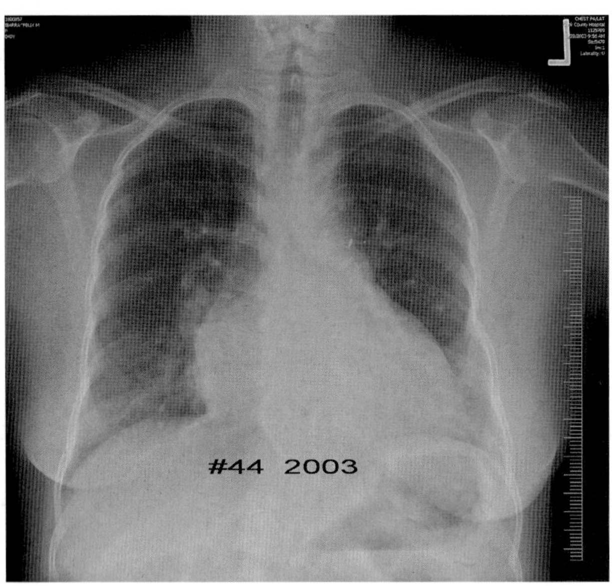

Figure 33.7 PA chest X ray 2003 showing a reduction in cardiac size and pulmonary plethora. Surgical clips are seen adjacent to where the ductus was ligated.

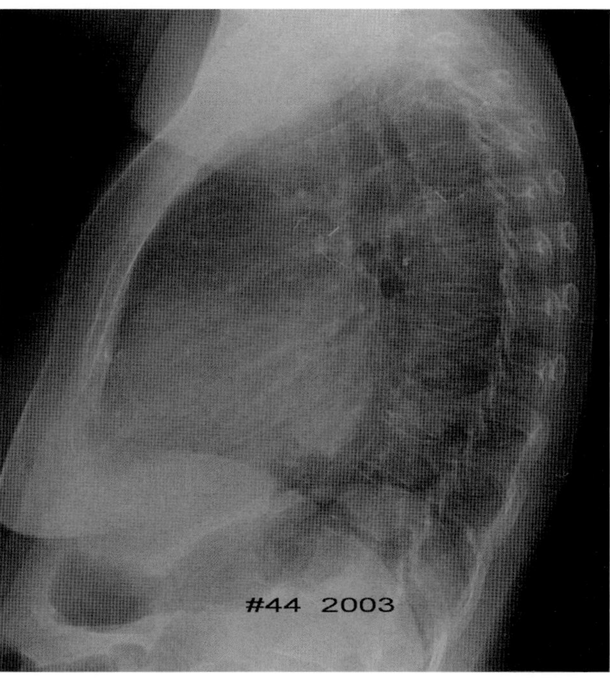

Figure 33.8 Lateral chest X ray 2003. Surgical clips at the site of PDA ligation are also seen.

Discussion

This patient had a PDA with severe pulmonary hypertension (PA systolic pressure > 2/3 of aortic systolic pressure) [2]. She had no change in PA or aortic pressures following 10 min of 100% oxygen, implying that hypoxemia was not a cause of her elevated pulmonary vascular resistance.

Patients with a PDA and severe pulmonary hypertension may require medical therapy (sildenafil or bosentan) and then PDA closure [3]. Transcatheter test occlusion of the PDA is first used to see if the patient is a suitable candidate for PDA closure. Patients who develop suprasystemic PA pressures and RV failure [3] during a test occlusion are not suitable candidates for PDA closure. A favorable response to transient PDA occlusion occurs when there is (i) a fall in PA pressure or no elevation [2, 4], (ii) no decrease in aortic pressure [4], and (iii) no worsening of signs and symptoms [4]. All these findings, when present, indicate that the PA hypertension is reversible [4]. A fall in the PA systolic pressure/aortic systolic pressure ratio to <0.8 during a test occlusion [3] also implies reversibility of the pulmonary hypertension.

This patient had no changes in PA and aortic pressures and remained asymptomatic during transient balloon occlusion of the PDA. She did, however, undergo successful ligation of the ductus in 1995 and was asymptomatic as of 2003.

Key points

1. Severe pulmonary hypertension occurs when the systolic PA pressure exceeds 2/3 of the aortic systolic pressure.
2. The diastolic component of the PDA murmur becomes shorter when significant pulmonary hypertension develops.
3. Balloon occlusion of the PDA is a useful test to see if patients with severe pulmonary hypertension can tolerate closure of the ductus.
4. Pre-surgical therapy with bosantan or sildenafil may be required to lower the PA pressure if it is severely elevated in patients with a PDA.

References

[1] Krichenko A, Benson LN, Burrows P et al. Angiographic classification of the isolated, persistently patent ductus arteriosus and implications for percutaneous catheter occlusion. *Am J Cardiol* 1989; 63: 877–880.
[2] Thanopoulos BD, Tsaousis GS, Djukic M et al. Transcatheter closure of high pulmonary artery pressure persistent ductus arteriosus with the Amplatzer muscular ventricular septal defect occluder. *Heart* 2002; 87: 260–263.
[3] Niu MC, Mallory GB, Justino H et al. Treatment of severe pulmonary hypertension in the setting of the large patent ductus arteriosus. *Pediatrics* 2013; 131: e1643–e1649.
[4] Yan C, Zhao S, Jiang S et al. Transcatheter closure of patent ductus arteriosus with severe pulmonary arterial hypertension in adults. *Heart* 2007; 93: 514–518.

34 PATIENT STUDY 34

Sequence of data presentation

1 12-lead ECG
↓
2 Chest X ray
↓
3 Oxygen sample run
↓
4 Intracardiac pressures
↓
5 Aortic, pulmonary and RV pressure curves
↓
6 Pressures and phonocardiogram
↓
7 RV angiogram
↓
8 Echocardiograms
↓
9 History and physical examination
↓
10 Diagnosis and treatment

1 12-lead ECG

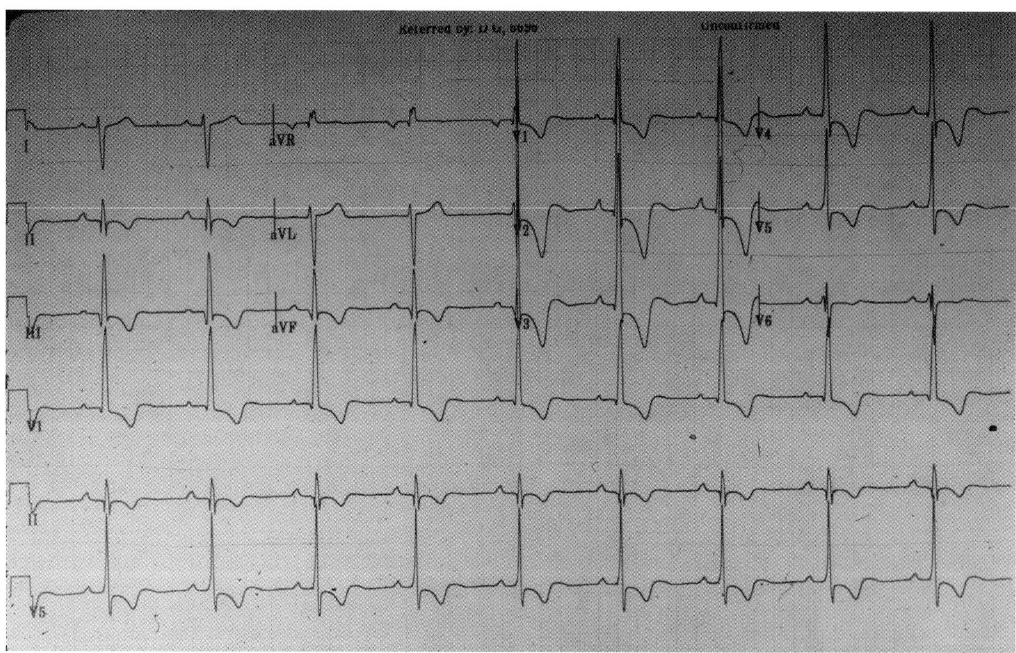

Figure 34.1 12-lead ECG.

What are the rate, rhythm, PR and QRS intervals, and QRS axis and impression?

Patient Studies in Valvular, Congenital, and Rarer Forms of Cardiovascular Disease: An Integrative Approach, First Edition. Franklin B. Saksena.

Companion Website: www.wiley.com/go/saksena/patientstudies

2 Chest X ray

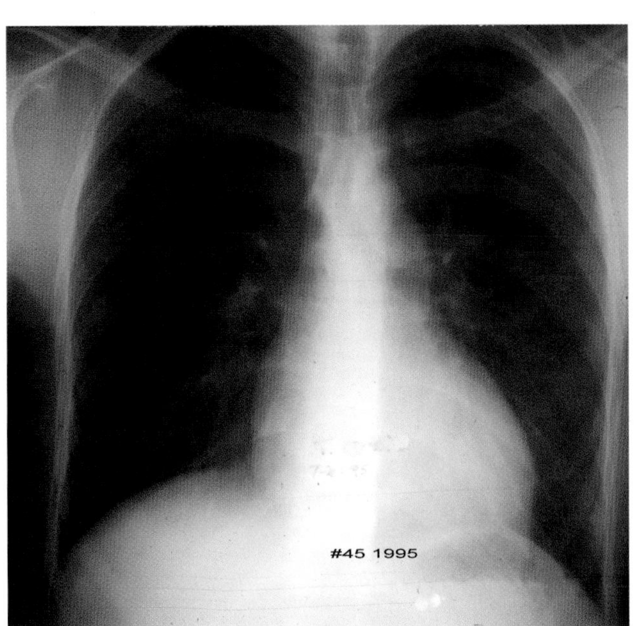

Figure 34.2 PA chest X ray.

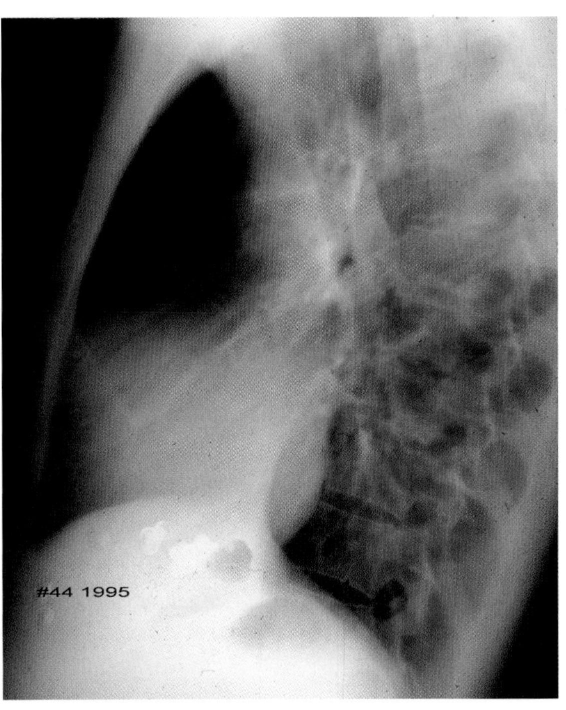

Figure 34.3 Lateral chest X ray.
Comment on the chamber size, C/T ratio, and lung fields.

3 Oxygen sample run

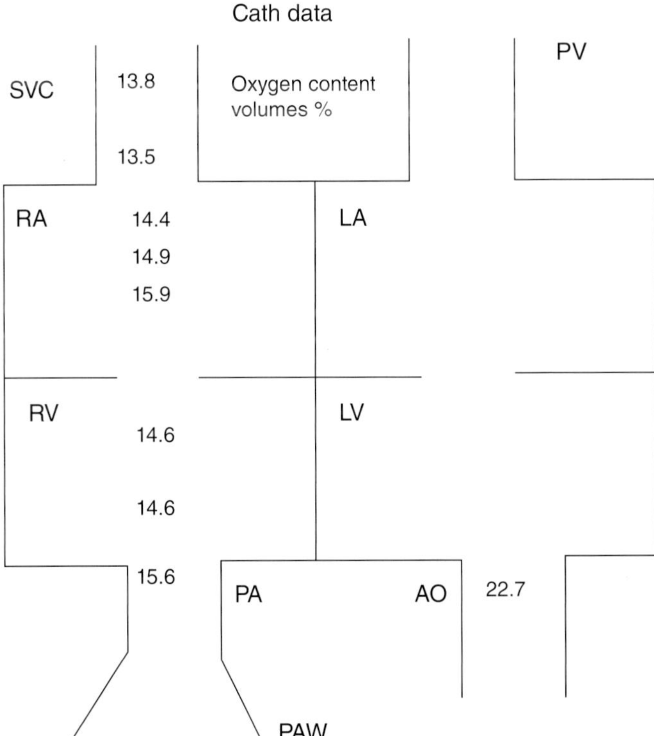

Figure 34.4 Oxygen sample run (oxygen content mL/100 mL blood).

4 Intracardiac pressures

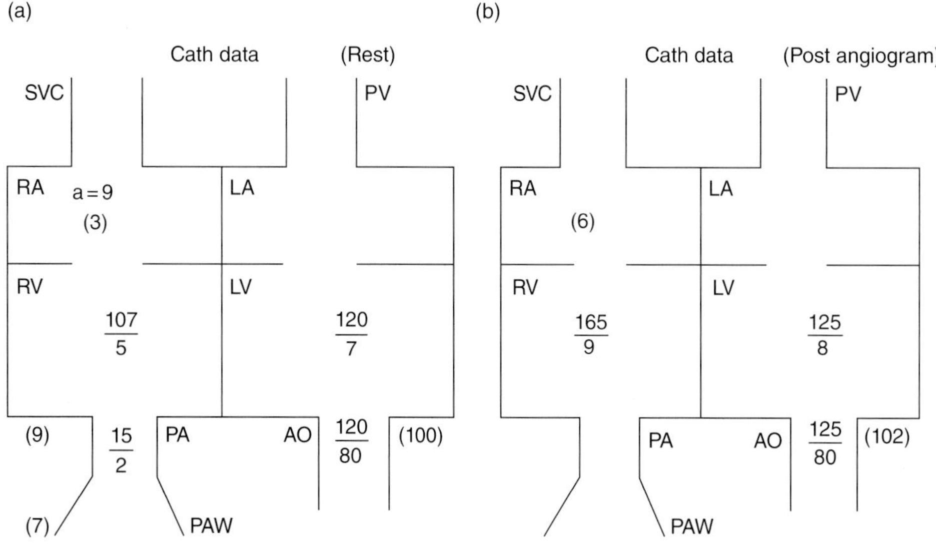

Figure 34.5 (a) Resting and (b) post-angiogram pressures.

5 Aortic, pulmonary and RV pressure curves

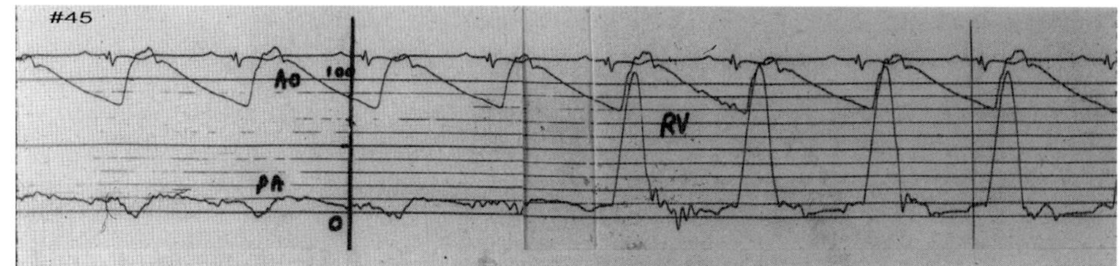

Figure 34.6 Simultaneous aortic pressure along with a withdrawal tracing from PA to RV.

6 Pressures and phonocardiogram

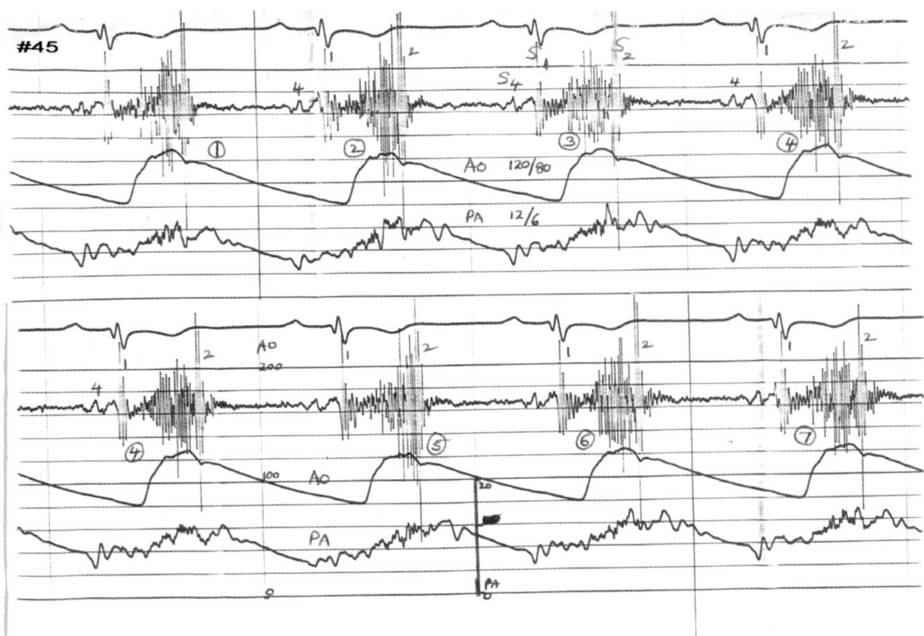

Figure 34.7 Simultaneous aortic and pulmonary pressures with a phonocardiogram recorded at the LLSB.

7 RV angiogram

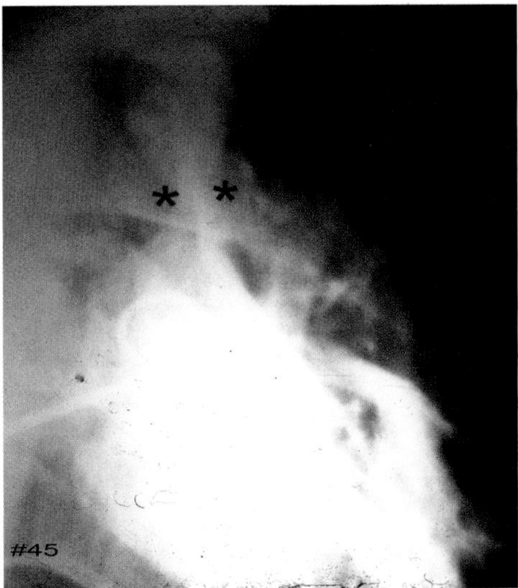

Figure 34.8 RV angiogram AP view. The RV outflow tract is seen between the two stars (*).

8 Echocardiograms

(a) (b)

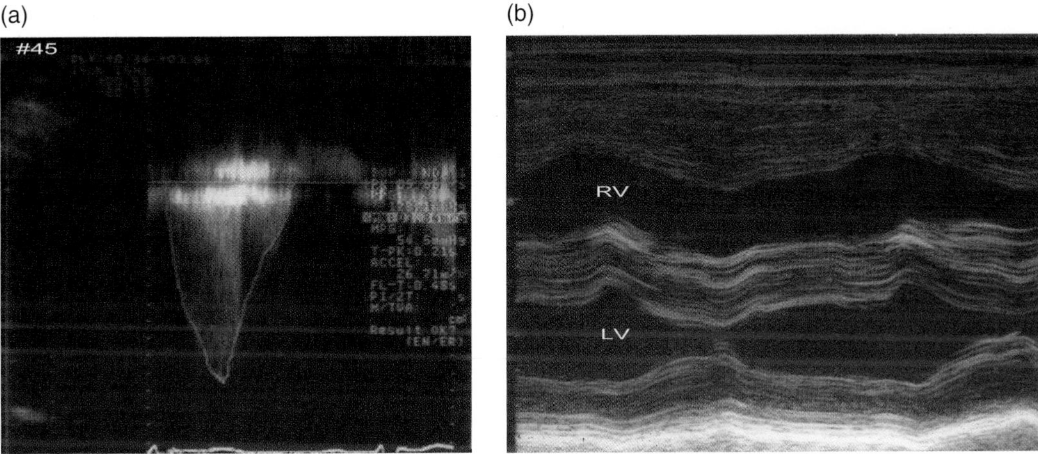

Figure 34.9 (a) The Doppler flow velocity across the pulmonary valve is 4.8 m/s. (b) M-mode echocardiogram showing RV and LV.

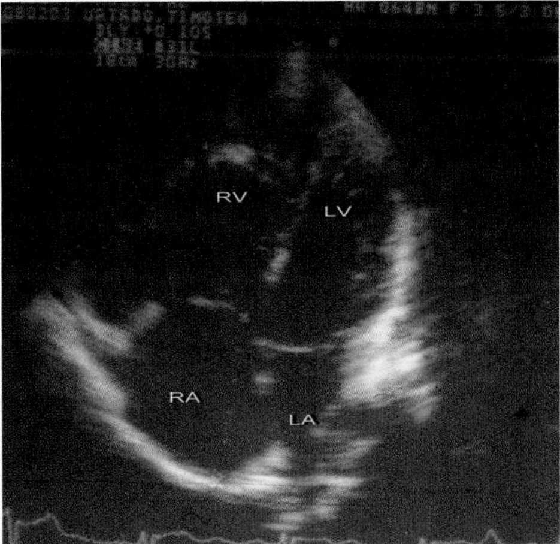

Figure 34.10 Four-chamber view echocardiogram.

Comment on each of the above findings.

9 History and physical examination

21-year-old male with a history of dyspnea and left upper chest pain (1995).
BP 110/70. HR 70/min regular.
Normal carotid upstroke. No elevation of jugular venous pressure.
Apex beat was in the 6th interspace 10 cm from the mid-sternal line.
The apical impulse was sustained and measured 5 × 5 cm.
Grade 4/6 late crescendo systolic murmur at LLSB.
S4 at LLSB.

10 Diagnosis and treatment

What are the diagnosis and treatment?

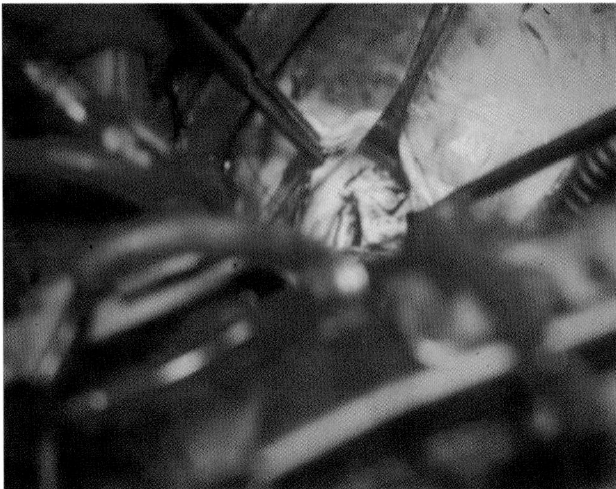

Figure 34.11 Operative appearance of pulmonic valve.

Answers and commentary

1 12-lead ECG

Sinus bradycardia, 56/min. PR 0.180 s. QRS 0.108 s. QRS axis +156°. RA enlargement. RV enlargement with strain pattern.

An R wave of 2 mv in V1 in a 21-year-old patient is very often due to pulmonic stenosis (normal R wave height in V1 in a 21-year-old male is 0.3 mv, range 0.03–0.9 mv).

2 Chest X ray

C/T ratio 14/29. The left PA is prominent with normal lung fields. In the lateral view the RV is enlarged.

Mitral stenosis or pulmonic stenosis are possible reasons for the above findings. The former is less likely as the LA is not enlarged and there is no upper lobe hyperemia or Kerley B lines discernible.

3 Oxygen sample run

This shows no significant step up, thus ruling out an ASD, VSD, or PDA.

An increase in oxygen content of 1.9 vol% from SVC to RA suggests an ASD, whereas an increase in oxygen content of 1 vol% from RA to RV suggests a VSD. An increase in oxygen content of 1.0 vol% from RV to PA suggests a PDA [1].

4 Intracardiac pressures

The RA pressure is normal with an 'a' wave that is not elevated. It is unclear why the 'a' wave was not increased in the face of such severe RV hypertension.

The RV pressure is severely elevated, with a large gradient in systole across the pulmonary valve, indicative of severe pulmonary stenosis. The mean pulmonary wedge pressure and the LVEDP are identical, thus excluding mitral stenosis. Left heart pressures are normal.

The RV pressure exceeded the systemic pressure after RV angiography.

5 Aortic, pulmonary and RV pressure curves

The PA pressure has a damped appearance and the dicrotic notch is not well seen. The peak-to-peak gradient across the pulmonic valve is 92 mmHg. No subpulmonic gradient was seen. The RV systolic pressure is only15 mmHg lower than the aortic pressure. The RV pressure contour shows a slow uprise and slow descent. These findings confirm the presence of pulmonary stenosis.

6 Pressures and phonocardiogram

Simultaneous phonocardiogram at the LLSB shows a low frequency sound preceding the QRS complex due to a right-sided S4. The aortic component of S2 corresponds to the aortic dicrotic notch, whereas the pulmonary component of S2 is not seen. The systolic murmur peaks in late systole. All these finding are indicative of severe pulmonary stenosis.

7 RV angiogram

AP view of RV angiogram show doming of the pulmonic valve indicative of pulmonic valvular stenosis. The AP view is the preferred view in assessing the pulmonic valve (I. Carr, personal communication). There is RV thickening.

8 Echocardiograms

The Doppler echocardiogram showed an increased velocity of 4.8 m/s across the pulmonic valve, yielding a peak-to-peak instantaneous gradient of $4(4.8 \times 4.8) = 88$ mmHg, which is similar to the systolic pressure gradient obtained at cardiac catheterization.

The M-mode echocardiogram showed significant RVH with marked septal thickening in the four-chamber view (Figure 34.10). The RV area is normally ≤2/3 of the LV area [2,3], but in this patient the RV area is about 1.5 times the LV area and is thus clearly enlarged. The LV has been displaced so that the RV now occupies the apex of the heart. The RA is also enlarged and encroaches on the LA.

9 and 10 History, physical examination, diagnosis, and treatment

The patient had severe pulmonic stenosis: RV lift, right-sided S4, systolic murmur with late peaking at LLSB.

In conclusion, the patient had severe pulmonic stenosis and no ASD or VSD. Operative intervention was recommended.

11 Course

At surgery (Figure 34.11) pulmonary valvotomy was successfully performed for a bicuspid valve. Nowadays balloon pulmonary valvuloplasty would have been the method of choice but this was not available to us at that time. Balloon valvuloplasty may occasionally fail if the leaflets are calcified or thickened and without commissural fusion (dysplasia) [4].

Discussion

Valvular pulmonic stenosis occurs in 1.5–6.5 per 10,000 live births and accounts for 2–13% of all patients with congenital heart disease [3]. There are three morphological types: acommissural dome-shaped, bicuspid (as in this patient), and dysplastic [5]. Noonan's syndrome is often associated with a dysplastic valve [5].

The severity of pulmonic stenosis is usually readily assessed at the bedside. Findings of a right-sided S4, pulmonary ejection murmur with late peaking, and RV lift all point to significant pulmonic stenosis, as was seen in this patient. If the pulmonic stenosis is mild then a pulmonary ejection click is heard, implying mobile leaflets, but as the pulmonary valve becomes more stiffer and stenotic the click disappears.

The chest X ray may show RV enlargement with normal pulmonary vasculature, as in this patient. Post-stenotic dilatation of the PA is also seen but does not correlate with the severity of the valvular stenosis [6]. There may be occasional chest deformities seen in young patients with pulmonic stenosis, such as pectus carinatum (pigeon chest) [7], as seen in the worked example in the prelims.

When the ECG shows a tall monophasic R wave in V1 and coved ST segments with inverted T waves in the precordial leads, there is severe RVH [8]. The amplitude of the R wave in V1 has a rough correlation to the severity of the RV systolic pressure according to some authors [6] but not others [9]. The amplitude of the R wave in lead V1 is more closely correlated with the inverse of the pulmonary valve area [9].

Grading of the severity of pulmonary stenosis [4] may be assessed as shown in Table 34.1.

Table 34.1 Grading of the severity of pulmonary stenosis [4]

Degree of obstruction	Peak systolic gradient (mmHg)*	RV systolic pressure (mmHg)
Trivial	<25	<50
Mild	25–49	50–74
Moderate	50–79	75–100
Severe	>80	>100

*Transvalvular gradient measured by Doppler, which corresponds closely with the peak-to-peak gradient measured at cardiac catheterization.

Echocardiographic and Doppler studies nowadays can delineate the morphology of the RV and the pulmonic valve, and measure the peak systolic gradient in systole across the pulmonic valve, thus obviating the need for cardiac catheterization in patients with suspected pure pulmonic stenosis. Cardiac catheterization and angiography still have a role (i) if the RV systolic pressure is 100–150 mmHg and RV infundibular stenosis needs to be excluded [6] and (ii) if pulmonary balloon angioplasty is being considered [4].

Key points

1. Patients with severe pulmonic stenosis have a late peaking ejection systolic murmur, soft P2, absence of a pulmonary ejection click as the valve becomes more rigid, a right-sided S4, and severe RVH.
2. The severity of the pulmonic stenosis may be assessed by measuring the transvalvular gradient either at catheterization or by Doppler echocardiography.
3. Pulmonic stenosis may be treated by either valvotomy or balloon valvuloplasty.

References

[1] Zimmerman HA. *Intravascular catheterization.* CC Thomas, Springfield, IL, 1966, pp 422–514 and pp 545–582.

[2] D'Oronzio U, Senn O, Biaggi P et al. Right heart assessment by echocardiography: Gender and body size matters. *J Am Soc Echocardiogr* 2012; 25: 1251–1258.

[3] Jiang L, Wiegers SE, Weyman AE. *Right ventricle. In: Principles of Echocardiography,* 2nd edn, Weyman AE (ed.). Lea and Febiger, Philadelphia, 1994, p. 905.

[4] Dore A. *Pulmonary stenosis.* In: Gatzoulis M, Webb G, Daubeney P (eds), Diagnosis and management of adult congenital heart disease. Churchill Livingstone, Philadelphia, 2003, pp 299–303.

[5] Waller BF, Howard J, Fess S. Pathology of pulmonic valve stenosis and pure regurgitation. *Clin Cardiol* 1995; 18: 45–50.

[6] Rudolph AM. *Congenital diseases of the heart: Clinical–physiological considerations. Pulmonary stenosis and atresia with intact ventricular septum,* 2nd edn. Futura, Armonk, NY, 2001, pp 551–616.

[7] Arosemena E, Elliott LP, Eliot RS. Chest deformity in adults with congenital heart disease. *Am J Cardiol* 1967; 20: 309–313.

[8] Perloff JK. *The clinical recognition of congenital heart disease,* 5th edn. WB Saunders, Philadelphia, 2003, pp 177–178.

[9] Bassingthwaighte JB, Parkin TW, DuShane JW, Wood EH, Burchell HB. The electrocardiographic and hemodynamic findings in pulmonary stenosis with intact ventricular septum. *Circulation* 1963; 28: 893–905.

Further reading

ACC/AHA. Guidelines for management of adults with congenital heart disease. *J Am Coll Cardiol* 2008; 52: 1890–1947.

35 PATIENT STUDY 35

Sequence of data presentation

1 Abdominal examination
↓
2 History
↓
3 Physical examination
↓
4 Laboratory data
↓
5 CT abdomen
↓
6 Course and treatment
↓
7 Pathology

1 Abdominal examination

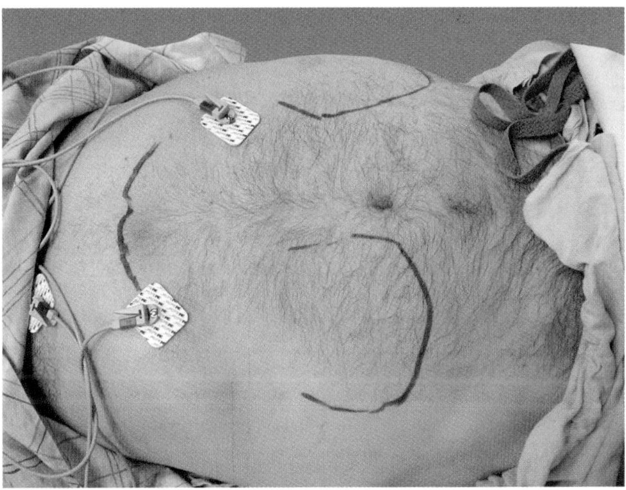

Figure 35.1 Abdominal examination showing two masses outlined by palpation in a patient with hypertension.

What are the possible diagnoses?

2 History

54-year-old man admitted in 2005 with chest pain probably of ischemic origin.
He had hypertension and PCK diagnosed in 1995. PTCA in 2003. At that time the LVEF was 67%.
He had smoked for 35 pack years. Father had PCK.

3 Physical examination

70 inches tall, 185 lb male with admitting BP of 164/107, which fell subsequently to 134/82. HR 70/min. Regular. Diagonal ear crease sign is present.

Patient Studies in Valvular, Congenital, and Rarer Forms of Cardiovascular Disease: An Integrative Approach, First Edition. Franklin B. Saksena.

Companion Website: www.wiley.com/go/saksena/patientstudies

Lungs were clear to auscultation and percussion.
No elevation of jugular venous pressure. Normal carotid upstroke.
Apex beat was in the 5th interspace, 12 cm from the mid-sternal line (= cardiomegaly).
Apical S4. Normal S1 and S2. Grade1/6 aortic systolic murmur.
Good peripheral pulses. No cyanosis, clubbing, or leg edema.
Abdominal findings are shown in Figure 35.1.

4 Laboratory data

Hb 12.6 g%. WBC 6050/mm^3. BUN 68 mg%. Cr 6.6 mg%. K 5.9 meq/L. Troponin levels normal. Normal ECG.

5 CT abdomen

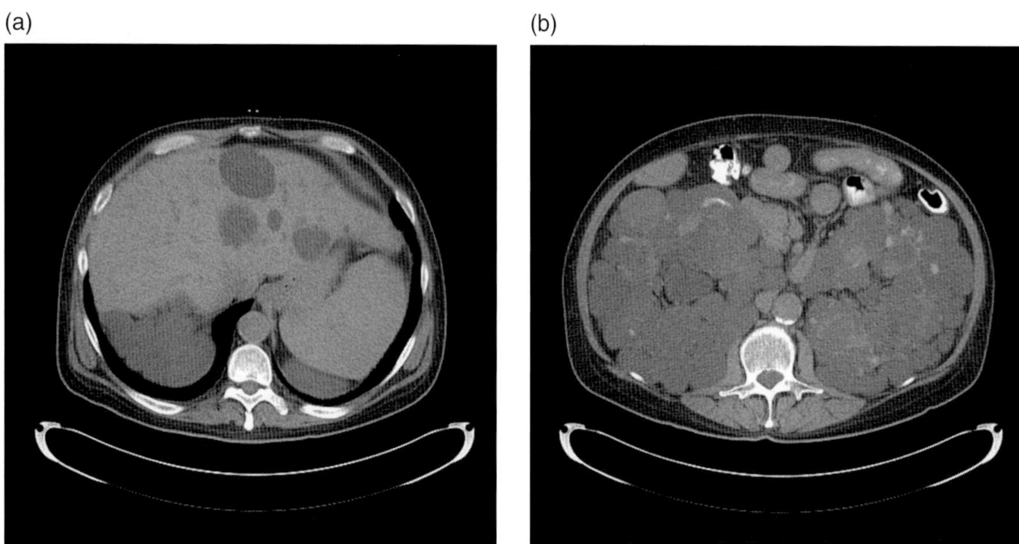

Figure 35.2 (a) CT of abdomen at the level of the liver. (b) CT of abdomen at the level of the kidneys.

6 Course and treatment

Table 35.1 Course of patient's renal function

	BUN mg%	Cr mg%	event
Jun 05	72	6	Chest pain
May 07			nephrectomy
Jun 07	49	7.3	
2007			Renal transplant
Dec 08	33	1.3	
Sep 2011	36	1.3	PTCA

Patient developed hematuria and severe abdominal pain in 2007.

What treatment would you recommend?

7 Pathology

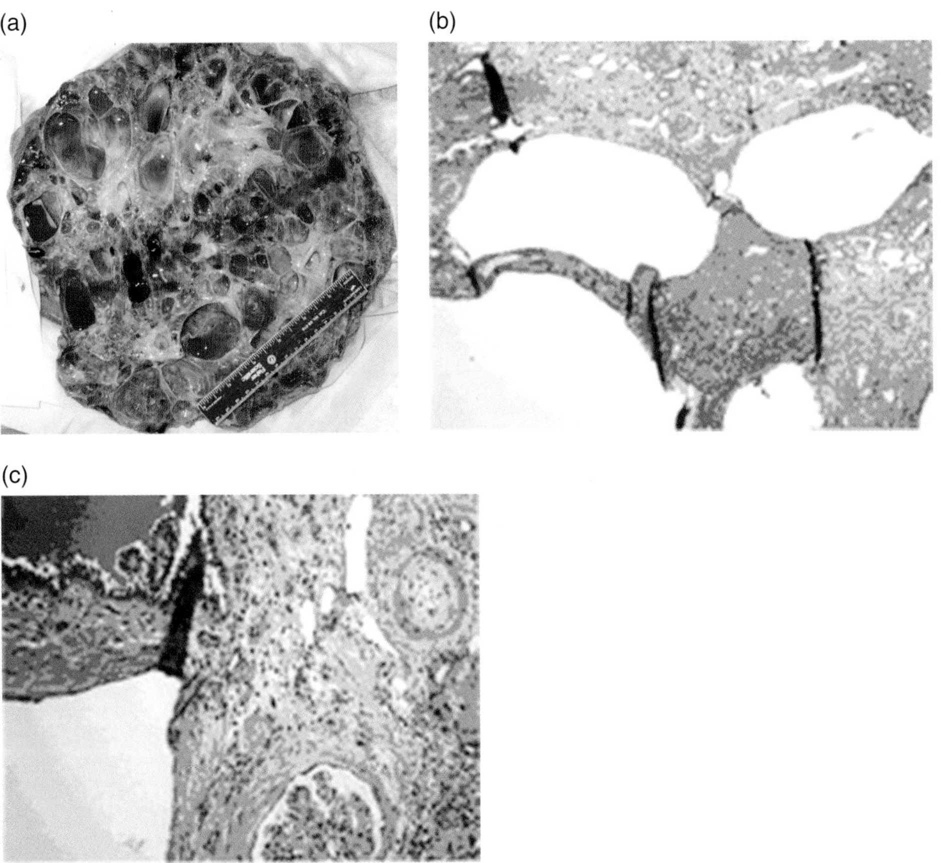

Figure 35.3 (a) Gross appearance of one of the surgically removed kidneys. (b) Microscopic examination of kidney. H and E stain. Low power. (c) Microscopic examination of kidney. H and E stain. High power.

Answers and commentary

1 Abdominal examination

There are two large lateral masses felt in the left and right side of the abdomen, probably due to enlarged kidneys, which could be due to polycystic kidneys or bilateral hydronephrosis. The former is more likely in view of the history of hypertension.

2 Additional history

The patient and his father had PKD, confirming the cause of his bilateral renal masses. The patient also had a history of coronary artery disease, but had no myocardial necrosis on his present admission (ECG and serum troponin were normal).

3 Physical examination

The patient initially had hypertension that responded to treatment. Hypertension would account for the patient's cardiomegaly and apical S4.

4 Laboratory data

Hb and WBC are normal but there is evidence of renal insufficiency.

5 CT of abdomen

There were liver cysts, of which the largest was 4.8 cm in diameter. The kidneys were markedly enlarged and measured 15 cm in cross-sectional diameter. The kidneys appeared to be composed of multiple small grape-like structures.

6 Course and treatment

The patient underwent bilateral nephrectomy and then received a renal transplant in 2007, which apparently malfunctioned. He has been on chronic hemodialysis from 2007 until at least 2011 (Table 35.1).

7 Pathology

The kidneys each weighed about 3000 g (normal weight 150 g). There are multiple small cysts on the renal surface, varying from 0.3 to 8 cm in diameter. Most of the cysts contained clear brown liquid with blood seen in some of them. The renal artery shows mild atherosclerotic changes.

Microscopically the renal parenchyma is mostly replaced by multiple cysts of varying sizes. A few glomeruli and tubules are seen, as well as some scattered areas of pyelonephritis. No malignant or atypical cells seen.

Discussion

The patient had PKD, hypertension, and coronary artery disease. PKD occurs in 1:500 to 1:1000 of the population [1, 2]. It is transmitted as an autosomal dominant trait and is the most common form of hereditary kidney disease [1, 2].

Symptoms consist of hematuria and flank pain [3], as in this patient. His extra-renal signs of PKD were only hypertension and benign liver cysts. Other extra-renal signs such as mitral valve prolapse or intracerebral aneurysms were not seen [1].

Hypertension often develops between the ages of 30 and 34, and may appear before significant renal dysfunction appears [1]. Despite its detection good BP control (≤130/80) is only attained in <30% of cases [1]. The pathogenesis of hypertension has been attributed in part to cystic compression of normal renal tissue producing renal ischemia, which then leads to an increase in angiotensin II levels [1].

Over 50% of patients with PKD develop end-stage renal disease by the fifth decade, as seen in this patient [1]. The only treatment for end-stage renal disease in PKD at present is dialysis or renal transplantation [3]. A height-adjusted kidney volume of over 600 mL/m predicts end-stage renal disease within 8 years [3].

In the post-dialysis era, patients with PKD usually die from coronary artery disease [1].

Key points

1. PKD is transmitted as an autosomal dominant trait.
2. PKD is a rare cause of hypertension that manifests itself in the third decade of life.
3. Other clinical manifestations of PKD are hematuria and abdominal masses, with renal failure occurring in about the fifth decade.
4. Bilateral nephrectomy followed by renal transplantation or hemodialysis may be required for severe abdominal pain (from the massively enlarged kidneys).

References

[1] Chapman AB, Stepniakowski K, Rahbari-Oskoui F. Hypertension in autosomal dominant polycystic kidney disease. *Adv Chronic Kidney Dis* 2010; 17: 153–163.

[2] Takiar V, Caplan MJ. Polycystic kidney disease: pathogenesis and potential therapies. *Biochim Biophys Acta* 2011; 1812: 1337–1343.

[3] Steinman TL. Polycystic kidney disease: a 2011 update. *Curr Opin Nephrol Hypertens* 2012; 21: 189–194.

Further reading

Ellison DH, Ingelfinger JR. A quest – Halting the progression of autosomal dominant polycystic kidney disease. *New Eng J Med* 2014; 371: 2329–2331.

36 PATIENT STUDY 36

Sequence of data presentation

1 ECG
↓
2 Chest X ray
↓
3 Oxygen saturation sample run
↓
4 Cardiac pressures
↓
5 Aortography
↓
6 Pressures and phonocardiogram
↓
7 History and physical examination
↓
8 Diagnosis
↓
9 Treatment
↓
10 Follow-up

1 ECG

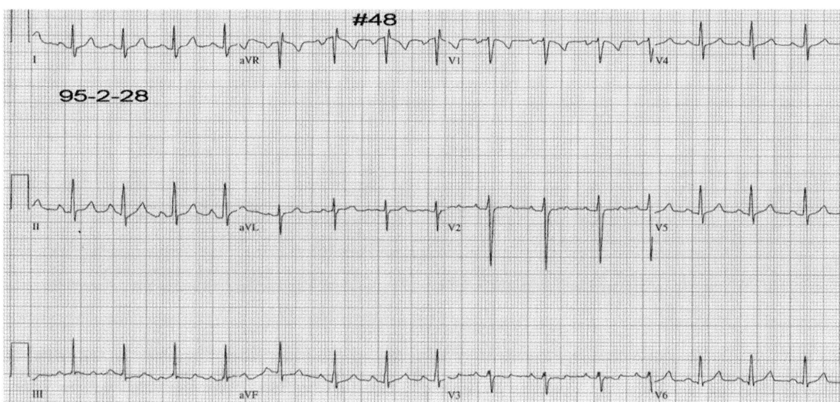

Figure 36.1 12-lead ECG 1995.

2 Chest X ray

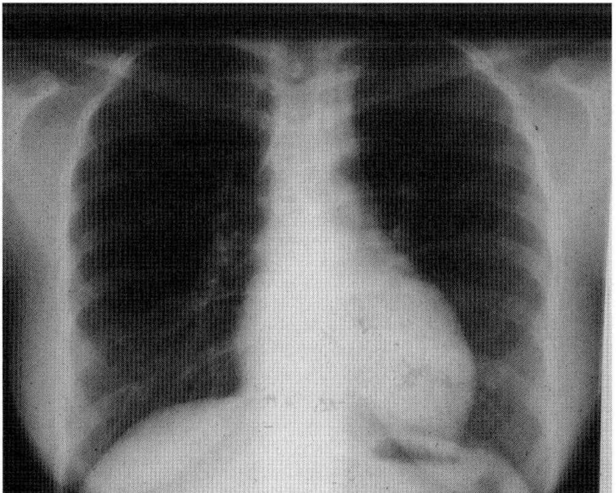

Figure 36.2 Chest X ray.

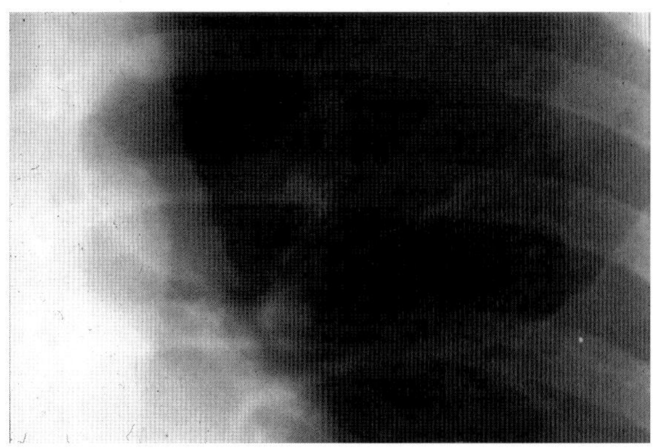

Figure 36.3 Chest X ray showing left upper lung field.

Patient Studies in Valvular, Congenital, and Rarer Forms of Cardiovascular Disease: An Integrative Approach, First Edition. Franklin B. Saksena.

Companion Website: www.wiley.com/go/saksena/patientstudies

3 Oxygen saturation sample run

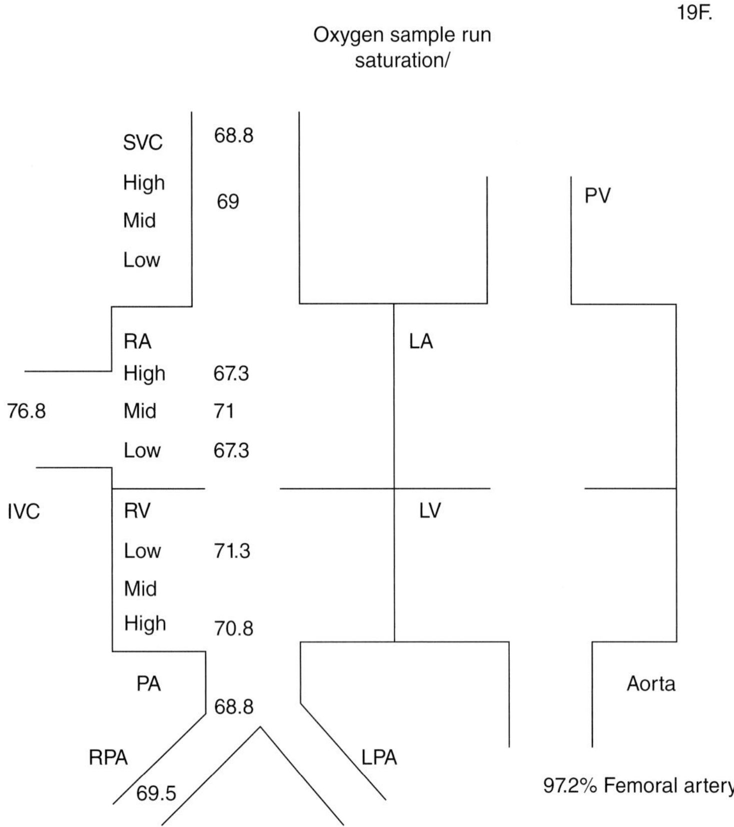

Figure 36.4 Oxygen saturation sample run.

4 Cardiac pressures

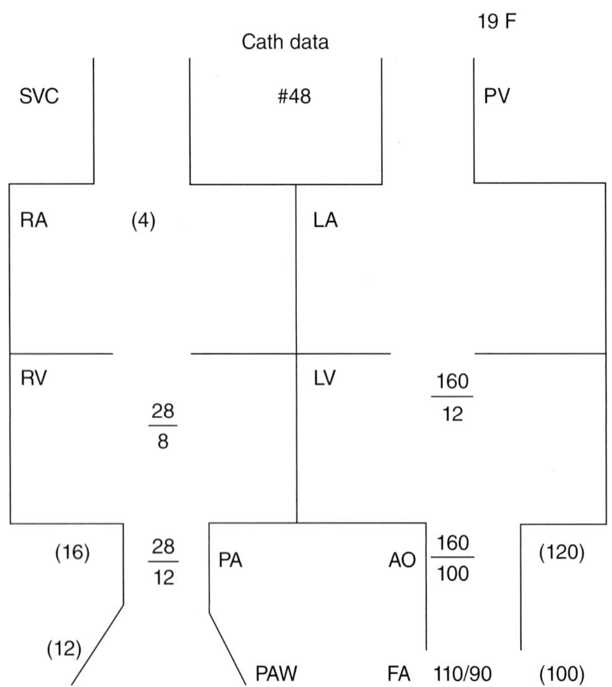

Figure 36.5 Intracardiac pressures.

5 Aortography

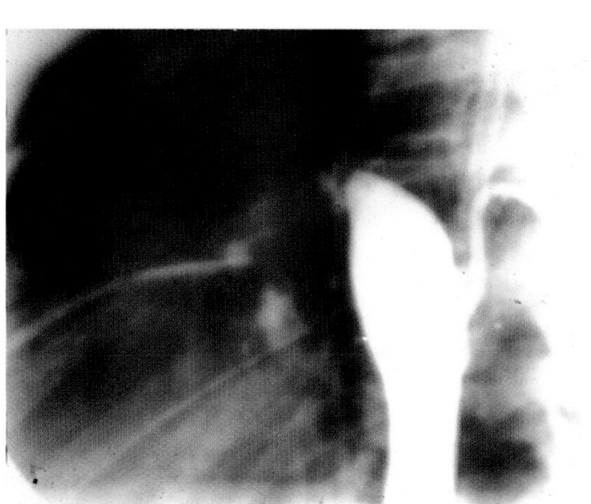

Figure 36.6 Descending aortogram.

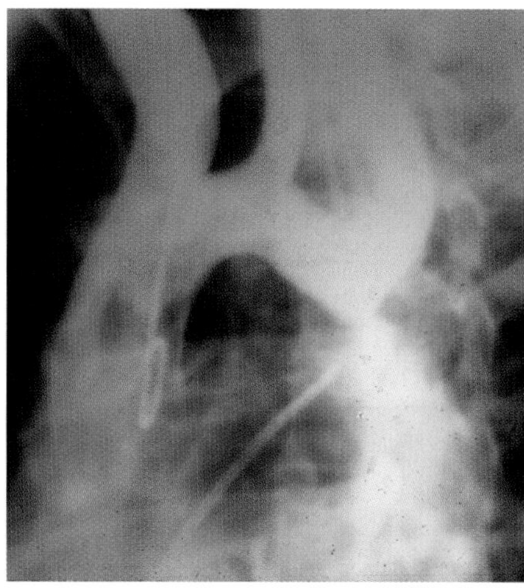

Figure 36.7 Ascending aortogram.

6 Pressures and phonocardiogram

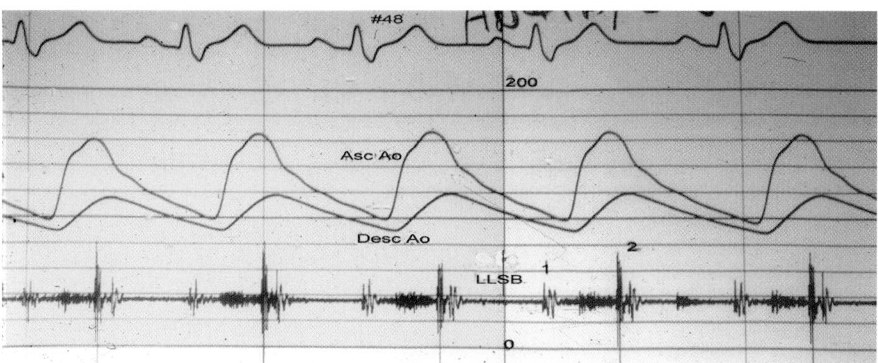

Figure 36.8 Simultaneous ascending and descending aortic pressure curves with phonocardiogram (loglog frequency) at LLSB. 0–200 mm Hg scale.

7 History and physical examination

History

19-year-old female admitted to hospital in 1996 with a long history of hypertension. A murmur was noted 5 years ago. She had aching in the legs on walking.

Physical examination

63 inches tall black female weighing 112 lb. BP 160/80. HR 57/min regular.

No elevation of jugular venous pressure. Suprasternal notch pulsations noted.

Apex beat was in the 5th interspace, 9 cm from the mid-sternal line.

S1 normal. S2 increased.

Grade 3/6 diamond-shaped systolic murmur maximum in left 3rd and 4th interspaces parasternally. No bruits heard in the back.

1+/4+ femoral pulses bilaterally. The femoral pulses were delayed compared to the brachial arteries.

Biphasic Doppler sounds heard over the femoral area, but none heard distally.

Feet and legs were cool to touch.

8 Diagnosis

What is your diagnosis?

9 Treatment

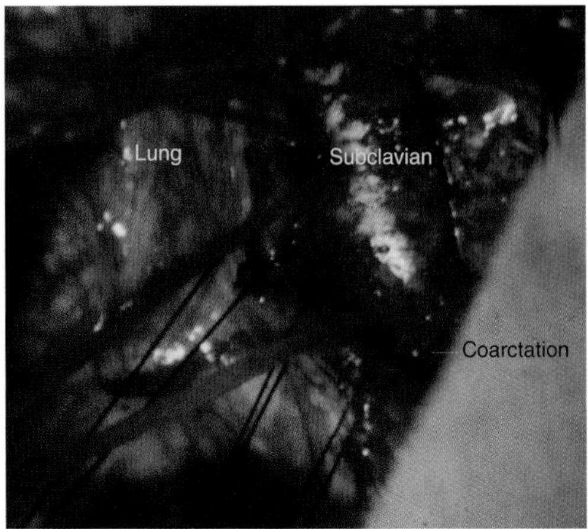

Figure 36.9 View of open chest at thoracotomy showing site of coarctation.

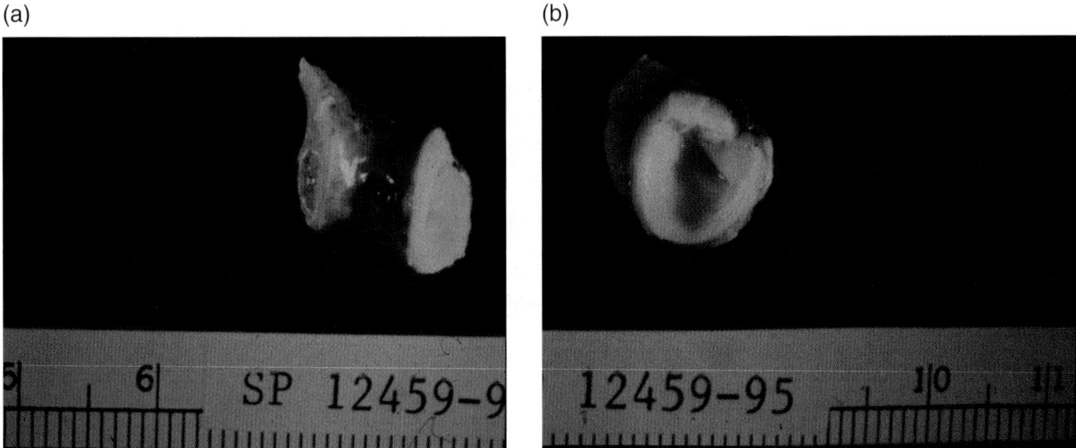

Figure 36.10 Two views of coarcted segment removed surgically 1995.

10 Follow-up

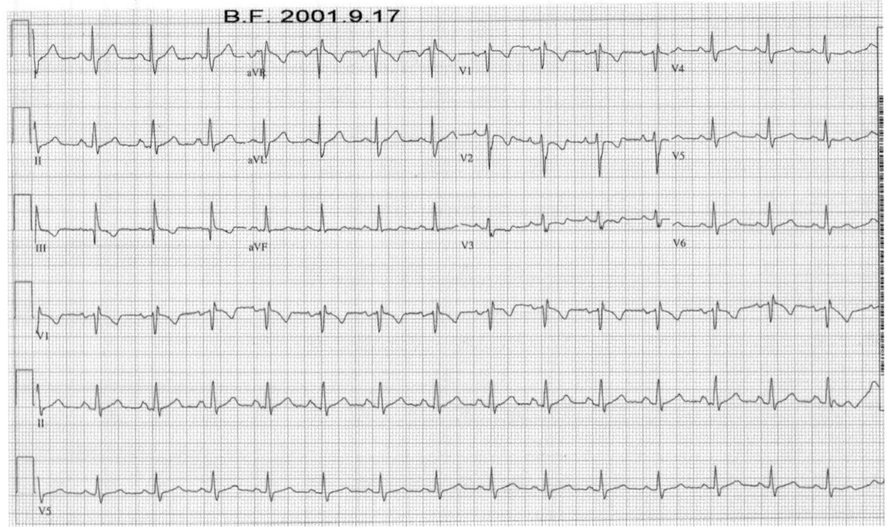

Figure 36.11 12-lead ECG 2001.

Answers and commentary

1 ECG

The rhythm is sinus. Rate 95/min. PR interval 0.16 s. QRS interval 0.09 s. QRS axis +75°. T biphasic in V3. Impression: normal ECG.

2 Chest X ray

No cardiomegaly. Lung fields appear normal.

Left subclavian artery is prominent (Baumgarten's sign).

Baumgarten's sign is often seen in coarctation of the aorta and is sometimes easier to detect than the 3 sign (formed by the dilated subclavian artery above the coarctation of the aorta and the dilated descending aorta below the coarctation of the aorta). Left 5th posterior rib is notched. Rib notching on right side not seen. The latter two findings are suggestive of coarctation of the aorta.

It is common to overlook rib notching and call the chest X ray (Figure 36.2) normal.

Rib notching is caused by the increased size and tortuosity of the intercostal arteries causing a groove in the inferior rib margin. In one series rib notching occurred in 50% of cases of coarctation of the aorta and correlated directly with age and inversely with the diameter of the coarctation [1].

In coarctation of the aorta the ribs are usually notched bilaterally from the 3rd to the 8th ribs, whereas if there is a left-sided subclavian artery stenosis the ribs are notched on the right side only. Left-sided notching in coarctation occurs if there is an aberrant right subclavian artery [2, 3].

Other causes of rib notching include SVC obstruction, neurofibromatosis, or a shunt procedure (Glenn or Blalock–Taussig) [3].

3 Oxygen saturation sample run

The right-sided sample run and the arterial saturation are normal, thus there is no evidence of an intracardiac shunt. A VSD is often seen with coarctation of the aorta [4].

4 Cardiac pressures

The right heart pressures are normal. There is borderline elevation of the LVEDP suggestive of some LV dysfunction. The absence of a systolic gradient across the aortic valve excludes aortic stenosis in this patient. Aortic stenosis is commonly seen in coarctation (see Figure 36.5) [4].

There is systolic and diastolic hypertension.

The ascending aortic pressure is 50 mmHg higher than the femoral arterial pressure, which may be seen in peripheral vascular disease or coarctation of the aorta. The latter is more likely in view of the age of the patient. Rib notching and a dilated left subclavian artery also support the diagnosis of coarctation.

5 Aortography

The descending aorta is tapered superiorly (Figure 36.6) and it was not possible to pass the guide wire across the coarcted site. A single intercostal collateral is also seen.

An ascending aortogram shows the site of coarctation at about T4. The coarctation is deemed significant if its diameter is ≤50% that of descending aorta at the level of the diaphragm [5]. The left subclavian artery is dilated, which is also seen on the plain chest X ray.

6 Pressures and phonocardiogram

The ascending aortic pressure exceeds the descending aortic pressure tracing by 50 mmHg, indicative of severe coarctation of the aorta. The descending aortic pressure tracing is delayed in onset, rises slower than the ascending aortic pressure, and has a narrower pulse pressure. This correlates well with the brachial femoral delay seen in coarctation.

The systolic murmur starts in mid systole and spills slightly into diastole in this patient. In coarctation of the aorta the longer the systolic murmur spills into diastole the more severe is the narrowing of the coarctation [6].

7 History and physical examination

A young patient with a history of long-standing hypertension may have renal disease or coarctation of the aorta.

Aching of the legs on walking suggests compromised blood flow to the legs, which favors coarctation of the aorta.

Physical examination showed evidence of coarctation of the aorta on the basis of (i) systolic hypertension and diminished pressures in the legs (by Doppler study), (ii) suprasternal notch pulsations (≡ dilated ascending aorta), and (iii) the femoral pulse is delayed in onset compared to the brachial artery (normally the onset of the femoral pulse precedes the brachial pulse) and is of reduced amplitude. The findings in (iii) are illustrated by the simultaneous tracings of the ascending and descending aorta in Figure 36.8.

All young patients with hypertension must be examined for any brachial–femoral pulse delay to see if coarctation might be the cause of their hypertension.

8 Diagnosis

Coarctation of the aorta.

9 Treatment

The narrowness of the coarcted site is seen at surgery in comparison to the enlarged aortic arch and subclavian artery (Figure 36.9).

The coarcted segment was removed surgically. Its lumen barely was 2 mm across, thus explaining why it was not possible to pass the guide wire across the coarcted site (Figure 36.10).

10 Follow-up

The patient did well after surgery. She was on no medications 1995–2001. In 2001 her BP was 135/79. The two-dimensional echocardiogram was normal.

ECG in 2001 showed sinus rhythm. Rate 90/min. PR 0.14 s. QRS 0.10 s. QRS axis +50°. Nonspecific anterior T wave changes were little changed from 1995.

She had an uneventful pregnancy in 200l.

Discussion

Coarctation of the aorta is a discrete constriction of the aorta usually immediately distal to the left subclavian artery near the insertion of the ductus arteriosus.

It is considered severe if the coarcted segment is <2.5 mm in diameter [6].

It accounts for 6–8% of live births with congenital heart diseases, with an estimated incidence of 1 in 2500 live births. Male/female ratio is about 1.7/1 [7].

Adult patients with coarctation of the aorta may be asymptomatic [4] but may present with symptoms due to hypertension or intermittent claudication, as was seen in this patient.

There is usually hypertension in the upper extremities and hypotension in the lower extremities. The systolic pressure in the legs may be ascertained using an appropriately sized thigh cuff and either a stethoscope or a hand-held Doppler device. The mean arterial pressure is also obtainable using the flush method [8]. This method could not be used in this patient as she was dark skinned, but was used in patient 12 (see website), who was light skinned (cf Figure 12.1).

Besides upper extremity hypertension the most important sign of coarctation of the aorta is the brachial–femoral delay. Several different murmurs have been noted in coarctation of the aorta: a delayed systolic ejection murmur spilling into diastole due to the coarcted segment, murmurs due to aortic valve disease (stenosis and regurgitation), and continuous murmurs heard over the back due to collateral circulation [6]. Occasionally extensive collateral circulation may even be visible over the chest, back, or abdomen [9]. A systolic ejection click may also be heard in coarctation of the aorta if there is a bicuspid aortic valve [4] (see legend for Figure 12.1).

Up to 50% of patients with coarctation of the aorta have associated cardiac lesions, the most common lesions being a VSD or valvular aortic stenosis (see Figure 12.1). Up to 85% of patients will have a bicuspid aortic valve [4].

Other vascular anomalies associated with coarctation are a right subclavian artery, arising aberrantly from the aorta just distal to the coarctation, and berry aneurysms in the Circle of Willis [4]. Collateral circulation develops between the subclavian artery above the coarctation (via the superior intercostal, scapular, and internal mammary arteries) to the intercostal arteries and epigastric artery, which then supply the descending aorta and its branches below the coarctation segment [10].

15–30% of patients with Turner's syndrome have coarctation of the aorta [4].

Cardiac catheterization and angiography, CT/MRI of chest, and MRA of the aorta are all useful methods in detecting coarctation of the aorta by assessing the severity of the aortic valve disease and the extent of the collateral circulation [4, 7]. Echocardiography and Doppler studies of the aorta also detect coarctation of the aorta and can quantitate the gradient across the coarcted segment [4, 7, 11].

Surgery or stenting of the coarctation of the aorta [5, 12] is required if there is angiographic evidence of a significant coarctation of the aorta (diameter of coarctation of the aorta/diameter of descending aorta ≤ 50%)

and a gradient across the coarctation of the aorta > 20 mmHg [4, 12]. However, surgical correction may still be required if the gradient is <20 mmHg because extensive collateral circulation, a large PDA, or LV dysfunction may attenuate the gradient across the coarcted site [7]. The usual surgical approach is to resect the coarcted site followed by end-to-end anastomosis, as was carried out in this patient. Other methods include patch aortoplasty, left subclavian patch aortoplasty, and bypass grafts between ascending and descending aorta [4].

Key points

1. The clinical manifestations of coarctation of the aorta are hypertension in the upper extremities, diminished and delayed femoral artery pulses, late aortic systolic murmur, and chest wall collateral circulation.
2. Chest X ray findings of coarctation of the aorta are rib notching from the 3rd to 8th ribs and a dilated left subclavian artery.
3. Surgical resection or stenting of the coarctation of the aorta is required if the narrowed site is ≤50% of descending aorta diameter and there is a gradient >20 mmHg across the coarcted site (in the absence of significant collateral circulation).

References

[1] Glancy DL, Roberts WC, Simon AL, Braunwald E. Coarctation of the aorta: hemodynamic, angiographic and anatomic correlations. (Abs) *Ann Int Med* 1968; 68: 1155.

[2] Boone ML, Swenson BE, Felson B. Rib notching: Its many causes. *Am J Roentgenol* 1964; 91: 1075–1088.

[3] Shapiro S, Schrire V. Unilateral notching of the ribs in cyanotic heart disease. *Br Heart J* 1964; 26: 620–624.

[4] Rothman A. Coarctation of the aorta: An update. *Curr Probl Pediatr* 1998; 28: 37–60.

[5] Thanopoulos BV, Eleftherakis N, Tzanos K et al. Stent implantation for adult aortic coarctation. *J Am Coll Cardiol* 2008; 52: 1815–1816.

[6] Spencer MP, Johnston FR, Meredith JH. The origin and interpretation of murmurs in coarctation of the aorta. *Am Heart J* 1958; 56: 722–737.

[7] Kenny D, Hijazi ZM. Coarctation of the aorta: from fetal life to adulthood. *Cardiol J* 2011; 18: 487–495.

[8] Constant J. *Bedside cardiology*, 5th edn. Lippincott, Williams and Wilkins, Philadelphia, 1999, p 55.

[9] Peters F, Essop R. Coarctation of the aorta with visible palpable collaterals over the scapular and anterior abdominal wall. *J Am Coll Cardiol* 2010; 56: 423.

[10] Edwards JE, Clagett OT et al. The collateral circulation in coarctation of the aorta. *Staff Meet Mayo Clin* 1948; 23: 333–339.

[11] Marx GR, Allen HD. Accuracy and pitfalls of Doppler evaluation of the pressure gradient in aortic coarctation. *J Am Coll Cardiol* 1986; 7: 1379–1385.

[12] Santoro G, Carminati M, Bigazzi MC et al. Primary stenting of native aortic coarctation. *Tex Heart Instit J* 2001; 28: 226.

Further reading

Agarwala BN, Bach E, Cao QL, Hijazi ZM. Clinical manifestations and diagnosis of coarctation of the aorta. www.uptodate.com, 2013 update.

37 PATIENT STUDY 37

Sequence of data presentation

1 ECG
↓
2 Chest X ray
↓
3 Hemodynamic and angiographic data
↓
4 History
↓
5 Physical examination
↓
6 Laboratory data
↓
7 Course and treatment

1 ECG

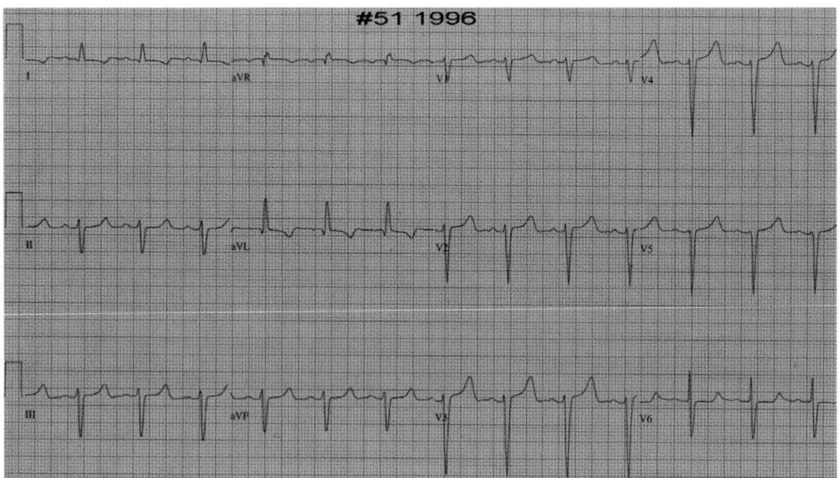

Figure 37.1 12-lead ECG.

2 Chest X ray

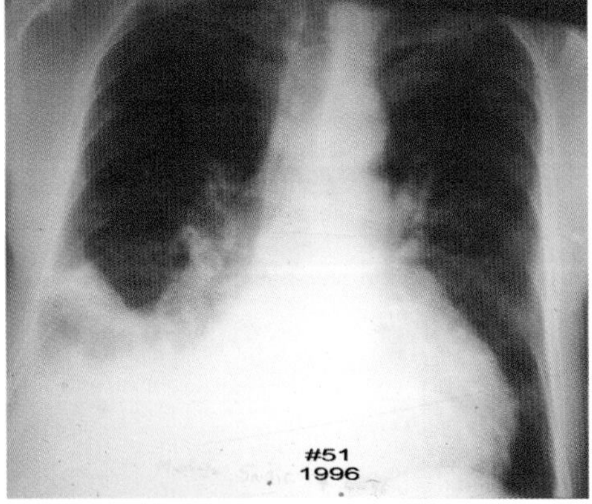

Figure 37.2 PA chest X ray.

Patient Studies in Valvular, Congenital, and Rarer Forms of Cardiovascular Disease: An Integrative Approach, First Edition. Franklin B. Saksena.

Companion Website: www.wiley.com/go/saksena/patientstudies

3 Hemodynamic and angiographic data

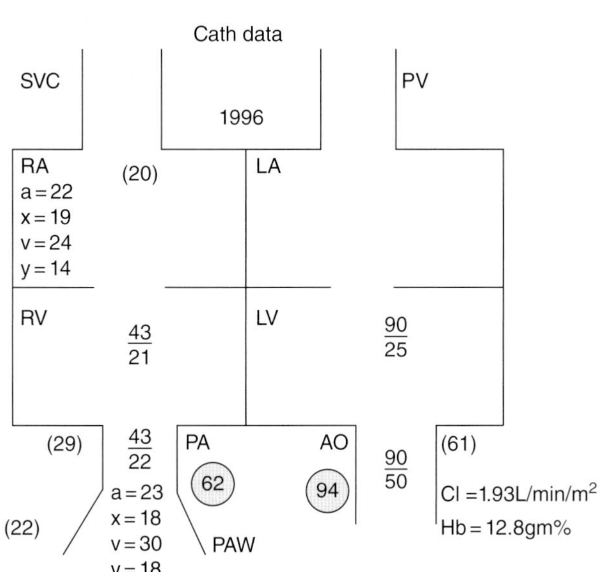

Figure 37.3 Hemodynamic and angiographic data. Numbers in circles are oxygen saturations.

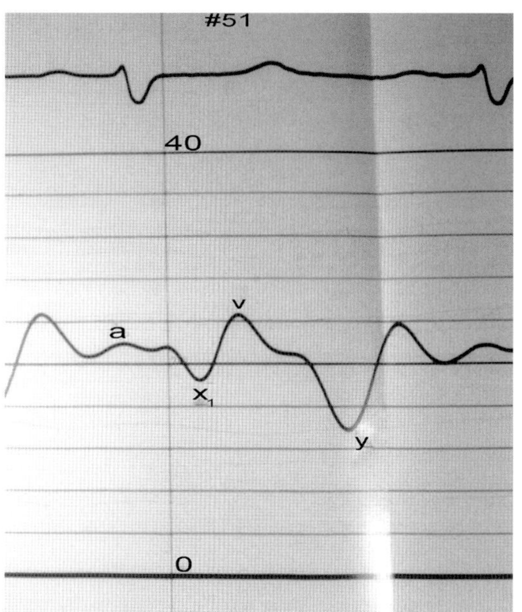

Figure 37.4 RA pressure tracing.

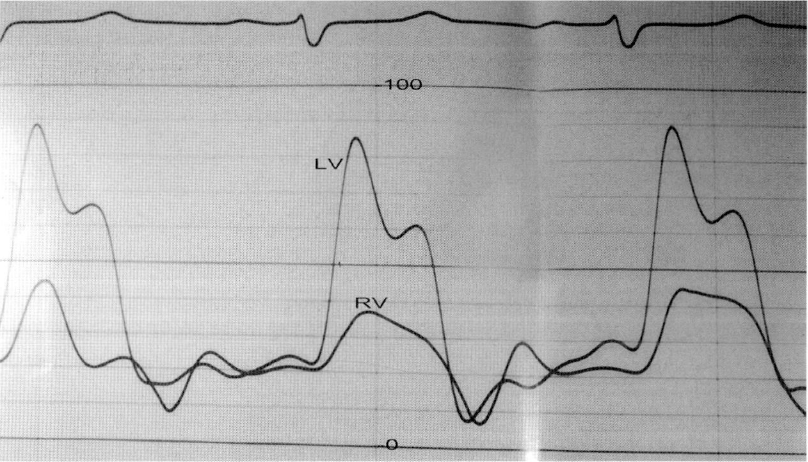

Figure 37.5 RV and LV pressure tracings.

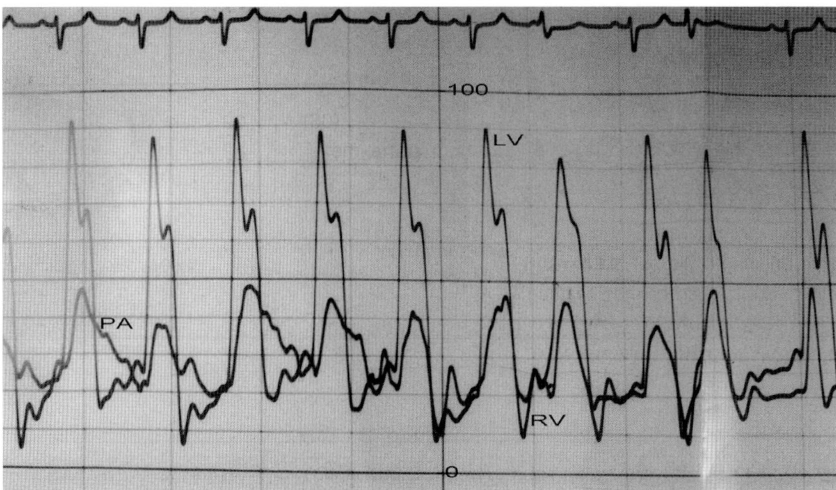

Figure 37.6 Withdrawal pressure tracings from PA to RV. Simultaneous RV and LV pressure tracings.

4 History

58-year-old man admitted to hospital in 1996 with exertional dyspnea and non-exertional chest pain for the last 8 months. He had a history of Sjorgren's syndrome.

5 Physical examination

72 inches tall male weighing 178 lb. BP 110/71. HR 70/min.
He had a positive ear crease sign.
The jugular venous pressure was elevated.
Breath sounds were diminished in the RLL.
Apex beat was in the 5th interspace, 13 cm from the mid-sternal line (cardiomegaly).
There was an apical S3.
The liver span was 13 cm. The spleen was felt 6 cm below the left costal margin.
No pedal edema.

6 Laboratory data

Hemoglobin 12.8 g%.
Chest X ray: C/T ratio was 15/29. RLL effusion. No pericardial calcification.
Two-dimensional echocardiography showed RV enlargement. Doppler studies were done, but were not available.
MUGA LV ejection fraction was 57%.
MUGA RV ejection fraction 44%.

7 Course and treatment

What is the likely course and treatment for this patient?

Answers and commentary

1 ECG

The rhythm was sinus. Rate 82/min. PR 0.16 s. QRS 0.09 s. QRS axis –45°.
Poor R wave progression V1–4. Deep S in V5.
Impression: left-axis deviation, possible old anteroseptal infarction or fibrosis.

2 Chest X ray

There is cardiomegaly, prominent proximal pulmonary vessels and RLL effusion. No pericardial calcification seen on this view.

3 Hemodynamic and angiographic data

There is a diastolic plateau seen in right heart pressures with $\overline{RA} \approx RVEDP \sim PADP \sim \overline{PAW}$, where $\overline{RA}$ and $\overline{PAW}$ are the mean RA and mean wedge pressures, respectively (Figure 37.3). This could be due to a restrictive cardiomyopathy or CCP. As the PA systolic pressure is >40 mmHg the former diagnosis is more likely [1].

The LVEDP is moderately elevated to 25 mmHg, mostly due to a stiff LV as the cardiac output was only slightly reduced.

A normal coronary angiogram indicates that his chest pain is of non-ischemic origin. The RA pressure tracing is shown in Figure 37.4. There is a rapid x_1.and y descent compatible with a restrictive filling pattern.

PA, RV, and LV pressures are shown in Figures 37.5 and 37.6. There is no gradient in systolic across the pulmonic valve. The RVEDP and LVEDP are increased and nearly identical, which also indicates a restrictive filling pattern.

4 History

Patients with Sjorgren's syndrome may be associated with an autoimmune disease such as lupus or rheumatoid arthritis, or very rarely with diastolic dysfunction [2].

5 Physical examination

Elevated jugular venous pressure, S3, cardiomegaly, and hepatomegaly suggest that there is RV failure. Splenomegaly may be seen in severe heart failure or possibly in CCP. The presence of a pleural effusion and an S3 point to LV dysfunction.

CCP is less likely as there was no paradoxical pulse, pericardial knock, or pericardial thickening/calcification either on X ray or echocardiogram [1].

6 Laboratory data

There is borderline cardiomegaly on chest X ray .The RLL effusion could be due to local pulmonary pathology or LV failure. As the LV ejection fraction is normal the patient has diastolic LV failure .He also has diastolic RV failure as the RV ejection fraction is still in the normal range.

Doppler studies are probably the best way of distinguishing between restrictive cardiomyopathy and CCP. Only in the latter is there marked respiratory variation in transvalvular flow and an increased expiratory reversal of diastolic hepatic vein flow [1].

7 Course and treatment

Patient was continued on an ACE inhibitor and diuretics.

Fat pad biopsy and rectal biopsy were negative for amyloid at our hospital.

At another hospital he was diagnosed with light chain amyloidosis as he had monoclonal immunoglobulins in the serum. However, a myocardial biopsy was non-diagnostic for amyloidosis. He was started on an alkalating agent, melpheran, without symptomatic improvement.

He was last seen in the ER in July 1997 for a scalp laceration. There was no mention of his cardiac status.

Discussion

The patient had diastolic heart failure from a restrictive cardiomyopathy rather than from a CCP as he had none of the features to suggest CCP [1]. Specific causes of a restrictive cardiomyopathy include amyloidosis, hemochromatosis, sarcoidosis, Loeffler's eosinophilic endomyocardial disease, and endomyocardial fibrosis [3]. This patient's cardiomyopathy was attributed to amyloidosis only on the basis of monoclonal immunoglobins found in the serum as the myocardial biopsy was inconclusive and the fat pad and rectal biopsies were negative.

Amyloidosis can be definitively diagnosed by myocardial biopsy or less invasively by subcutaneous skin biopsy [4]. Takashio et al. [4] reported a sensitivity of 80% in diagnosing cardiac amyloidosis by subcutaneous skin biopsy.

Amyloid appears microscopically as interstitial hyaline material that stains metachromatically with crystal violet stain and Congo red positivity with apple green birefringence under cross-polarized light [5].

Indirect methods of diagnosing amyoidosis include echocardiography [6, 7], late gadolinium-enhancement cardiac magnetic resonance [4], or ^{99m}Tc-DPD scintigraphy [8].

Untreated amyloid heart disease has a poor prognosis, with most patients dying within 6–12 months after the onset of heart failure [5–7]. High-dose chemotherapy and autologous stem cell transplantation show promise in patients with light-chain amyloidosis [6, 7]. The long-term follow-up in this patient is unknown.

Key points

1. The right heart pressures showed a diastolic plateau, which can be seen in CCP or a restrictive cardiomyopathy.
2. The distinction between these two entities is not always easy, as hemodynamic studies can be inconclusive. However, Doppler echocardiography can make the distinction as only in CCP is there marked respiratory variations in transvalvular flow.
3. Amyloid heart disease is best diagnosed with a biopsy of the heart. Indirect methods of diagnosing amyloid heart disease include MRI and nuclear studies. Amyloid heart disease can also be detected on fat pad or rectal biopsy.

References

[1] Kronzon I, Fedor M, Schwartz D et al. A 56 year old man with shortness of breath, ascites, and leg edema. Clinicopathological Conference. *Circulation* 1996; 94: 1483–1488 (discussion of λ light-chain amyloidosis of the myocardium).

[2] Knockaert DC. Cardiac involvement in systemic inflammatory diseases. *Eur Heart J* 2007; 38: 1797–1804.

[3] Benotti JR, Grossman W, Cohn PF. Clinical profile of restrictive cardiomyopathy. *Circulation* 1980; 61: 1206–1212.

[4] Takashio S, Izumiya Y, Jinnin M et al. Diagnostic and prognostic value of subcutaneous tissue biopsy in patients with cardiac amyloidosis. *Am J Cardiol* 2012; 110: 1507–1511.

[5] Ruberg FL, Berk JL. Transthyretin (TTR) cardiac amyloidosis. *Circulation* 2012; 126: 1286–1300.

[6] Falk RH. Cardiac amyloidosis. A treatable disease, often overlooked. *Circulation* 2011; 124: 1079–1085.

[7] Seward JB, Casaclang-Verzosa G. Infiltrative cardiovascular diseases. Cardiomyopathies that look alike. *J Am Coll Cardiol* 2010; 55: 1769–1779.

[8] Perugini E, Guidalotti PL, Salvi F et al. Noninvasive etiologic diagnosis of cardiac amyloidosis using ^{99m}Tc-3, 3-diphosphono-1,2-propanodicarboxylic acid scintigraphy. *J Am Coll Cardiol* 2005; 46: 1076–1084.

Further reading

Esplin BL, Gertz MA. Current trends in diagnosis and management of cardiac amyloidosis. *Curr Probl Cardiol* 2013; 38: 47–96.

38 PATIENT STUDY 38

Sequence of data presentation

1 History
↓
2 ECG 1998
↓
3 Laboratory data
↓
4 Hemodynamics
↓
5 Angiography
↓
6 Physical examination
↓
7 Phonocardiogram
↓
8 Diagnosis and course

1 History

37-year-old man admitted to hospital in 1998 with a history of dyspnea on walking half a mile or up two flights of stairs for the last 6 months.

He used to run 6 miles without difficulty.

He had scarlet fever as a child but was not restricted from playing sports.

He was noted to have a heart murmur 13 years ago when he was in the navy.

No chest pain, syncope, or pedal edema.

There is a long-standing history of asthma. He used cocaine up until 6 months ago. No alcoholism.

2 ECG 1998

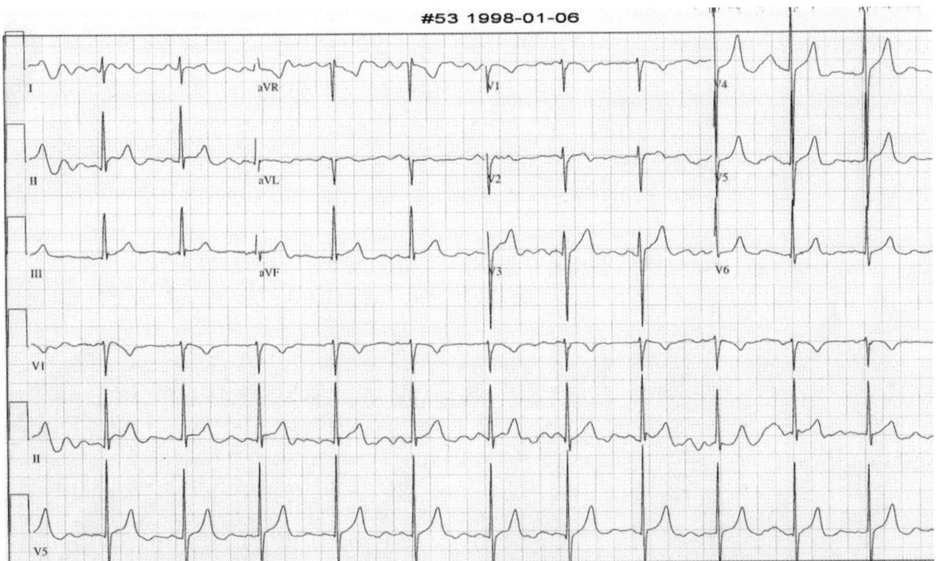

Figure 38.1 12-lead ECG.

Patient Studies in Valvular, Congenital, and Rarer Forms of Cardiovascular Disease: An Integrative Approach, First Edition. Franklin B. Saksena.

Companion Website: www.wiley.com/go/saksena/patientstudies

3 Laboratory data

Chest X ray C/T = 12/26. The lung fields were hyperinflated. There was no pulmonary congestion. An echocardiogram was done in 1997.

4 Hemodynamics

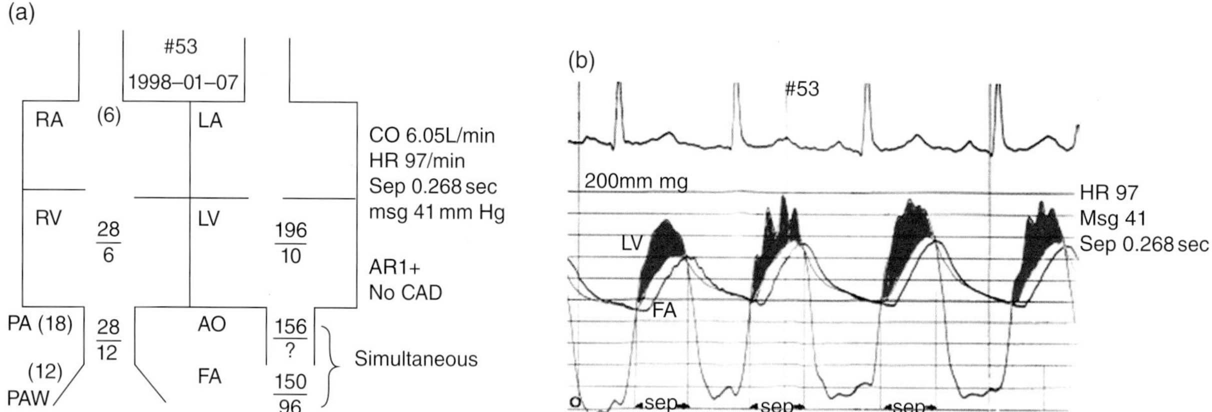

Figure 38.2 (a) Hemodynamic data. (b) LV and FA pressures. 0–200 mmHg scale. AR aortic regurgitation; CAD, coronary artery disease; CO, cardiac output; FA, femoral artery; HR, heart rate; msg, mean systolic gradient; sep, systolic ejection period.

What is the aortic valve area?

5 Angiography

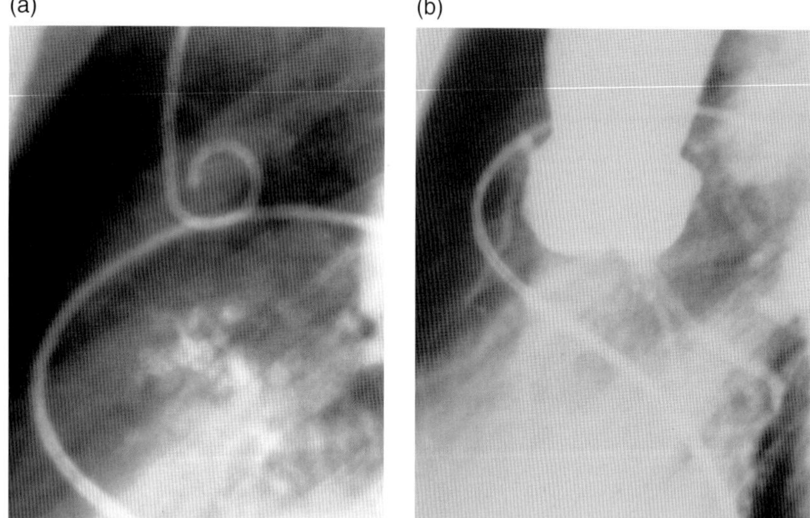

Figure 38.3 (a) LAO view showing aortic catheter position prior to aortography. (b) LAO view of aortogram.

6 Physical examination

67 inches tall black male weighing 140 lb. BP 118/64. HR 75/min regular.

Delayed carotid upstroke. No elevation of jugular venous pressure.

Apex beat is in the 6th interspace, 9 cm from the mid-sternal line.

S1 normal. S2 −1 decreased. S4 + 1 at apex.

Grade 2/6 crescendo decrescendo systolic murmur best heard in the right 3rd interspace parasternally. No diastolic murmur noted.

Decreased air entry bilaterally.

No abdominal masses noted.

No pedal edema. 2+/4+ foot pulses.

7 Phonocardiogram

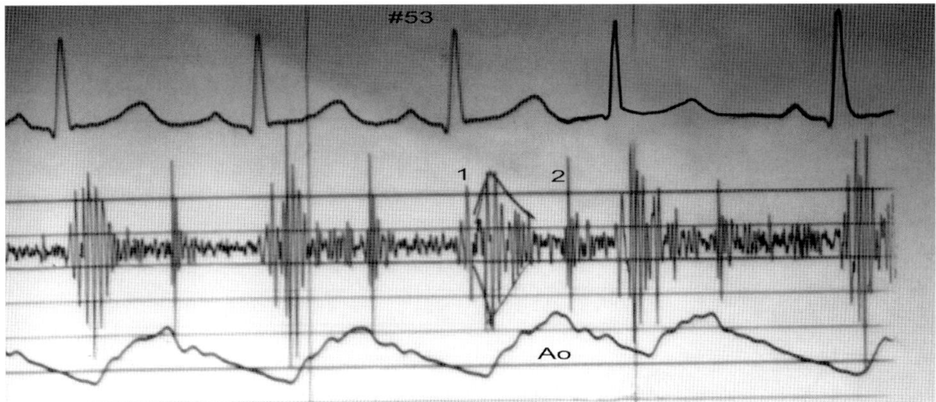

Figure 38.4 Phonocardiograms showing aortic pressure tracing and recording of murmur at the 3rd interspace parasternally.

8 Diagnosis and course

What is the diagnosis?
What treatment would you advise and what is the likely course?

Answers and commentary

1 History

The new onset of dyspnea in a man who has a heart murmur and previously had normal exercise tolerance could be due to progression of a left-sided valvular disease or a cardiomyopathy. The long-standing history of asthma could be due to underlying heart failure or chronic lung disease. The chest X ray showed no evidence of heart failure and was more in favor of chronic lung disease.

2 ECG 1998

Sinus rhythm. Rate 70/min. PR 0.20 s. QRS 0.08 s. QRS axis +90°.

R wave in lead AVF = 1.2 mv.

Impression: LVH by voltage criterion.

Addendum: The R wave in AVF has increased from 0.5 to 1.2 mv since 1997, indicating that LVH has become more evident since 1997.

3 Laboratory data

The heart size is normal. The lung findings are compatible with chronic obstructive lung disease.

An echocardiogram done in 1997 showed aortic stenosis.

4 Hemodynamics

The patient had normal right-sided pressures. There was a mean gradient (msg) in systolic across the aortic valve of 41 mmHg due to aortic stenosis. The delayed upstroke of the femoral artery (also seen in the aortic pressure tracing on the phonocardiogram in Figure 38.4) favors valvular stenosis.

Calculation of the AVA using the Gorlin formula yielded a valve area of only 0.81 cm^2, as shown below.

Data

Cardiac output (CO) 6050 mL/min, mean systolic gradient (msg) 41 mmHg, HR 97/min, systolic ejection period (sep) 0.268 s.

$$\text{AVA} = \frac{\dfrac{\text{CO}}{\text{HR} \times \text{sep}}}{44.1\sqrt{\text{msg}}} = \frac{\dfrac{6050}{97 \times 0.268}}{44.1\sqrt{41}} = 0.81\ \text{cm}^2$$

5 Angiography

Prior to aortic root angiography calcification is seen in the AVA (Figure 38.3a). Aortic root angiography shows that the aortic valve is bicuspid and that there is trace aortic regurgitation (Figure 38.3b). There was no coronary artery disease.

6 Physical examination

The patient had the features of significant aortic stenosis on the basis of a delayed carotid upstroke, inferiorly displaced apex beat, diminished S2, an S4, and a diamond-shaped systolic murmur best heard in the right 3rd interspace parasternally [1,2]. The intensity of the murmur could have been attenuated by the presence of COPD. However, the loudness of the murmur correlates poorly with the severity of aortic stenosis [1]. An aortic ejection click is often heard in patients with a bicuspid aortic valve. The absence of an aortic ejection click in this patient reflects the loss of mobility of the aortic valve leaflet from calcification. Calcification of a bicuspid aortic valve is often present by 40 years of age [3].

LVH seen on the ECG without coexisting hypertension also favors significant aortic stenosis.

7 Phonocardiogram

The delay in the aortic pressure upstroke and the diamond-shaped systolic murmur corroborate the physical finding described previously.

8 Diagnosis and course

The patient had a calcified bicuspid aortic valve with moderately severe aortic stenosis.

He underwent successful aortic valve replacement in 1998. In 2005 his BP remained within normal limits (119/66). No further CVS symptoms as of 2007.

Discussion

A bicuspid aortic valve is seen in 1–2% of the adult population, with a male/female ratio of 3/1 [1]. Symptoms usually arise as a result of calcification and subsequent stenosis of the aortic valve, as in this patient. The onset of symptoms occurs on the average between 44 and 52 years of age [3], which is earlier than for trileaflet degenerative aortic disease [3]. Additional complications of a bicuspid aortic valve are aortic regurgitation, infective endocarditis, and aortic dissection [1].

A bicuspid aortic valve is often associated with a dilated aorta or coarctation of the aorta [3], neither of which this patient had.

The diagnosis of a bicuspid aortic valve in this patient was made on aortography rather than on the echocardiography as details of the latter were not available.

Echocardiography (two-dimensional and/or TEE) is of great value in diagnosing the anatomical type of aortic valve present, the presence of LVH, an aortopathy, or coarctation of the aorta. The severity of aortic stenosis may be assessed by the Doppler aortic velocity jet. A peak velocity jet of 4 m/s indicates severe aortic stenosis corresponding to a peak systolic gradient of 64 mmHg or a mean systolic gradient of about 40–45 mmHg [4]. Calculation of the aortic valve area may also be done using the continuity equation. Critical aortic stenosis occurs when the area is $<0.5\,cm^2/m^2$ [1].

Echocardiographic examples from other patients showing a bicuspid valve are seen in Figures 38.5 and 38.6.

This patient underwent successful aortic valve replacement and was doing well 7 years later. The operative mortality for replacing the aortic valve without an underlying aortopathy is very low, but increases in the presence of an aortopathy [1,5].

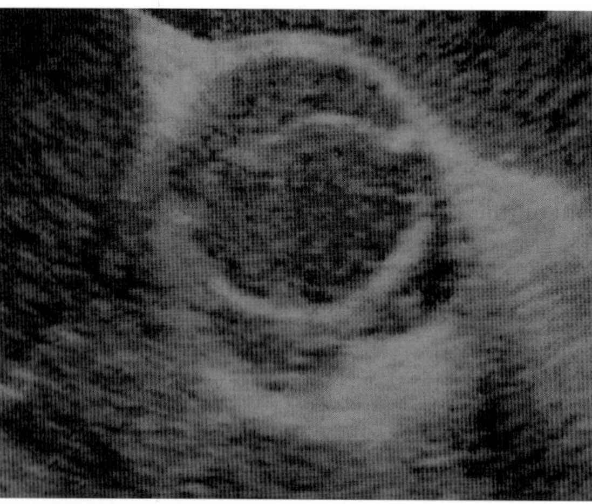

Figure 38.5 TEE in a 46-year-old man with a bicuspid aortic valve. No gradient across the aortic valve.

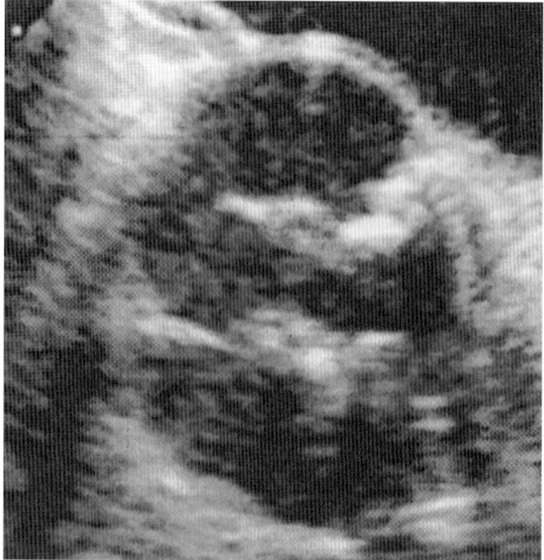

Figure 38.6 TEE in a 62-year-old man with a bicuspid aortic valve that was calcified and stenotic.

Key points

1. A congenital bicuspid aortic valve is a common cause of severe aortic stenosis in the younger patient.
2. Physical examination in conjunction with echocardiography and Doppler studies is able to assess the severity of the aortic stenosis.
3. Associated features of a bicuspid aortic valve include an aortopathy and coarctation of the aorta.
4. Replacement of the aortic valve in pure severe bicuspid aortic stenosis can be carried out with a low mortality rate.

References

[1] Olson LJ, Edwards WD, Tajik AJ. Aortic valve stenosis: Etiology, pathophysiology, evaluation, and management. *Curr Probl Cardiol* 1987; 12: 453–508.
[2] Ranganathan N, Sivaciyan V, Saksena FB. *The Art and Science of Cardiac Physical Examination*. Humana Press, Totowa, NJ, 2006, p 333.
[3] Siu SC, Silversides CK. Bicuspid aortic valve disease. *J Am Coll Cardiol* 2010; 55: 2789–2800.
[4] Munt B, Legget ME, Kraft CD et al. Physical examination in valvular aortic stenosis: Correlation with stenosis severity and prediction of clinical outcome. *Am Heart J* 1999; 137: 298–306.
[5] Tzemos N, Therrien J, Yip J et al. Outcomes in adults with bicuspid aortic valves. *JAMA* 2008; 300: 1317–1325.

Further reading

Braverman AC, Guven H, Beardslee MA. The bicuspid aortic valve. *Curr Probl Cardiol* 2005; 30: 470–522 (164 references).
Verna S, Siu SC. Aortic dilation in patients with bicuspid aortic valve. *New Eng J Med* 2014; 370: 1920–1929 (discusses pathophysiology and management of bicuspid aortopathy).

39 PATIENT STUDY 39

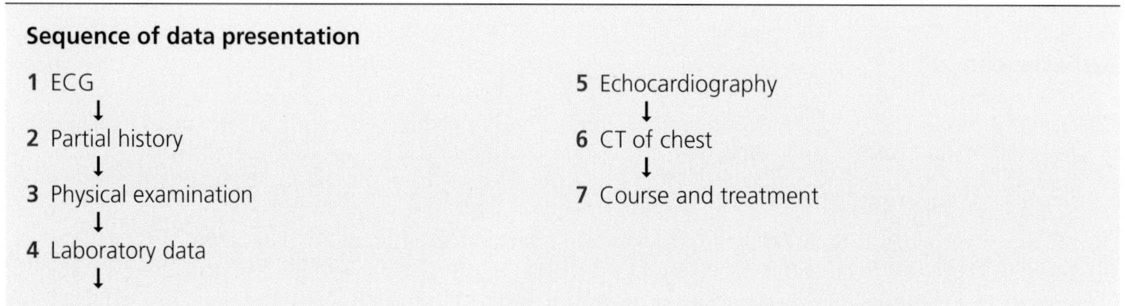

Sequence of data presentation

1 ECG
↓
2 Partial history
↓
3 Physical examination
↓
4 Laboratory data
↓
5 Echocardiography
↓
6 CT of chest
↓
7 Course and treatment

1 ECG

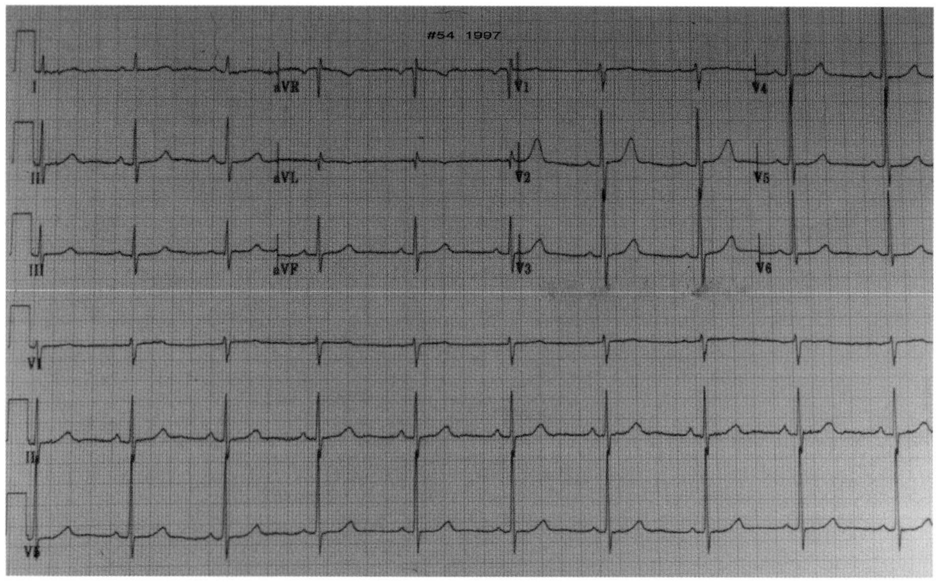

Figure 39.1 ECG.

2 Partial history

24-year-old female with history of cardiovascular disease since age 5.
She is asymptomatic. She does not drink alcohol or smoke or use drugs.

3 Physical examination

She is 73 inches tall and has an arm span of 71 inches (Figure 39.2). She has long thin fingers (Figure 39.3). Weight 143 lb. BP 102/60. HR 72/min regular. T 98.5 °F.

Patient Studies in Valvular, Congenital, and Rarer Forms of Cardiovascular Disease: An Integrative Approach, First Edition. Franklin B. Saksena.

Companion Website: www.wiley.com/go/saksena/patientstudies

No elevation of jugular venous pressure. Normal carotid upstroke.

Apex beat is in the 5th interspace, 8 cm from the mid-sternal line. S1 normal. S2 normal.

Mid-systolic click at the apex. There is a grade 2/6 diastolic decrescendo blowing murmur heard at LLSB. There was no apical systolic murmur.

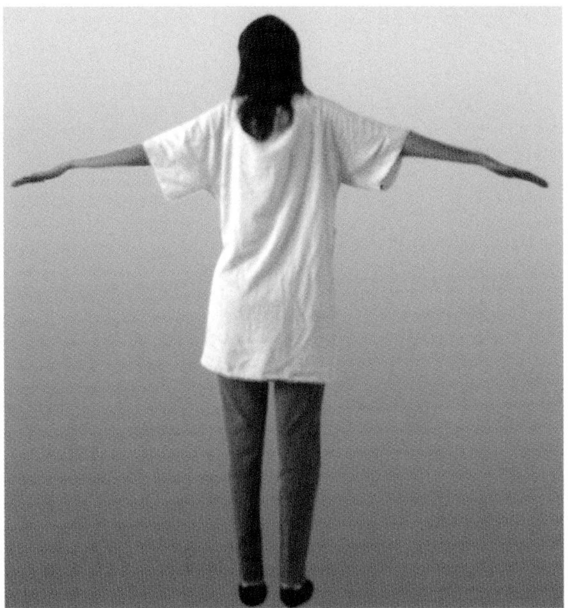

Figure 39.2 Physical appearance of patient.

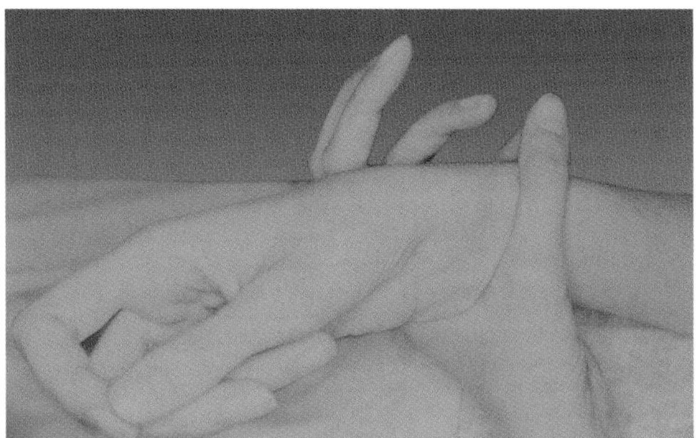

Figure 39.3 Wrist sign. The thumb and fifth finger can encircle the wrist and touch each other.

4 Laboratory data

Normal chest X ray in 1997.

Table 39.1 Aortic root dimensions 1997–2001

Year	Aortic root size (cm)	Aortic root index (cm/m²)
1997	5.0	2.7
2000	5.7	2.8
2001	6.0	2.9

5 Echocardiography

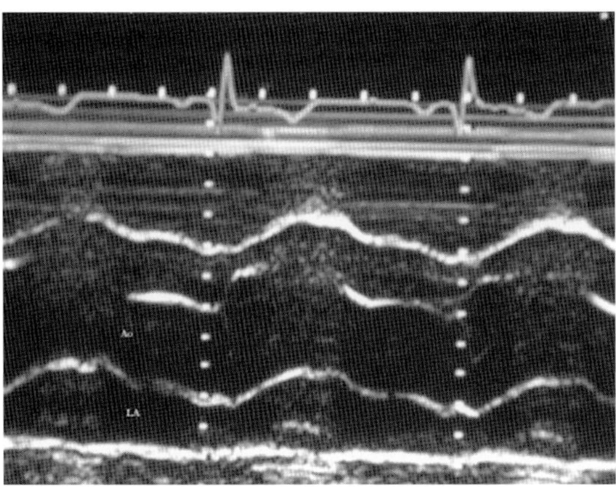

Figure 39.4 M-mode echocardiogram showing aorta and LA.

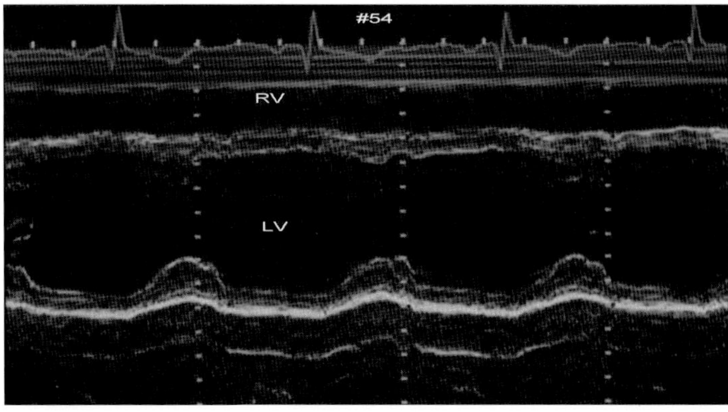

Figure 39.5 M-mode echocardiogram showing LV and RV.

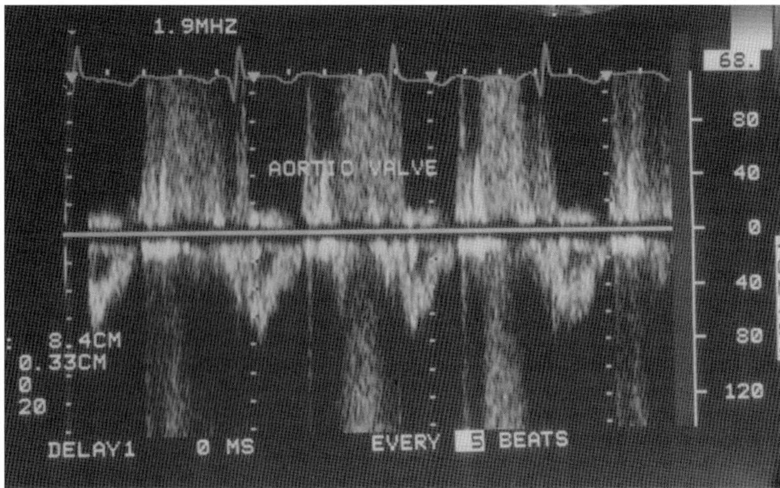

Figure 39.6 Doppler flow velocity across the aortic valve.

6 CT of chest

(a)

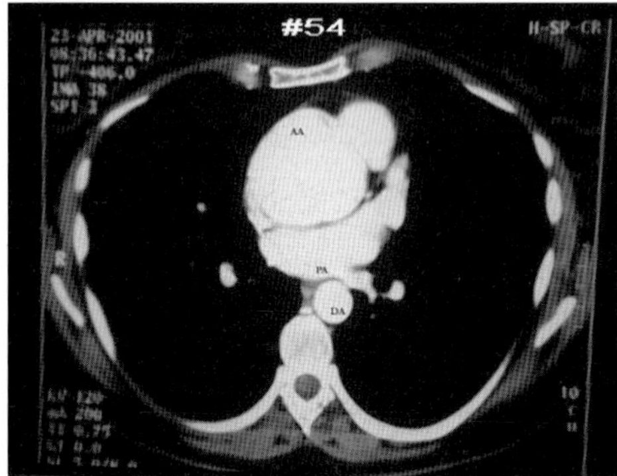

(b)

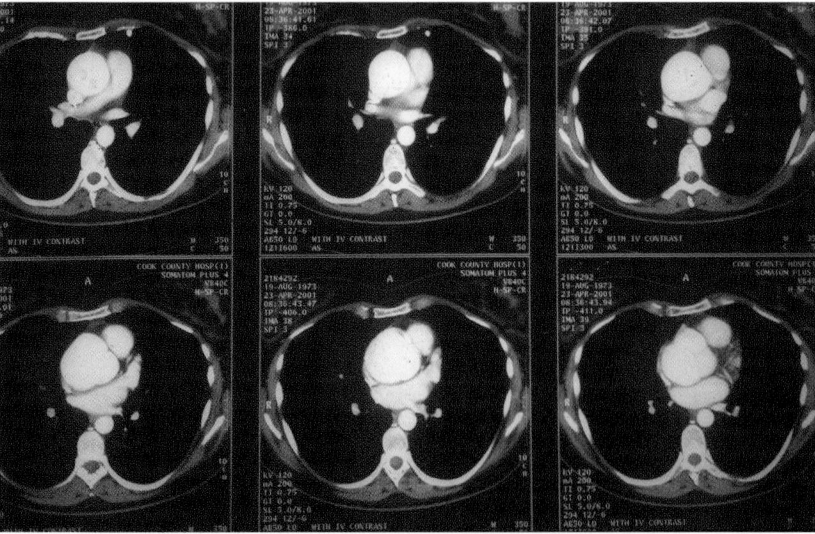

Figure 39.7 (a) CT of chest showing ascending aorta (AA), PA and descending aorta (DA) 2001. (b) CT of chest showing six successive sections from above downwards of which Figure 39.7a is image 38 (middle of lower panel) 2001.

7 Course and treatment

What is your diagnosis?

What is the likely course if untreated?

What is the treatment?

Answers and commentary

1 ECG

Sinus rhythm. Rate 62/min. PR 0.16 s. QRS 0.06 s. QRS axis +60°.
Impression: normal ECG.

2 Partial history

The patient had a history of Marfan syndrome since the age of 5.
She has been on beta-blockers for the last 4 years and now wishes to become pregnant.

3 and 4 Physical examination and laboratory data

She had the physical features of Marfan syndrome, with arm span ≈ height, polydactyly (positive wrist and thumb signs), mitral valve prolapse, and aortic regurgitation. There is no cardiomegaly either on physical examination or on chest X ray.

5 Echocardiography

In Figure 39.4 the aortic root is dilated to at least 5 cm (upper limit of normal = 3.7 cm).

In Figure 39.5 the LV is slightly enlarged as the LV end-diastolic dimension is 6 cm. The LV end-systolic dimension of 4 cm and the RV end-diastolic dimension of 1.8 cm are within normal limits.

In Figure 39.6 the Doppler flow velocity study across the aortic valve show aortic regurgitation.

Table 39.1 shows a gradual increase in aortic root diameter from 5 to 6 cm, placing the patient in the moderate risk category (8% risk of aortic rupture per year) [1].

The use of the BSA to index the aortic root diameter may be subject to some error as the patient gained weight from 143 lb in 1997 to 189 lb in 2001.

6 CT of chest

The diameter of the aortic root is dilated to 6 cm.

7 Course and treatment

The patient had Marfan syndrome with a critically dilated aortic root, mild aortic regurgitation, and mitral valve prolapse without mitral regurgitation.

Untreated the ascending aortic aneurysm may develop aortic dissection or rupture.

Pregnancy will increase the risk of aortic rupture [2].

The patient underwent a David procedure (Figure 39.8) in 2001. The risks of aortic rupture during pregnancy will be considerably reduced in this patient. However, for the newborn there is still a 50% chance of developing Marfan syndrome [2].

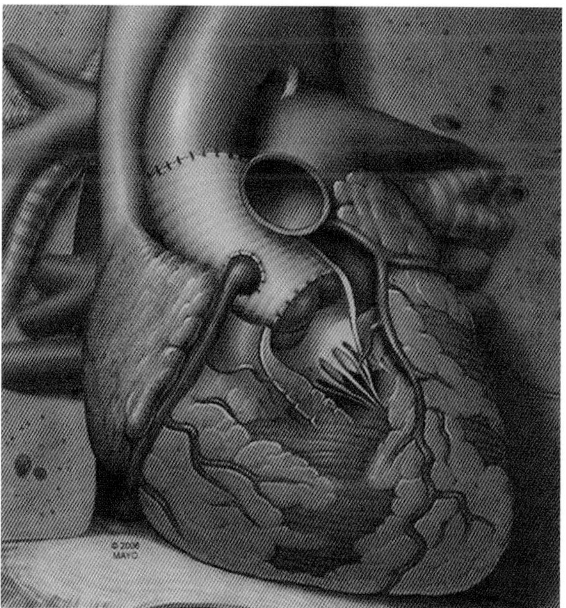

Figure 39.8 David-type procedure showing the ascending aorta has been replaced by a tube graft, the native aortic valve preserved, and the coronary arteries reimplanted into the graft . Source: Ammash NM, Connolly HM. (2007). Reproduced with permission of Mayo Foundation for Medical Education and Research, all rights reserved. © the Mayo Clinic.

In 2003 the chest X ray showed that the heart size remained normal (Figure 39.9) and a repeat CT of the chest (Figures 39.10 and 39.11) showed a normal sized aortic root (2.7 cm). She no longer had any aortic regurgitation on physical examination. She was continued on beta-blockers and was asymptomatic when last seen in 2004.

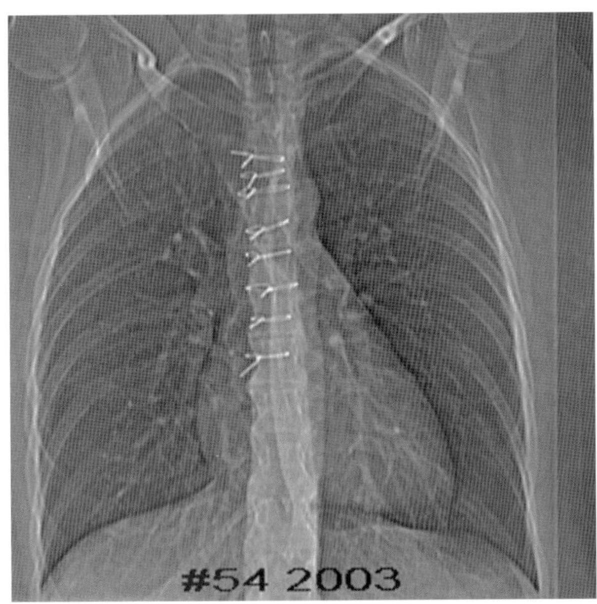

Figure 39.9 Scout chest X ray 2003.

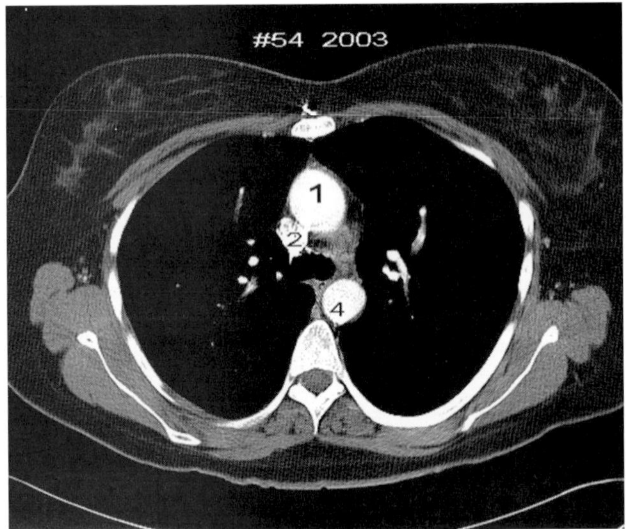

Figure 39.10 CT of chest 2003 at T5-6 level. 1, ascending aorta; 2, SVC; 4, descending aorta.

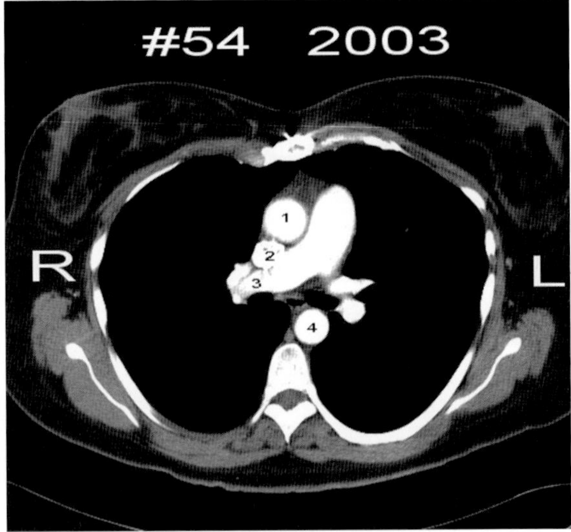

Figure 39.11 CT of chest 2003 at T6-7 level. 1, ascending aorta; 2, SVC; 3, right PA; 4, descending aorta.

Discussion

Marfan syndrome occurs in 1:5000 of the general population [2]. It is an autosomal dominant disorder of connective tissue that may involve abnormalities of the cardiovascular, skin, and skeletal, ocular, pulmonary, and dura mater. About a third of patients have a negative family history of Marfan syndrome [2, 3]. Untreated patients with Marfan syndrome have a life span of about 32 years [2].

This patient fulfilled the criteria for Marfan using the Ghent criteria, namely long thin extremities (positive wrist and thumb signs), a dilated ascending aorta at the level of the aortic sinuses, aortic regurgitation and mitral valve prolapse.

Occasionally some patients may present with massive dilatation of the ascending aorta that on angiography resembles an Erlenmeyer flask (Figure 39.12).

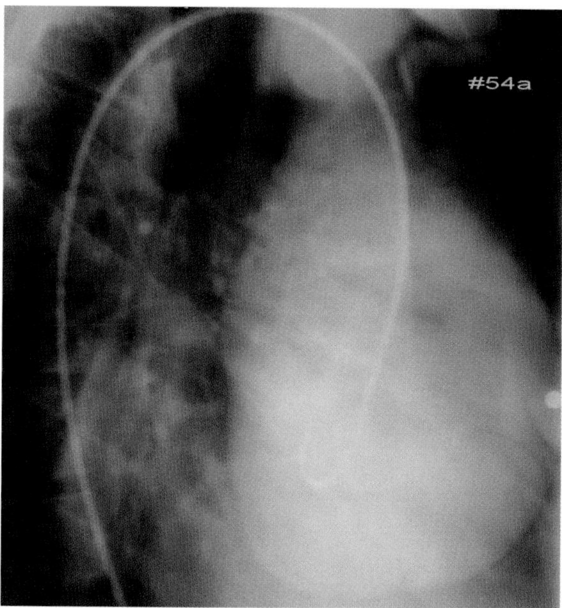

Figure 39.12 Aortic angiogram in RAO view of a 30-year-old man with Marfan syndrome showing marked enlargement of the ascending aorta (>6 cm in diameter) resembling an Erlenmeyer flask.

Ectopia lentis occurs in 60% of patients with Marfan syndrome but this was not present in this patient.

Despite the use of beta-blockers (to decrease the arterial stiffness) our patient's aortic root diameter continued to enlarge, placing her at a moderate risk of aortic rupture (aortic root index = 2.75–4.24 cm/m^2) and she was deemed ready to undergo a David procedure.

The main complication of Marfan syndrome is aortic dissection and aortic rupture. Both of these have a higher incidence should the patient become pregnant. The incidence of annual rupture increases with increasing aortic root size, i.e. 4% for an aortic root index of <2.75 cm/m^2 and 20% for an aortic root index >4.25 cm/m^2 [1].

Serial echocardiographic measurements of the aortic root are useful in determining the progress of the disease and when to consider surgery. Elective operative repair is recommended at an aortic root index of ≥2.75 cm/m^2 [1]. Following operative repair (David procedure) patients have a near-normal life expectancy [2, 4].

Key points

1. Marfan syndrome may be diagnosed on the basis of ectopia lentis, long thin extremities (positive wrist and thumb signs, arm span > height), aortic root enlargement, and aortic regurgitation. Two-thirds of patients will have a positive family history of Marfan syndrome.
2. Serial echocardiograms are a useful way of detecting progressive aortic root enlargement.
3. Beta-blockers may slow the progress of the aortic root enlargement. Pregnancy should be advised against.
4. Elective operative repair is recommended for an aortic root ≥2.75 cm/m^2, resulting in a near-normal life expectancy.

References

[1] Davies RR, Gallo A, Coady MA et al. Novel measurement of relative aortic size predicts rupture of thoracic aortic aneurysms. *Ann Thorac Surg* 2006; 81: 169–177. (315 patients had ascending aortic aneurysms with women having a higher likelihood of rupture and dissection. BSA was measured using the Dubois formula.)

[2] Ammash NM, Sundt TM, Connolly HM. Marfan syndrome – diagnosis and management. *Curr Probl Cardiol* 2008; 33: 7–39.

[3] Paterick TE, Humphries JA, Ammar KA et al. Aortopathies: etiologies, genetics, differential diagnosis, prognosis and management. *Am J Med* 2013; 126: 670–678.

[4] Ammash NM, Connolly HM. Marfan syndrome diagnosis and management. *South African Heart* 2007; 4: 10–17.

40 PATIENT STUDY 40

Sequence of data presentation

1 ECG 7 February 2001
↓
2 Echocardiogram 9 February 2001
↓
3 Holter monitor report
↓
4 Chest X rays
↓
5 Physical examination 2001
↓
6 History 2001
↓
7 Hands 2003
↓
8 ECG
↓
9 Course 2001–2003

1 ECG 7 February 2001

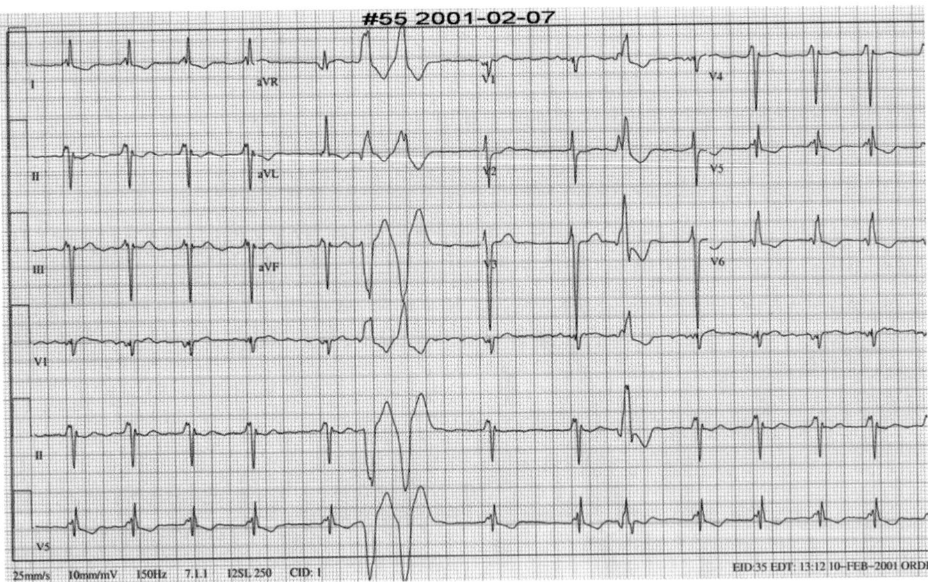

Figure 40.1 12-lead ECG 7 February 2001.

Patient Studies in Valvular, Congenital, and Rarer Forms of Cardiovascular Disease: An Integrative Approach, First Edition. Franklin B. Saksena.

Companion Website: www.wiley.com/go/saksena/patientstudies

2 Echocardiogram 9 February 2001

Table 40.1 Two-dimensional echocardiogram report 9 February 2001

Dimensions (cm)	
Aortic root	2.8
LA	4.3
LV end-diastolic dimension	6.0
LV end-systolic dimension	4.0
Additional data	
LV ejection fraction	20-25%
RV systolic pressure(calc.)	40-45 mm Hg
Moderate tricuspid regurgitation, mild mitral, and pulmonic regurgitation	
Normal valve morphology	
No pericardial effusion	

3 Holter monitor report

Table 40.2 Holter monitor report 20 February 2001

Atrial fibrillation with intraventricular conduction disturbance QRS duration 0.146 s
Frequent PVCs (50 per hour)
Asymptomatic ventricular tachycardia (140/min)

4 Chest X rays

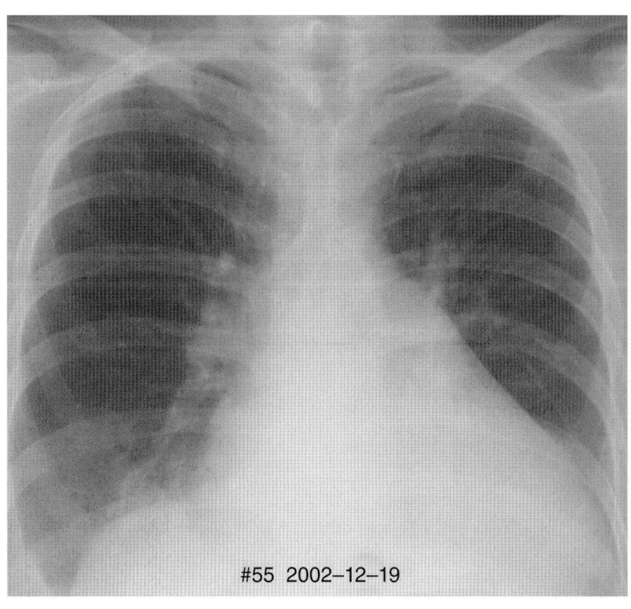

Figure 40.2 PA chest X ray 19 December 2002.

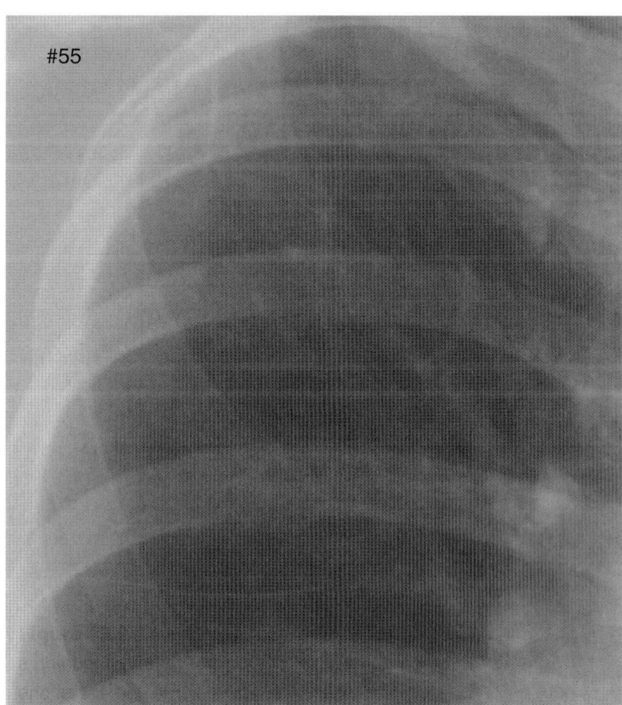

Figure 40.3 Enlarged right lower zone lung field 19 December 2002.

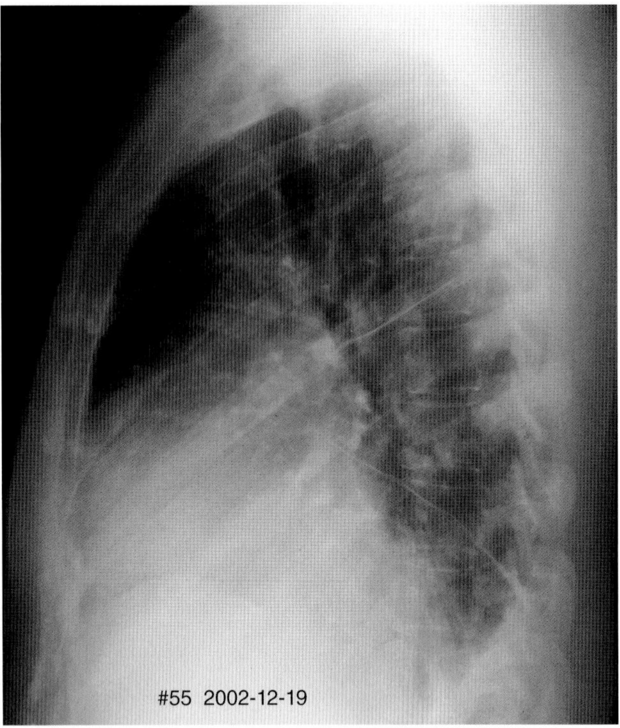

Figure 40.4 Lateral chest X ray 19 December 2002.

5 Physical examination 2001

62 inches tall, 114 lb female. BP 95/60. HR 80/min irregular. T 98.4 °F.
No elevation of jugular venous pressure.
Apex beat is in the 6th interspace, 9 cm from the mid-sternal line.
RV lift 1+. S1 and S2 normal. Lungs clear.
Grade 2/6 systolic murmur at LLSB, increasing with inspiration.
No hepatosplenomegaly.
No edema, cyanosis, or clubbing.

6 History 2001

34-year-old female admitted to hospital in Korea 1 month after delivery with dyspnea and edema in 1998.
She was first seen in Chicago in 2001 with three-block dyspnea and occasional paroxysmal nocturnal dyspnea. She was already on anticongestive measures.
No history of rheumatic fever, diabetes, hypertension, or CVA.
No history of smoking, drinking alcohol, or drug use.

7 Hands 2003

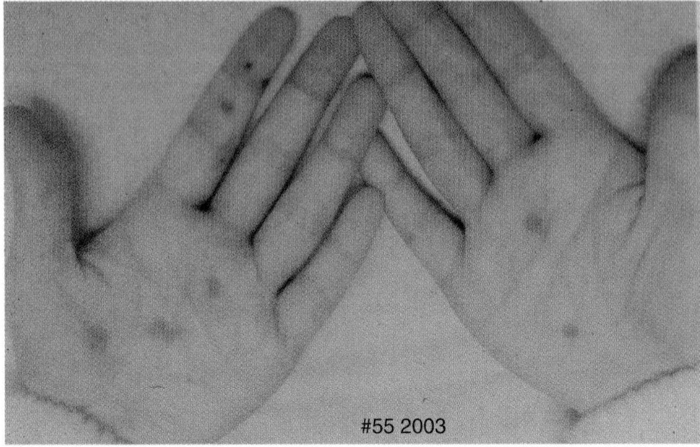

Figure 40.5 Hands 2003.

8 ECG

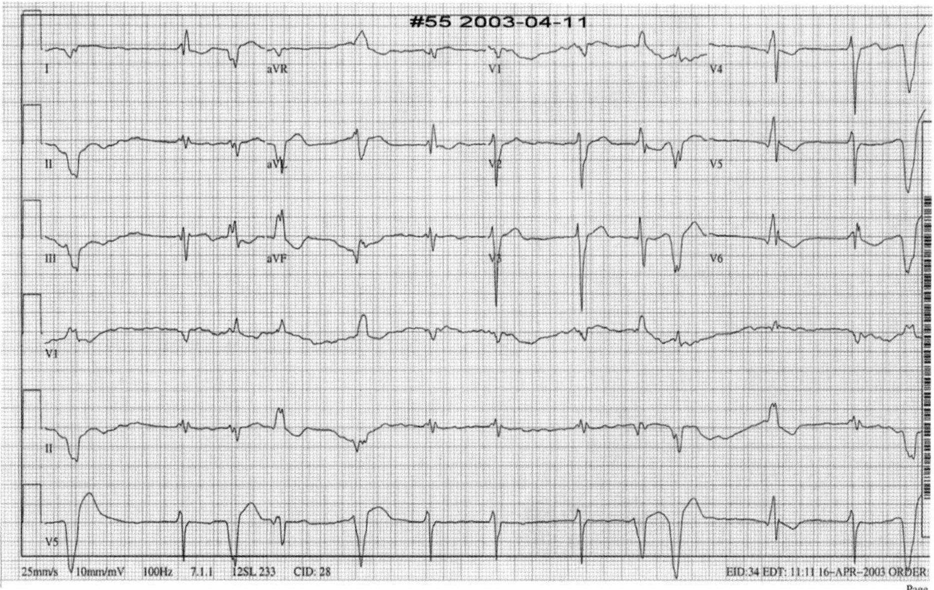

Figure 40.6 12-lead ECG 11 April 2003.

9 Course 2001–2003

The patient was treated with digoxin, captopril furosemide, warfarin, and spironolactone from 2001.

She was admitted for 2 days in heart failure in December 2002 after running out of medicine.

In January 2003 she was able to walk two blocks slowly. She had some leg edema.

Physical examination: BP 80/?, HR 84/min irregular. There was cardiomegaly, an S3, and 1+ leg edema.

In February 2003 two-dimensional echocardiogram showed four-chamber enlargement, LV ejection fraction of 20–25% and a calculated RV systolic pressure that had now risen to 70 mmHg.

In April 2003 she again ran out of medicine and now had 3+ leg edema and marked cardiomegaly (apex beat 12 cm from the mid-sternal line).

She had some hand lesions at this time (Figure 40.5)

What is the diagnosis for the hand lesions?

She died suddenly later that year (2003).

Answers and commentary

1 ECG 7 Febraury 2001

P waves are not seen. QRS complexes are mostly regular, suggesting a junctional rhythm. Some of the QRS complexes occur irregularly so an underlying atrial fibrillation cannot be excluded. One PVC couplet is seen. The ventricular rate is 90/min. The QRS duration is prolonged to 0.150 s due to an IVCD (or an atypical LBBB). There is left-axis deviation with a frontal QRS axis of –60° (or +300°).

The findings of an IVCD and marked left-axis deviation could represent a form of bifascicular block. Common causes of a bifascicular block include coronary artery disease, hypertensive heart disease, aortic valve disease, and cardiomyopathy. Less common causes are primary conduction disturbances (Lev/Lenegre diseases) or endocardial cushion defects [1].

2 Echocardiogram 9 February 2001

The LA and LV are enlarged with a very low LV ejection fraction. There is no LVH. There is mild to moderate pulmonary hypertension. In the absence of valvular heart disease a cardiomyopathy is a consideration, especially in the presence of an IVCD and left-axis deviation.

3 Holter monitor report 20 February 2001

The frequent PVCs and short run of ventricular tachycardia represent further evidence of LV dysfunction. As the patient had no symptoms at this time during the Holter recording anti-arrhythmic drugs were not used.

4 Chest X rays 19 December 2001

The PA chest X ray shows cardiomegaly, enlarged proximal PAs, and pulmonary congestion.

An enlargement of the right lung field shows increased pulmonary markings that do not extend to the lung periphery.

The lateral chest X ray shows probable RV enlargement with fluid seen in the minor and major fissures.

Impression: heart failure of unknown cause, probable pulmonary hypertension.

5 Physical examination 2001

The patient had borderline cardiomegaly with RV dysfunction. No overt LV failure. The systolic murmur at the apex could be due to tricuspid regurgitation but co-existent mitral regurgitation cannot be excluded. The echocardiogram suggests that tricuspid regurgitation was the more dominant lesion.

6 History 2001

The patient developed heart failure 1 month after delivery so she was diagnosed with postpartum cardiomyopathy in the absence of any other causes of heart failure (i.e. no hypertension, valvular heart disease, alcoholism, or coronary artery disease). It is unlikely that a Korean female would have had asymptomatic coronary artery disease at age 29.

7 Hands 2003

Several echymotic areas are seen on both hands, which might suggest a vasculitis. She was afebrile and had no pain, which makes a vasculitis less likely. The numerous echymotic areas were attributed to acupuncture of the hands in a patient on warfarin. She underwent acupuncture because she was not feeling well.

8 ECG 11 April 2003

The rhythm is atrial fibrillation with frequent PVCs. HR 75/min. QRS 0.150 s. QRS axis −35°. IVCD (atypical LBBB?). Ventricular tachycardia is no longer seen as compared to a previous ECG done on 24 January 2003.

9 Course 2001–2003

Despite anticongestive measures and anticoagulants the patient gradually developed progressive heart failure. Her low BP and an S3 indicated a low output state. Her sudden death in 2003 could have been due to an arrhythmia.

Discussion

This patient fulfilled the criteria for a peripartum cardiomyopathy, namely idiopathic heart failure in the last trimester of pregnancy or 5 months postpartum [2] as well as having an LV fraction <45% on echocardiography [3]. This occurs in 1:3200 live births and usually in women over the age of 30. The incidence is slightly higher in Asian patients [4].

Recovery occurs in >50% of patients within 2–6 months of the onset of peripartum cardiomyopathy [3,4].

Complications include severe heart failure, cardiogenic shock, cardiac arrest secondary to heart failure or arrhythmias, thromboembolism, and sudden death [4].

Patients with an LV ejection fraction less than 25% (as in this patient) are at increased risk of these complications [4]. In the USA the mortality rate can vary from 0 to 19% [4]. Patients who do recover from the cardiomyopathy are at increased risk of recurrence of heart failure in subsequent pregnancies [4].

Key points

1. Postpartum or peripartum cardiomyopathy usually occurs in women over the age of 30. It is slightly more common in Asians than Caucasians.
2. It may present with heart failure, cardiogenic shock, cardiac arrest thromboembolism, or sudden death.
3. Prognosis is worse if the LV ejection fraction is <25%. About 50% of patients will recover in 2–6 months, but the recurrence rate is high in subsequent pregnancies.

References

[1] Chou T-C. *Electrocardiography in Clinical Practice*. Adult and Pediatric, 4th edn. WB Saunders, Philadelphia, 1996, p 112.

[2] Demakis JG, Rahimtoola SH, Sutton GC et al. Natural course of peripartum cardiomyopathy. *Circulation* 1971; 44: 1053–1061 (all 27 patients were from Cook County Hospital).

[3] Elkayam U, Akhter MW, Singh H et al. Pregnancy associated cardiomyopathy. Clinical characteristics and a comparison between early and late presentation. *Circulation* 2005; 111: 2050–2055 (123 patients).

[4] Elkayam U. Clinical characteristics of peripartum cardiomyopathy in the United States. *J Am Coll Cardiol* 2011; 58: 659–670.

41 PATIENT STUDY 41

Sequence of data presentation

1 ECG 23 December 2001
↓
2 Chest X rays
↓
3 Laboratory data
↓
4 TEE report 23 December 2001
↓
5 CT of chest 23 December 2001
↓
6 History
↓
7 Physical examination
↓
8 Course

1 ECG 23 December 2001

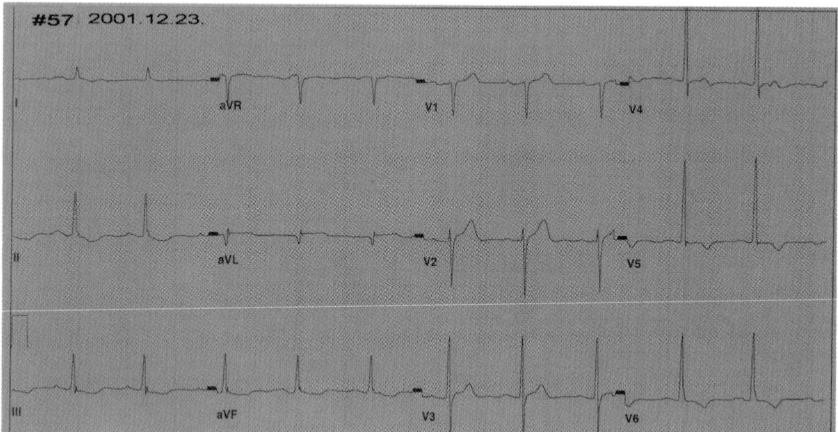

Figure 41.1 12-lead ECG.

2 Chest X rays

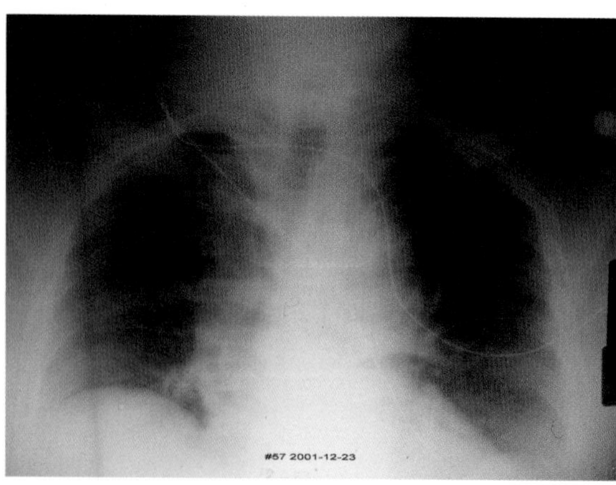

Figure 41.2 Portable chest X ray 23 December 2001.

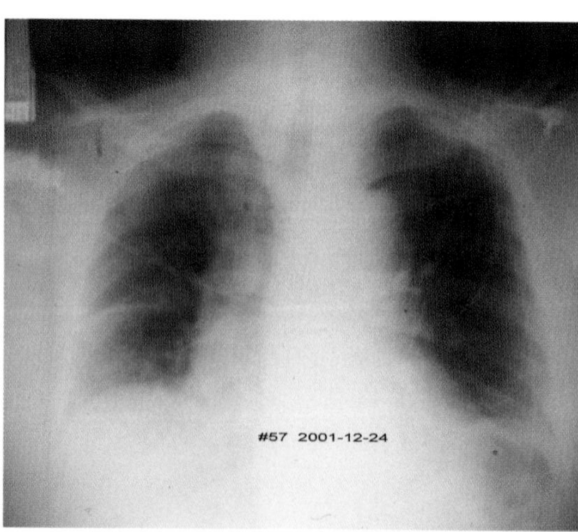

Figure 41.3 Portable chest X ray 24 December 2001.

Patient Studies in Valvular, Congenital, and Rarer Forms of Cardiovascular Disease: An Integrative Approach, First Edition. Franklin B. Saksena.

Companion Website: www.wiley.com/go/saksena/patientstudies

3 Laboratory data

Hemoglobin 13 g%, which fell to 10.9 g% 2 days later. WBC 9800/mm^3 and 1 day later rose to 11,400/mm^3. Glucose 139–152 mg%. BUN 11–19 mg%. Good urine output.

Three successive troponin levels were normal.

4 TEE report 23 December 2001

Severe LVH with normal LV systolic function.

AD beginning in descending aorta and extending to below the diaphragm.

Descending aorta diameter is 3–3.3 cm.

Ascending aorta is normal.

Mild aortic regurgitation.

No thrombosis or stasis in atria or aorta.

5 CT of chest 23 December 2001

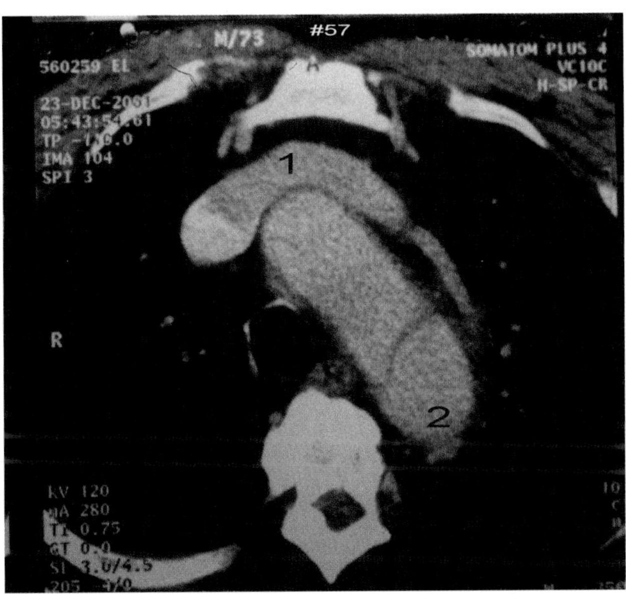

Figure 41.4 CT of chest at T3–4 level showing aortic arch and brachiocephalic vein.

Name the structures labeled 1 and 2.

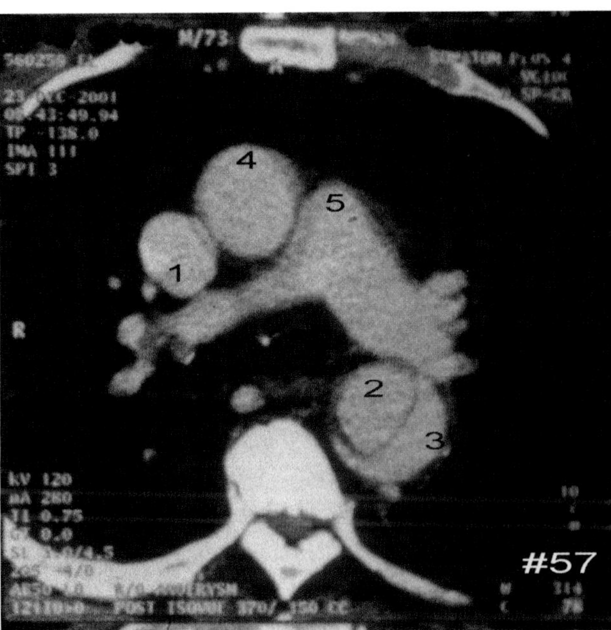

Figure 41.5 CT of chest at T5–6 level showing ascending aorta and descending aorta.

Name the structures labeled 1–5.

6 History

73-year-old male admitted with low back pain radiating to the left anterior chest and arms, and lasting for 40 min. He drove himself to the hospital. In the ER he had epigastric pain (10/10) and nausea. BP 227/123. He was given IV nitroglycerine and his BP fell to 180/80.

The patient has had hypertension for 20 years. He was non-compliant with his antihypertensive medication. No history of diabetes or myocardial infarction. He has smoked for 50 pack years, but does not drink alcohol.

7 Physical examination

74 inches tall man weighing 250 lb. BP 180/80 (R), 180/90 (L). Systolic BP in both legs was 150 mmHg. HR 103/min. RR 36/min. Temperature 97.8 °F.

No elevation of jugular venous pressure.

Apex beat in the 5th interspace, 12 cm from the mid-sternal line (cardiomegaly).
S1 normal. S2 loud A2.
Grade 2/6 aortic systolic murmur. No diastolic murmur or pericardial friction rub.
Lungs clear to auscultation and percussion. Slight decrease in air entry bilaterally.
No edema, cyanosis, or clubbing.
Bounding peripheral pulses.
No abdominal masses or abdominal tenderness.

8 Course

The patient was diagnosed as having type 3 AD (Stanford type B). He was seen by the cardiovascular surgeon, who recommended surgery but the patient refused to have surgery.

The patient was treated with intravenous nitroprusside, atenolol, and then captopril and furosemide, and his BP fell to 146–173 systolic and 58–72 diastolic. He became pain free. No aortic regurgitant murmur was noted.

On 25 December 2001 he had an occasional wheeze on chest examination but denied any dyspnea or chest pain. Later that day he had a sudden cardiac arrest and died despite CPR measures.

Why do you think the patient died?

Answers and commentary

1 ECG 23 December 2001

Sinus rhythm with first degree heart block. Rate 63/min. PR 0.22 s. QRS 0.09 s. QRS axis +75°.
LVH with repolarization abnormalities.
Addendum: ST sagging in V5–6, 2, 3, F have appeared since 27 February 1994.

2 Chest X rays

Mediastinal widening noted on 23 December 2001. Cardiomegaly may or may not be present.

On 24 December 2001 the mediastinum had widened further and there was a small left-sided pleural effusion. Such findings suggest AD.

3 Laboratory data

The normal troponin levels ruled out myocardial necrosis. In retrospect the drop in hemoglobin reflected an aortic leak. He maintained a normal BUN and urine output throughout his hospital stay.

4 TEE report 23 December 2001

The TEE was diagnostic for acute AD starting distal to the left subclavian artery (type 3 De Bakey or type B Stanford). The ECG and TEE both noted the presence of LVH, which was attributed to long-standing hypertension.

5 CT of chest 23 December 2001

Figure 41.4 shows an AD that begins slightly inferior to the left subclavian artery. An intimal flap is seen at the level of the aortic arch.
1 = brachiocephalic vein
2 = true lumen of aorta

Figure 41.5 shows that the intimal flap extends to the level of T12.
1 = superior vena cava
2 = true lumen of aorta
3 = false lumen
4 = ascending aorta
5 = main pulmonary artery

Subsequent films showed that the AD extended to the renal arteries.
There was no evidence of an aortic leak on 23 December 2011.

6 History

The patient had long-standing hypertension but was not compliant with his medications. The low back pain, left chest pain, and epigastric pain of sudden severe onset favor the diagnosis of AD rather than myocardial infarction (note that troponin levels were normal).

7 Physical examination

The patient had hypertensive heart disease. The wide pulse pressure accounted for his bounding pulses. As the systolic BP in the legs was similar to the arms, it is unlikely that the AD had extended to the iliac vessels or even the renal arteries (as the laboratory data showed no compromise of renal function).

Significant aortic regurgitation and pericardial involvement are usually seen when the ascending aorta is involved (type A AD) rather than the descending aorta (type B).

8 Course

The patient died suddenly because of aortic rupture, as shown by the following autopsy results (Figures 41.6, 41.7, and 41.8).

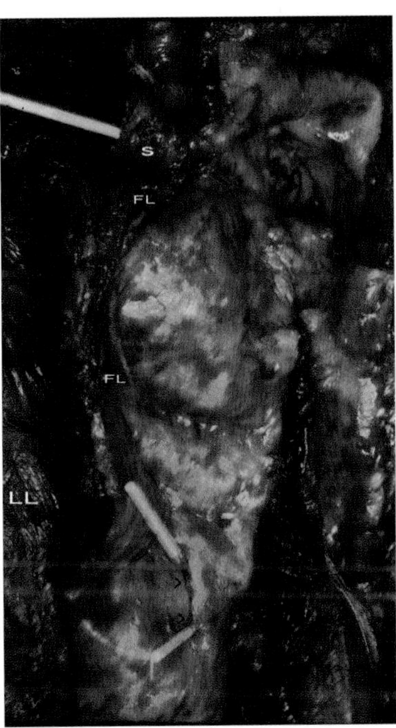

Figure 41.6 Gross appearance of descending aorta. FL, false lumen; LL, left lung with clotted blood around it; S, subclavian artery with white probe. Site of intimal tear shown by arrow heads and the two probes.

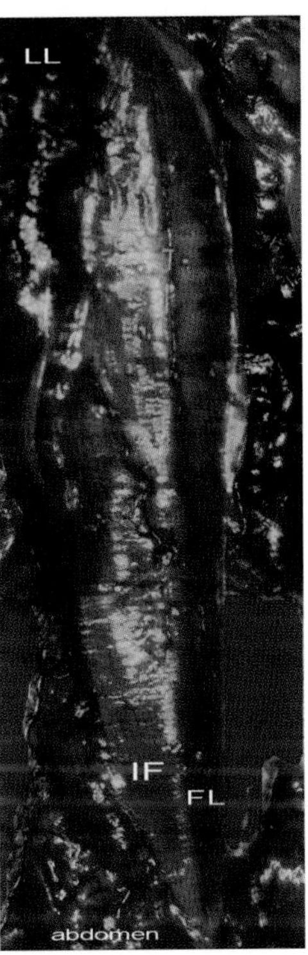

Figure 41.7 Gross appearance of descending aorta showing false lumen (FL), a long intimal flap (IF), and left lung with blood clot (LL).

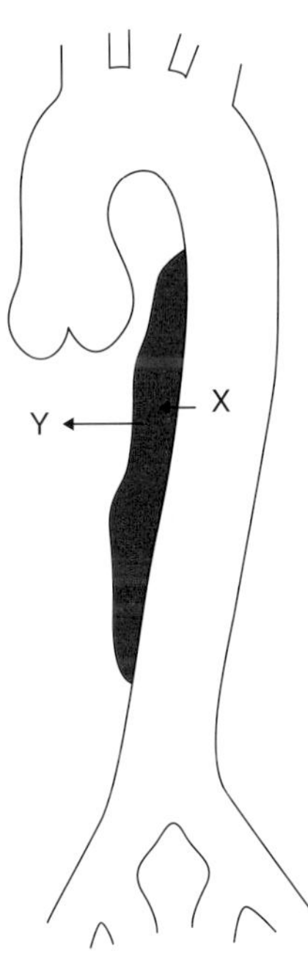

Figure 41.8 Diagram of site of intimal tear (x) and site of aortic rupture (y). The red color shows the dissecting hematoma.

Hypertensive heart disease with LV thickness of 2.3 cm. Heart weighed 550 g.
No significant coronary artery disease.
Mild to moderate atherosclerosis of the aorta.
Type 3 dissection (Figures 41.4 and 41.5), with a 1.5 cm intimal tear in descending aorta.
The AD extended to slightly superior to the renal arteries.
Rupture of aorta with 2800 mL of blood and blood clot in left pleural cavity (Figures 41.6 and 41.7). The left lung was collapsed.

Discussion

The patient had a type B AD with severe hypertension, chest pain, and a widened mediastinum. Treatment relieved his chest pain but despite antihypertensive treatment the BP failed to reach the ideal goal of 135/80 [1]. Uncomplicated type B AD is treated medically with an early (first 2 weeks) mortality rate of 6.4% [2], whereas acute complicated AD undergoing surgical repair has an early mortality rate of 17.5% [2]. Complications may occur in 15–25% of patients presenting with AD [2,3] and consist of refractory hypertension, shock, hypotension (<90 mmHg systolic), organ malperfusion, and impending rupture (detected on serial CT by progressive enlargement of false lumen and/or hemothorax) [2,4]. This patient might have benefited from surgery because his BP was only partially controlled and there had been further widening of the mediastinun. As he had refused surgery the only option was continued medical treatment.

About 20–30% of patients with AD die before reaching hospital [5].

Death from type B dissection commonly occurs when the aorta ruptures, leading to a hemothorax or a hemomediastinum. This patient's aorta ruptured, resulting in a massive hemothorax and death.

Key points

1. Hypertension is the most common preventable cause of AD.
2. It is not uncommon for patients with AD to be mistaken for a myocardial infarction and given anticoagulants, with disastrous results. The pattern of AD pain is different from myocardial infarction, often occurring in the back and is severe at the onset.
3. Type B AD still carries a significant mortality rate.
4. Chest X rays are usually portable in critically ill patients and may be technically suboptimum in diagnosing mediastinal widening.
5. TEE or CT of the chest is the preferred way of making a rapid diagnosis of AD.
6. Early surgical consultation is essential in all patients suspected of having an acute AD.

References

[1] Mukherjee D, Eagle KA. Aortic dissection – an update. *Curr Probl Cardiol* 2005; 30: 281–326 (excellent review article).

[2] Fattori R, Mineo G, Di Eusanio M. Acute type B aortic dissection: Current management strategies. *Curr Opin Cardiol* 2011; 26: 488–493.

[3] Hughes GC, Andersen ND, McCann RL. Management of acute type B aortic dissection. *J Thorac Cardiovasc Surg* 2013; 145: S202–S207.

[4] Umana JP, Lai DT, Mitchell S et al. Is medical therapy still the optimal treatment strategy for patients with acute type B aortic dissections? *J Thorac Cardiovasc Surg* 2002; 124: 896–891.

[5] Fattori R, Cao P, De Rango P et al. Interdisciplinary expert consensus document on management of type B aortic dissection. *J Am Coll Cardiol* 2013; 61: 1661–1678 (reviews 63 studies totaling 6711 patients between 2006 and 2012).

42 PATIENT STUDY 42

Sequence of data presentation

1 Chest X ray
↓
2 ECG
↓
3 Hemodynamics 29 August 2001
↓
4 History and physical examination
↓
5 Aortogram
↓
6 CT of chest
↓
7 PA angiogram 12 October 2001
↓
8 Echocardiogram reports 2002
↓
9 Diagnosis
↓
10 Treatment and course

1 Chest X ray

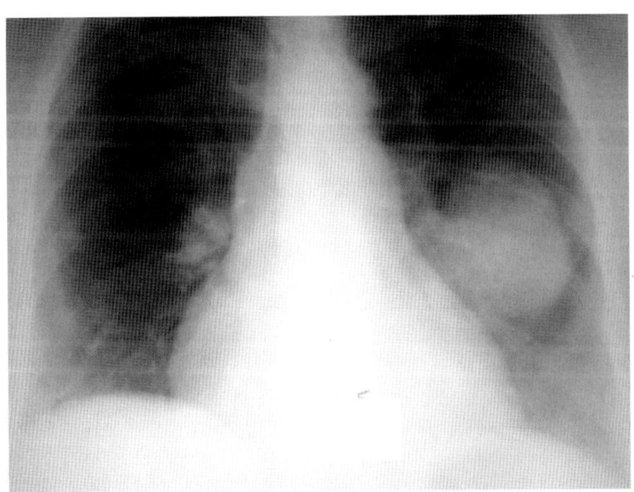

Figure 42.1 PA chest X ray.

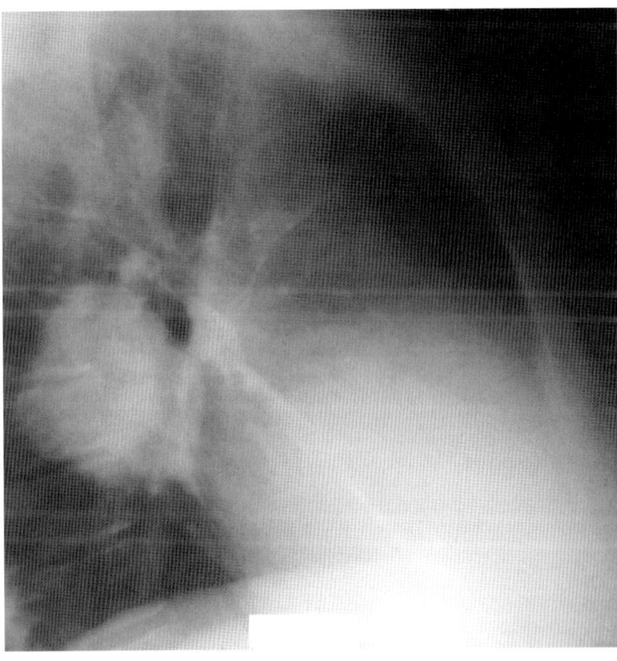

Figure 42.2 Lateral chest X ray.

Patient Studies in Valvular, Congenital, and Rarer Forms of Cardiovascular Disease: An Integrative Approach, First Edition. Franklin B. Saksena.

Companion Website: www.wiley.com/go/saksena/patientstudies

2 ECG

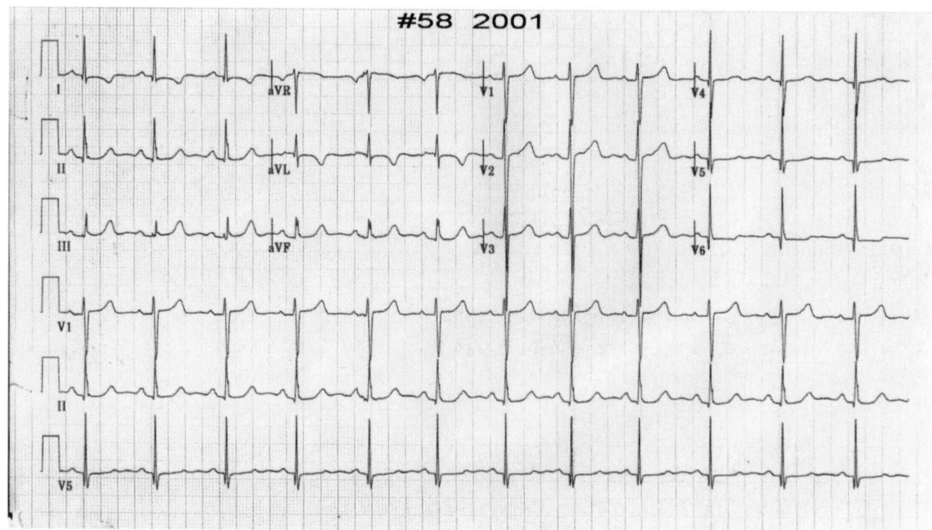

Figure 42.3 ECG.

3 Hemodynamics 29 August 2001

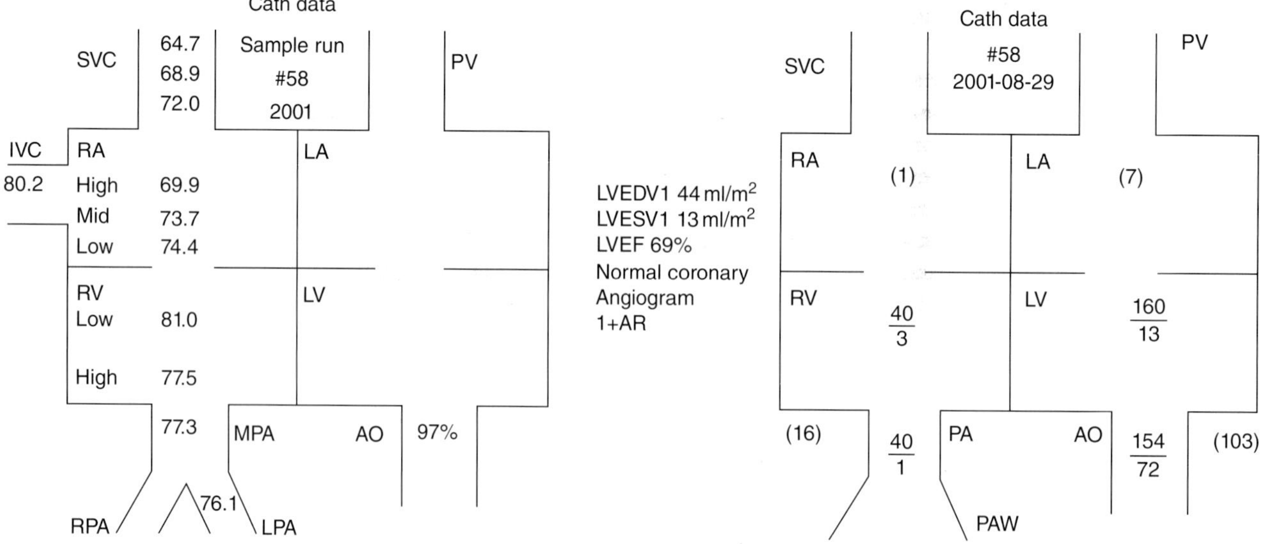

Figure 42.4 Oxygen saturation sample run.

Figure 42.5 Pressures and angiography results.

4 History and physical examination

History

42-year-old female with a history of hypertension for 10 years, admitted to hospital with dyspnea on walking one block for the last 6 months. She has a history of a heart murmur.

The patient does not drink alcohol, smoke, or use drugs.

Physical examination

The patient is 64 inches tall and weighs 140 lb. BP 127/73. HR 59/min.

There was no elevation of jugular venous pressure. Normal carotid upstroke.

Apex beat was in the 5th interspace, 10 cm from the mid-sternal line. No RV lift.

S1 normal. S2 –1 decreased. Single.

There was a grade 3/6 pansystolic murmur, best heard at the LLSB.

There was a grade 3/6 diastolic decrescendo blowing murmur best heard at the left 3rd nterspace parasternally.

Lungs were clear.

No edema, cyanosis, or clubbing. Normal peripheral pulses.

5 Aortogram

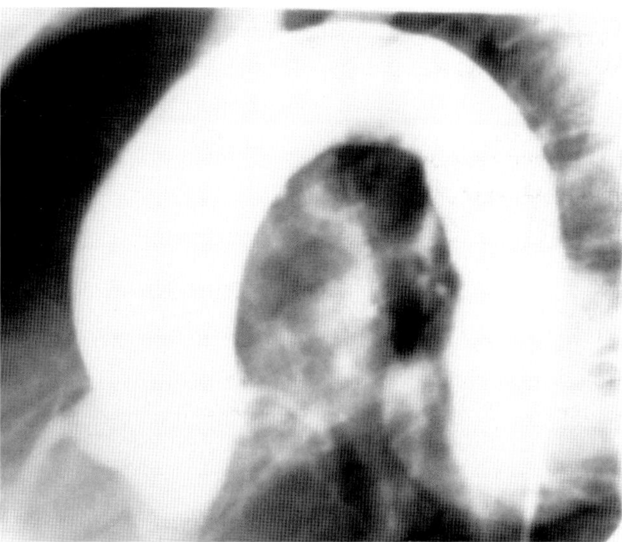

Figure 42.6 Aortogram lateral view.

6 CT of chest

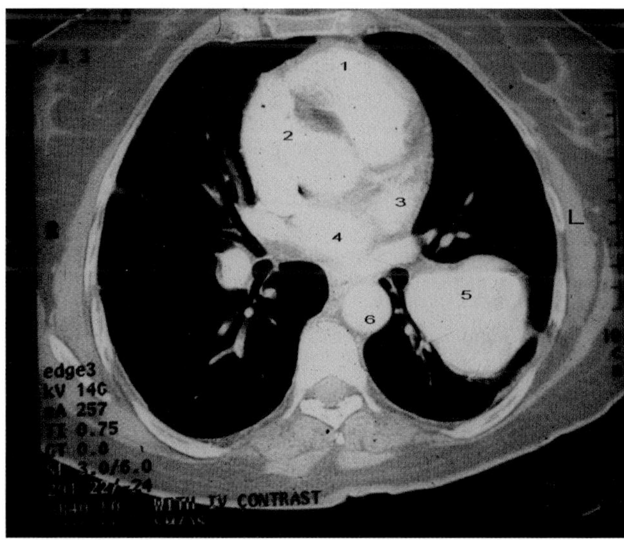

Figure 42.7 CT of heart at level ~T5.
What are the names of the structures labeled 1–6?

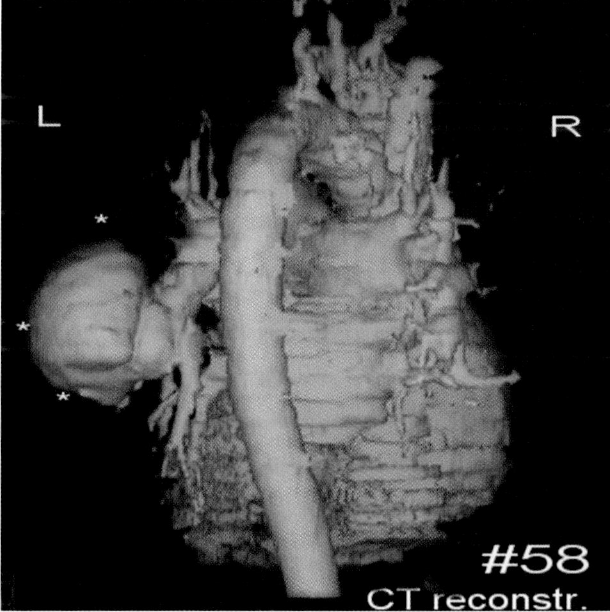

Figure 42.8 Three-dimensional reconstruction of CT of chest structures.
What is the structure surrounded by stars?

7 PA angiogram 12 October 2001

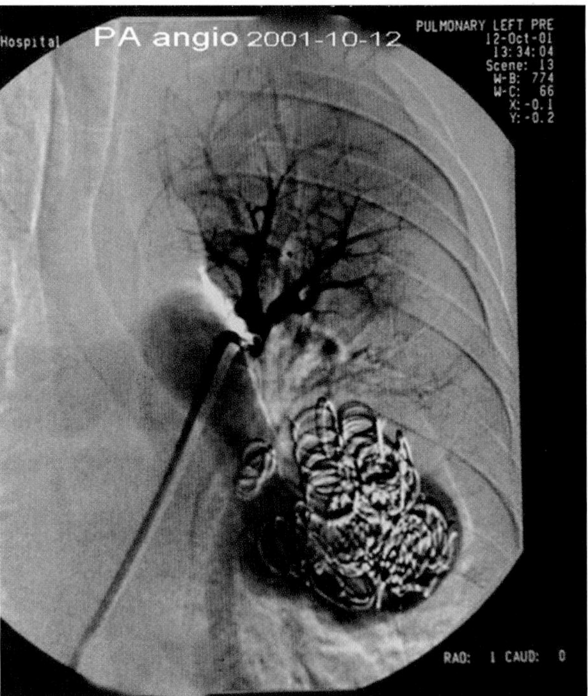

Figure 42.9 Selective left PA angiogram 12 October 2001.

8 Echocardiogram reports 2002

TEE 3 April 2002

RA and RV enlargement unchanged from 2001.
Normal LV size and systolic function.
Supracristal infundibular VSD with left to right blood flow.
Mild aortic regurgitation.

TEE 4 April 2002 (post operative)

VSD is now closed. Minimal pulmonic regurgitation. (Table 42.1)

Table 42.1 Echocardiogram reports 2002

a) TEE 2002-04-03
RA and RV enlargement, unchanged from 2001
Normal LV size and systolic function
Supracristal infundibular VSD with to right blood flow
Mild aortic regurgitation
b) TEE 2002-04-04 (post op)
VSD is now closed. Minimal pulmonic regurgitation

9 Diagnosis

What is the diagnosis?

10 Treatment and course

What treatment did the patient receive?

Answers and commentary

1 Chest X ray

PA view: The right heart is enlarged. There is a 4 cm sized globular mass noted in the left mid and lower lung field. No pulmonary congestion or plethora.

Lateral view: The globular mass is seen posterior to the cardiac shadow and has a height two and a half times that of the thoracic vertebrae.

2 ECG

Sinus rhythm. Rate 75/min. PR 0.16 s. QRS 0.07 s. QRS axis +20°.

T inverted in 1 and L. T low or biphasic in V5–6.

Impression: non-specific T wave abnormalities, no chamber enlargement.

3 Hemodynamics 29 August 2001

There is a small step up in oxygen saturation on entering the RV from the RA: Q_p/Q_s = 1.8/1 (Figure 42.4).

Figure 42.5 shows the pressures and angiographic results. The PA pressure was normal. The wide pulse pressure seen in the PA pressure tracing suggests pulmonary regurgitation.

Borderline elevation of LVEDP. Mild systolic hypertension.

Normal LV systolic function and volumes. No coronary artery disease.

The LV angiogram showed a small subpulmonic VSD (not shown).

4 History and physical examination

The pansystolic murmur at the LLSB was due to a VSD.

The left to right shunt from the VSD is not large as there was no RV lift or loud P2 or pulmonary plethora on chest X ray, and the LV was not enlarged or hypertrophied. The diastolic murmur at the left 3rd interspace was due to pulmonary and aortic regurgitation (verified on catheterization and angiography).

5 Aortogram

There is 1+/4+ aortic regurgitation. The aortic arch and descending aorta are normal.

6 CT of chest

The globular structure measuring 6 cm in diameter is a large saccular aneurysm of the left PA in the left lower lobe (superior segment) connected to the main PA by a narrow neck (Figure 42.7; 1, RV; 2, RA; 3, LV; 4, LA; 5, PA aneurysm; 6, descending aorta).

CT reconstruction shows a saccular aneurysm of the left PA (surrounded by stars) about 6 × 9 cm (Figure 42.8).

7 PA angiogram 12 October 2001

Shows 57 coils placed in the PA aneurysm with partial occlusion of neck of aneurysm.

Addendum: A further 124 coils were placed in the PA aneurysm on 8 January 2002 with subsequent near obliteration of the PA aneurysm.

8 Echocardiogram reports 2002

The patient's right heart enlargement seen on chest X ray was also confirmed on echocardiography. The VSD was small. The Q_p/Q_s flow was 1.8/1 at catheterization.

9 Diagnosis

PA aneurysm.

Small VSD.

Mild aortic regurgitation.

10 Treatment and course

The patient underwent embolotherapy in October 2001 and January 2002 with >90% volume occlusion of the PA aneurysm. She then underwent successful VSD closure on 4 April 2002. This dual approach obviated the need to do two thoractomies on the patient.

Postoperatively, the patient was able to walk two blocks without dyspnea. Her physical findings were unchanged as of 14 June 2002. She then returned to her country of origin in 2002 only on antihypertensive medications.

Discussion

The patient had a large left-sided aneurysm involving the main pulmonary branch to the left lobe. There was probably an associated dilatation of the pulmonary annulus [1] or an abnormality of the pulmonary valve [2], which would account for pulmonary regurgitation and thence right heart enlargement.

A PA aneurysm is very rare, occurring 1 in 13,696 autopsies [3]. The aneurysm in this patient measured 6 cm in diameter. The normal diameter of the main PA on chest CT is ≤2.9 cm [4].

The complications of a PA aneurysm are rupture, dissection [1, 3], pulmonary embolism [5], and sudden death [1, 3]. Patients with PA aneurysm often have coexistent pulmonary hypertension [3, 6], which in the face of an intrinsic weakness of the vessel wall (e.g. vasculitis, medial cystic necrosis) results in rupture or dissection [3]. Thus patients with high pulmonary flow states such as due to a left to right shunt are at risk of rupturing a PA aneurysm if there is also some intrinsic wall weakness.

This patient did have a VSD but the PA pressure was normal so that the cause of her PA aneurysm is unknown [3, 5].

Treatment of the PAA involves treating the underlying cause and surgical removal if the diameter is >6 cm [1]. PAA may also be treated with embolotherapy coils [3], as in this patient.

A conservative strategy may be considered in low-pressure PA aneurysm in the absence of pulmonary valve dysfunction [2].

Key points

1. PA aneurysm is very rare. It may idiopathic or due to high PA flow associated with an intrinsic weakness of the PA wall.
2. PA aneurysm may be associated with a left to right shunt and/or pulmonary valve dysfunction.
3. Surgical removal is recommended if the PA aneurysm is >6 cm in diameter to prevent its rupture.
4. Embolotherapy is an alternative way of treating a PA aneurysm by gradually occluding the neck of the aneurysm with coils.

References

[1] Seguchi M, Wada H, Sakakura K et al. Idiopathic pulmonary artery aneurysm. *Circulation* 2011; 124: e369–e370.

[2] Veldtman GR, Dearani JA, Warmes CA. Low pressure giant pulmonary artery aneurysms in the adult: natural history and management strategies. *Heart* 2003; 89: 1067–1070. (Four patients with PA aneurysm were surgically treated. All four had abnormal pulmonary valves.)

[3] Graham JK, Shehata B. Sudden death due to dissecting pulmonary artery aneurysm. A case report and review of the literature. *Am J Forensic Med Pathol* 2007; 28: 342–344 (extensive table of causes and pathogenesis of PA aneurysm).

[4] Nguyen ET, Silva CIS, Seely JM et al. Pulmonary artery aneurysms and pseudoaneurysms in adults: findings at CT and radiography. *Am J Roentgenol* 2007; 188: W126–W134 (12 illustrated examples given).

[5] Serasli E, Antoniadou M, Steiropoulos P et al. Low pressure pulmonary artery aneurysm presenting with pulmonary embolism: a case series. *J Med Case Reports* 2011; 5: 163–166.

[6] Shankarappa RK, Moorthy N, Chandrasekaran D et al. Giant pulmonary artery aneurysm. Secondary to primary pulmonary hypertension. *Tex Heart Instit J* 2010; 37: 244–245.

43 PATIENT STUDY 43

Sequence of data presentation

1 Partial history
↓
2 Hemodynamics 1963 and 1977
↓
3 Hemodynamics 1999
↓
4 ECG 1999
↓
5 Chest X ray 1999
↓
6 Additional history 1963–1999
↓
7 Physical examination 1999
↓
8 Diagnosis
↓
9 Course

1 Partial history

37-year-old P1 G1 admitted in 1999 with dyspnea and orthopnea for the last month. She was a 'blue baby' at birth and underwent cardiac surgery in 1963 and 1977.

2 Hemodynamics 1963 and 1977

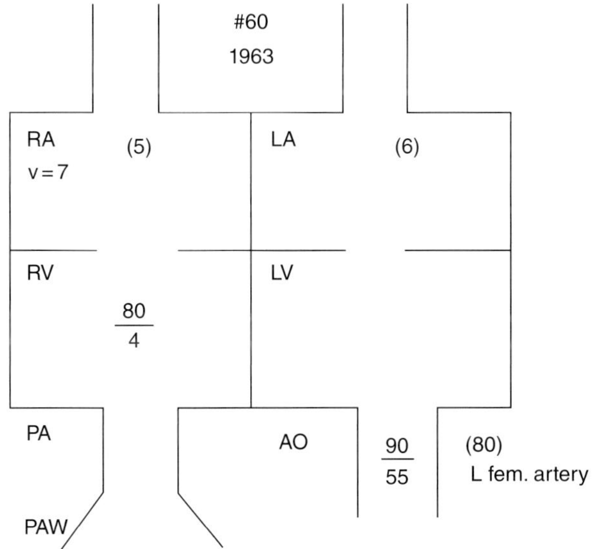

Figure 43.1 Intracardiac pressures 1963.

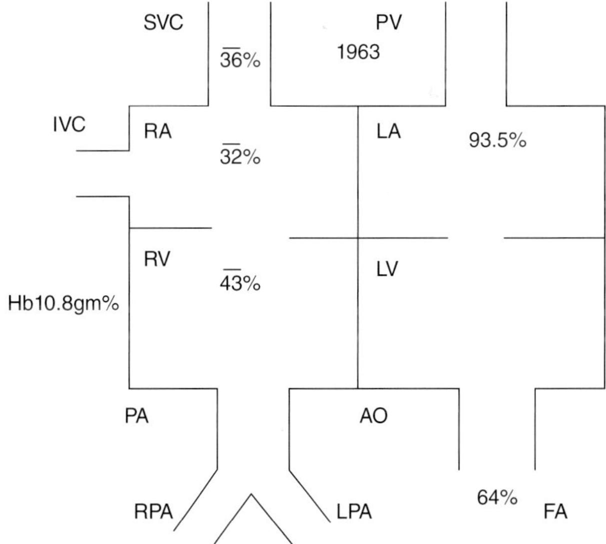

Figure 43.2 Oxygen saturation sample run 1963. Values with M̄ over a number represents an average of three readings in the SVC and RA, and an average of two readings in the RV.

What is the pulmonary/systemic flow ratio?

Patient Studies in Valvular, Congenital, and Rarer Forms of Cardiovascular Disease: An Integrative Approach, First Edition. Franklin B. Saksena.

Companion Website: www.wiley.com/go/saksena/patientstudies

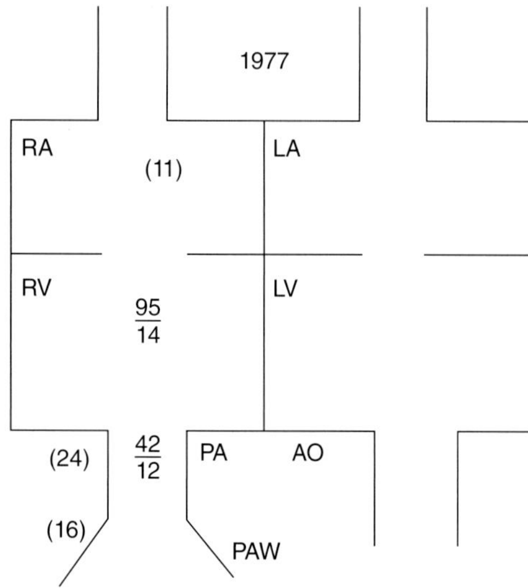

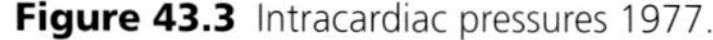
Figure 43.3 Intracardiac pressures 1977.

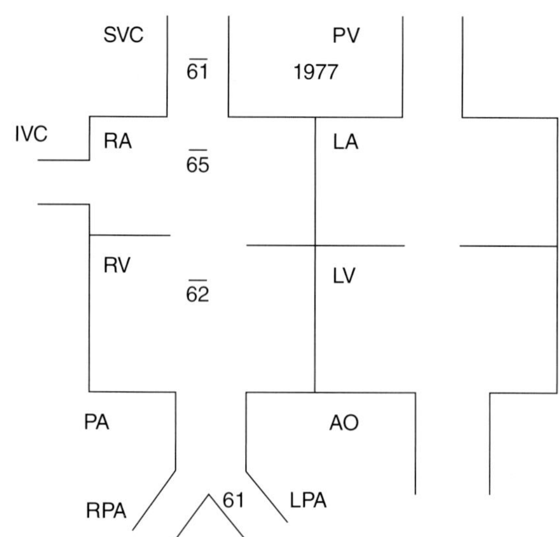

Figure 43.4 Oxygen saturation sample run 1977.

3 Hemodynamics 1999

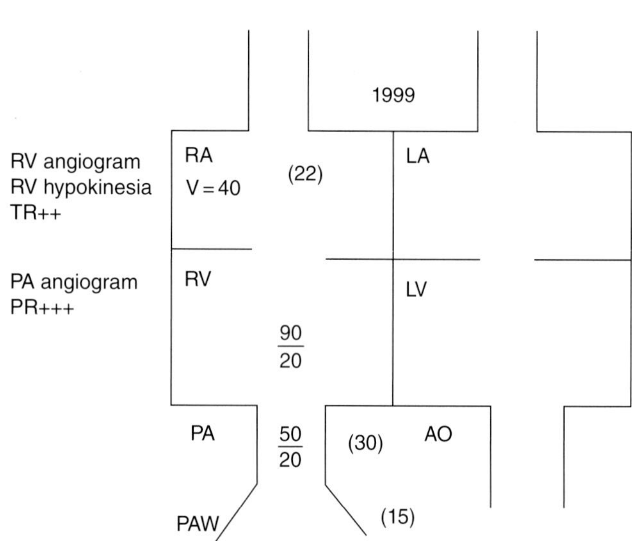

Figure 43.5 Intracardiac pressures and angiographic results 1999.

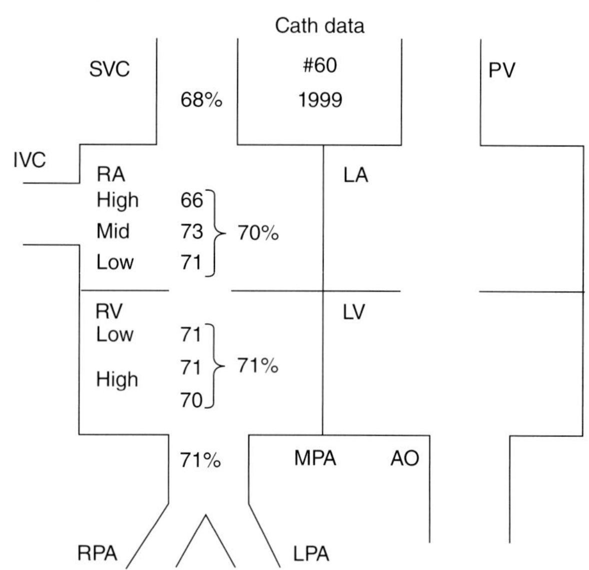

Figure 43.6 Oxygen saturation sample run 1999.

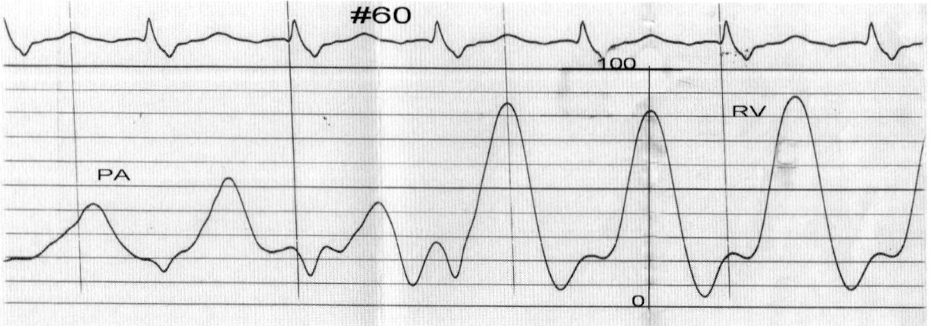

Figure 43.7 Withdrawal pressures from PA to RV 1999. 0–100 mmHg scale.

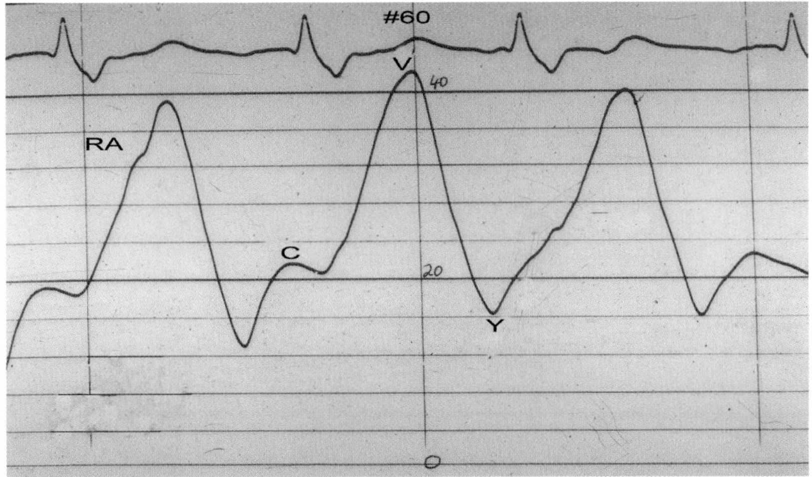

Figure 43.8 RA pressure curve 1999. 0–40 mmHg.

4 ECG 1999

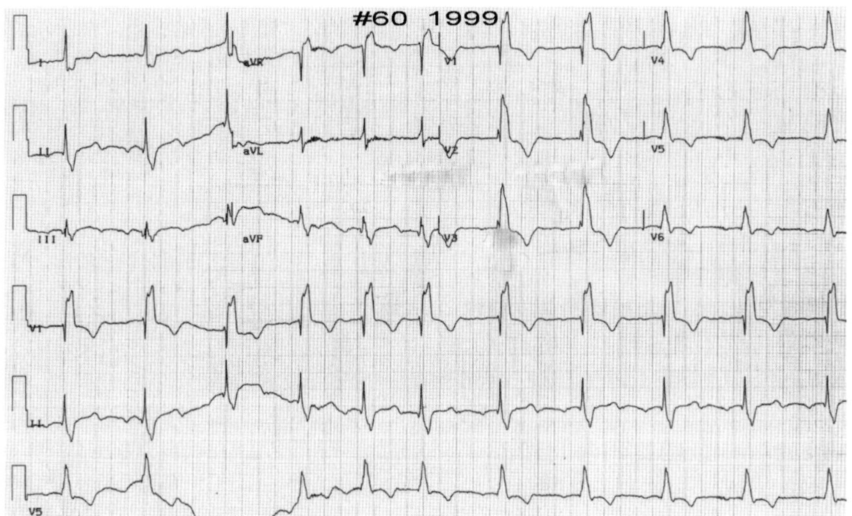

Figure 43.9 12-lead ECG 1999

5 Chest X ray 1999

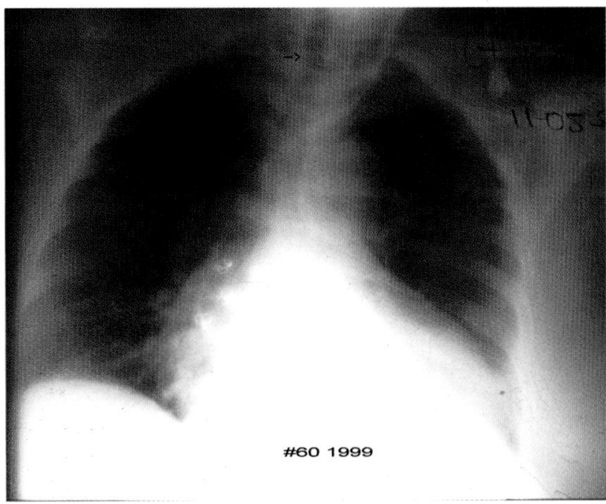

Figure 43.10 Chest X ray 1999.

6 Additional history 1963–1999

The patient underwent a Blalock–Taussig procedure in 1963 and then underwent a total corrective procedure (VSD closure and pulmonary valvotomy) in 1977 at another hospital. She was lost to follow-up until 1990, when she was noted to have pulmonary regurgitation and tricuspid regurgitation in the pediatric cardiology department. An echocardiogram at that time showed a dilated RV with paradoxical septal motion. Arterial oxygen saturation was 96%.and Hb 12 gm%.

She was admitted to adult cardiology in 1999 with dyspnea on exertion.

7 Physical examination 1999

70 inches tall, 200 lb female. BP 115/48. HR 100/min.
Normal jugular venous pressure. Decreased carotid artery amplitude.
RV lift 2+/3+.
S1 normal. S2 single.
*Grade 3/6 pulmonary systolic murmur.
*Grade 2/6 pulmonary diastolic murmur.
Left thoracotomy and medians sternotomy scars.
Bilateral femoral artery cutdown sites.
2+/4+ femoral artery pulses.
*Note: similar findings had been noted in 1990.

8 Diagnosis

What is the diagnosis?

9 Course

What is the course and treatment?

Answers and commentary

1 Partial history

Cyanotic heart disease at birth is most commonly due to TOF. Less common causes include transposition of the great vessels, tricuspid atresia or truncus arteriosus [1].

2 Hemodynamics 1963 and 1977

Hemodynamics 1963

The patient had marked elevation of the RV pressure that was near systemic levels.

There was a step up in oxygen saturation on entering the RV from the RA, indicative of a VSD. The presence of arterial oxygen desaturation indicates that the shunt is right to left.

The pulmonary (Q_p) to systemic (Q_s) blood flow ratio is 0.63, as shown below.

Given: Hb 10.8 gm%, BSA 0.34 m², oxygen consumption (VO_2) 51.8 mL/min

Step 1 Convert oxygen saturations to oxygen content, assuming 1 gm Hb combines with 1.34 cc of oxygen.

Total oxygen content = 1.34 × 10.8 = 14.53 vol%
Femoral arterial content (C_{fa}) = 64% × 14.53 = 9.33 mL/100 mL blood or vol%
Preshunt (SVC) content (C_{svc}) = 36% × 14.53 = 4.66 mL/100 mL blood
LA content (C_{LA}) = 93.5% × 14.53 = 13.59 mL/100 mL blood
RV oxygen content (C_{RV}) = 43% × 14.53 = 6.24 mL/100 mL blood

Step 2 Find the systemic blood flow (Q_s)

$$Q_s = \frac{Vo_2}{C_{fa} - C_{svc}} = \frac{51.8 \text{ mL/min}}{10(9.33 - 4.66)} = 1.1 \text{ L/min}$$

where C_{la} = arterial O_2 content and C_{SVC} is the preshunt blood content.

Step 3 Find the pulmonary blood flow (Q_p)

$$Q_p = \frac{Vo_2}{C_{la} - C_{rv}} = \frac{51.8 \text{ mL/min}}{10(13.59 - 6.24)} = 0.7 \text{ L/min}$$

Assuming that the LA oxygen content (C_{LA}) = pulmonary venous oxygen content (C_{PV}) and that RV oxygen content (C_{RV}) = PA oxygen content (C_{PA}).

Step 4 Find the pulmonary/systemic flow ratio

$$\frac{Q_p}{Q_s} = \frac{0.7}{1.1} = 0.63$$

Thus the patient had a right to left shunt.

Hemodynamics 1977 (postoperative)

There is a 53 mmHg gradient in systole between the RV apex and the RV outflow tract, indicative of a mild infundibular stenosis. The mean PA pressure is mildly elevated to 24 mmHg. The PAW pressure was slightly elevated for unclear reasons. The femoral artery could not be entered because of scar tissue.

The oxygen sample run shows no step up in the RV, indicating that the VSD has been successfully closed.

3 Hemodynamics 1999

There is no evidence of a VSD based on the sample run. The femoral artery could not be entered for technical reasons.

The RA mean pressure had increased to 22 mmHg with a prominent v wave (Figure 43.8). The v wave was only 7 mmHg in 1963 and in 1999 it had risen to 40 mmHg. These findings indicate that tricuspid regurgitation has developed. The elevated RVEDP (20 mmHg) suggests the development of RV failure.

The gradient between the RV apex and outflow tract is about the same as it was in 1977 (Figure 43.7). The borderline elevation in PAW was unchanged from 1977.

Angiography confirmed the presence of severe RV hypokinesia with delayed emptying of the RV, moderate tricuspid regurgitation, and severe pulmonary regurgitation. The RV ejection fraction was not measured.

4 ECG 1999

Atrial fibrillation with RBBB. HR 60/min. QRS 0.12 s. QRS axis indeterminate.

Atrial fibrillation has appeared since 1990.

5 Chest X ray 1999

Cardiomegaly. Right heart enlargement.

6 Additional history 1963–1999

The patient did well after total correction of the tetralogy, but did not come for annual follow-ups until she became symptomatic with RV failure in the 1990s.

7 Physical examination 1999

The decreased carotid amplitude suggests a low output state. The prominence of the RV lift indicates significant RV dysfunction, which is supported by the presence of RV enlargement on chest X ray and an elevated RVEDP of 20 mmHg.

The murmurs are due to pulmonic infundibular stenosis and regurgitation.

8 Diagnosis

Post-operative surgical correction of TOF. VSD is closed, residual infundibular pulmonary stenosis.

Severe RV failure due to pulmonary regurgitation.

Tricuspid regurgitation secondary to RV failure.

Atrial fibrillation.

9 Course

Pulmonary valve replacement was recommended to the patient, which she refused. On 20 October 2000 she was noted to be in significant RV failure. She was lost to further follow-up to either adult or pediatric cardiology.

Discussion

The patient had TOF diagnosed in infancy and underwent a Blalock–Taussig procedure followed by a complete repair in 1977. In 1990 she had developed pulmonary regurgitation and RV dysfunction, which 9 years later had progressed to severe RV failure. The RV failure was aggravated by the development of atrial fibrillation after 1990. Reoperation for pulmonary valve dysfunction [2,3] may have benefited this patient to prevent further deterioration in RV dysfunction.

Annual follow-ups are recommended for patients who have been operated on for TOF [4], but unfortunately did not occur in this case.

An annual follow-up would encompass at least a detailed physical examination, ECG, and echocardiography to detect any residual VSD, residual RV outflow tract obstruction or the development of pulmonary regurgitation, RV failure, aortic valve disease, or arrhythmias [4].

Patients with a QRS duration of >0.180 s or a QT dispersal > 0.06 s are at a high risk for ventricular tachycardia and sudden death [4]. The incidence of sudden death in the post-operative TOF is 5% [5].

The RV size and function can be determined by echocardiography or better still by MRI [3, 4]. A severely dilated RV is also a risk factor for ventricular tachycardia [5].

All patients operated on for TOF will need life-long endocarditis prophylaxis [5].

The diagnosis of TOF is now being made in utero or in the neonatal period (see Figures 43.11 and 43.12), but such an option was not available to this patient in 1963.

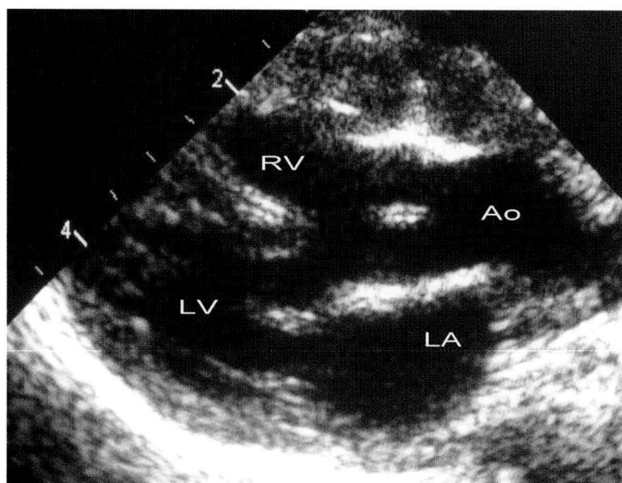

Figure 43.11 Echocardiogram of a newborn infant with TOF, long axis view. There is a VSD and an overriding aorta. Flow across the pulmonic valve is absent, implying pulmonary atresia. A PDA was also noted in the study, supplying hypoplastic PA branches.

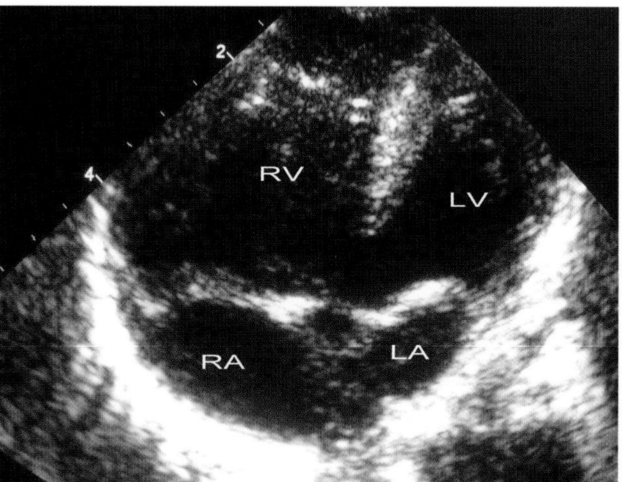

Figure 43.12 Echocardiogram of the same patient as in Figure 43.11, four-chamber view. The RV is larger than the LV and there is a VSD.

Key points

1. TOF is the most common congenital heart disease, presenting as a 'blue baby' at birth.
2. Successful treatment often requires a palliative left to right shunt in infancy followed by complete correction.
3. Pulmonary regurgitation and RV failure are late complications of surgical correction.
4. At least annual follow-up visits are required in patients following corrective surgery, with adult cardiologists working hand in hand with pediatric cardiologists.

References

[1] Flanagan MF, Yeager SB, Weindling SN. In: *Neonatology. Pathophysiology and management in the newborn*, 5th edn. Avery GB, Fletcher MA, MacDonald MG (eds). Lippincott, Williams and Wilkins, Philadelphia, 1999, pp 603–604.

[2] Geva T. Indications for pulmonary valve replacement in repaired tetralogy of Fallot. The quest continues. *Circulation* 2013; 128: 1855–1857.

[3] Therrien J, Provost Y, Merchant N, Williams W, Colman J, Webb G. Optimal timing for pulmonary valve replacement in adults after Tetralogy of Fallot repair. *Am J Cardiol* 2005; 95: 779–782 (RV function was determined using multiplanar MRI pre and post pulmonary valve replacement in 17 patients).

[4] Phillips SD, Bonnichsen CR, Mcleod CJ et al. Adults with congenital heart disease and previous intervention. *Curr Probl Cardiol* 2013; 38: 285–358.

[5] Gatzoulis MA. *Tetralogy of Fallot*. In: Diagnosis and management of Adult Congenital Heart disease. Gatzoulis MA, Webb GD, Daubeney PEF (eds). Edinburgh: Churchill Livingstone 2003, pp 315–326.

44 PATIENT STUDY 44

Sequence of data presentation

1 ECG
↓
2 Chest X ray
↓
3 Laboratory data
↓
4 Hemodynamic data
↓
5 Biplane LV angiography
↓
6 Cardiogreen dye curves
↓
7 History
↓
8 Physical examination
↓
9 Phonocardiogram
↓
10 Course

1 ECG

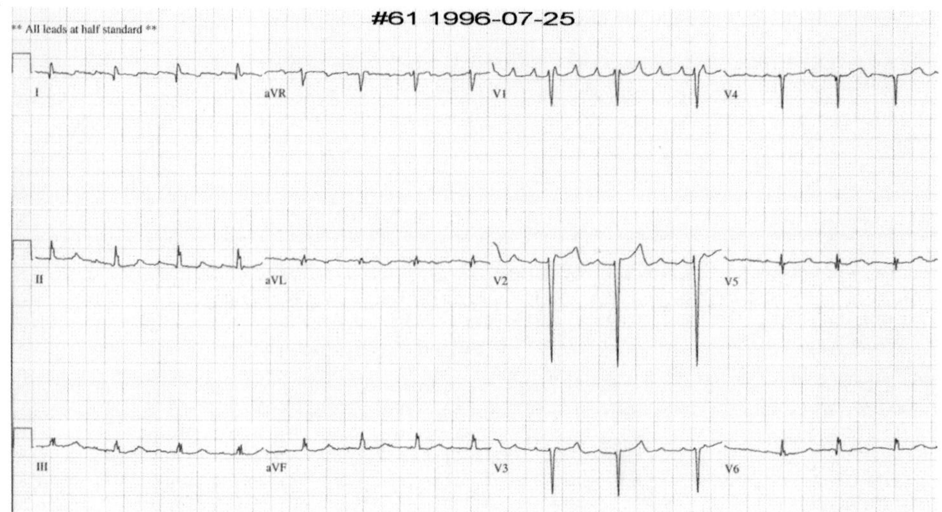

Figure 44.1 12-lead ECG 26 July 1996.

Patient Studies in Valvular, Congenital, and Rarer Forms of Cardiovascular Disease: An Integrative Approach, First Edition. Franklin B. Saksena.

Companion Website: www.wiley.com/go/saksena/patientstudies

2 Chest X ray

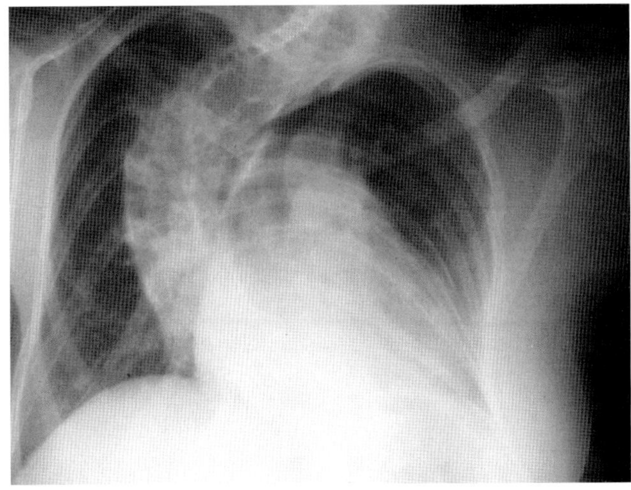

Figure 44.2 Chest X ray PA view.

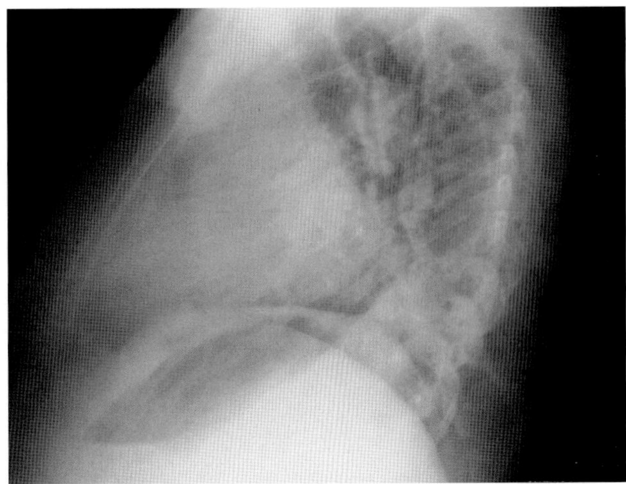

Figure 44.3 Chest X ray lateral view.

3 Laboratory data

Hemoglobin 13 g%.
Two-dimensional echocardiogram: possible LVH, technically poor quality.
TEE not technically feasible.

4 Hemodynamic data

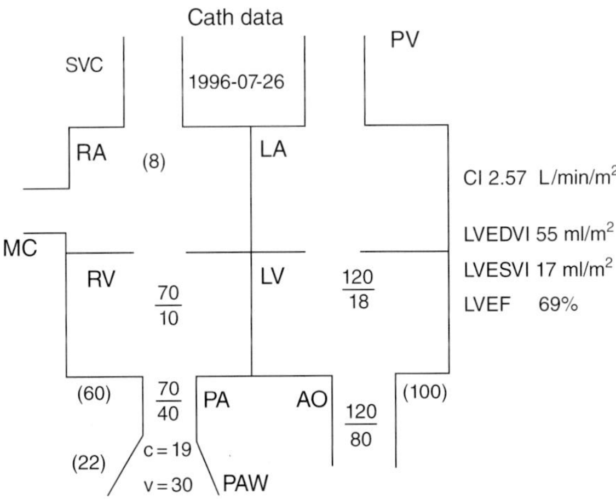

Figure 44.4 Hemodynamics 26 July 1996.

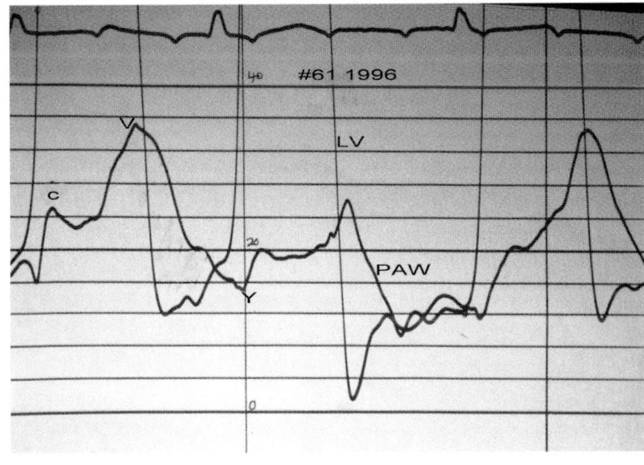

Figure 44.5 LV and PAW pressures. 0-40 mmHg scale.

5 Biplane LV angiography

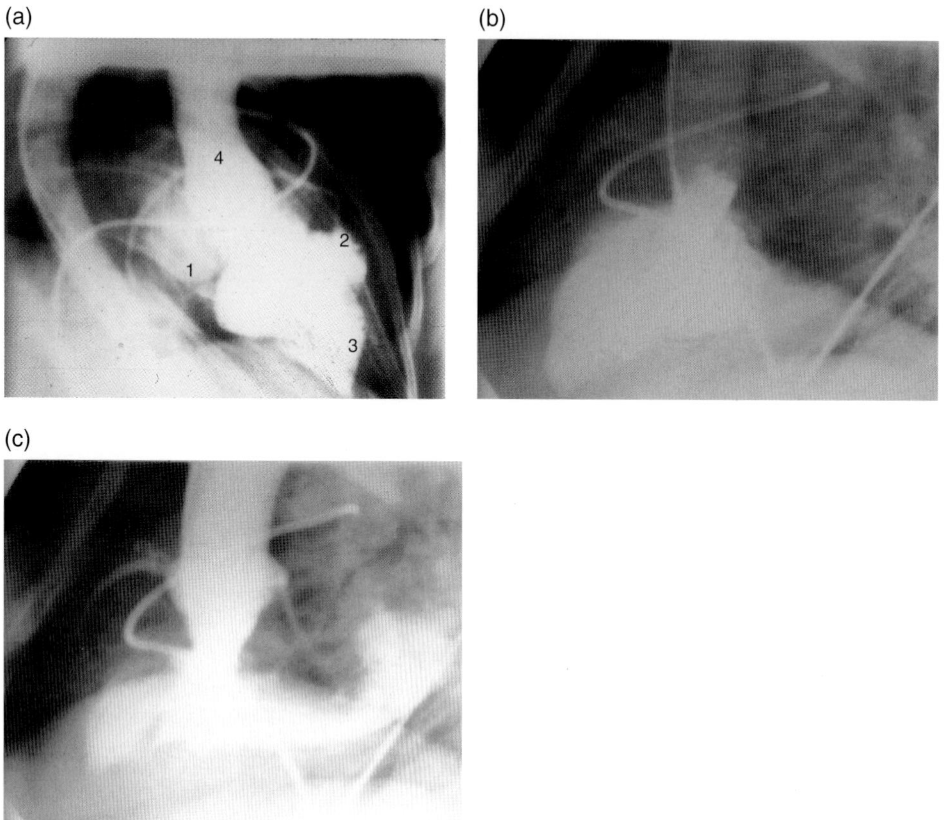

Figure 44.6 (a) LV angiography AP view. (b) LV angiography lateral view (early). (c) LV angiography lateral view (late).
Identify the structures labeled 1–4 in Figure 44.6a.

6 Cardiogreen dye curves

Table 44.1 Cardiogreen dye curves showing injection site, sampling site, and appearance time

Site of injection	Sampling site	Appearance time (s)
RA	LV	14
LV	PA	∞
PA	Ao	13

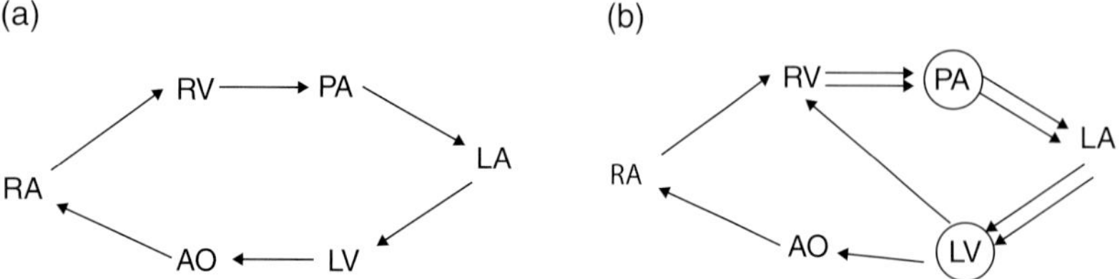

Figure 44.7 (a) Normal blood flow pattern. (b) Blood flow pattern in a VSD.

7 History

27-year-old female admitted to hospital in 1996 with new onset of dyspnea and paroxysmal nocturnal dyspnea for the last 2 months. Two months ago she was noted to have had a heart murmur and atrial flutter on the ECG.

8 Physical examination

48 inches tall female weighing 103 lb. She has webbing of the neck and kyphoscoliosis.
BP 110/64 (right arm), 110/? (right leg). HR 92/min irregular.
No elevation of jugular venous pressure.
Apex beat was in the 5th interspace, 10 cm from the mid-sternal line.
S1 +1 increased. S2 +l increased. No S3.
Grade 3/6 diamond-shaped systolic murmur maximally heard at the left 2nd interspace parasternally, radiating to the right 3rd interspace parasternally and less well heard at the apex.
Femoral pulse were 1+/4+ bilaterally.

9 Phonocardiogram

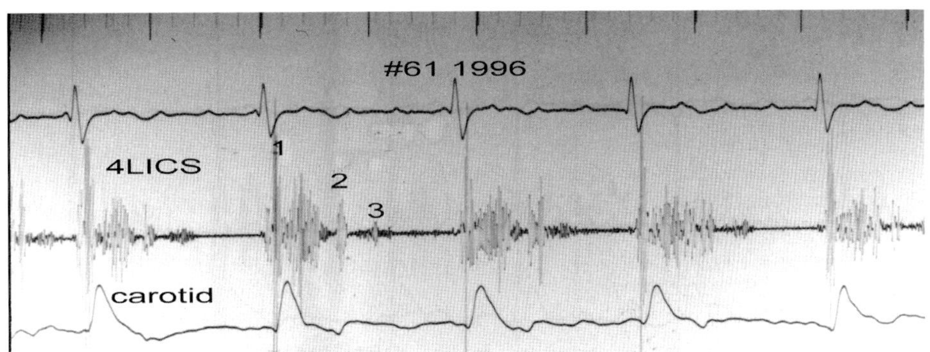

Figure 44.8 Phonocardiogram recorded at the 4th left interspace parasternally (4LICS) with ECG and carotid pulse tracing. 1, 2, and 3 represent the first, second, and third heart sounds, respectively.

10 Course

What is the course of treatment?

Answers and commentary

1 ECG

Atrial flutter with variable block. HR 85/min.
QRS 0.08 s. QRS axis +60°. Poor R wave progression V1–4 suggest a pseudo-infarction pattern.
Atrial arrhythmias in a young patient favors mitral valvular disease rather than a VSD.

2 Chest X ray

The PA view shows an S-shaped kyphoscoliosis.
The lateral view shows an enlarged heart.

3 Laboratory data

Echocardiography was not feasible in this patient because of severe kyphoscoliosis.

4 Hemodynamic data

There is severe pulmonary hypertension (mean PA = 60 mmHg).
There is mild RV dysfunction with RVEDP of 10 mmHg.
There is moderate elevation of the wedge pressure with a prominent 'v' wave.
In some patients with acute mitral regurgitation the 'v' wave may be two or three times that of the mean PA wedge pressure [1] but this was not the case here, probably because the LA had enlarged and was more compliant.
There is a small gradient in early diastole across the mitral valve, which with a normal y descent is against the diagnosis of mitral stenosis (Figure 44.5). The LVEDP is moderately elevated to 18 mmHg, which is most likely due to a non-complaint LV as the cardiac output and LVEF are normal.

LV systolic function and dimensions are normal.

Normal biplane aortography indicates that there was no PDA, aortic regurgitation, or coarctation of the aorta.

5 Biplane LV angiography

Figure 44.6a shows the LV angiogram in AP view with complete filling of the LA. It has slightly less opacification than the aorta, implying that there is significant mitral regurgitation. 1, LA; 2, LA appendage; 3, LV; 4, aorta.

Figures 44.6b and 44.6c show 4+ mitral regurgitation with a counterclockwise jet entering the LA and reflux of contrast into the pulmonary veins. In this view the opacification of the LA is about the same as in the aorta, also indicating severe mitral regurgitation.

The LV is not enlarged, implying that the mitral regurgitation is of recent origin. The direction of the jet suggests a flail mitral leaflet (? anterior). There was no evidence of a VSD. The LA was twice normal size.

6 Cardiogreen dye curves

An LV to PA dye curve failed to show any early appearance in the PA, thus excluding a VSD or PDA (see Table 44.1) .The injection of dye into the LV would appear in a few seconds in the PA if there was a VSD (see Figure 44.7).

7 and 8 History and physical examination

The new onset of symptoms and the location of the murmur were initially attributed to a VSD. A suboptimal echocardiogram showed LVH, which can be seen either in VSD or mitral regurgitation. Kyphoscoliosis distorts the normal anatomy so that the diagnosis of a murmur by location alone is unreliable.

Angiography was required to make the correct diagnosis as it was technically impossible to obtain a reliable echocardiogram.

Webbing of the neck may be seen in coarctation of the aorta, which can be excluded on clinical grounds (leg and arm pressures are the same) and a normal aortogram. In this patient the reason for the webbing is unknown. The femoral pulses were unaccountably diminished.

9 Phonocardiogram

This showed a diamond-shaped systolic murmur at the 4th left interspace parasternally. As noted previously, the shape of the murmur in acute mitral regurgitation can be quite variable [1,2]. An S3 was recorded on the phonocardiogram but was not detected on physical examination.

10 Course

Mitral valve replacement was recommended, but the patient was lost to follow-up.

Discussion

This 27-year-old patient had severe mitral regurgitation of recent onset, presumably due to a flail mitral valve leaflet from myxomatous disease. Other causes of a flail leaflet such as infective endocarditis or trauma [1,2] were absent in this patient. This recent onset of mitral regurgitation could account for the normal size LV, elevated LVEDP, high normal LVEF, LA enlargement, and severe pulmonary hypertension.

Patients with kyphoscoliosis may also develop pulmonary hypertension, probably as a result of a restrictive lung pattern and hypoxemia [3].

Key points

1. Severe kyphoscoliosis can distort the normal anatomy so that the diagnosis of a murmur based on location is unreliable.
2. The diagnosis of mitral regurgitation was only obtainable by angiography as echocardiography could not be performed because of severe kyphoscoliosis.
3. Severe pulmonary hypertension was attributed to acute mitral regurgitation and kyphoscoliosis.
4. Webbing of the neck can be idiopathic and is not always associated with coarctation of the aorta.

References

[1] Carabello BA. Progress in mitral and aortic regurgitation. *Curr Probl Cardiol* 2003; 28: 549–584.

[2] Otto CM. *Acute mitral regurgitation in adults*. www.uptodate.com. 2013.

[3] Naeye RL. Kyphoscoliosis and cor pulmonale. *Am J Pathol* 1961; 38: 561–573 (nine patients with kyphoscoliosis whose lungs were studied at necropsy).

45 PATIENT STUDY 45

Sequence of data presentation

1 History
↓
2 ECG 23 April 2002
↓
3 Chest X ray
↓
4 Oxygen sample run
↓
5 Pressures
↓
6 Angiograms
↓
7 Physical examination
↓
8 Phonocardiogram
↓
9 Diagnosis
↓
10 Surgery

1 History

41-year-old man who first developed dyspnea on exertion 1 year ago (2001). He developed leg edema 6 months ago and had episodes of paroxysmal nocturnal dyspnea 2 months ago. He had to stop working as a food vendor 1 month ago because of progressive dyspnea on walking half block or climbing up one flight of stairs.

He was told he had had a hole in his heart at birth but was able to participate in sports at school without any dyspnea.

There is no history of rheumatic fever, diabetes, CVA, or myocardial infarction. He has had hypertension since 1992. He had smoked for 10 pack years and drinks six 12-ounce cans of beer per weekend and one bottle of whiskey every 3 days.

2 ECG

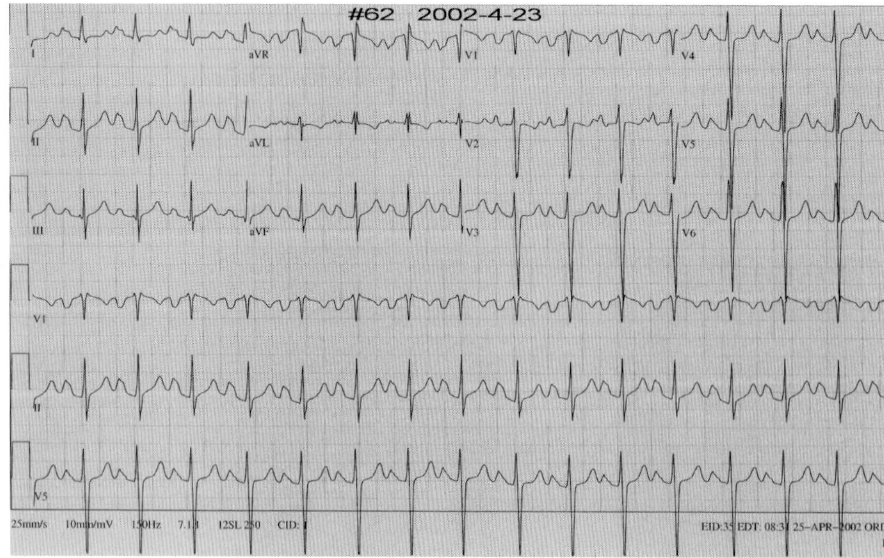

Figure 45.1 ECG.

Patient Studies in Valvular, Congenital, and Rarer Forms of Cardiovascular Disease: An Integrative Approach, First Edition. Franklin B. Saksena.

Companion Website: www.wiley.com/go/saksena/patientstudies

3 Chest X ray

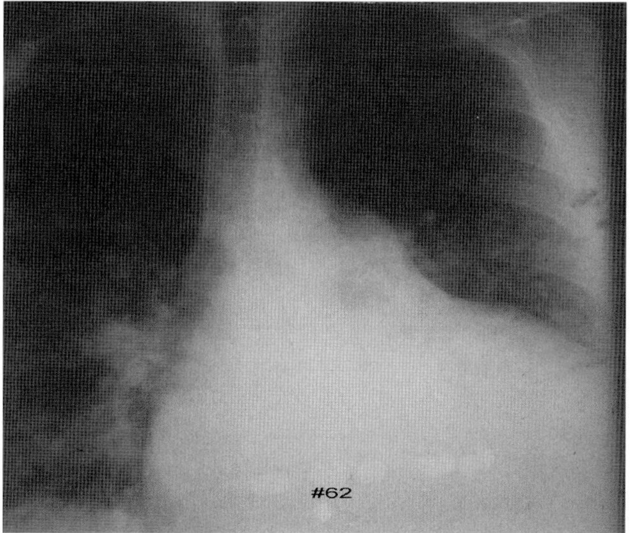

Figure 45.2 Chest X ray.

4 Oxygen sample run

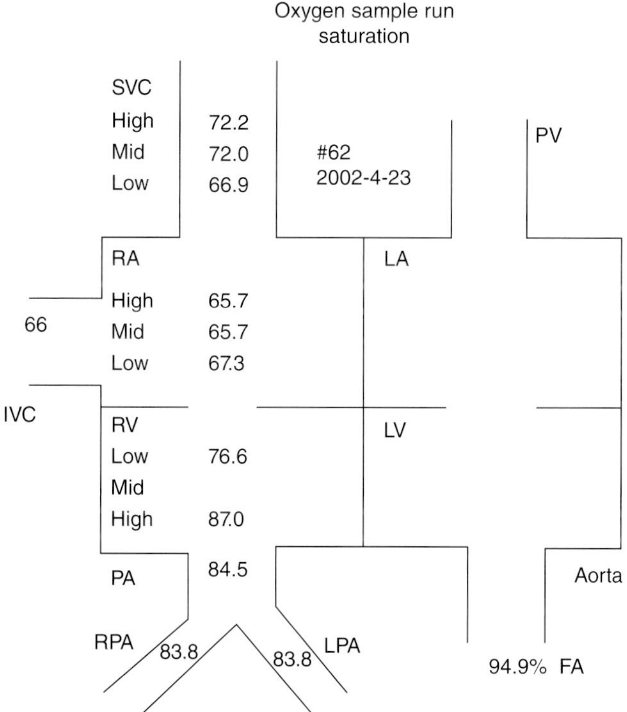

Figure 45.3 Oxygen sample run.

5 Pressures

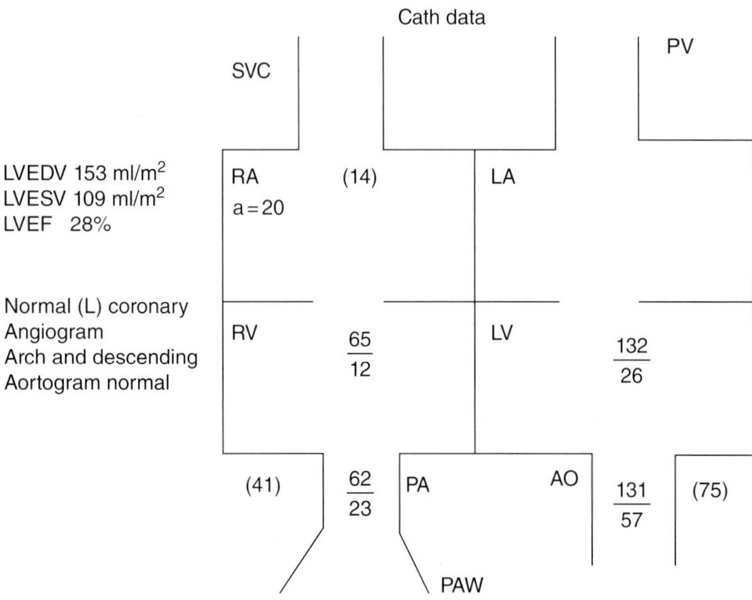

Figure 45.4 Pressure measurements.

6 Angiograms

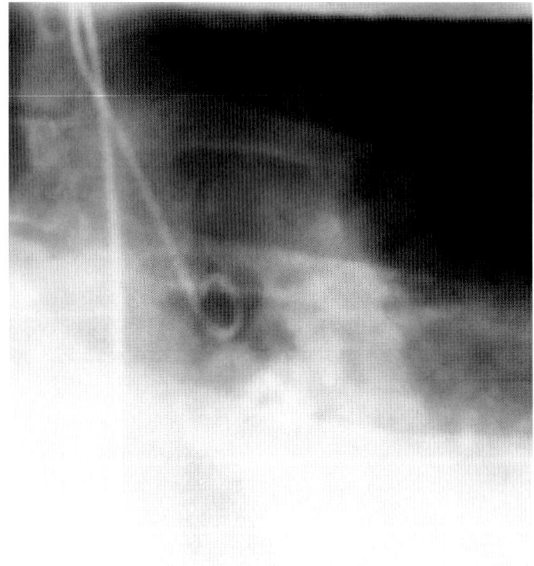

Figure 45.5 Catheter in ascending aorta AP view, prior to aortography.

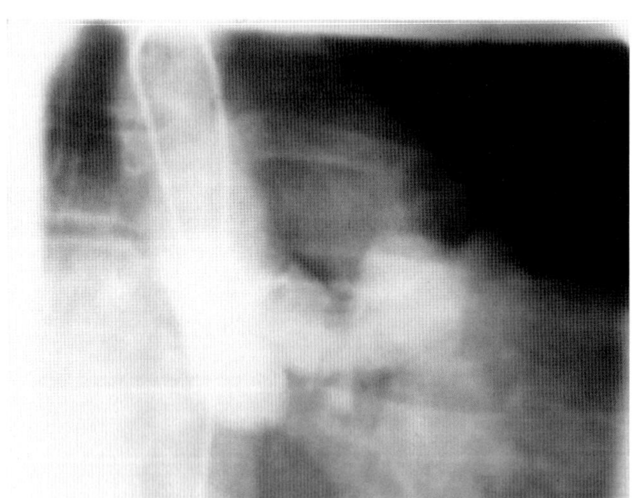

Figure 45.6 Aortic root angiography AP view.

7 Physical examination

The patient is 69 inches tall and weighs 258 lb. BP 160/40/0. HR 70/min. He has bounding peripheral pulses. No elevation of jugular venous pressure.

The apex beat was in the 5th and 6th interspaces, 15 cm from the mid-sternal line (marked cardiomegaly). There was 1+ RV lift.

S1 –1 decreased. S2 –1 decreased.

There was a grade 4/6 continuous murmur best heard in the 3rd left interspace parasternally, which did not radiate to the neck and faded towards the apex.
Liver span 15 cm. There were systolic liver pulsations.
1+ leg edema.

8 Phonocardiogram

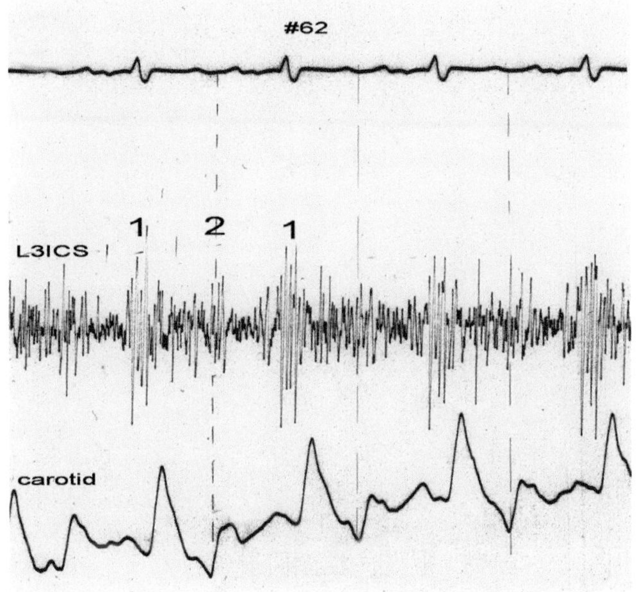

Figure 45.7 Phonocardiogram recorded at the left 3rd interspace parasternally and the carotid pulse.

Table 45.1 Causes of continuous murmurs

1 Systemic to right heart connection
(a) aorta → PA: AP window, PDA, surgical shunts
(b) aorta → RV: RSV
(c) aorta → bronchial aa → PA: TOF, truncus
(d) coronary a → right heart
2 Pulmonary arteriovenous fistula
3 Arterial narrowing: coarctation of aorta, PA, branch stenosis
4 Mimics of continuous murmurs: VSD + AR, AS + AR, MS + ASD
5 Innocent: venous hum, mammary soufflé

a, artery; aa, arteries; AP, aorto-pulmonary; AR, aortic regurgitation; AS, aortic stenosis; MS, mitral stenosis;

9 Diagnosis

What is your diagnosis and treatment plan?

10 Surgery

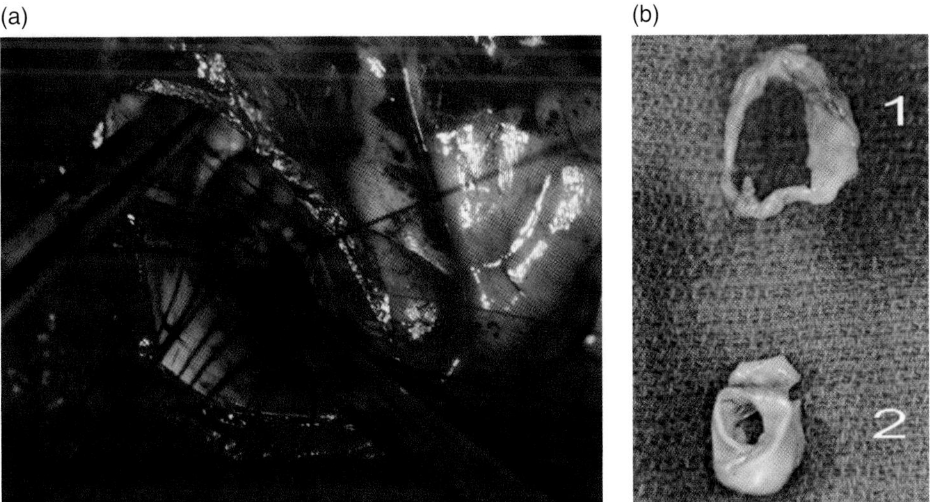

Figure 45.8 (a) Surgery showing VSD via aortotomy site. (b) Fragments of the aneurysm that were removed surgically. 1, rim of aneurysm; 2, aneurysm en face showing rupture.

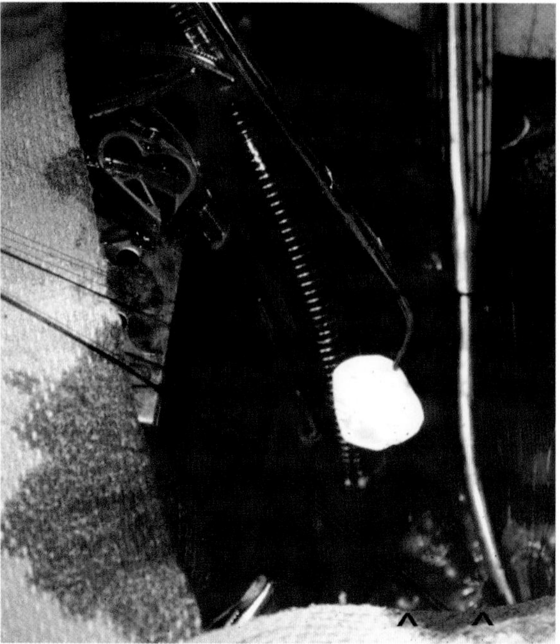

Figure 45.9 Surgery showing placement of patch over the VSD (just above the two arrow heads).

Answers and commentary

1 History

The history indicates the gradual onset of progressive congestive heart failure, which has a myriad of causes (e.g. hypertension). The patient's alcoholism could suggest an underlying cardiomyopathy.

2 ECG 23 April 2002

Sinus rhythm. Rate 100/min. PR 0.22 s. QRS 0.12 s. QRS axis + 60°. Deep S in V5–6.
Tall broad P in 2, 3, F. Biphasic P in V1 with prominent negative deflection.
Impression: biatrial enlargement, intraventricular conduction disturbance, possible RVH.

3 Chest X ray

There is marked cardiomegaly (RV and LV), with prominence of proximal pulmonary arteries and pulmonary plethora. Fluoroscopy showed a hilar dance and a calcified aortic valve.
A hilar dance is often seen in left to right shunts associated with an increased pulmonary blood flow.
The history, ECG, and chest X ray suggest biventricular failure with a left to right shunt.

4 Oxygen sample run

There is a step up in oxygen saturation on entering the RV indicative of a left to right shunt, such as a VSD, RSV, PDA with pulmonary regurgitation or a coronary-RV fistula. As the PA saturations are similar to the RV samples, a PDA can be excluded. The arterial saturation is normal, which excludes a significant right to left shunt.
The pulmonary flow/systemic flow ratio (Q_p/Q_s) was 2.6/1, as shown below.
Given:
average RA saturation (S_{ra}) = 66.2%, average PA saturation (S_{pa}) = 84%
arterial saturation (S_a) = 94.9%
we have:

$$\frac{Q_p}{Q_s} = \frac{S_a - S_{ra}}{S_a - S_{pa}} = \frac{94.9 - 66.2}{94.9 - 84} = 2.6/1$$

This is a moderate sized left to right shunt.

5 Pressures

The RA pressure is moderately elevated to 14 mmHg, with a dominant 'a' wave of 20 mmHg. These findings are compatible with the patient's moderately severe pulmonary hypertension (PA mean of 41 mmHg). The RVEDP is elevated to 16 mmHg, indicative of RV dysfunction. The LVEDP is also elevated, indicating LV dysfunction.

There is a wide pulse pressure that is seen in patients having aortic regurgitation or an AV fistula or a high output state. As the stroke volume was not increased (44 mL/m^2) and there was no aortic regurgitation on angiography, the wide pulse pressure must be attributed to an arterio-venous fistula, which in this case is an aortic–RV connection.

LV volumes showed a dilated LV (3× normal volume) with a reduced ejection fraction that reflects the severe volume overload from the left to right shunt. It is also possible that the patient may have a coexistent alcoholic cardiomyopathy.

6 Angiograms

Aortography showed a dilated right sinus of valsalva about 3 cm in diameter protruding into the RV (Figures 45.5 and 45.6). There was no evidence of a PDA or aortic regurgitation.

The left coronary artery was normal but the right coronary artery could not be entered because of the aneurysm.

7 Physical examination

The presence of liver pulsations suggests that the patient has tricuspid regurgitation. He would be expected to have an elevated jugular venous pressure with a prominent 'v' wave but this was not detected on physical examination as he was quite obese.

A continuous murmur maximal at the 3rd left interspace is said to be more compatible with an RSV than a PDA [1, 2].

See Table 45.1 for other causes of a continuous murmur.

8 Phonocardiogram

There is a continuous murmur recorded at the left 3rd interspace parasternally. The systolic component is louder than the diastolic component.

9 Diagnosis

1 RSV of right coronary cusp into the RV.
2 VSD with pulmonary/systemic flow ratio of 2.6/1.

10 Surgery

The aneurysm of the right sinus of valsalva was removed, the VSD closed, and the aortic valve repaired.

Discussion

The patient had an RSV, a left to right shunt between the aorta and RV, and, based on the prior history, a VSD.

The three sinuses of valsalva are small outpouchings of the aortic wall just superior to the three aortic cusp margins (right, left, and non-coronary).

Congenital aneurysms of the sinus of valsalva are rare, with an estimated incidence of 0.1–3.5% of all congenital heart anomalies [3]. The male/female ratio is 3/1 and they commonly rupture in the third decade of life [4].

The right coronary sinus of valsalva is the most common site for an aneurysm (Figure 45.11) to form [5–8], as in this patient. The aneurysm gradually enlarges and elongates like a windsock, protruding into the RV (Figure 45.12). Rupture of the aneurysm must have occurred gradually in this patient, producing a left to right shunt that led to progressive biventricular volume overload. If the patient had had an acute rupture he would have presented in acute congestive heart failure [6].

The continuous murmur heard in RSV is usually maximally heard at the 3rd or 4th left interspace parasternally [1, 2], whereas the continuous murmur of a PDA is usually heard best in the 2nd left interspace parasternally [1]. However, slight variations in the anatomy of the thoracic cage may make the distinction between a PDA and an RSV difficult based only on where the murmur is maximally heard. A PDA murmur tends to have a late crescendo systolic component, whereas the RSV murmur tends to be of uniform intensity throughout systole and becomes softer in diastole, especially at the higher thoracic sites [1, 6].

Associated features of an RSV include aortic regurgitation, a VSD, or a bicuspid aortic valve in 44%, 31%, and 9% of cases, respectively [5]. This patient only had a VSD.

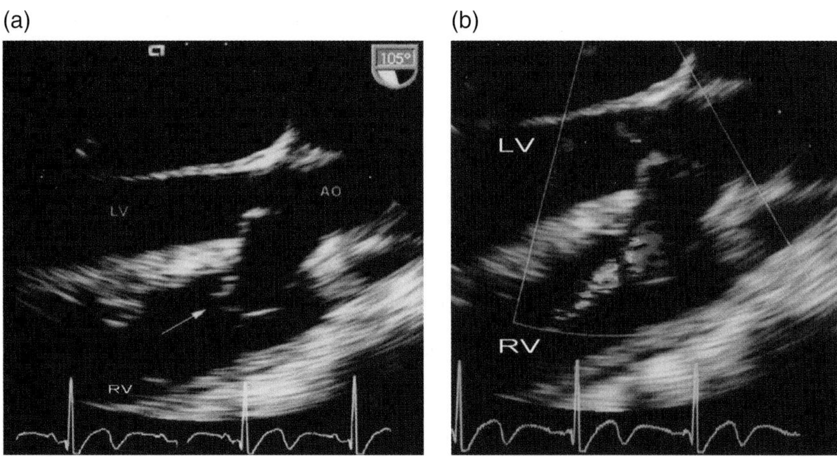

Figure 45.10 (a) TEE showing rupture of the aneurysm of the RSV into the RV outflow tract (arrow). (b) TEE showing color Doppler study of the same patient as in (a). There is turbulent flow through the ruptured aneurysm and trivial aortic regurgitation. Source for (a) and (b): Cullen S, Vogel M, Deanfield JE, Redington AN. (2002). Reproduced with permission of Wolters Kluwer Health.

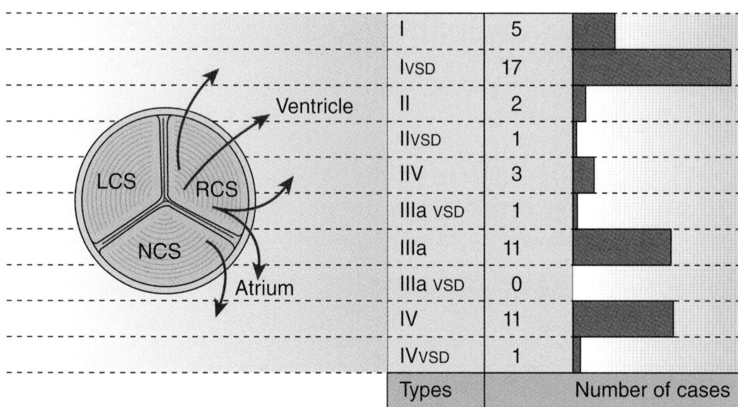

Figure 45.11 Routes of RSV aneurysms. Type 1 is the most common cause of congenital aneurysms of the sinus of valsalva. LCS, left coronary cusp; NCS, non-coronary cusp; RCS, right coronary cusp. Source: Sakakibara S, Konno S. (1962). Reproduced with permission of Elsevier.

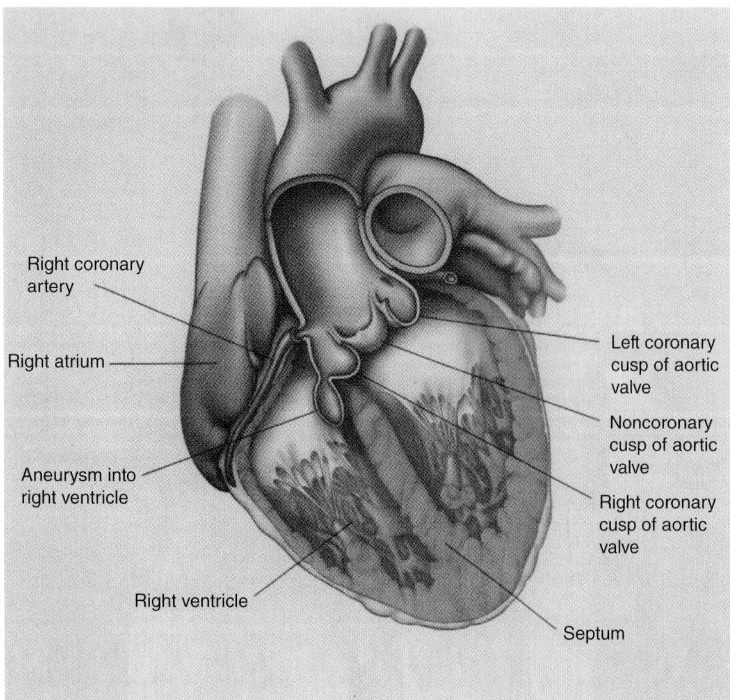

Figure 45.12 Aneurysm of sinus of valsalva of right coronary cusp protruding into the RV. Source: Mikielski K, Brechtken J, Lever H. (2002). Reproduced with permission of the *Cleveland Clinic Journal of Medicine*.

The diagnosis of RSV can be established at cardiac catheterization or on TEE [8, 9] (Figure 45.10a and b).

The treatment of choice is surgery [2, 4, 5, 8], although some have advocated percutaneous closure of an RSV [9, 10].

Surgical treatment involves resection of the aneurysm, closure of the VSD, and aortic valve repair/replacement with 10-year survival rates between 63 and 92% [5].

Key points

1. A ruptured aneurysm of the right coronary sinus of valsalva may be suspected in a patient with a continuous murmur maximum at the left 3rd or 4th interspace parasternally along with acute or chronic biventricular failure.
2. The right coronary sinus of valsalva is the most common site for an aneurysm to occur.
3. Rupture of the right coronary sinus of valsalva usually occurs into the RV, producing a left to right shunt between the aorta and the RV.
4. Associated features of an RSV are aortic regurgitation, a VSD, or a bicuspid aortic valve.
5. Surgical resection of the RSV is the treatment of choice.

References

[1] Constant J. *Bedside Cardiology*, 5th edn. Lippincott Williams and Wilkins, Philadelphia, 1999, pp 271–278.

[2] Morch JE, Greenwood WF. Rupture of the sinus of valsalva. A study of 8 cases with discussion on the differential diagnosis of continuous murmurs. *Am J Cardiol* 1966; 18: 827–836.

[3] Michiels V, Salgado R, Vrints C et al. Sinus of valsalva aneurysm. *J Am Coll Cardiol* 2009; 54: 876 (reconstructed CT angiogram showing a right coronary sinus aneurysm).

[4] Mikielski K, Brechtken J, Lever H. A 23 year old man with a continuous heart murmur. *Clev Clin J Med* 2002; 69: 128–137 (good discussion of continuous murmurs).

[5] Moustafa S, Mookadam F, Cooper L et al. Sinus of valsalva aneurysms – 47 years of a single center experience and systemic overview of published reports. *Am J Cardiol* 2007; 99: 1159–1164 (results of surgical repair of 86 patients).

[6] Perloff JK. *The clinical recognition of congenital heart disease*, 5th edn. WB Saunders, Philadelphia, 2003, pp 457–470.

[7] Sakakibara S, Konno S. Congenital aneurysm of the sinus of valsalva. Anatomy and classification. *Am Heart J* 1962; 63: 405–424.

[8] van Son JAM, Danielson GK, Schaff HV et al. Long-term outcome of surgical repair of ruptured sinus of valsalva aneurysm. *Circulation* 1994; 90 [part 2]: II-20–II-29 (good TEE and pathology pictures)

[9] Cullen S, Vogel M, Deanfield JE, Redington AN. Rupture of aneurysm of the right sinus of valsalva into the right ventricular outflow tract. Treatment with amplatzer atrial septal occluder. *Circulation* 2002; 105: e1–e2.

[10] Jayaranganath M, Subramanian A, Manjunath CN. Retrograde approach for closure of ruptured sinus of valsalva. *J Invasive Cardiol* 2010; 22: 343–345 (a muscular VSD intracardiac patch occluder was used).

46 PATIENT STUDY 46

Sequence of data presentation

- **I** First admission 31 August 2002–3 September 2002
  - **I.1** Clinical data
  - **I.2** ECG 1 September 2002
- **II** Second admission 4 September–21 September 2002
  - ↓
  - **II.1** History
  - ↓
  - **II.2** Physical examination 4 September 2002
  - ↓
  - **II.3** Laboratory data 4–7 September 2002
  - ↓
  - **II.4** ECGs
  - ↓
  - **II.5** Echocardiogram report 4 September 2002
  - ↓
  - **II.6** Cardiac catheterization 4 September 2002
  - ↓
  - **II.7** Diagnosis
  - ↓
  - **II.8** Course

I First admission 31 August 2002–3 September 2002

I.1 Clinical data

78-year-old female admitted to hospital on 31 August 2002 with palpitations. She had atrial fibrillation with a ventricular rate of 166/min. No history of smoking, alcohol use, or illicit drugs. She has had hypertension in the past.

BP 118/68. HR 166/min.

Lungs clear. No leg edema.

Echocardiogram showed a normal LV ejection fraction.

Troponin <0.09 ng/mL.

She responded to cardizem, digoxin, and anticoagulants. She was sent home on 3 September 2002.

I.2 ECG 1 September 2002

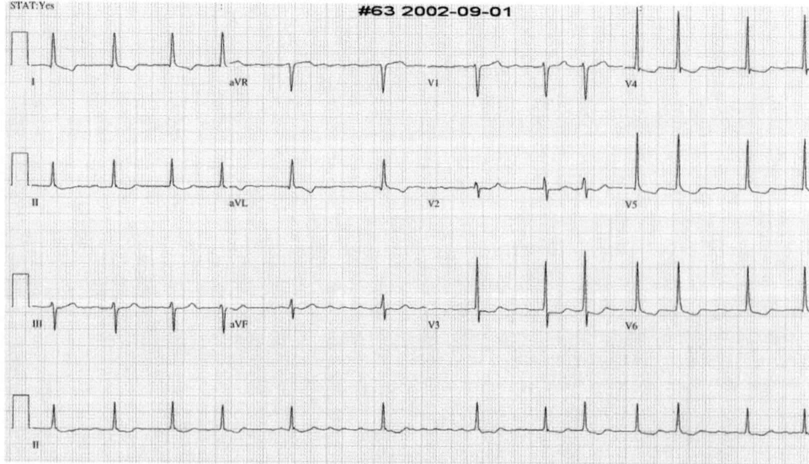

Figure 46.1 ECG 1 September 2002.

Patient Studies in Valvular, Congenital, and Rarer Forms of Cardiovascular Disease: An Integrative Approach, First Edition. Franklin B. Saksena.

Companion Website: www.wiley.com/go/saksena/patientstudies

II Second admission 4–21 September 2002

The second admission include history, physical exam, etc.

II.1 History

On 4 September 2002 the patient returned to hospital with dyspnea and exertional central chest pain. The chest pain was relieved with a nitroglycerine drip.

II.2 Physical examination 4 September 2002

The patient is 63 inches tall and weighs 163 lb.
BP 108/66. HR 88 sinus. R 18, T 97°F.
No elevation of jugular venous pressure. No carotid bruits.
No cardiomegaly. S1 normal. S2 normal.
Grade 3/6 apical systolic murmur radiating to the axilla.
Some crackles noted in the basal lung fields.

II.3 Laboratory data 4–7 September 2002

On admission Hb 10.9 g%, WBC 10,850, and chest X ray showed mild pulmonary congestion.
Serum troponin levels (ng/mL) were:
4 September: 1.96 and then 2.62
5 September: 3.30
6 September: 2.25
7 September: 1.45

II.4 ECGs

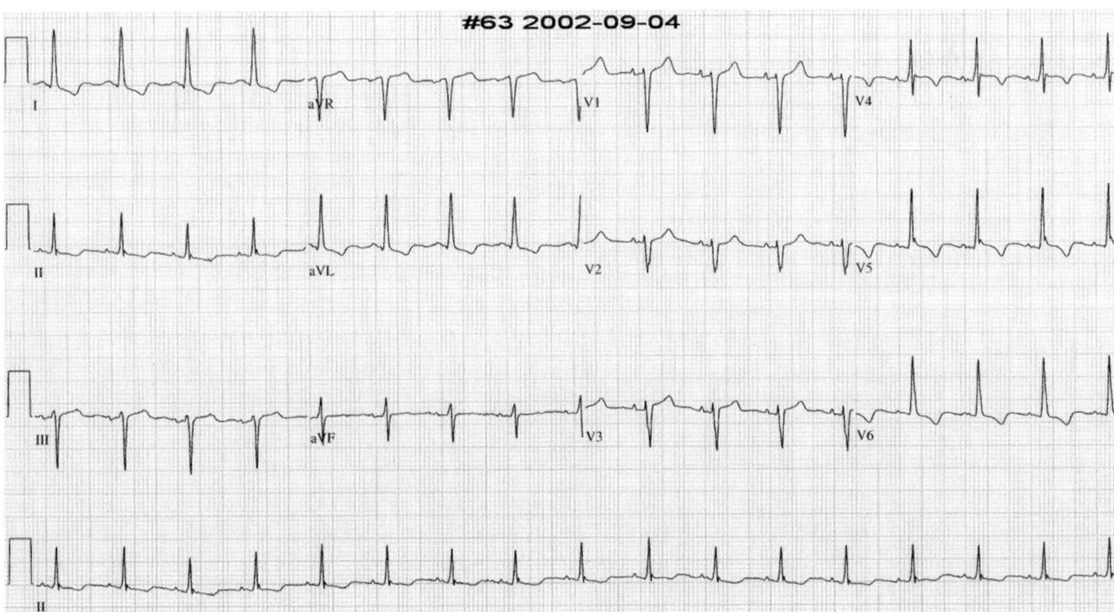

Figure 46.2 ECG 4 September 2002.

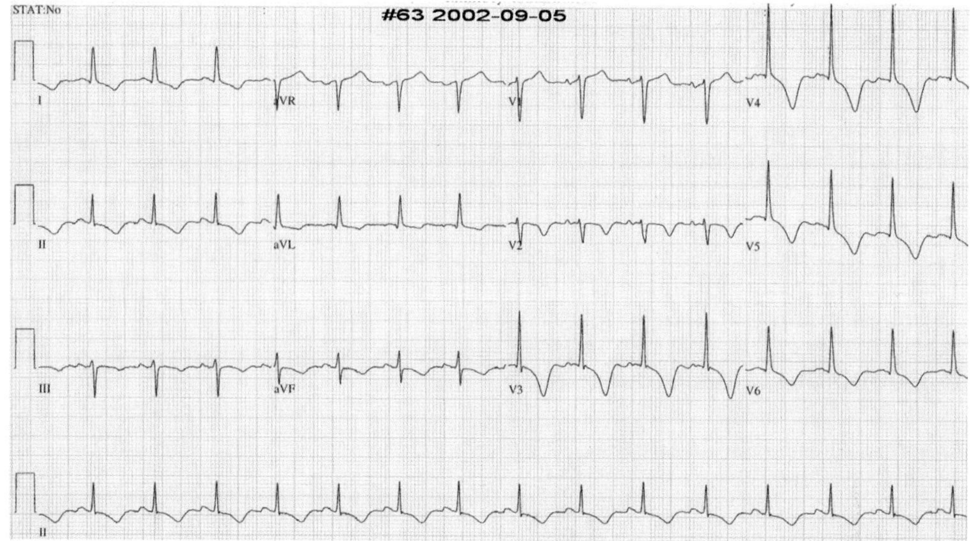

Figure 46.3 ECG 5 September 2002.

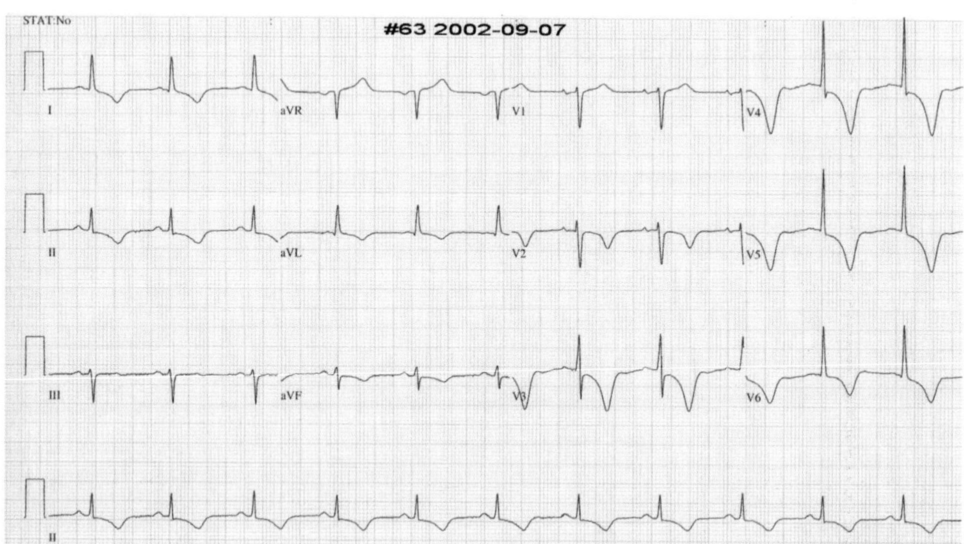

Figure 46.4 ECG 7 September 2002.

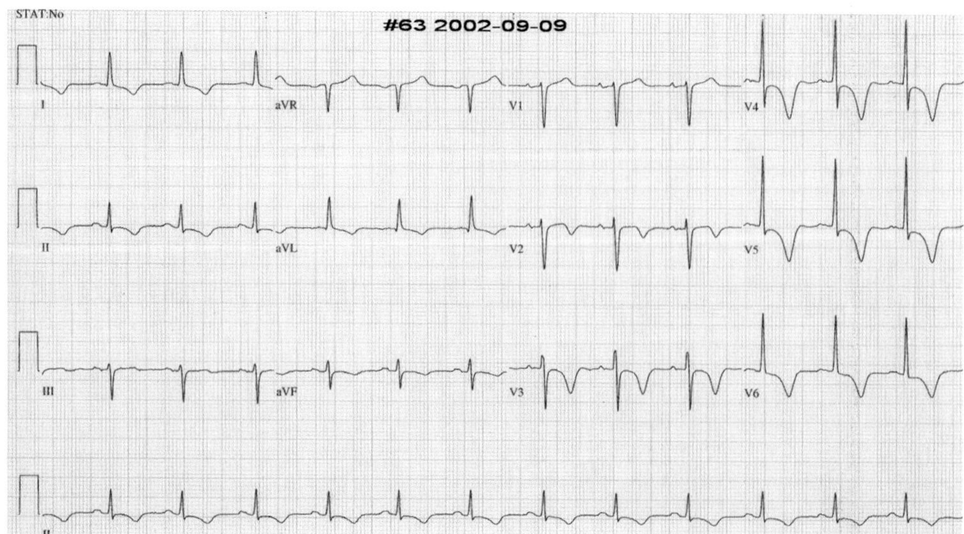

Figure 46.5 ECG 9 September 2002.

II.5 Echocardiogram report 4 September 2002

There is a large anteroseptal and apical akinetic region occupying one half of the distal LV. The base of the heart is hyperdynamic.

There is LVH. The estimated LV ejection fraction is 40–45%.

There is mitral regurgitation, systolic anterior motion of the mitral valve, and an estimated systolic gradient across the LV outflow tract ~100 mmHg.

II.6 Cardiac catheterization 4 September 2002

There was no significant coronary artery disease.

LV 155/30. Aortic pressure 97/43 (65).

Peak systolic gradient across the LV outflow tract was at least 60 mmHg. There was mitral regurgitation.

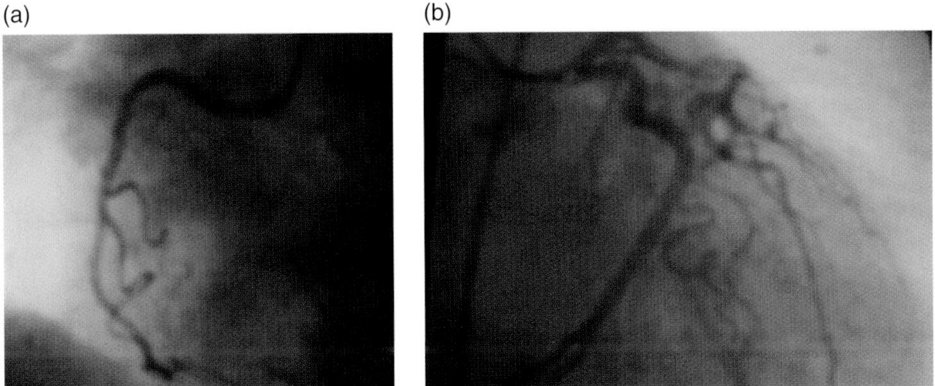

Figure 46.6 (a) Coronary angiography (right). (b) Coronary angiography (left).

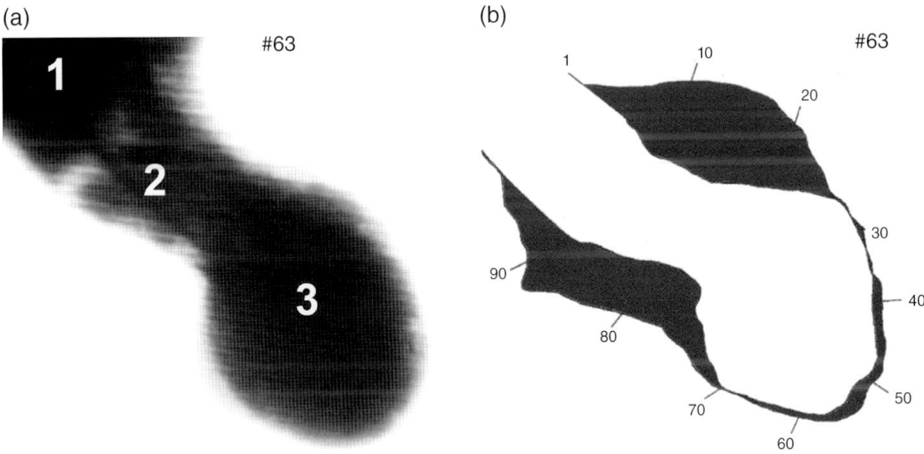

Figure 46.7 (a) LV angiography (end systole). (b) LV silhouette with end diastole shown in red.

Name the labelled structures 1, 2, 3.

II.7 Diagnosis

What is your diagnosis?

II.8 Course

What is the patient's likely course?

Answers and commentary

I First admission 31 August 2002–3 September 2002

I.1 Clinical data

The patient was admitted with atrial fibrillation with rapid ventricular response. Her heart rate was controlled with digoxin and cardizem, and she was placed on warfarin.

I.2 ECG 1 September 2002

Atrial fibrillation. HR 75/min. QRS 0.08 s. QRS axis 0°. ST sagging V4–6, 1, L due to either digoxin effect or lateral wall ischemia. QTc 0.38 s.

The heart rate has slowed from 127/min to 75/min since 31 August.

She was pain free at this time.

II Second admission 4–21 September 2002

II.1–3 History, physical examination, and laboratory data 4–7 September 2002

The patient had new onset angina and was in mild LV failure. She had a slight increase in her serum troponin levels, indicating some myocardial necrosis.

II.4 ECGs

ECG 4 September 2002

Sinus rhythm. Rate 100/min. PR 0.12 s. QRS 0.08 s. QRS axis 0°. QTc 0.4 s.

LVH with further ST sagging in 1, L, V4–6 since 1 September.

ECG 5 September 2002

Sinus rhythm. Rate 90/min. PR 0.14 s. QRS 0.08 s. QRS axis 0°. QTc 0.48 s.

Deeply inverted T waves are now seen in 1, 2, V2–6, indicative of anterolateral ischemia with prolongation of QTc.

ECG 7 September 2002

Sinus rhythm. Rate 68/min. PR 0.15 s. QRS 0.08 s. QRS axis 0°. QTc 0.48 s.

Further deepening of T waves in anterolateral leads as compared to 5 September, indicating further ischemia.

ECG 9 September 2002

Sinus rhythm. Rate 78/min. PR 0.16 s. QRS 0.09 s. QRS axis −10°. QTc 0.47 s.

T waves are slightly less deeply inverted in the anterolateral leads.

II.5 Echocardiogram 4 September 2002

There has been a sudden deterioration in LV function with anteroseptal and apical akinesia that correlates well with the anterior wall ischemic changes on the ECG.

There has been a sudden increase in the LVOT obstruction compared to the echocardiogram done on 3 September.

II.6 Cardiac catheterization 4 September 2002

1. There is a significant systolic gradient across the LV outflow tract .The LV ejection fraction has also fallen, as seen on the echocardiogram.
2. Normal coronary angiograms are seen (Figures 46.6a and b). The LV angiogram in end systole (Figure 46.7a) shows anterolateral, apical, and inferior wall akinesia (ballooning of the LV) labeled 3. There is hypercontractility of the basal portion of the LV labeled 2. The LV end-systolic contour resembles a Japanese octopus pot (Tako-tsubo). With the addition of some mitral regurgitation labeled 1, the LV and LA silhouettes resemble a dumbbell [1].

   Figure 46.7b shows superimposed computer generated contours of the LV in end systole and in end diastole, confirming the akinesia of the mid and distal LV with a highly expansile basal portion. The red area shows how much the LV enlarges in end diastole. These findings are indicative of Tako-tsubo cardiomyopathy (TC).

II.7 Diagnosis

1. TC.
2. Dynamic LV outflow tract obstruction.
3. Mitral regurgitation.
4. No significant coronary artery disease.

II.8 Course

Course in hospital 4–21 September 2002

The patient was treated with lopressor furosemide and warfarin with symptomatic improvement. The mitral regurgitation murmur became less audible. By 19 September she was walking 500 ft without difficulty. She was discharged on 21 September.

Further course

The patient's anterolateral T wave abnormalities gradually regressed towards normal (Figure 46.8), as did the echocardiographic findings (Table 46.1).

She was readmitted in 2004 with atrial fibrillation. Her LV ejection fraction remained normal. An ECG in 2010 was essentially unchanged from 2004.

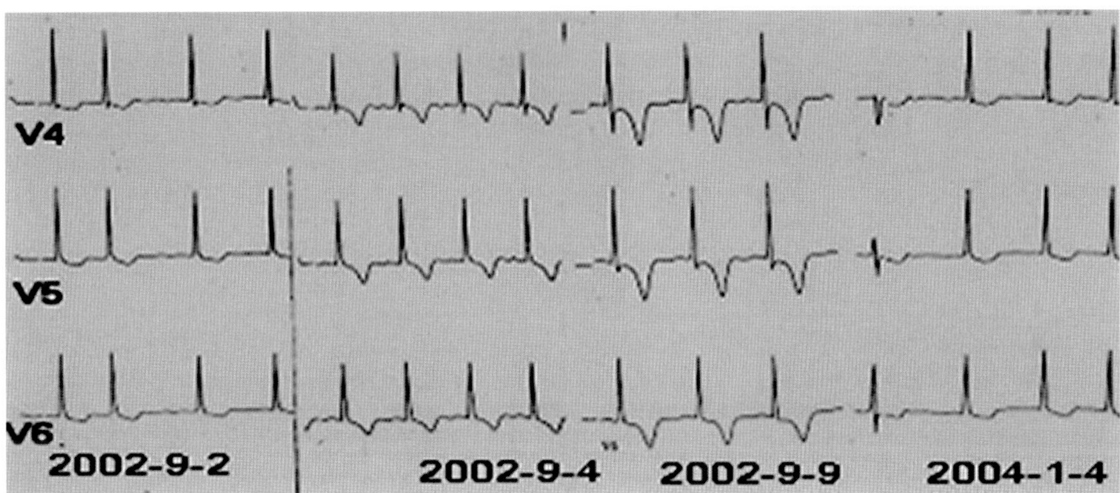

Figure 46.8 Serial ECGs of V4–6 2002–2004.

Table 46.1 Serial two-dimensional echocardiograms 2002–2004

Date	LVEF	LV systolic function	Mitral regurgitation	LVOT gradient (mmHg)
3 September 2002	N	N	Mild	15
4 September 2002	40%	Anterosep ↓ Basal ↑	Moderate	100
10 September 2002	↓	Anterosept ↓ Basal ↑	Mild to moderate	60
2 December 2002	N	N	Mild	0
4 January 2004	N	N	Mild	0
13 January 2004	65%	N	Trace	0

↓, decreased; ↑, increased; N, normal.

Discussion

This post-menopausal woman had angina, marked subendocardial ischemia on ECG, modest elevation of the serum troponin, reversible ballooning of the lower half of the LV, and normal coronary angiography. All of the above findings and the absence of a pheochromcytoma or myocarditis fulfill the Mayo Clinic criteria for diagnosing TC [2]. In addition she had LV outflow obstruction and mitral regurgitation, both of which resolved over the next few weeks.

Over 90% of patients with TC are post-menopausal women. TC is somewhat more frequent in Asians than Caucasians [1–3].

Two thirds of patients give a history of severe emotional or physical stress but one third will have no definite precipitating factor, as in this patient [1, 4, 5].

16% of patients may have associated LV outflow tract obstruction attributed to excessive contractility of the basal part of the LV, which resolves with normalization of LV function [1, 4], as seen in this patient.

The LV ejection fraction is considerably reduced when TC patients are admitted with chest pain and dyspnea. On average the LV ejection fraction recovers in about 18 days [4].

The quantitation of the LV ejection fraction in TC using the area-length method is subject to some error as the LV end-systolic contour is quite unlike an ellipsoid. Ideally a MUGA or MR ejection fraction should be obtained, but as this may not be feasible in an acutely ill patient, a bedside echocardiogram will at least qualitatively demonstrate LV dysfunction.

Of patients presenting as an acute myocardial infarction 1–2% may have TC [3, 5]. The diagnosis of TC may be considered if the patient has ST elevation or deeply inverted T waves out of proportion to the relatively modest rise in serum troponin levels and confirmed when there is apical ballooning of the LV without significant CAD [1–5].

About 20% of patients will have complications such as LV failure, arrhythmias, shock, LV outflow tract obstruction, mitral regurgitation, free wall rupture, and LV apical thrombi [1, 2, 4]. The in-hospital mortality rate is about 2% [2] to 8% [1].

Catecholamines play a role in TC but the exact pathophysiology remains elusive [1].

The management of TC follows the usual treatment of an acute myocardial infarction, which includes early coronary angiography [4].

Key points

1. TC may present as an acute coronary syndrome, usually in post-menopausal women following a significant stress.
2. It may be suspected if there are disproportionate ischemic changes in the ECG with only a modest elevation of serum troponins.
3. Confirmatory diagnosis requires a normal coronary angiography and reversible apical LV ballooning.
4. Complications are similar to an acute myocardial infarction but are less common. Prognosis is usually good.

References

[1] Kurisu S, Kihara Y. Tako-tsubo cardiomyopathy: Clinical presentation and underlying mechanism. *J Cardiol* 2012; 60: 429–437.

[2] Madhaven M, Prasad A. Proposed Mayo Clinic criteria for the diagnosis of Tako-Tsubo cardiomyopathy and long term prognosis. *Herz* 2010; 35: 240–244. © Urban & Vogel 2010.

[3] Akashi YJ, Goldstein DS, Barbaro G et al. Takosubo cardiomyopathy. A new form of acute, reversible heart failure. *Circulation* 2008; 118: 2754–2762.

[4] Pernicova I, Garg S, Bourantas CV et al. Takotsubo cardiomyopathy: A review of the literature. *Angiology* 2010; 61: 166–173.

[5] Reeder GS, Prasad A. *Stress-induced (takotsubo) cardiomyopathy*. www.uptodate.com ©2013, pp 1–12.

Further reading

Citro R, Lyon AR, Meimoun P et al. Standard and advanced echocardiography in Takostsubo (Stress) Cardiomyopathy: Clinical and Prognostic Implications. *J Am Soc Echocardiogr* 2015; 28: 57–74.

47 PATIENT STUDY 47

Sequence of data presentation

1 History, physical examination, and laboratory data 1967
↓
2 Hemodynamic data 1967–1968
↓
3 Angiograms 1967
↓
4 Physical examination and laboratory data 1968
↓
5 Hemodynamic data 1968
↓
6 History and physical examination 1973
↓
7 Hemodynamic data 1973
↓
8 Course 1994
↓
9 Laboratory data 1994–1997
↓
10 History and physical examination 1998
↓
11 Phonocardiograms 1998
↓
12 ECG 1998
↓
13 Chest X ray 1998
↓
14 Hemodynamic data 1998
↓
15 Angiography 1998
↓
16 Diagnosis

1 History, physical examination, and laboratory data 1967

History

The patient was first seen in 1967 at 11 months of age. He had a heart murmur at 1 month of age and heart failure at 10 months. He had circumoral cyanosis when he cried. His heart failure improved on digitalis and he was referred for cardiac catheterization in August 1967.

Physical examination

Height 27 inches, 13 lb infant. BP 130/80.
No elevation of jugular venous pressure.
Lungs clear.
Apex beat 6th intercostal space lateral to the mid-clavicular line.
S2 was single.
Grade 3/6 high-pitched systolic regurgitant murmur at LLSB.
Continuous murmur noted in right anterior axillary line.
Good peripheral pulses.

Laboratory data 1994–1997

1. Hemoglobin 13.2 g%
2. EKG: Sinus rhythm, LA enlargement, LVH
3. Chest X ray: cardiomegaly and increased pulmonary markings

Cardiac catheterization data are shown in Figures 47.1 and 47.2.
Note that the PA could not be entered.

Patient Studies in Valvular, Congenital, and Rarer Forms of Cardiovascular Disease: An Integrative Approach, First Edition. Franklin B. Saksena.

Companion Website: www.wiley.com/go/saksena/patientstudies

2 Hemodynamic data 1967–1968

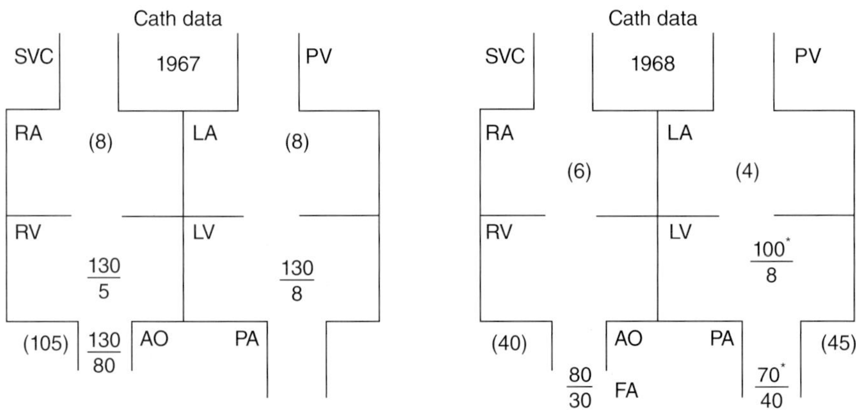

Figure 47.1 Intracardiac pressure measurements 1967 and 1968.

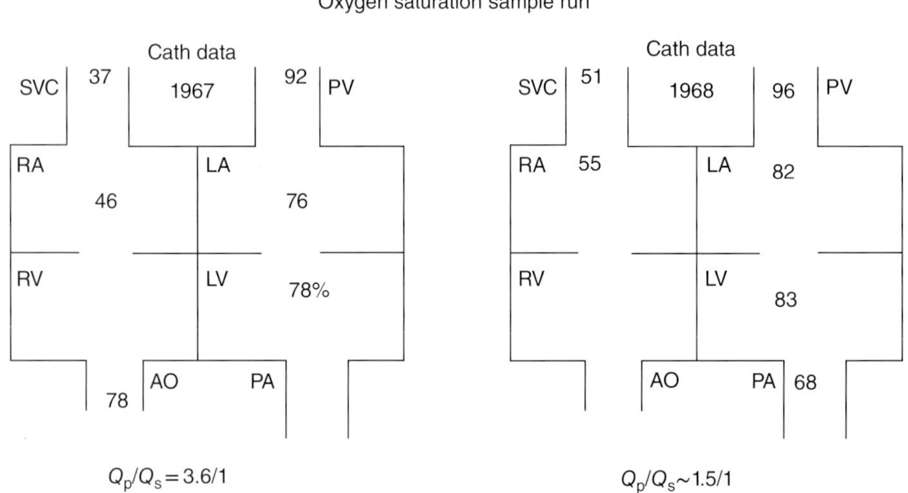

Figure 47.2 Oxygen saturation sample runs 1967 and 1968.

3 Angiograms 1967

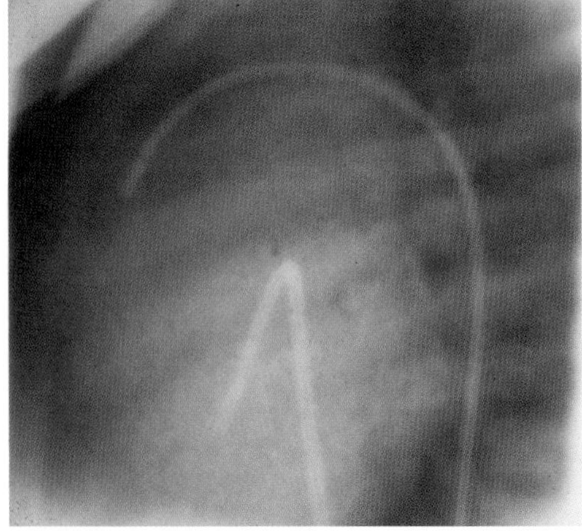

Figure 47.3 Lateral view of aortic and right atrial catheters 1967.

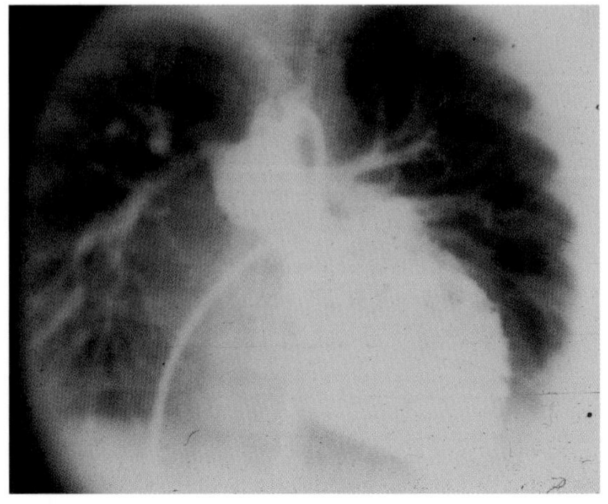

Figure 47.4 AP view of LV angiogram 1967.

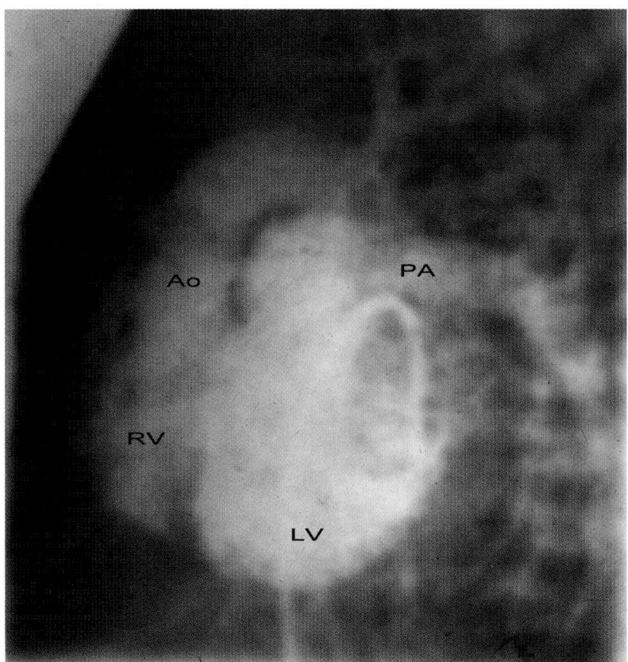

Figure 47.5 LAO view of LV angiogram 1967.

4 Physical examination and laboratory data 1968

Physical examination

2 years old. Height 28 inches. Weight 18 lb (<3rd percentile).
1+ clubbing of fingers. 2+ central cyanosis.
S1 increased. S2 single and increased. LV lift.
Grade 3/6 harsh ejection systolic murmur heart along mid and upper left sternal border.
Grade 4/6 continuous murmur heard along RUSB and all over right side of chest.
Hepatomegaly.

Laboratory data

1. Hemoglobin 12.4 g%
2. ECG unchanged from 1967
3. Chest X ray: cardiomegaly and increased lung markings.

5 Hemodynamic data 1968

Cardiac catheterization data are shown in Figure 47.3.
Note that the RV could not be entered via the RA.

6 History and physical examination 1973

History 1973

7-year-old male with increased fatigue as compared to other children while playing.

Physical examination

The patient is in no acute distress.
2+ clubbing of fingers and toes. 2+ central cyanosis.
Physical examination is otherwise unchanged from 1968.

7 Hemodynamic data 1973

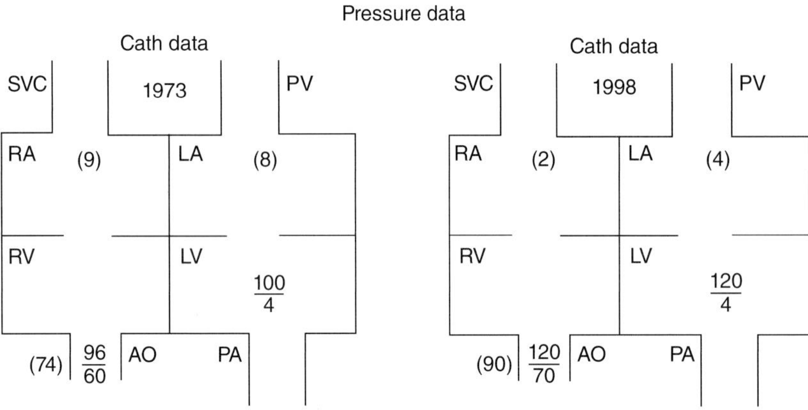

Figure 47.6 Intracardiac pressure measurements 1973 and 1998.

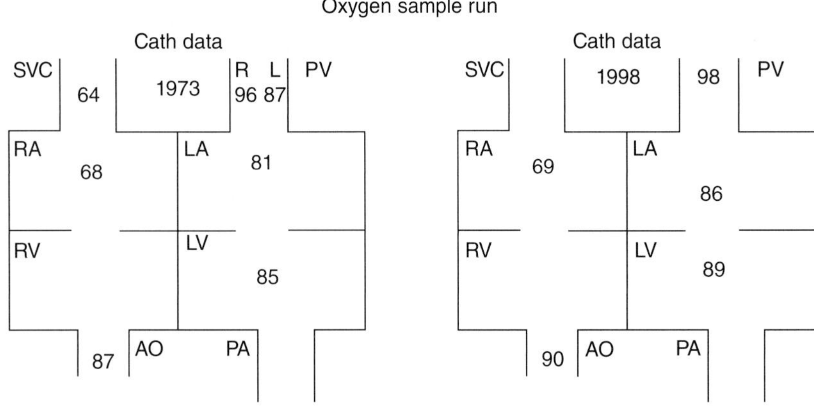

Figure 47.7 Oxygen saturation sample runs 1973 and 1998.

8 Course 1994

29-year-old man admitted to hospital in 1994 with chest pain and dyspnea on exertion.
At cardiac catheterization he had mild mitral regurgitation, a dilated LV, and normal coronary angiography.
The patient refused any surgical intervention for his cyanotic heart disease.

9 Laboratory data 1994–1997

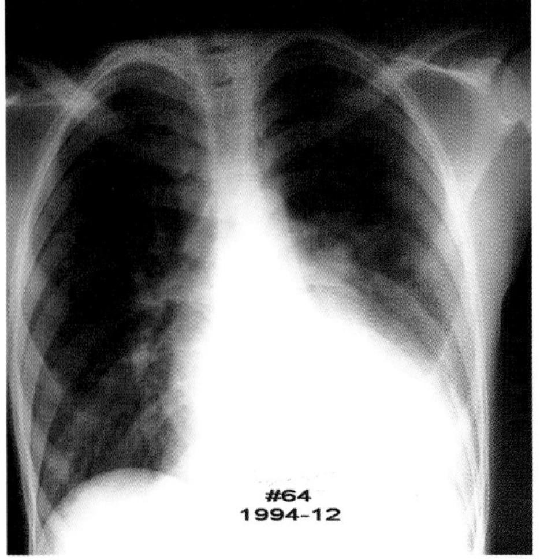

Figure 47.8 PA chest X ray 1994.

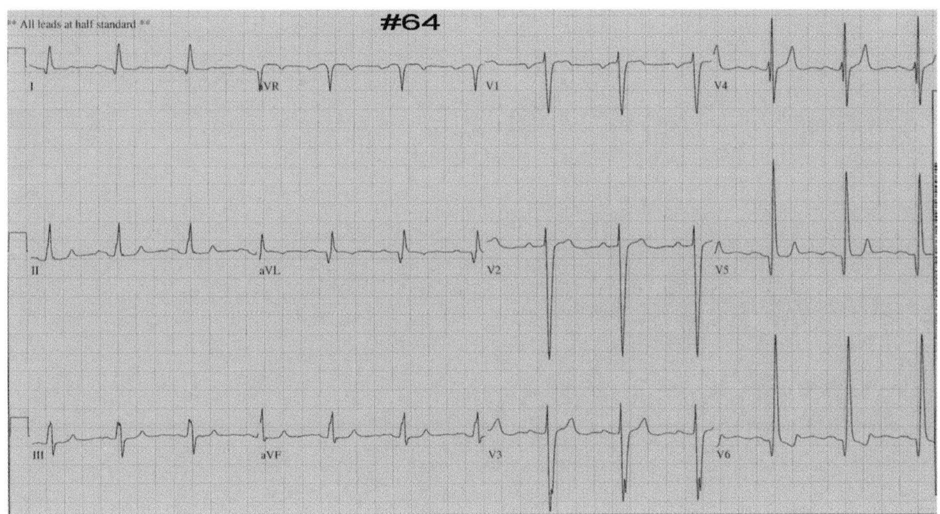

Figure 47.9 12-lead ECG 1994.

Table 47.1 Two-dimensional echocardiogram data 1997

Site	Measurement (cm)	Normal values
Aortic root	3.6	2–3.7
LA	2.8	2.3–3.8
LV end diastolic	6.4	3.7–5.7
LV end systolic	4.8	3.1–4.6
LV septum	1.5	0.5–1.1
LV posterior wall	1.5	0.5–1.1
RA	6.0	2.3–5.2

10 History and physical examination 1998

History

In 1998 he returned with dyspnea, fatigue, and headaches. He had a lifelong history of clubbing and did not play sports as a child.

Physical examination

64 inches tall, 101 lb male. BP 120/75. HR 72/min regular.
Hands are depicted in Figure 47.10.

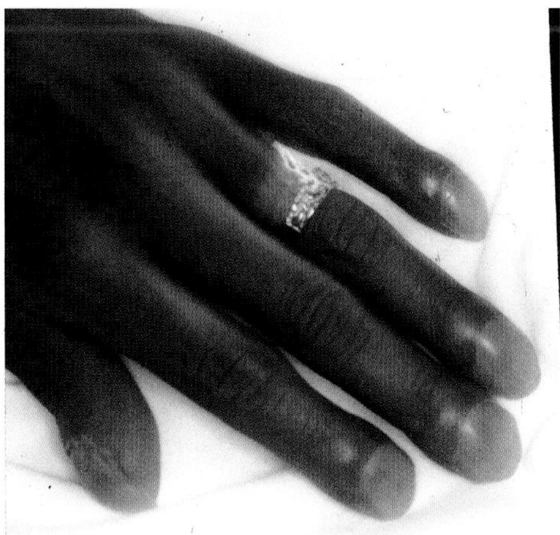

Figure 47.10 Hands of patient 1998.

No elevation of jugular venous pressure.
Apex beat 6–7th interspace is in the anterior axillary line, 14 cm from the mid-sternal line.
LV thrust. No RV lift.
S1 is increased and palpable. S2 is narrowly split.
Grade 2/6 diamond-shaped murmur maximum at left 2nd interspace parasternally.
Grade 3/6 holosystolic murmur best heard along right sternal border.
No hepatomegaly.

11 Phonocardiograms 1998

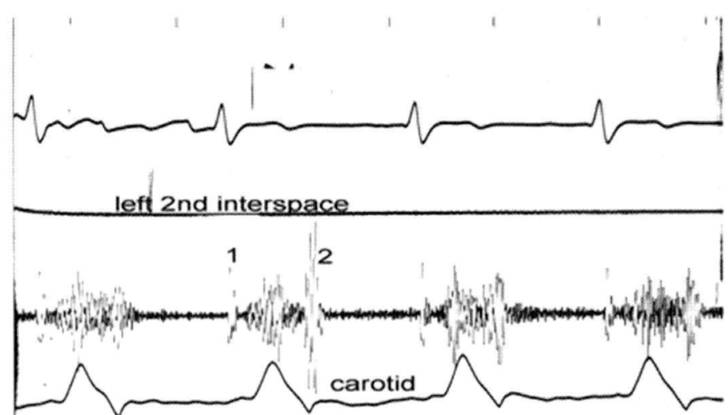

Figure 47.11 Phonocardiogram, left upper sternal border.

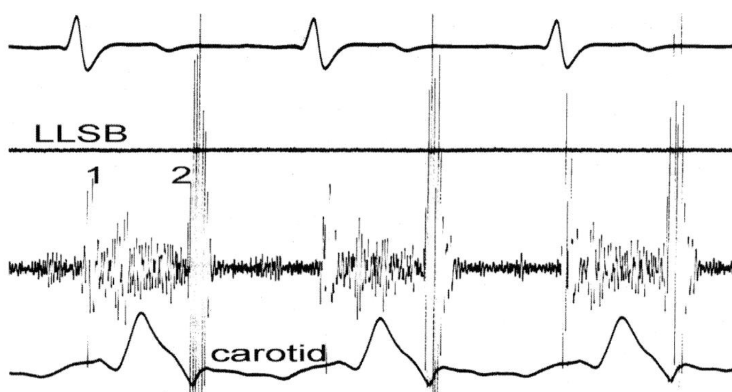

Figure 47.12 Phonocardiogram, left lower sternal border.

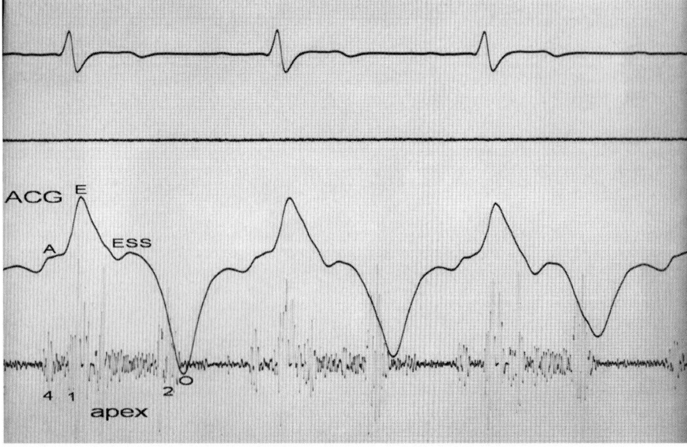

Figure 47.13 Phonocardiogram at apex.

12 ECG 1998

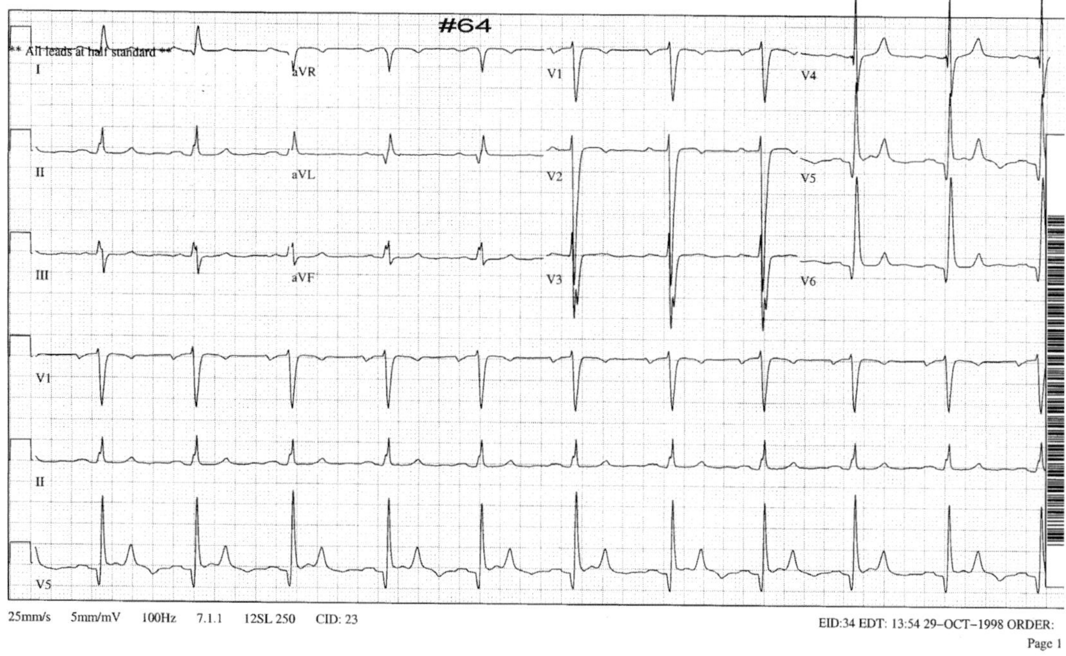

Figure 47.14 12-lead ECG 1998.

13 Chest X ray 1998

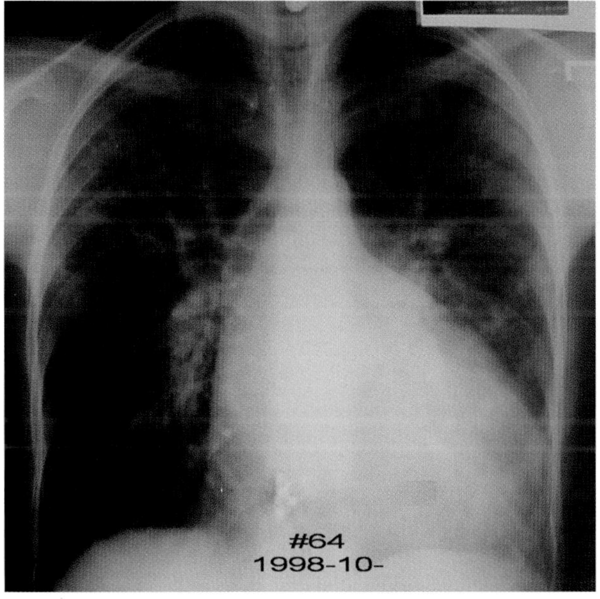

Figure 47.15 Chest X ray PA 1998.

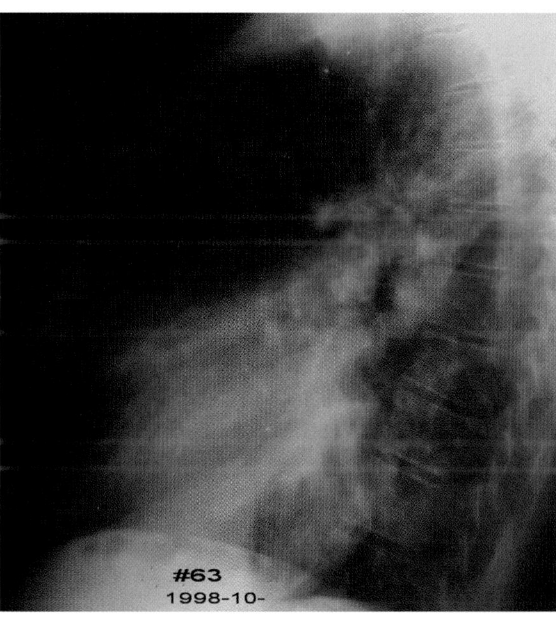

Figure 47.16 Chest X ray lateral 1998.

14 Hemodynamic data 1998

Table 47.2 Additional hemodynamic data 1998

LV end-diastolic volume index	174 mL/m^2
LV end-systolic volume index	72 mL/m^2
LV ejection fraction	58%

15 Angiography 1998

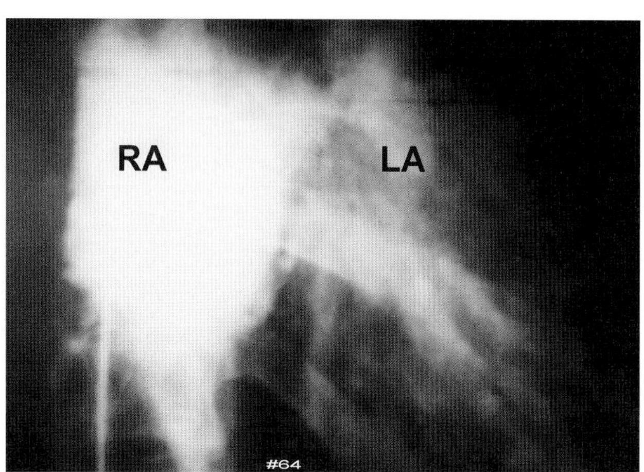

Figure 47.17 RA angiogram RAO view 1998.

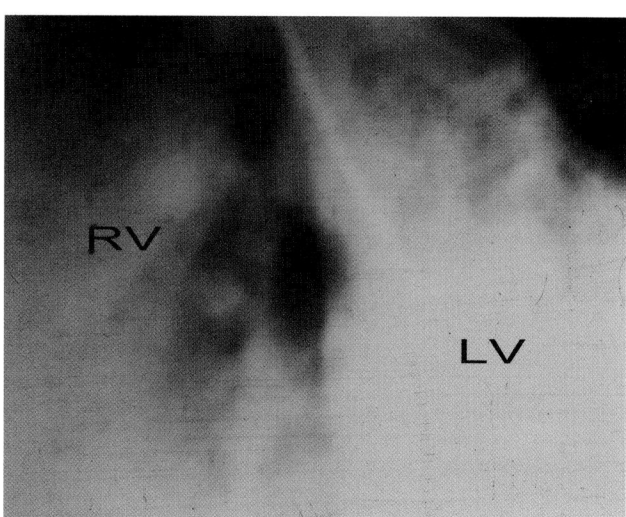

Figure 47.18 LV angiogram LAO view 1998.

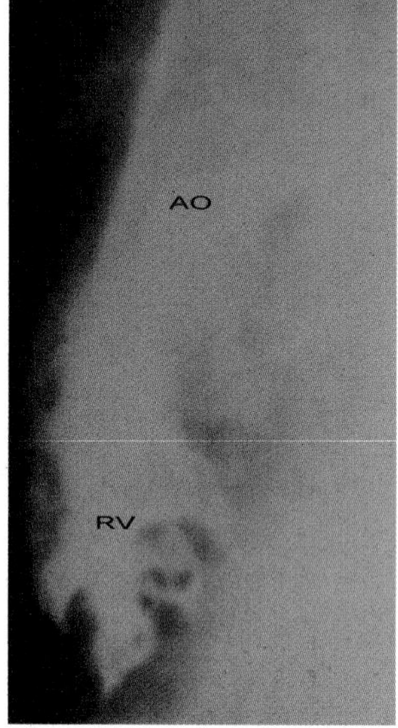

Figure 47.19 RV angiogram LAO view 1998.

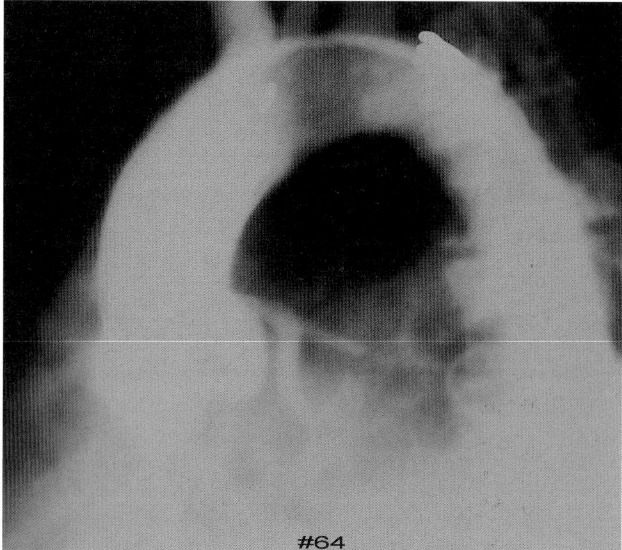

Figure 47.20 Aortic root angiogram LAO view 1998.

16 Diagnosis

What is the diagnosis?

Answers and commentary

1 History, physical examination, and laboratory data 1967

The patient had a history of heart failure, cyanosis, cardiomegaly, and a systolic murmur at LLSB, raising the possibility of a VSD. The child is underdeveloped. The continuous murmur in the right anterior axillary line could be due to pulmonary AV fistula or multiple areas of peripheral pulmonic stenosis.

Laboratory data show a normal hemoglobin level and LVH.

2 Hemodynamic data 1967–1968

The mean RA and LA pressures are the same as the LVEDP of 8 mmHg, indicative of an ASD.

The RV and LV systolic pressures are identical and indicate severe RV hypertension.

The RV was entered via the aorta and not by the RA.

There is evidence of a right to left shunt at atrial level because of the step down in oxygen saturation on entering the LA from the pulmonary vein and because of arterial oxygen desaturation.

3 Angiograms 1967

Figure 47.3 shows an anteriorly located aortic catheter, implying the presence of transposition of the great vessels. The other catheter is in the RA.

Figure 47.4 shows an AP view of a LV angiogram. The LV fills a dilated main PA. The peripheral PAs show areas of narrowing in the secondary and tertiary branches, indicative of peripheral pulmonary stenoses.

Figure 47.5 is an LAO view of a LV angiogram. The RV is small and fills via a VSD. The RV is connected to the ascending aorta.

4 Physical examination and laboratory data 1968

At 2 years of age the child is still underdeveloped and now has clubbing and cyanosis.

There was LVH but no mention of RV involvement. The murmurs were unchanged from 1967.

5 Hemodynamic data 1968

The absence of a systolic gradient between the LV and the PA excludes pulmonary valvular stenosis. A right to left shunt is still present across the ASD.

The inability to enter the RV via the RA as noted previously points to TA.

Surgical correction was recommended but not carried out.

6 History and physical examination 1973

The patient's fatigue is a non-specific finding but may be seen in patients with a low output state. The physical examination was essentially unchanged.

7 Hemodynamic data 1973

The pressures in the RA and left heart are unchanged. The RV could not be entered via the RA due to TA. The right to left atrial shunt is unchanged.

At this time a PDA was excluded.

8 Course 1994

The patient was admitted with chest pain.

9 Laboratory data 1994–1997

Chest X ray showed cardiomegaly (C/T ratio 0.66) with pulmonary plethora (Figure 47.8). The 1994 ECG is shown in Figure 47.9.

Sinus rhythm. Rate 75/min. PR 0.20 s. QRS 0.12 s. QRS axis +45°. P biphasic in V1.

Impression: LVH with QRS widening and LA enlargement.

There was no evidence of coronary artery disease in 1994 as his ECG remained unchanged and he had normal coronary arteriography.

His mitral regurgitation probably reflects a dilated LV.

Echocardiogram in 1997 (Table 47.1) showed RA and LV enlargement. A bubble study confirmed the right to left shunt at atrial level.

10 History and physical examination 1998

The patient returned with dyspnea and fatigue. He had cyanosis and clubbing (Figure 47.10). There had been a further increase in heart size on physical examination. The absence of an RV lift in the presence of cyanosis and clubbing along with LV hypertrophy all point to TA.

11 Phonocardiograms 1998

The systolic ejection murmur recorded at the LUSB could be due to peripheral pulmonary stenosis (Figure 47.11).

The systolic murmur at LLSB and apex could be due to a VSD (Figures 47.12 and 47.13) and mild mitral regurgitation. The previously described continuous murmur heard in the right axilla is most likely due to peripheral pulmonic stenoses.

The phonocardiogram (Figure 47.13) recorded an apical S4 indicative of a stiff LV.

12 ECG 1998

The rhythm is now back in sinus (patient had atrial fibrillation in 1997).

Rate 68/min. PR 0.22 s. QRS 0.12 s. QRS axis + 30°. P biphasic in V1.

S in V1+ R in V6 > 2.5 mv.
Impression: sinus rhythm with first-degree heart block, LVH with widening of QRS, LA enlargement.

13 Chest X ray 1998

Marked cardiomegaly (C/T ratio 0.65). The proximal PAs are enlarged.
The lateral film shows a small gap between the sternum and the RV, perhaps indicating a small RV.

14 Hemodynamic data 1998

The intracardiac pressures are about the same as in 1973 with a similar degree of arterial desaturation (Figures 47.5 and 47.6).
Table 47.2 shows marked enlargement of the LV volumes with a normal LV ejection fraction.

15 Angiography 1998

Figure 47.17 shows an RA injection (RAO) with prompt filling of the LA. The absence of RV filling is suggestive of TA.
Figure 47.18 shows the LV angiogram in LAO view with filling of the RV via a VSD.
Figure 47.19 shows a small trabeculated RV filling from the aorta, thus confirming the presence of transposition of the great vessels.
Figure 47.20 shows a normal aortogram, thus ruling out a PDA and coarctation of the aorta.

16 Diagnosis

TA.
Right to left shunt at atrial level.
VSD.
Peripheral pulmonic arterial stenosis.
Transposition of the great vessels.

Discussion

The patient had TA, transposition of the great vessels, an ASD, a VSD, and peripheral pulmonary stenosis.
TA has a prevalence of 1 in 10,000 live births or about 2% of all patients with congenital heart disease [1]. The diagnosis may be considered in any patient with cyanotic heart disease with LVH and without any RVH [2].
Type 1 TA has normal anatomical great vessels whereas type 2 has d-transposition of the great vessels [3].
Type 2 d-transposition of the great vessels TA occurs in 20–42% of patients [1, 3, 4], as in this patient. Patients with type 2 may also have PDA and coarctation of the aorta [3], but these were not present in this patient.
As a result of TA, blood entering the RA must communicate with the left side via an ASD. This right to left shunt is necessary for survival and accounts for the patient's long-standing cyanosis and clubbing.
Blood then enters the LV, which acts as a single pumping chamber for systemic and pulmonary circulation as the hypoplastic RV is essentially non-functioning.
In this patient the LV pumps blood into the aorta via a VSD and also directly into the pulmonary circulation. The amount of blood entering the pulmonary circuit is limited by the multiple areas of peripheral pulmonic stenoses (Figure 47.21), which accounts for the long survival of the this patient.
The hemodynamics of the patient had mostly been worked out by the pediatric cardiologists in 1973. The patient's relatives refused surgery at that time. He was lost to follow-up until seen in adult cardiology in 1994 with chest pain. His coronary angiogram was normal and free of coronary artery anomalies. Patients with TA may rarely have an anomalous coronary artery [1].
A repeat study in 1998 confirmed the results of earlier studies but unfortunately the patient again decided against surgery and has not been seen since. It is likely that his LV will continue to become more and more dilated until he develops irreversible LV failure.
Nowadays the diagnosis of TA is often made by echocardiography (Figure 47.22) as this can detect the absence of a tricuspid valve, an ASD with a right to left shunt, a VSD RVOT obstruction, and the position of the great vessels. Pulmonary angiography would be required to detect peripheral pulmonic stenosis.
Palliative surgery consists of redirecting systemic venous blood to the PA by (i) having the SVC blood drain directly into the PA and (ii) directing IVC blood to the PA using a conduit that is created inside a right atrial baffle or via an extracardiac interposition graft [5–7].

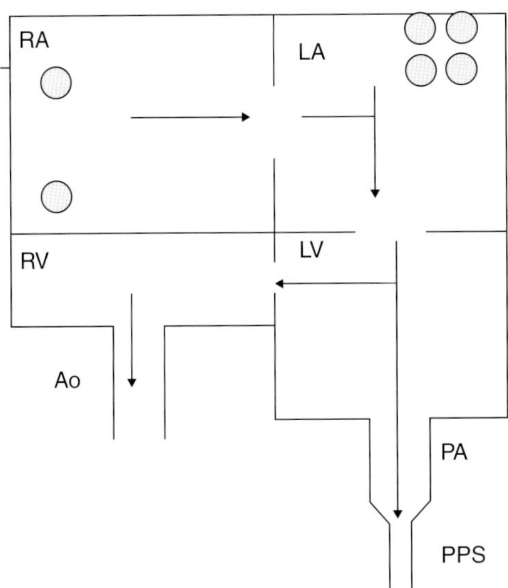

Figure 47.21 Diagram of blood flow in this patient with TA, ASD, VSD, transposition of great vessels, and peripheral pulmonic stenosis.

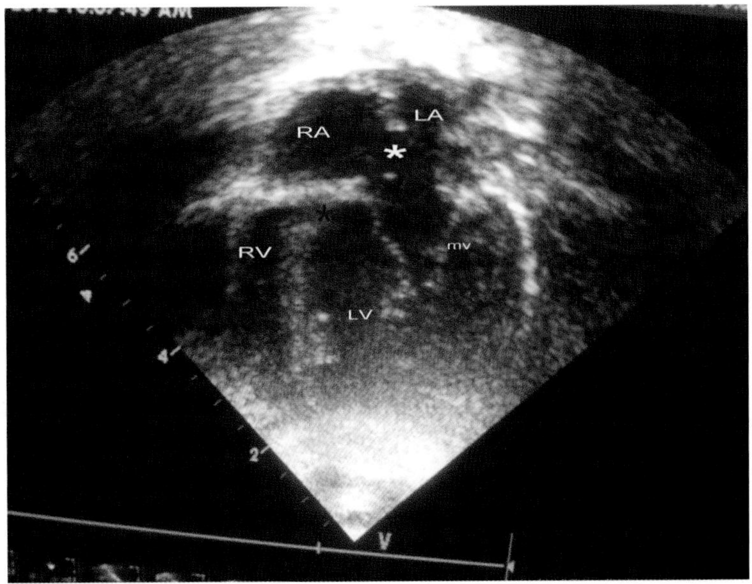

Figure 47.22 Two-dimensional echocardiography in a 3-month-old infant in 2013 with TA with a hypoplastic RV. There is a thickened band of scar tissue replacing the tricuspid valve. The mitral valve (mv) is opening normally into a somewhat dilated LV. The LA is normal. There is an ASD (*) and the red * is pointing to a VSD. The patient also had a PDA and normally positioned great vessels.

Key points

1. TA should be considered if the patient has cyanotic heart disease with LVH and no RVH.
2. There is an obligatory right to left shunt at atrial level in TA for the patient to survive.
3. LV failure usually occurs in TA as the LV has to pump blood into the systemic and pulmonary circulation.
4. Long-term survival in TA is possible if the amount of blood that enters the pulmonary circulation is limited by either pulmonic stenosis or peripheral pulmonic stenosis.
5. Palliative surgery consists of redirecting caval blood to the PA.

References

[1] Rao PS. Tricuspid atresia. *Curr Treat Opt Cardiovasc Med* 2000; 2: 507–520.
[2] Perloff JK. *The clinical recognition of congenital heart disease*, 5th edn. WB Saunders, Philadelphia, 2003, p 488.
[3] Dick M, Fyler DC, Nadas AS. Tricuspid atresia: Clinical course in 101 patients. *Am J Cardiol* 1975; 36: 327–337.
[4] Tandon R, Edwards JE. Tricuspid atresia. A re-evaluation and classification. *J Thorac Cardiovasc Surg* 1974; 67: 530–542.
[5] d'Undekem Y, Iyengar AJ, Cochrane AD et al. The Fontan Procedure. Contemporary techniques have improved long-term outcomes. *Circulation* 2007; 116(suppl I) I-157–I-164.
[6] Kanakis MA, Petropoulos AC, Mitropoulos FA. Fontan operation. *Hellenic J Cardiol* 2009; 50: 133–141.
[7] Khairy P, Poirer N, Mercier L-A. Univentricular heart. *Circulation* 2007; 115: 800–812.

48 PATIENT STUDY 48

Sequence of data presentation

1 History 1992
↓
2 Physical examination 1992
↓
3 12-lead ECG 1992
↓
4 Chest X rays 1990 and 1992
↓
5 Echocardiography 1992
↓
6 Nuclear medicine data 1992
↓
7 Hemodynamic data 1992
↓
8 Course 1992–1995
↓
9 History 1995
↓
10 Physical examination 1995
↓
11 Additional laboratory data 1995
↓
12 Chest X ray 1995
↓
13 ECG 1995
↓
14 Hemodynamic data 1995
↓
15 Echocardiographic data 1995 (pre- and postoperative)
↓
16 Course 1995–1999

1 History 1992

76-year-old man admitted to another hospital in 1992 with half-block dyspnea, leg edema, and 20 lb weight gain all in the last 2 weeks.

2 Physical examination 1992

77 inches tall male weighing 198 lb.
BP 130/80. P 111/min irregular.
Cardiomegaly.
No murmurs recorded. 3+ leg edema.

Patient Studies in Valvular, Congenital, and Rarer Forms of Cardiovascular Disease: An Integrative Approach, First Edition. Franklin B. Saksena.

Companion Website: www.wiley.com/go/saksena/patientstudies

3 12-lead ECG 1992

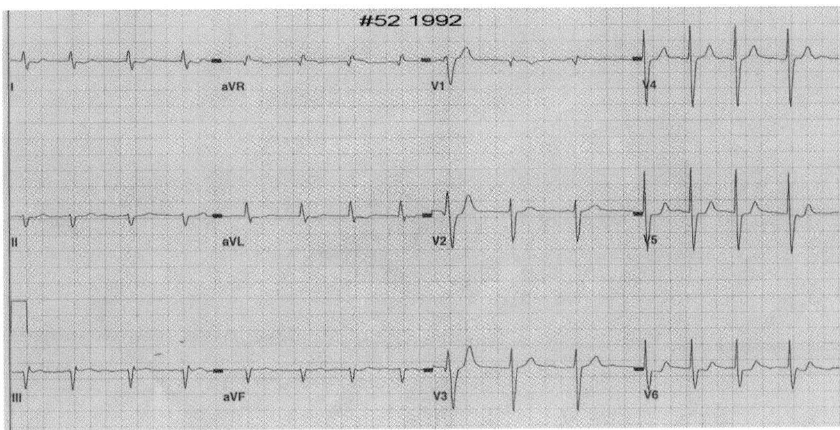

Figure 48.1 ECG 1992.

4 Chest X rays 1990 and 1992

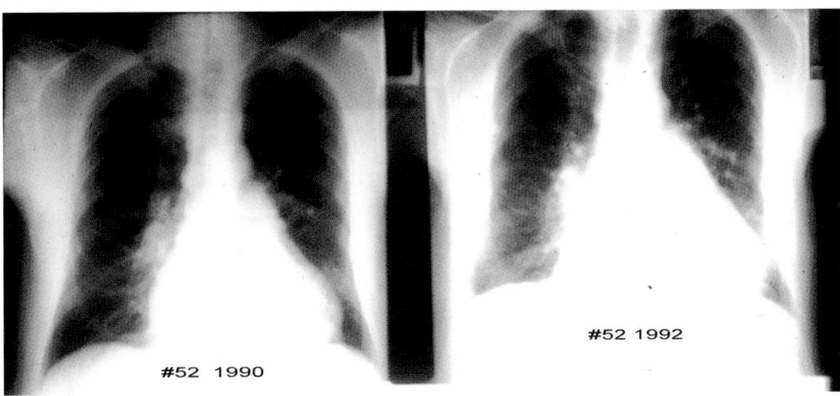

Figure 48.2 PA chest X rays 1990 and 1990.

5 Echocardiography 1992

Table 48.1 Echocardiographic data 1992

Marked enlargement of RA and RV	
Dimensions	
LA	5.8 cm
LV end-diastolic dimension	4.4 cm
LV end-systolic dimension	3.8 cm
Normal LV septal thickness	
Reduced LV ejection fraction	
ASD diameter	2.5 cm
1+/4+ tricuspid regurgitation	
1+/4+ mitral regurgitation	
Doppler flow velocity across tricuspid valve	2.8 m/sec

6 Nuclear medicine data 1992

Table 48.2 Nuclear medicine data 1992

MUGA LV ejection fraction	41%
LV septal hypokinesia	

7 Hemodynamic data 1992

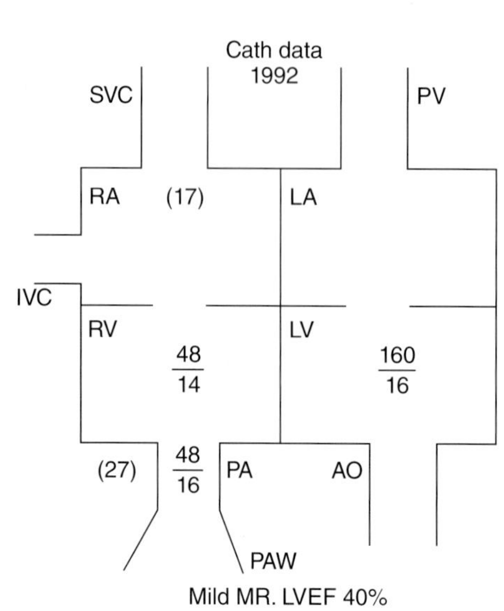

Figure 48.3 Hemodynamic data 1992.

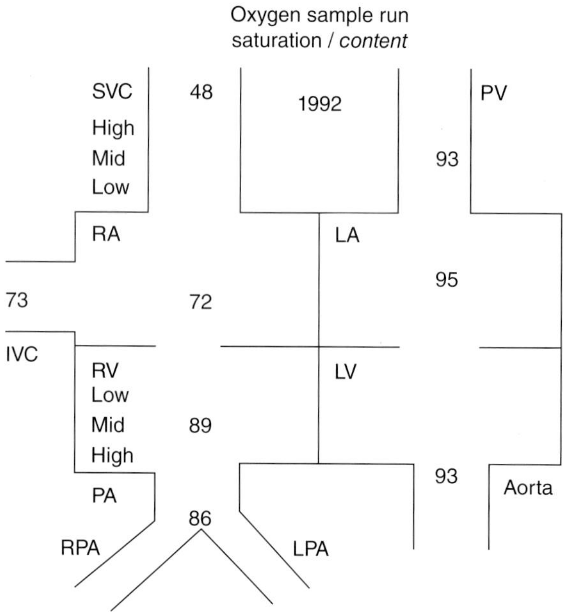

Figure 48.4 Oxygen sample run 1992.

What is your diagnosis?

8 Course 1992–1995

The patient's heart failure in 1992 was treated with digoxin and diuretics.

A 3 × 5.5 cm ASD was closed by direct suture and he underwent successful three-vessel coronary artery bypass surgery.

9 History 1995

The patient was admitted to our hospital with dyspnea and edema for 2 months.

10 Physical examination 1995

79-year-old, 74 inches tall, 190 lb male.
BP 150/80. HR 70/min irregular.
Prominent 'v' wave in jugular venous pulse.
Apex 6th interspace, 14 cm from mid-sternal line (cardiomegaly).
S1 +1 increased. S2 is widely split and varied with respiration.
Grade 2/6 pulmonary ejection systolic murmur.
Grade 2/6 apical pan systolic murmur.
Trace leg edema.

11 Additional laboratory data 1995

He exercised for only 4 min on the Bruce protocol ~ functional class 3.

12 Chest X ray 1995

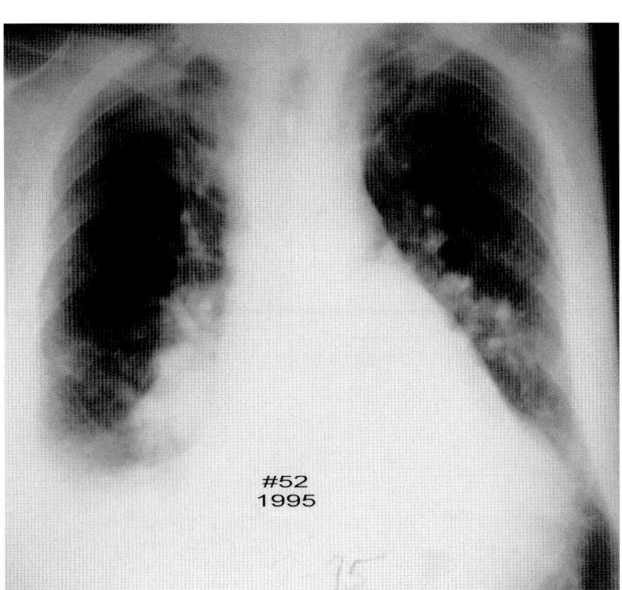

Figure 48.5 Chest X ray PA view 1995.

Figure 48.6 Right lung field of Figure 48.5 1995.

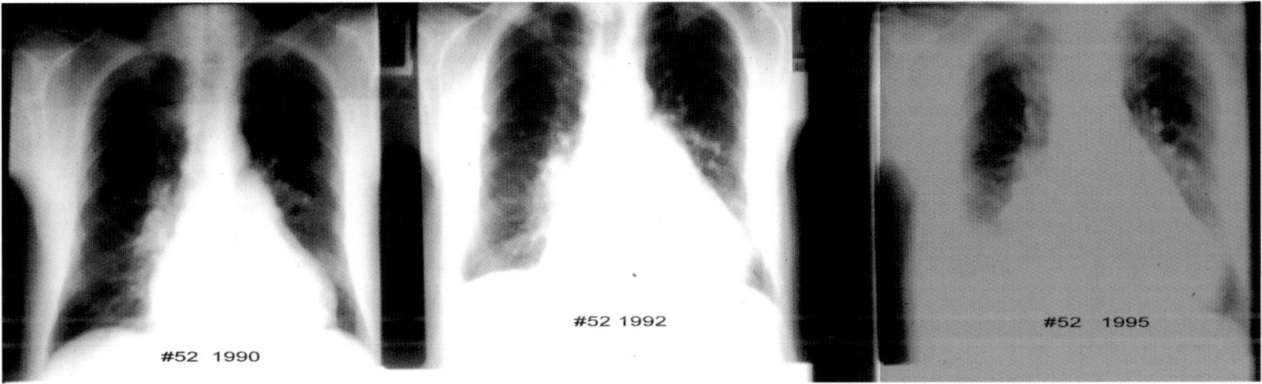

Figure 48.7 Chest X rays PA view: 1990, 1992, and 1995 compared.

13 ECG 1995

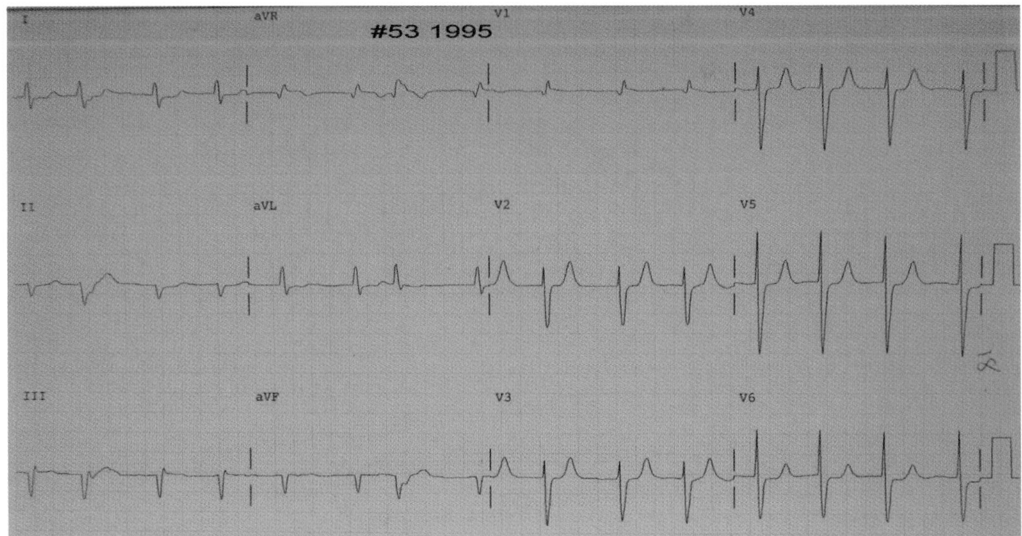

Figure 48.8 ECG 1995.

14 Hemodynamic data 1995

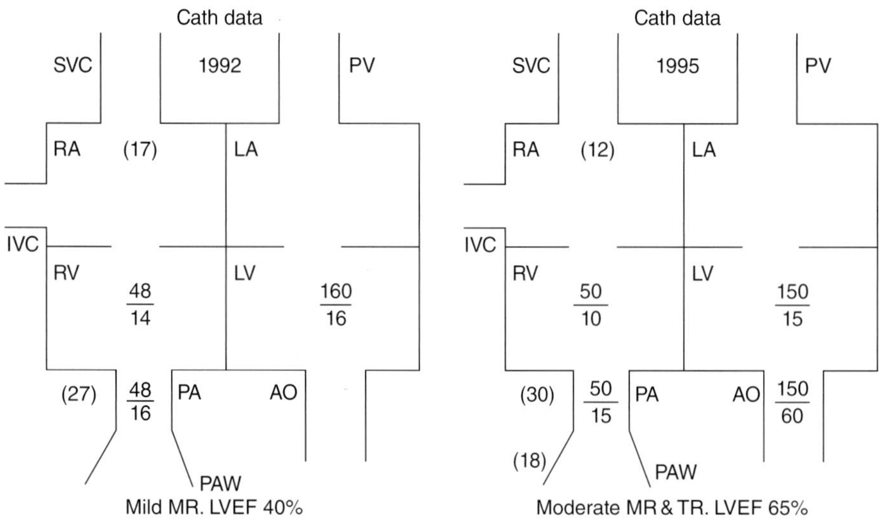

Figure 48.9 1992 and 1995 pressures compared. MR, mitral regurgitation; TR, tricuspid regurgitation; EF, LV ejection fraction.

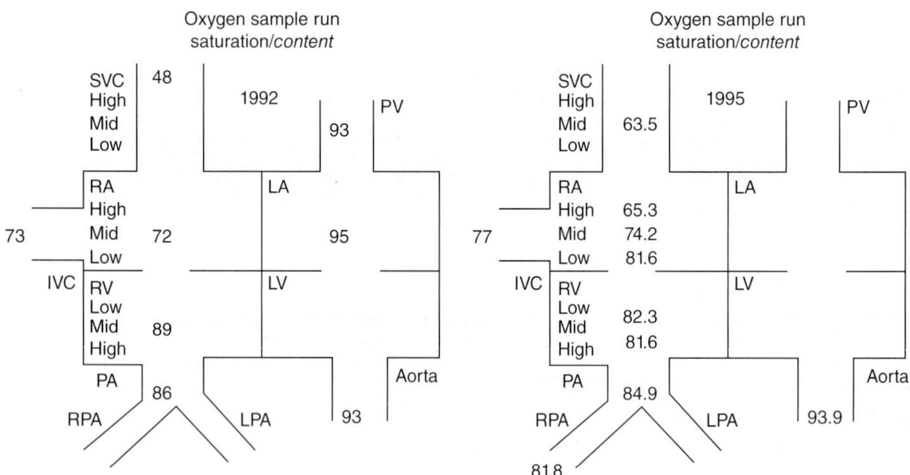

Figure 48.10 1992 and 1995 oxygen sample runs compared

15 Echocardiographic data 1995 (pre- and postoperative)

Table 48.3 Echocardiographic data 1992–1998

Measurement	1992	Feb 1995	Oct 1995	1996	1998
RA and LV	↑↑	↑↑	↑↑	↑↑	↑↑
LA (cm)	5.8	5.9	5.6	6.2	6.8
LVEDD (cm)	4.4		5.0	5.4	6.0
LVESD (cm)	3.8				
LV septum (cm)	normal		1.4	1.4	1.2
Ejection fraction	↓↓		normal	normal	↓
ASD diameter (cm)	2.5	1.4	0	0	0
Doppler data					
TR	+	++			++
TV_v (m/s)	2.8	3.5			3.5
MR	+	++	++	+	+++

LVEDD, LV end-diastolic dimension; LVESD, LV end-systolic dimension; MR, mitral regurgitation; TR, tricuspid regurgitation; TV_v, peak tricuspid flow velocity jet across tricuspid valve; ↑↑, very enlarged; +, mild; ++, moderately severe; ↓↓, moderately decreased; ↓, mildly decreased.

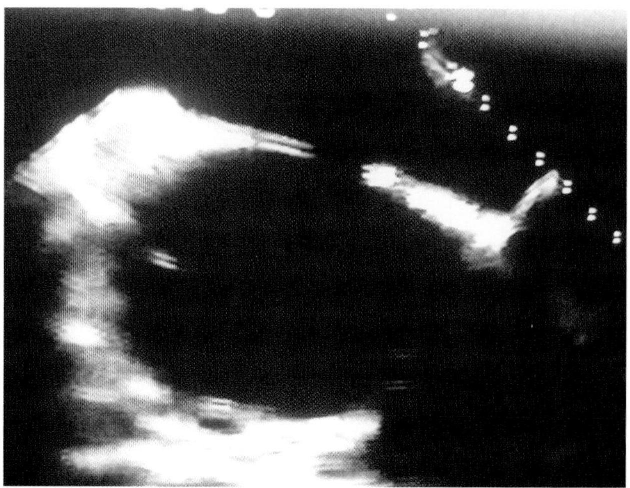

Figure 48.11 TEE 1995 showing ASD.

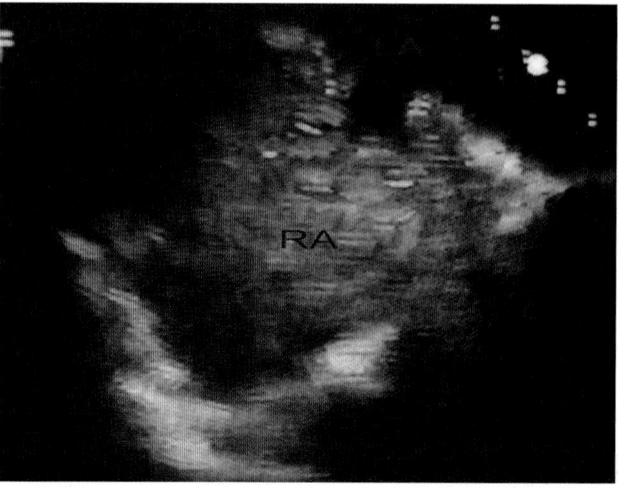

Figure 48.12 Same TEE as in Figure 48.11 showing microbubbles in RA with negative contrast entering RA from LA, indicative of an ASD. The RA is enlarged.

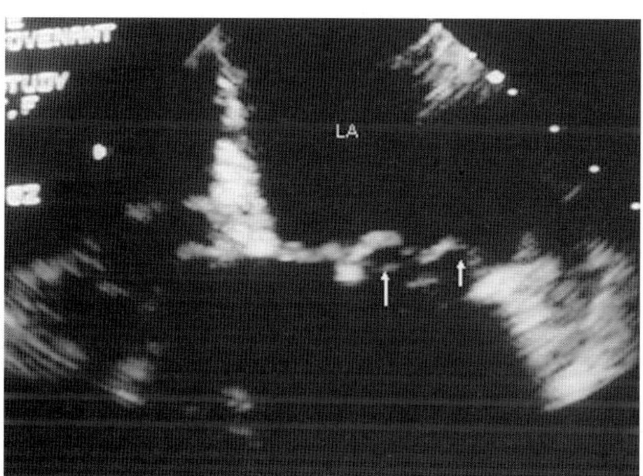

Figure 48.13 TEE 1995 (postoperative) showing enlarged LA with mitral valve prolapse (arrows).

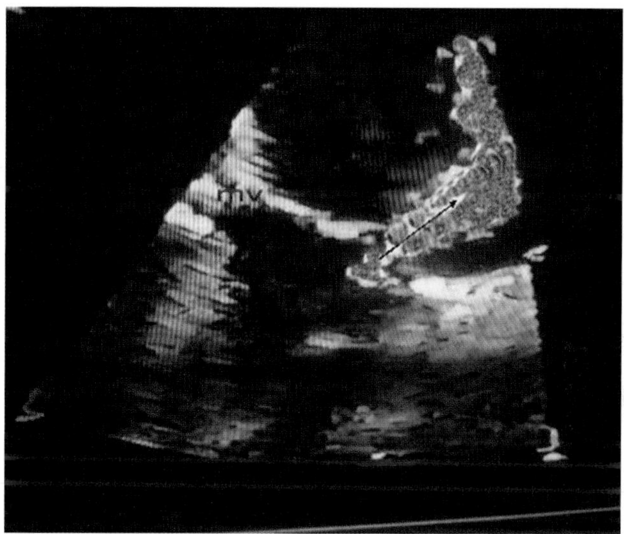

Figure 48.14 TEE 1995 (postoperative) showing an eccentric mitral regurgitant jet (arrow).

16 Course 1995–1999

At surgery in March 1995 a 1 × 2 cm ASD was sutured closed and the mitral valve ring was plicated.

Answers and commentary

1 and 2 History and physical examination 1992

The physical findings of an ASD were initially overlooked at the other hospital, probably because the patient was in severe heart failure. Only when the echocardiogram was performed was it realized that he had an ASD.

3 12-lead ECG 1992

Atrial fibrillation and a single PVC. Rate 75/min. QRS 0.11 s. QRS axis –60°. Deep S in V5.

Impression: above rhythm with IRBBB and left-axis deviation, inferior wall MI.

Incomplete RBBB and left-axis deviation may be seen in primum ASD or secundum ASD with coronary artery disease.

A secundum ASD may be suspected in an elderly patient with atrial fibrillation and RBBB, provided that there is no underlying chronic obstructive lung disease.

4 Chest X rays 1990 and 1992

There is an increase in heart size from 1990 to 1992. The proximal pulmonary arteries are prominent and there is pulmonary plethora (Figure 48.2), which could be due to heart failure and/or a left to right shunt.

5 Echocardiography 1992

This confirmed the presence of a large ASD with RV volume overload, mild tricuspid and mitral regurgitation, and a reduced LV ejection fraction.

6 Nuclear medicine data 1992

The LV ejection fraction is moderately reduced based on the MUGA scan and there was LV septal hypokinesia, reflecting underlying coronary artery disease.

7 Hemodynamic data

In 1992 there is mild pulmonary hypertension (PA mean 27 mmHg) and biventricular dysfunction. The LV systolic function is moderately reduced (LVEF 0.40) with mild mitral regurgitation (Figure 48.3). He had three-vessel coronary artery disease.

In 1992 there is a step up in oxygen saturation in RA compared to SVC.

As the arterial saturation is normal, the likeliest diagnosis is an ASD with a left to right shunt. Calculated Q_p/Q_s ratio = 6/1 (Figure 48.4).

8 Course 1992–1995

The patient did well initially and was in functional class 1 but became symptomatic in 1995.

9 and 10 History and physical examination 1995

The patient returned with symptoms that were compatible with heart failure. On physical examination he had evidence of an ASD with cardiomegaly and widely split S2. The systolic apical murmur could be due to mitral regurgitation and /or tricuspid regurgitation.

11 Additional laboratory data 1995

The patient's exercise tolerance had deteriorated to functional class 3.

12 Chest X ray 1995

The heart size remained enlarged in 1995 compared to 1992 with prominent pulmonary arteries. C/T ratio 0.64.

13 ECG 1995

There is atrial fibrillation with left-axis deviation and IRBBB, as in 1992.

14 Hemodynamic data 1995

In 1995 the mean PA pressure has risen slightly to 30 mmHg compared to 1992. There is still biventricular dysfunction (? diastolic). The LV systolic function is now normal (LVEF 65%) with moderately severe mitral and tricuspid regurgitation.

The improvement in LV ejection fraction in 1995 compared to 1992 reflects an improvement in myocardial perfusion following coronary artery bypass surgery.

There is evidence of a left to right shunt at atrial level with a pulmonary/systemic flow ratio of 3/1 (Figure 48.10).

15 Echocardiographic data 1995

Preoperatively (1995) there is a 1.4 cm sized ASD, and moderate mitral and tricuspid regurgitation. The LA is moderately enlarged.

Impression: the ASD has reopened.

Postoperatively in March 1995 (Figures 48.13 and 48.14) there is evidence of mitral valve prolapse and Doppler flow evidence of mitral regurgitation.

16 Course 1995–1999

The patient was discharged on bumex, digoxin, and warfarin, and followed in the office from 1995 to 1999. His exercise tolerance improved and he was walking 1–2 miles a day without dyspnea or chest pain.

On physical examination he still had cardiomegaly (CT ratio 0.63 in 1995 and 0.56 in 1997), absence of a pulmonary flow murmur, a widely split S2 that was occasionally fixed, and a grade 1–2/6 apical systolic murmur.

After a successful closure of an ASD, the pulmonary flow murmur usually is less intense rather than disappearing altogether. The splitting of the second sound remains wide but not fixed and cardiomegaly lessens [1].

This patient developed incipient heart failure in 1997 that improved when enalapril was added as an afterload reducing agent.

Serial echocardiograms (Table 48.3) showed persistence of pulmonary hypertension (based on tricuspid Doppler flow velocity studies) and some increase in mitral regurgitation. Despite these findings the patient remained in functional class 1.

In 1999 the patient at age 84 went into a retirement center still in functional class 1.

Discussion

When an ASD is detected in patients over 65 years old they usually present with dyspnea (as in this patient) and less often with angina [2]. They usually have atrial fibrillation, RBBB, and rarely pulmonary hypertension [2]. The patient's ASD at surgery was very large (3 × 5.5 cm) and part of the lower sutured area probably gradually dehisced because of his large RA. An ASD may reopen after surgical closure in 2–6% of patients [3, 4] but not always [5].

Significant mitral regurgitation may occur in patients with an ASD due to either mitral valve prolapse [6] or non-specific thickening of the mitral valve [7, 8].

Non-specific thickening of the mitral valve leaflets may be because friction develops between the anterior and posterior mitral leaflets due to abnormal LV motion secondary to RV volume overload [8].

In this patient the mitral regurgitation was due to mitral valve prolapse. Mitral regurgitation temporarily improved after surgical plication of the valve but then became worse based on the development of mild dyspnea, a gradual increase in the grade of the mitral systolic murmur, and an increase in the LA and ventricular dimensions.

Up to 27% of patients (20 out of 74) had an increase in severity or new onset of mitral regurgitation following ASD repair [9] .One explanation of worsening of mitral regurgitation following an ASD repair is that there was poor coaptation and tethering of the mitral valve due to the restricted motion of the posterior leaflet (? fibrosis) in addition to further geometric changes of the LV after ASD closure [10].

Key points

1. An ASD can be overlooked in elderly patients in the presence of severe heart failure.
2. Patch closure of an ASD may be preferable to direct suture closure in the presence of a large RA.
3. Reopening of a surgically closed ASD can occur in 2–6% of cases.
4. Mitral regurgitation may occur or become more severe after ASD closure.

References

[1] Saksena FB, Aldridge HE. Atrial septal defect in the older patient: a clinical and hemodynamic study in patients over the age of 35. *Circulation* 1970; 42: 1009–1019.

[2] Rodstein M, Zeman FD, Gerber IE. Atrial septal defect in the aged. *Circulation* 1961; 23: 665–674.

[3] Fiore AC, Naunheim KS, Kessler KA et al. Surgical closure of atrial septal defect in patients older than 50 years of age (51 patients operated on age range 50–77). *Arch Surg* 1988; 123: 965–967.

[4] Valdes-Cruz LM, Pieroni DR, Jones M et al. Residual shunting in the early postoperative period after closure of atrial septal defect: echocardiographic comparison of patch materials. *J Thorac Cardiovasc Surg* 1982; 84: 73–76.

[5] Horvath KA, Burke RP, Collins Jr JJ. Surgical treatment of adult atrial septal defect. *J Am Coll Cardiol* 1992; 20: 1156–1159 (166 patients, mean age 44 years, 20-year follow-up).

[6] Kestelli M. Mitral valve prolapse in atrial septal defect. *Internet J Cardiol* 2002; 1.DOI:10.5580/1eb5.

[7] Boucher CA, Liberthson RR, Buckley MJ. Secundum atrial septal defect and significant mitral regurgitation: incidence, management and morphologic basis. *Chest* 1979; 75: 697–702.

[8] Furuta S, Wanibuchi Y, Aoki K. Etiology of mitral regurgitation in secundum atrial septal defect. *Jpn Circ J* 1982; 46: 346–351.

[9] Yoshida S, Numata S, Tsutsumi Y et al. Mitral valve regurgitation after atrial septal defect repair in adults. *J Heart Valve Dis* 2014; 23: 310–315 (20 of 74 patients had new onset or worsening of mitral regurgitation following ASD repair. These patients' preoperative risk factors: age >50, atrial fibrillation and $Qp/Qs > 2.89$.)

[10] Nishiga M, Izumi C, Matsutani H et al. A case of significantly increased mitral regurgitation early after atrial septal defect closure. *J Echocardiography* 2012; 10: 69–71.

Further reading

Webb G, Gatzoulis MA. Atrial septal defects in the adult. *Circulation* 2006; 114: 1645–1653.

49 PATIENT STUDY 49

Sequence of data presentation

1 History 1982
↓
2 Physical examination 1982
↓
3 Laboratory data 1982
↓
4 Course May to July 1984
↓
5 Echocardiogram July 1984
↓
6 Chest X ray July 1984
↓
7 Hemodynamic data July 1984
↓
8 Diagnosis
↓
9 Surgery and outcome

1 History 1982

This 37-year-old Asian female had an episode of dyspnea and chest pain in 1974 that subsided spontaneously. She had her first syncopal episode in 1979. In 1982 she was hospitalized because of several episodes of syncope each associated with chest pain, dyspnea, and dizziness.

2 Physical examination 1982

BP 130/80. Pulse 70/min. R 18/min. T 98.7°F.
Apex beat was in the 5th interspace just medial to the left mid-clavicular line.
S1 normal. S2 normal. No S3.
Grade 2/6 high-pitched apical systolic murmur.

3 Laboratory data 1982

Non-specific ST T wave changes on ECG.
No abnormalities found on M-mode or two-dimensional echocardiography.
Normal cardiac enzymes, 24 Holter monitor, upper GI X rays, V/Q lung scan, and CT of brain.

4 Course May to July 1984

1. The patient was hospitalized in May 1984 with exertional dyspnea that was attributed to congestive heart failure. M-mode echocardiogram showed only mitral valve thickening and a small pericardial effusion.
2. She was rehospitalized in June 1984 with exertional dyspnea.

Physical examination June 1984

BP 108/78. HR 90/min. R 40 /min. T 99.2°F.
The jugular venous pressure was increased.

Patient Studies in Valvular, Congenital, and Rarer Forms of Cardiovascular Disease: An Integrative Approach, First Edition. Franklin B. Saksena.

Companion Website: www.wiley.com/go/saksena/patientstudies

Apex beat was 2 cm to the left of the mid-clavicular line in the 6th interspace.
Apical S3.
Grade 3/6 apical systolic murmur that radiated to the axilla.
No pericardial friction rub. Crackles heard over both lung fields.

Laboratory data June 1984

Hemoglobin 10.9 g%. WBC 7400 mm^3. ESR 60 mm/h. Platelets 106,000 mm^{-3}.
EKG: non-specific ST T wave changes.
Chest X ray: cardiomegaly and pulmonary congestion.
Two-dimensional echocardiogram ? LV mass.

What is the diagnosis?

3. She was transferred to our hospital on 20 July 1984 for further evaluation.

What is the course of treatment?

Comment on what was found at surgery (Figure 49.5).

---

5 Echocardiogram July 1984

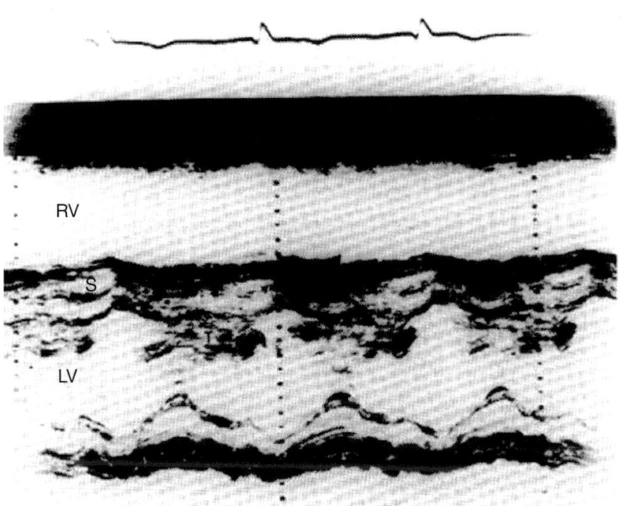

Figure 49.1 M-mode echocardiogram. Source: Ghali J, Saksena FB, Santhanam V et al. (1988). Reproduced with permission of Mary Ann Liebert Inc.

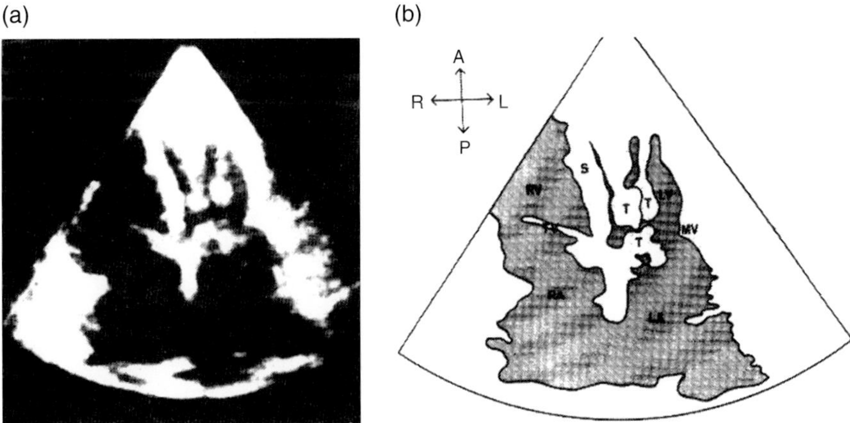

Figure 49.2 (a) Two-dimensional echocardiogram showing the four-chamber view. (b) Diagram of two-dimensional echocardiogram shown in (a). MV, mitral valve; S, septum; TV, tricuspid valve. Source: Ghali J, Saksena FB, Santhanam V et al. (1988). Reproduced with permission of Mary Ann Liebert Inc.

What is T?

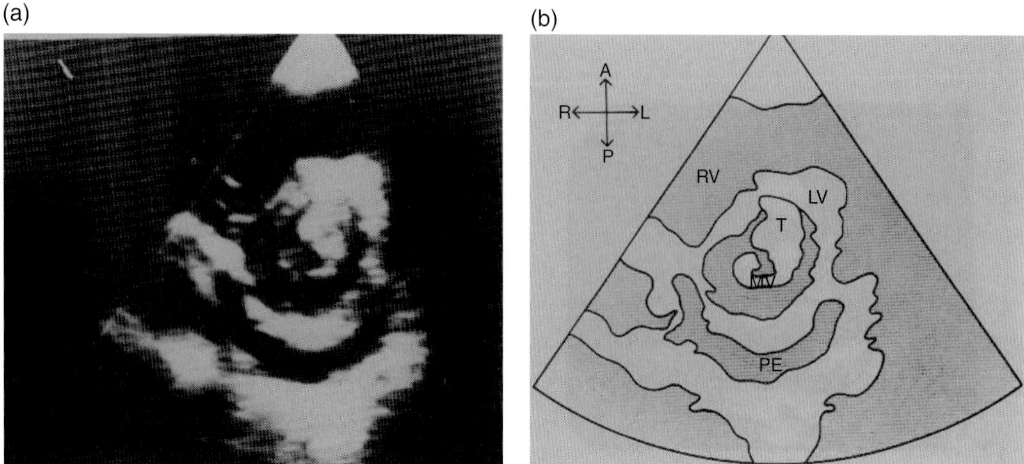

Figure 49.3 (a) Two-dimensional echocardiogram showing short-axis view of the LV. T, tumor mass. (b) Diagram of the two-dimensional echocardiogram depicted in (a). Source: Ghali J, Saksena FB, Santhanam V et al. (1988). Reproduced with permission of Mary Ann Liebert Inc.

Table 49.1 Echocardiographic measurements

Site	Measurement (cm)	Normal values
Aortic root (diastole)	3.1	2.0–3.7
LA	4.5	1.9–4.0
RV end-diastolic dimension	2.5	0.7–2.3
LV end-diastolic dimension	5.0	3.6–5.6
LV end-systolic dimension	3.5	1.8–4.2
LV septum	1.5	0.6–1.1
LV posterior wall	1.4	0.6–1.1

6 Chest X ray July 1984

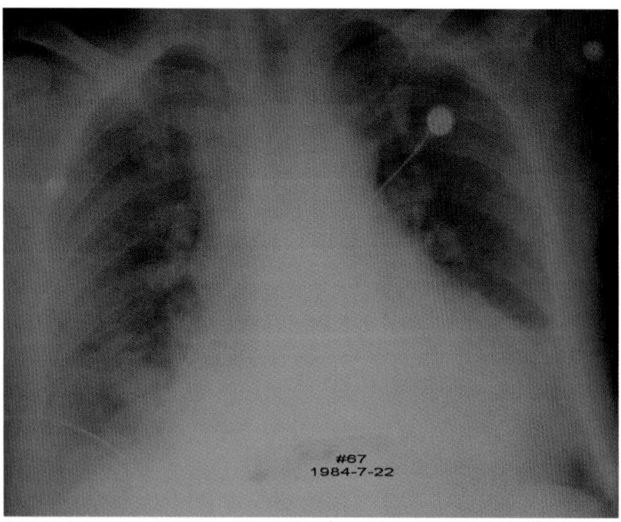

Figure 49.4 Chest X ray 22 July 1984.

7 Hemodynamic data July 1984

Table 49.2 Hemodynamics July 1984

	Pressures (mmHg)
RA	(12)
RV	90/8
PA	86/53
PA wedge	(23)
Cardiac output	1.4 L/min

8 Diagnosis

What is the diagnosis?

What is the treatment?

9 Surgery and outcome

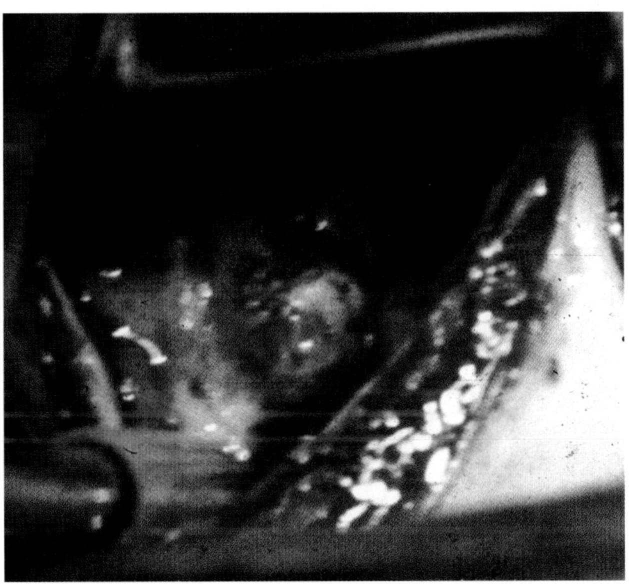

Figure 49.5 The LA has been opened and a large cauliflower-shaped tumor is seen filling it. Source: Ghali J, Saksena FB, Santhanam V et al. (1988). Reproduced with permission of Mary Ann Liebert Inc.

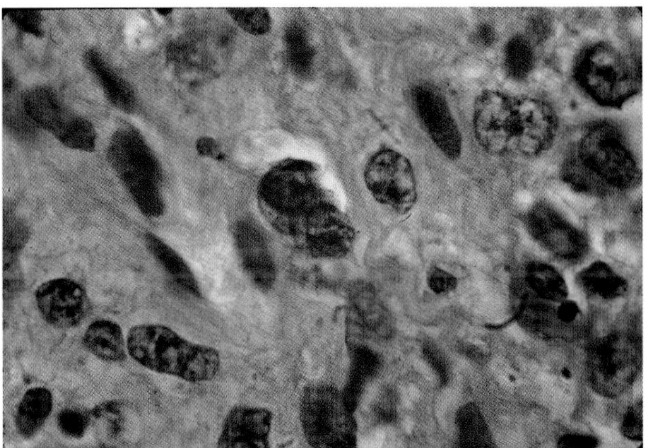

Figure 49.6 Microscopic appearance of tumor. Source: Ghali J, Saksena FB, Santhanam V et al. (1988). Reproduced with permission of Mary Ann Liebert Inc.

Answers and commentary

1–3 History, physical examination, and laboratory data 1982

The patient had recurrent syncope between 1979 and 1982 but no cause for this was initially found. Physical examination and echocardiographic data pointed to mitral valvular disease.

4 Course May to July 1984

She was admitted in May and July 1984 for heart failure based on the high jugular venous pressure, S3, cardiomegaly, and probable worsening of her mitral regurgitation.

She was mildly anemic and had a very high unexplained ESR.

5 Echocardiogram July 1984

Table 49.1 shows an enlarged LA and a mildly enlarged RV. The LV size is normal.

Figure 49.1 is an M-mode echocardiogram showing a tumor (T) in the cavity of a normal sized LV. The RV is dilated.

Figure 49.2a is a two-dimensional echocardiogram showing the four-chamber view of the heart.

Two tumor masses appear to hang down from the LV apex-like stalactites. Another mass appears to blend in with the mitral valve. The LA is enlarged and appears free of tumor.

Figure 49.2b is a diagram of the two-dimensional echocardiogram depicted in Figure 49.2a.

Figure 49.3a is a two-dimensional echocardiogram showing the short-axis view of the LV. Tumor mass is seen blending in with the mitral valve. There is a moderately enlarged pericardial effusion posteriorly.

Figure 49.3b is a diagram of the two-dimensional echocardiogram depicted in Figure 49.3a.

6 Chest X ray July 1984

There is cardiomegaly and some pulmonary vascular congestion.

7 Hemodynamic data July 1984

The patient has severe pulmonary hypertension and a low cardiac output. These findings may be attributed to mitral valve obstruction or LV failure.

8 Diagnosis

An LV tumor causing mitral valve obstruction leading to syncope and severe pulmonary hypertension.

9 Surgery and outcome

At surgery the patient had a large fleshy tumor occupying the entire LA and LV, obstructing the mitral valve and the LV outflow tract.

A frozen section of the tumor was suggestive of a sarcoma. Microscopically the tumor consisted of spindled cells, polygonal cells, and multinucleated giant cells haphazardly arranged in a densely collagenous stroma (Figure 49.6). Most of the tumor cells by electron microscopy were fibroblastic and contained alpha-antichymotrypsin (via immunohistochemical staining). These features are diagnostic of a malignant fibrous histiocytoma.

In an attempt at palliation some of the tumor was excised from the LV outflow tract. It was difficult to wean the patient from the cardiopulmonary bypass machine despite the use of an intra-aortic balloon pump. She died several hours postoperatively. No autopsy was obtained.

Discussion

MFH accounts for 1% of primary malignant tumors of the heart [1]. It usually involves the LA [2, 3] and occasionally the LV, the RV [4] or the pericardium, rarely it spreads to the jejunum [5]. The age ranges from 14 to 77 years old [4].

This patient had MFH that severely encroached on both the LA and the LV, producing severe LV outflow and LV inflow obstruction. These findings accounted for the patient's recurrent syncope and intractable heart failure.

A high ESR has been reported in MFH [3] and was present in this patient.

Two-dimensional echocardiography failed to detect the LA involvement by the tumor. This may be because the vascularity of the tumor may have a similar echogenicity to the blood in the LA [5, 6].

In this patient two-dimensional echocardiography provided the first clue to the diagnosis of a cardiac tumor in the LV. Delineation of an MFH has also been reported with the use of TEE, CT, and MRI [2–4].

MFH is radioresistant, but does respond transiently to chemotherapy [4]. Surgical removal of the tumor is usually followed by recurrence [3].

Key points

1. MFH is a rare cardiac malignancy that may present as syncope or heart failure.
2. MFH usually presents with mitral valve obstruction and/or LV outflow obstruction. It is readily diagnosed by two-dimensional echocardiography or by TEE.
3. MFH is radioresistant and often recurs following surgical removal.

References

[1] McAllister MA, Fenoglio JJ. *Tumors of the cardiovascular system*. In: Atlas of Tumor Pathology, Second Series Fasc 15. Armed Forces Institute of Pathology, Washington DC, 1978, pp 95–98.
[2] Rashidi A, Silverberg ML, McCray RD. Malignant fibrous histiocytoma of the heart. *Echocardiography* 2011; 28: E217–E218.
[3] Yuan S-M, Shinfeld A, Lavee J et al. Imaging morphology of cardiac tumors. *Cardiol J* 2009; 16: 26–35.
[4] Balaceanu A, Mateescu D, Diaconu C et al. Primary malignant fibrous histiocytoma of the right ventricle. Case report and review of the Literature. *J Ultrasound Med* 2010; 29: 655–658.
[5] Ghali J, Saksena FB, Santhanam V et al. Echocardiographic findings in a malignant fibrous histiocytoma of the heart. *J Cardiovasc Ultrason* 1988; 7: 353–358.
[6] Fyke FE III, Seward JB, Edwards WD et al. Primary cardiac tumors: Experience with 30 consecutive patients since the introduction of two-dimensional echocardiography. *J Am Coll Cardiol* 1985; 5: 1465–1473.

Further reading

Felner JM, Knoff WD. Echocardiographic recognition of intracardiac and extracardiac masses. *Echocardiography* 1985; 2: 3–55 (212 references).

50 PATIENT STUDY 50

Sequence of data presentation

1 Echocardiogram
↓
2 Laboratory data
↓
3 History
↓
4 Physical examination
↓
5 Course and treatment
↓
6 Surgical findings and follow-up

1 Echocardiogram

(a)

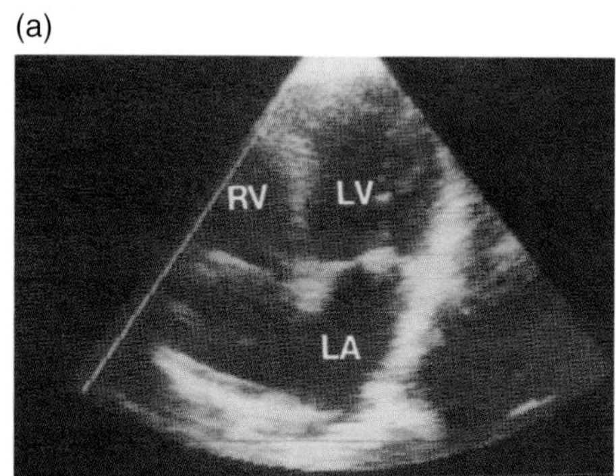

(b)

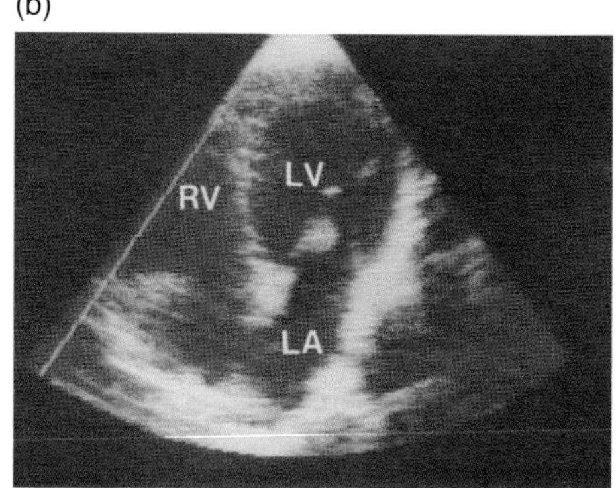

Figure 50.1 Two-dimensional echocardiogram showing an apical four-chamber view of the heart: (a) systolic; (b) diastole. There is a mobile nodule attached to the anterior leaflet of the mitral valve. Source: Saksena FB, Ghali J, Chomka EV, Brundage BL. (1993). Reproduced with permission of Mary Ann Liebert Inc.

2 Laboratory data

Normal ECG.
Six blood cultures failed to grow any organisms.
CT of head did not show any intracranial bleeding.

3 History

33-year-old man admitted to hospital following a grand mal seizure (1985).

4 Physical examination

The patient was stuporose. BP 130/94. Pulse 64/min. Respiratory rate 24/min. T 97.7°F.
No cardiac abnormalities noted. Peripheral pulses were normal.
There was a left-sided facial weakness, left hemiplegia, and subsequently an expressive aphasia.

Patient Studies in Valvular, Congenital, and Rarer Forms of Cardiovascular Disease: An Integrative Approach, First Edition. Franklin B. Saksena.

Companion Website: www.wiley.com/go/saksena/patientstudies

5 Course

The patient was placed on anticoagulants and his neurological deficits cleared in 2 days.

6 Surgical findings and follow-up

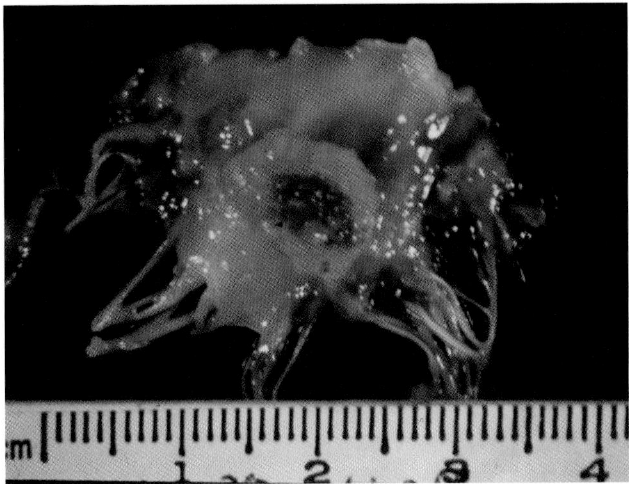

Figure 50.2 There is a 1.2 × 0.9 × 0.8 cm yellow mass and a thrombus attached to the surgically excised mitral valve. Source: Saksena FB, Ghali J, Chomka EV, Brundage BL. (1993). Reproduced with permission of Mary Ann Liebert Inc.

Answers and commentary

1 Echocardiogram

A mobile 5 mm echo-dense nodule was seen on the atrial side of the anterior mitral valve leaflet that was initially diagnosed as a vegetation (31 August 1985).

2 Laboratory data

The diagnosis of endocarditis appeared less likely as the patient had no murmurs, was afebrile, and had six negative blood cultures. He could have a tumor or a thrombus on the mitral valve.

3 and 4 History and physical examination

A stroke in a young patient could be due to an embolism arising from (i) the left heart due to a thrombus or a tumor or (ii) a blood clot from the leg entering the systemic circulation via a patent foramen ovale.

5 Course and treatment

His rapid response to anticoagulants implied that his hemiplegia was due to thrombo-embolism.

6 Surgical findings and follow-up

A 1.2 × 0.9 × 0.8 cm mass was removed from the mitral valve (13 September 1985), consisting of a polyp and fresh thrombus. Histologically the polyp was a papillary fibroma.

The mitral valve was replaced with a 29 mm Hemex Duromedics valve. He had an uneventful recovery.

Discussion

Papillary fibroma is the second most common benign tumor of the heart, occurring in 1–8% of all cardiac tumors [1]. It is usually pedunculated and is attached to the aortic or mitral valves. Rarely it may involve the right and left heart valves [2] or be localized to the LV septum [3]. Papillary fibroma may occur at any age and the sex ratio is about equal [4].

While this tumor is often found incidentally either at autopsy or operation its presence should be considered in the setting of an echo dense nodule on a left-sided valve and peripheral embolism (brain, coronary artery, leg).

This patient had a cerebral embolism originating from a thrombus on the mitral valve since his neurologic deficit cleared rapidly on anticoagulant therapy. Cerebral emboli of tumor origin are uncommon in papillary fibroma, as the latter are more firmly adherent to the valve than are thrombi [1].

Two-dimensional echocardiography can detect a nodule ≤2 mm in diameter and as such is a very sensitive method of detecting a papillary fibroma. However, echocardiography cannot distinguish such a nodule from a thrombus or an atrial myxoma. Other modalities such as ultrafast cine CT, TEE, three-dimensional echocardiography, or MRI may also play a role in evaluating cardiac masses [1, 4].

Early surgical removal is warranted as a papillary fibroma has a high incidence of embolism [1, 3–5].

The prognosis is excellent and recurrences have not been reported so far [3, 5].

Key points

1. Papillary fibroelastoma is the second most common benign tumor of the heart.
2. It usually involves the mitral or aortic valves as a small pedunculated mass.
3. Papillary fibroelastoma is readily detected by two-dimensional echocardiography. A tissue diagnosis is required to distinguish a papillary fibroelastoma from a vegetation or a blood clot.
4. Early surgical removal is warranted as papillary fibroelastoma has a tendency to embolize.

References

[1] Saksena FB, Ghali J, Chomka EV, Brundage BL. The diagnosis of papillary fibroma of the mitral valve by two-dimensional echocardiography and ultrafast cine-computed tomography. *J Cardiovasc Diagn and Proc* 1993; 11: 135–140.

[2] Vittala SS, Click RL, Challa S et al. Multiple papillary fibroelastomas. *Circulation* 2012; 126: 242–243.

[3] Saxena P, Shehatha J, Naran A et al. Papillary fibroelastoma of the interventricular septum. Mimicking a cardiac myxoma. *Tex Heart Inst J* 2010; 37: 119–120.

[4] Jha NK, Khouri M, Murphy DM et al. Papillary fibroelastoma of the aortic valve – a case report and literature review. *J Cardiothorac Surg* 2010; 5: 84–88.

[5] Sun JP, Asher CR, Yang XS et al. Clinical and echocardiographic characteristics of papillary fibroelastomas. A retrospective and prospective study in 162 patients. *Circulation* 2001; 103: 2687–2693.

51 PATIENT STUDY 51

Sequence of data presentation

1 History
↓
2 Physical examination
↓
3 Laboratory data
↓
4 ECG
↓
5 Chest X ray
↓
6 Echocardiogram
↓
7 CT of chest
↓
8 Cardiac catheterization
↓
9 Surgical results
↓
10 Follow-up

1 History

44-year-old female with a history of chest pain and dyspnea for 2 days. No history of deep vein thrombosis in the legs.

No history of drug, alcohol, or tobacco misuse.

2 Physical examination

65 inches tall female weighing 165 lb. BP 160/90. HR 100/min. T 97.9°F.

Lungs clear to percussion and auscultation.

No cardiomegaly or murmurs.

Trace of leg edema.

3 Laboratory data

Normal CBC and complete metabolic profile.

pO_2 58 mmHg. Arterial saturation 90%. pH 7.41. pCO_2 35 mmHg.

Troponin 0.03. D-dimer 855.

Patient Studies in Valvular, Congenital, and Rarer Forms of Cardiovascular Disease: An Integrative Approach, First Edition. Franklin B. Saksena.

Companion Website: www.wiley.com/go/saksena/patientstudies

4 ECG

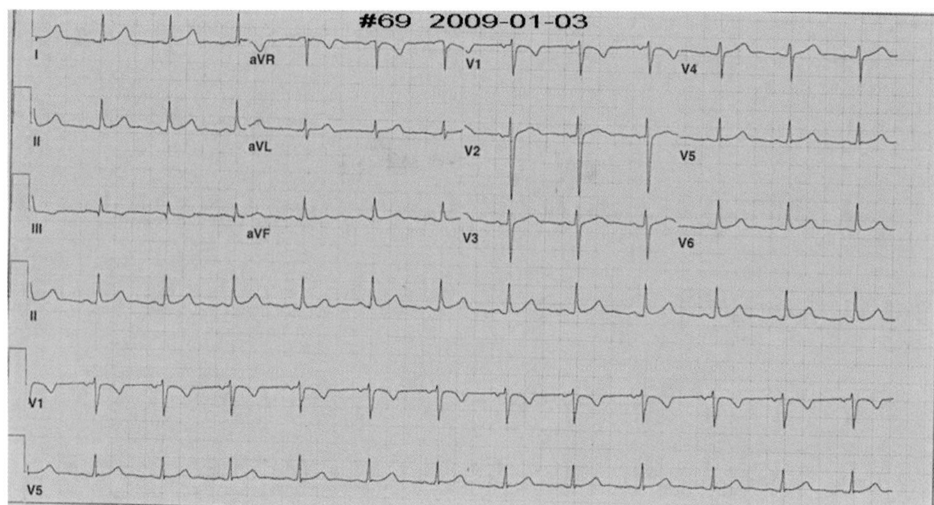

Figure 51.1 12-lead ECG 3 January 2009.

5 Chest X ray

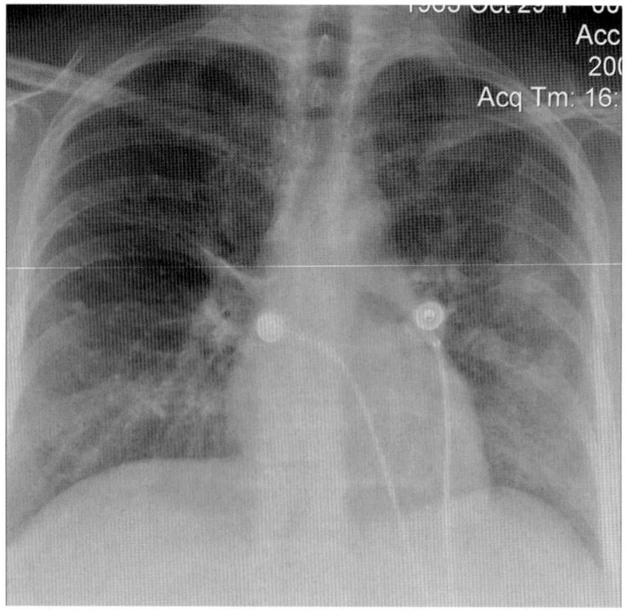

Figure 51.2 Chest X ray 30 December 2008.

6 Echocardiogram

Table 51.1 Echocardiographic data 31 December 2008 (pre-operative) and 16 January 2009 (postoperative)

(a) Pre-operative and postoperative dimensions (cm)

Site	Pre-operative	Postoperative	Normal values
Aortic root	3.21	3.13	2.0–3.7
LA	4.03	4.13	1.9–4.0
LV septum (diastole)	1.14	1.20	0.6–1.1
LV end diastolic	4.29	4.47	3.6–5.6
LV post wall	1.14	1.07	0.6–1.1

Table 51.1 *(Continued)*

(b) Additional data

Measurement	Pre-operative	Postoperative	Normal value
RV systolic pressure	45 mmHg	29 mmHg	<30 mmHg
LV ejection fraction	64%	57%	>55%
HR	86/min	80/min	60–100/min

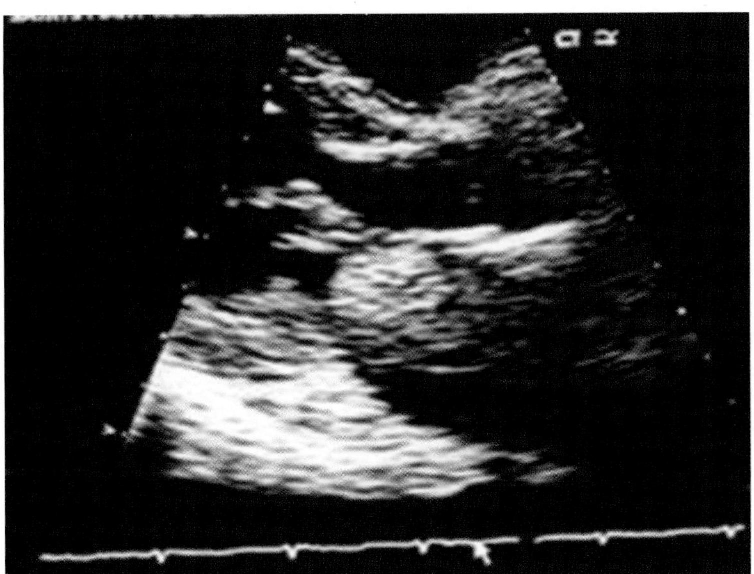

Figure 51.3 Two-dimensional echocardiography long-axis view 31 December 2008.

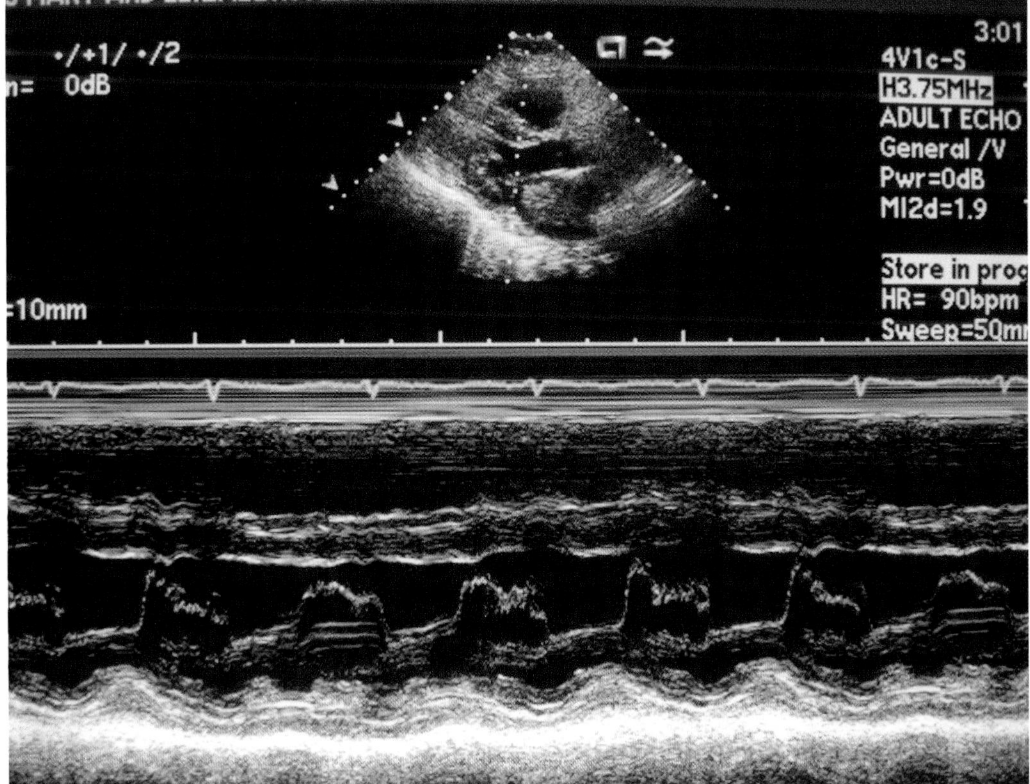

Figure 51.4 Mitral valve echogram 31 December 2008.

7 CT of chest

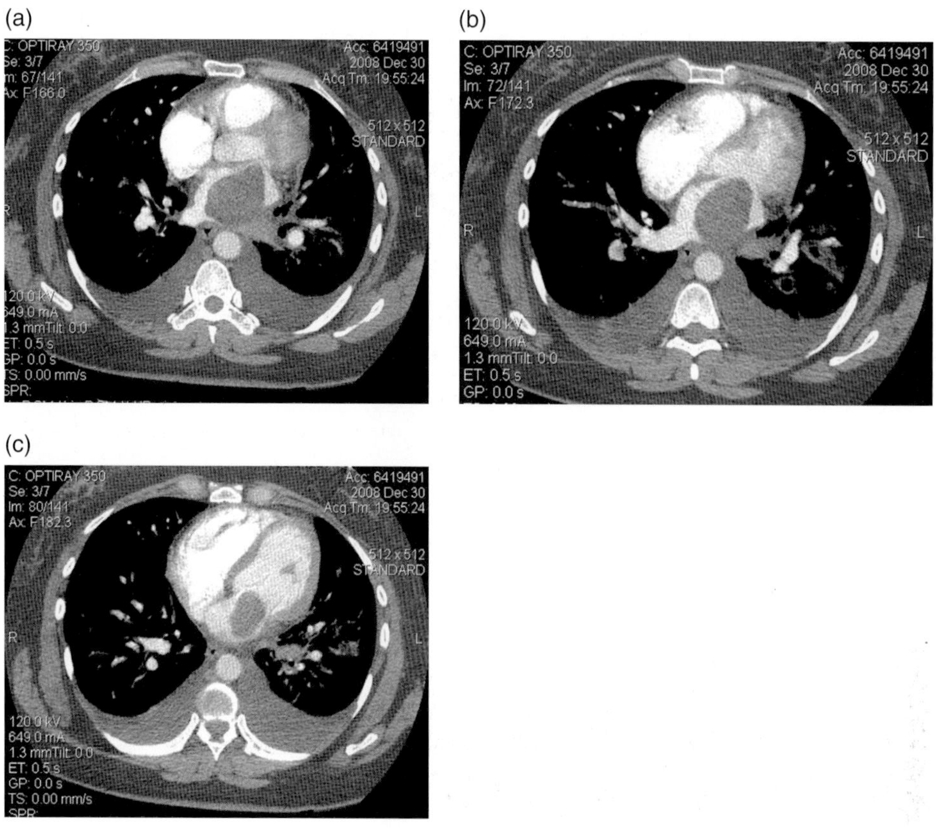

Figure 51.5 CT of chest showing three successive slices from above downwards (Panels a, b, and c).

8 Cardiac catheterization

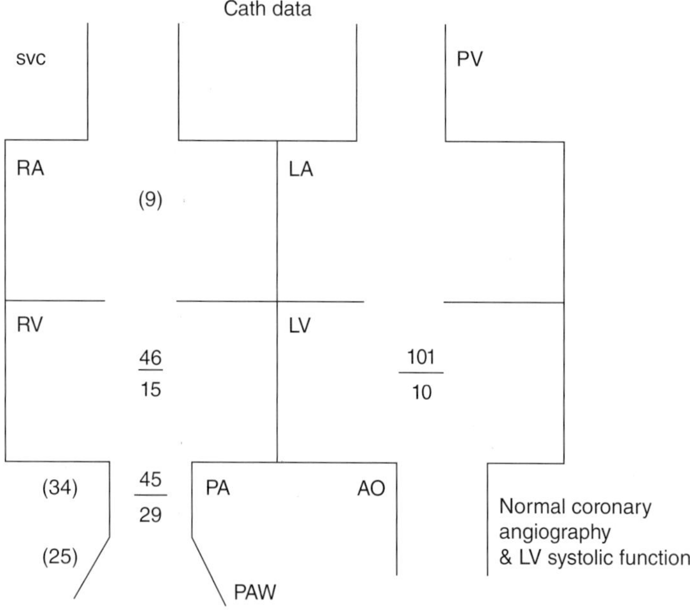

Figure 51.6 Hemodynamic data. Numbers in brackets are mean values in mmHg.

9 Surgical results

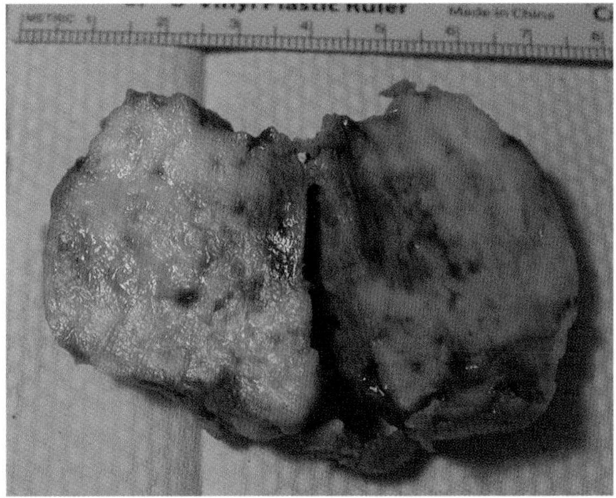

Figure 51.7 Gross appearance of surgically removed tumor.

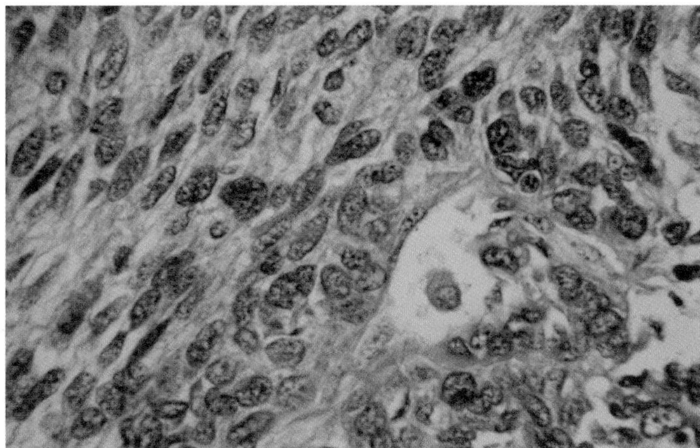

Figure 51.8 Microscopic appearance of tumor.

10 Follow-up

What is the treatment?

Answers and commentary

1 and 2 History and physical examination

The findings are compatible with either a pulmonary embolism or pneumonia.

3 Laboratory data

The arterial blood gases show hypoxemia. The elevation of the d-dimer is a non-specific finding.

4 ECG

Sinus rhythm. Rate 75/min. PR 0.14 s. QRS 0.09 s. QRS axis +40°.
Impression: normal ECG.

5 Chest X ray

Normal heart size with bilateral pulmonary infiltrates compatible with either congestion or pneumonia.

6 Echocardiogram

Preoperatively in Table 51.1 there is borderline LA enlargement, a normal LV ejection fraction, and moderate elevation of the estimated RV systolic pressure.

In Figure 51.3 there is a large mass in the LA that partially blocks the mitral valve. A tissue diagnosis is required to determine the pathology of the mass. The LV is not dilated.

In Figure 51.4 there are linear densities within the mitral valve echogram on the third and seventh beats due to the mass impinging on the mitral leaflets.

7 CT of chest

There is a dense slightly irregular shaped mass occupying most of the LA. It appears to be partially blocking the mitral valve. Panels A and B show the mass extending to the left pulmonary vein, implying that the mass is malignant. No pulmonary embolism was seen on the remainder of the CT examination.

8 Cardiac catheterization

There was moderately severe pulmonary hypertension. The gradient across the mitral valve in diastole was attributed to narrowing of the mitral valve orifice by the tumor.

9 Surgical results

A hard gray yellow mass measuring 5.0 × 3.5 × 3.2 cm and weighing 32 g was removed from the LA. It was attached to the dome of the LA and pulmonary vein. As some of the mass involved the full thickness of the atrial wall not all the tumor could be removed.

There was no tumor involvement of the LA appendage or the mitral valve.

Microscopic examination of the tumor showed pleomorphic spindle-shaped cells consistent with a high-grade undifferentiated sarcoma not further classifiable by extensive immunohistochemical staining techniques.

10 Follow-up

Postoperative echocardiogram

Figure 51.9 shows the disappearance of the linear densities within the mitral valve echogram due to the removal of the tumor. The mitral valve appears normal. There is a small posterior pericardial effusion (PE).

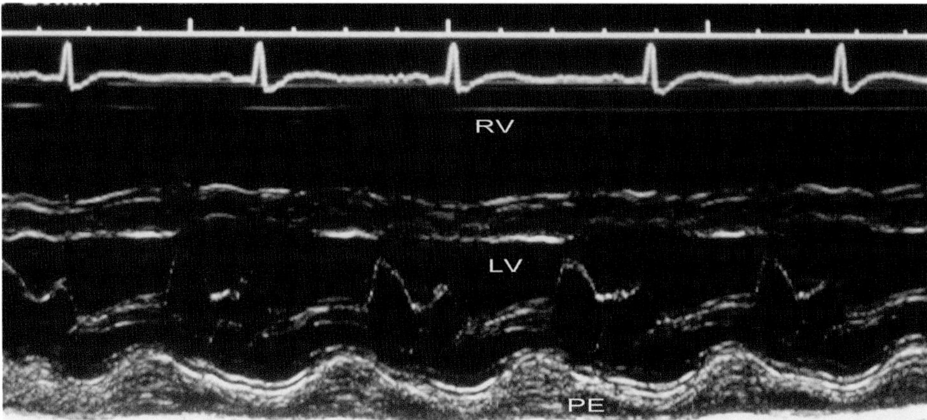

Figure 51.9 Postoperative mitral valve echogram.

Table 51.1 shows that the RV systolic pressure has now fallen to normal limits following the removal of the tumor. The LV ejection fraction remains normal.

The patient remained asymptomatic over the next 9 weeks. MRI of the heart showed residual tumor in the LA. The LV ejection fraction was 60%. The patient was referred to a radiation oncologist, who concluded that she would not benefit from radiation therapy.

Discussion

Primary tumors of the heart are benign in 70% of cases and malignant in 30% of cases [1]. A sarcoma is the most common malignant tumor of the heart. The two most common histological types are an angiosarcoma and an undifferentiated sarcoma [2].

Sarcomas usually occur in the fourth decade of life with an equal sex ratio [2].

The most common sites of an undifferentiated sarcoma are the LA, the pericardium, the RA, and the LV [2]. Thus the patient may present with signs of mitral valve obstruction, pericardial tamponade, heart failure, systemic emboli, or distant metastases [1]. This patient had evidence of mitral valve obstruction, pulmonary hypertension, and pulmonary vascular congestion.

The patient's LA mass was malignant as it was invading the pulmonary veins, as seen on the CT of the chest. This latter finding excludes an LA myxoma [1]. At surgery this mass was an undifferentiated sarcoma. Undifferentiated sarcomas may also invade the renal veins and vena cavae, and spread to the lungs, liver, and bone [2].

Two-dimensional echocardiography is the method of choice in detecting a cardiac tumor [1]. TEE and CT of the chest may be required to better delineate such tumors.

Chemotherapy, radiation, and surgical excision have been attempted in patients with an undifferentiated sarcoma but the results have been dismal. The mean survival time is 10 months [2].

Key points

1. A sarcoma is the most common malignancy of the heart. It has a poor prognosis.
2. A sarcoma is commonly seen in the LA and may metastasize widely, thus distinguishing it from a benign tumor such as a myxoma.
3. A sarcoma may cause mitral valve obstruction, heart failure, or pericardial tamponade.
4. Echocardiography is the definitive way to detect such tumors, but the type of tumor requires a tissue diagnosis.

References

[1] Hsieh P-L, Lee D, Chiou K-R et al. Echocardiographic features of primary cardiac sarcoma. *Echocardiography* 2002; 19: 215–220.
[2] Burke AP, Cowan D, Vermani R. Primary sarcomas of the heart. *Cancer* 1992; 69: 387–395 (75 primary cardiac sarcoma cases).

52 PATIENT STUDY 52

Sequence of data presentation

1 History 2008 → 2 Physical examination → 3 Two-dimensional echocardiogram → 4 Chest X rays → 5 CT of chest → 6 Diagnosis

1–3 History 2008, physical examination, and two-dimensional echocardiogram

80-year-old female diabetic with peripheral vascular disease.
63 inches tall, 158 lb female. BP 127/63. HR 80/min.
Rapid carotid upstroke. No increase in jugular venous pressure.
Apex beat is in the 5th interspace, 10 cm from the mid-sternal line.
No murmurs.
ECG normal.

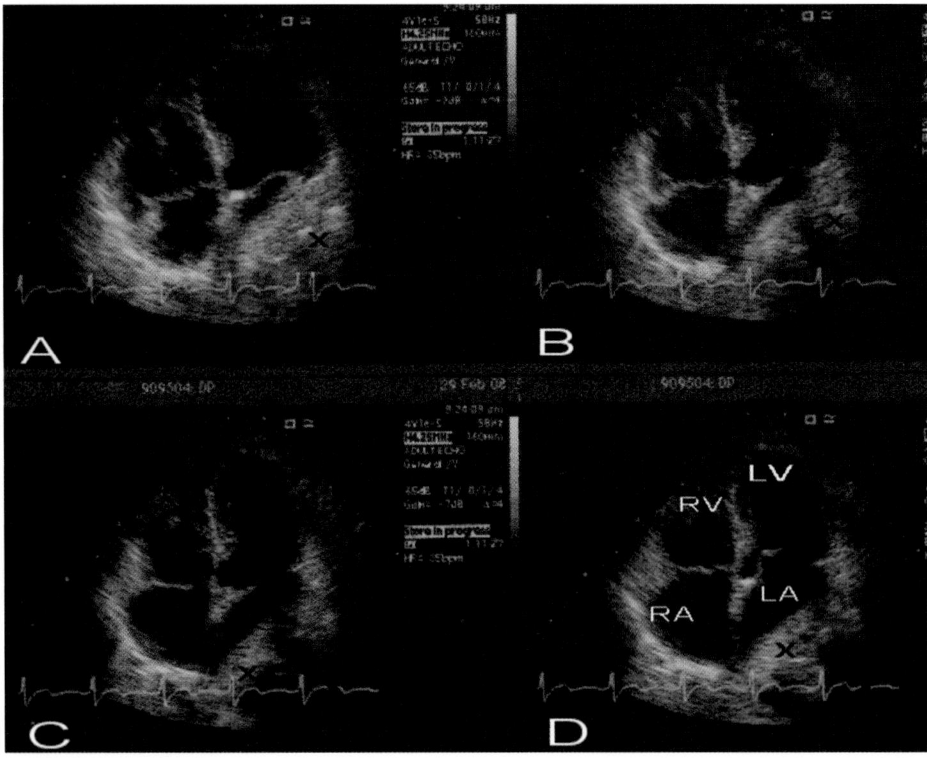

Figure 52.1 Two-dimensional echocardiogram showing four-chamber view of the heart. Panels A to D are four successive frames.
Name the structure labeled x.

Patient Studies in Valvular, Congenital, and Rarer Forms of Cardiovascular Disease: An Integrative Approach, First Edition. Franklin B. Saksena.

Companion Website: www.wiley.com/go/saksena/patientstudies

4 Chest X rays

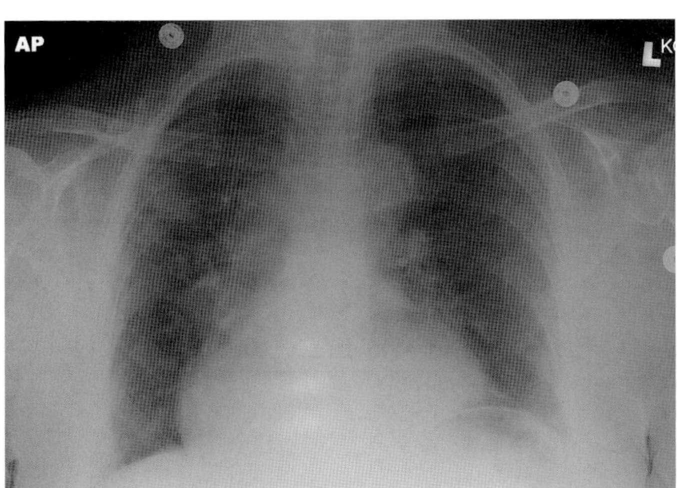

Figure 52.2 PA view of chest.

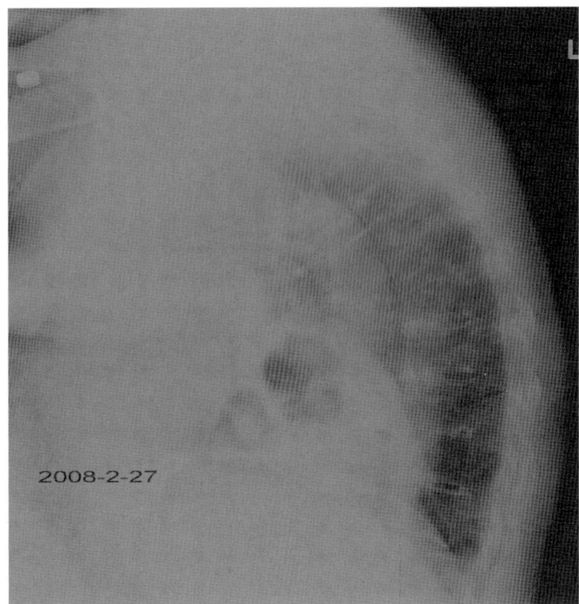

Figure 52.3 Lateral view of chest.

5 CT of chest

(a)

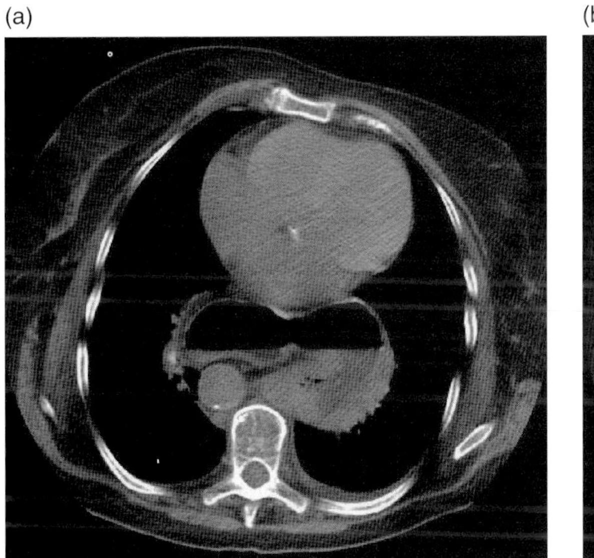

(b)

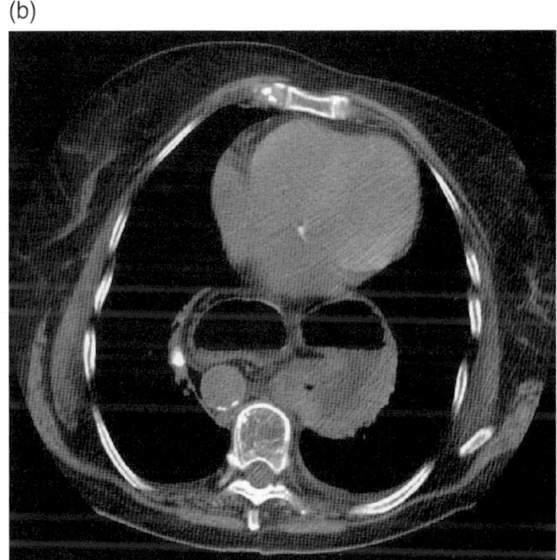

Figure 52.4 Two successive frames of CT of chest.

6 Diagnosis

What is the diagnosis?

Answers and commentary

1 and 2 History 2008 and physical examination

The patient had no cardiac symptoms. Physical examination showed only borderline cardiomegaly.

3 Two-dimensional echocardiogram

In the four-chamber view there is a mass (x) in the LA that is more prominent in systole (panel A) than in diastole (panel D). This mass could be mistaken for an LA tumor. The RA, RV, LV and LA are not enlarged. Normal LV systolic function.

4 Chest X rays

PA view

The heart is shifted to the right and the left diaphragm is higher. The right lung fields are clear. A gastric or bowel shadow is seen under the left diaphragm.

Lateral view

There is a gastric air bubble level in the mid thorax, indicative of a large hiatus hernia.

5 CT of chest

There is a large hiatus hernia pressing on the LA wall and simulating a mass in the LA cavity, as seen in the four-chamber view.

6 Diagnosis

Large hiatus hernia encroaching on the LA, simulating an LA mass.

Discussion

The patient had a large intrathoracic diaphragmatic hiatus hernia encroaching the LA cavity on echocardiography and simulating an LA mass. Carcinoma of the esophagus, metastatic lung cancer, or a descending aortic aneurysm may also appear as masses pressing on the posterior LA wall [1] but are unlikely to be present on clinical grounds and the fact that the patient is alive and well 5 years after the intrathoracic findings were first noted.

In this patient the diagnosis of a hiatus hernia pressing on the LA was confirmed by the lateral chest X ray and CT of the chest.

Other diagnostic echocardiographic features of an intrathoracic hiatus hernia are (i) a slow swirling motion in the hiatus hernia when the patient drinks a carbonated drink, (ii) respiratory variation in the degree of encroachment on the LA, (iii) partial or complete obscuration of the normally sharp sonolucency of the descending aorta in the four-chamber and long-axis views, and (iv) encroachment of the posterobasal LV wall [1].

Some patients with a large hiatus hernia compressing the heart may develop dyspnea on exertion [2] but this was not the case in this patient.

Key points

1. The encroachment of the posterior LA wall by a large hiatus hernia was an incidental finding on echocardiography.
2. The de Cruz criteria help to confirm the diagnosis of a hiatus hernia compressing the LA.
3. The use of a lateral chest X ray and CT of the chest are also useful in excluding other causes of extrinsic compression of the LA (e.g. tumor or aneurysm).

References

[1] D'Cruz IA, Hancock HL. Echocardiographic characteristics of diaphragmatic hiatus hernia. *Am J Cardiol* 1995; 75: 308–310 (20 patients).

[2] Naoum C, Falk GL, Austin CC et al. Left atrial compression and the mechanism of exercise impairment in patients with a large hiatal hernia. *J Am Coll Cardiol* 2011; 58: 1624–1634 (25 of 30 patients with a large hiatal hernia had exertional dyspnea despite normal mean baseline respiratory function. All had relief of symptoms following surgical repair of the hiatal hernia).

53 PATIENT STUDY 53

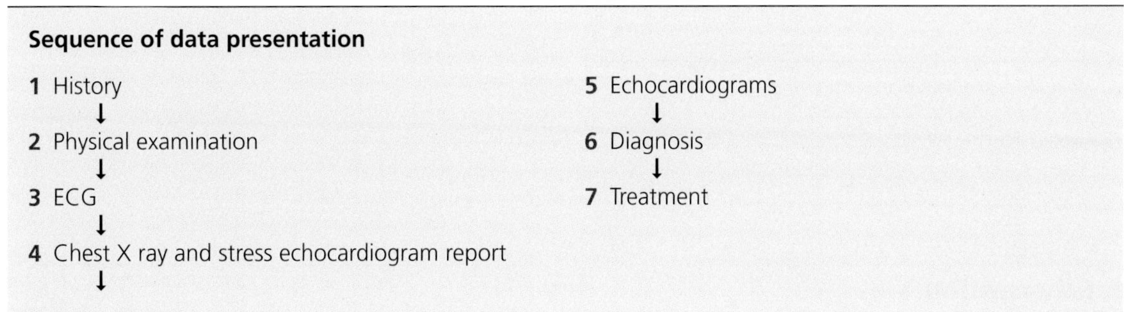

Sequence of data presentation

1 History
↓
2 Physical examination
↓
3 ECG
↓
4 Chest X ray and stress echocardiogram report
↓
5 Echocardiograms
↓
6 Diagnosis
↓
7 Treatment

1 History

42-year-old female with history of palpitations and an abnormal echocardiogram in 2006.

2 Physical examination

67 inches tall, 212 lb female. BP 108/72. HR 76/min regular.
No cardiovascular abnormalities found in 2006 and in 2012.

3 ECG

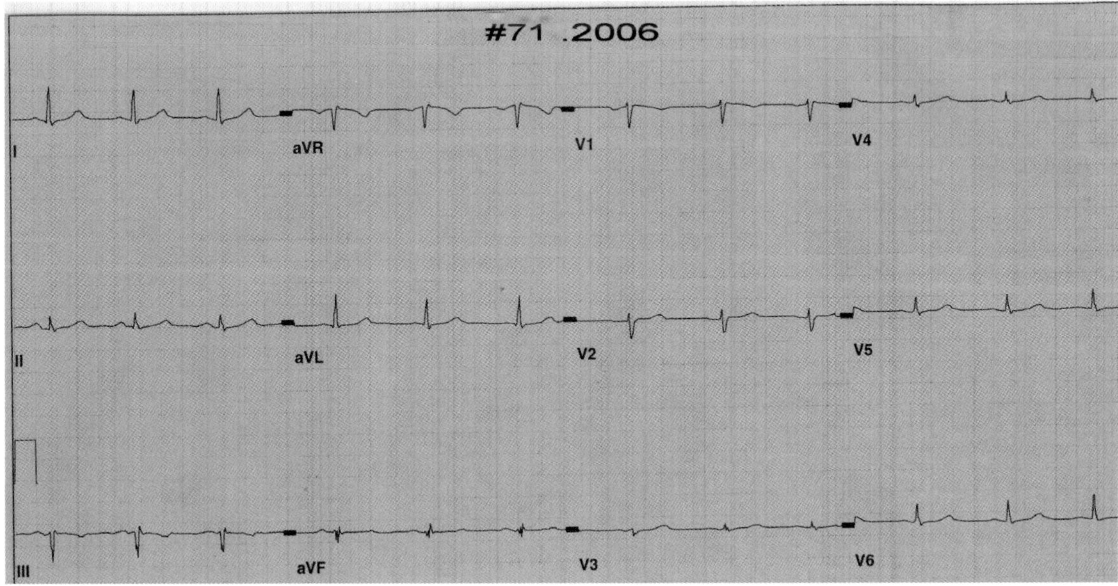

Figure 53.1 12-lead ECG.

Patient Studies in Valvular, Congenital, and Rarer Forms of Cardiovascular Disease: An Integrative Approach, First Edition. Franklin B. Saksena.

Companion Website: www.wiley.com/go/saksena/patientstudies

4 Chest X ray and stress echocardiogram report

Table 53.1 Chest X ray and stress echocardiographic results

	Rest	Exercise
HR	76/min	160/min
BP	108/72	164/80
ECG	normal	normal
LVEF	70%	>70%

1 Chest X ray normal 2006
2 Exercise stress-echocardiogram 2011
Patient exercised for 9 min on Bruce protocol without any ischemic ST changes or regional wall abnormalities

5 Echocardiograms

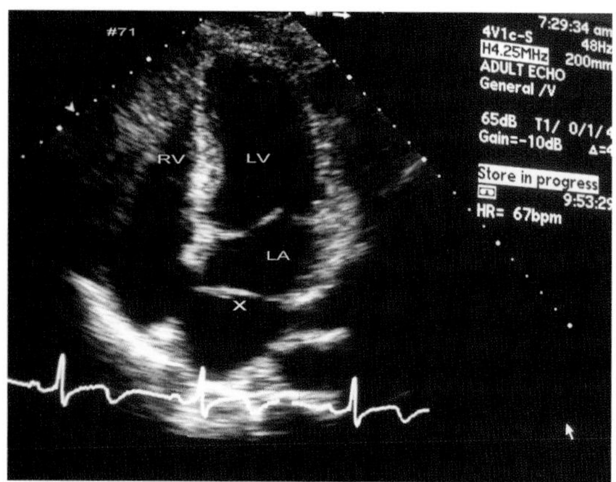

Figure 53.2 Echocardiogram showing four-chamber view. *What is x?*

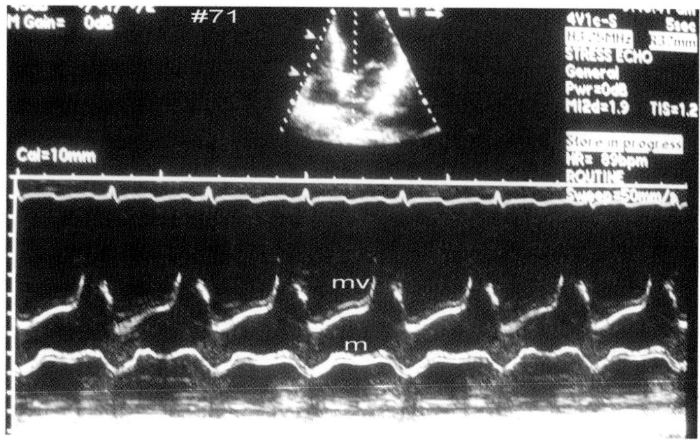

Figure 53.3 Mitral valve (mv) and a left atrial structure (m).

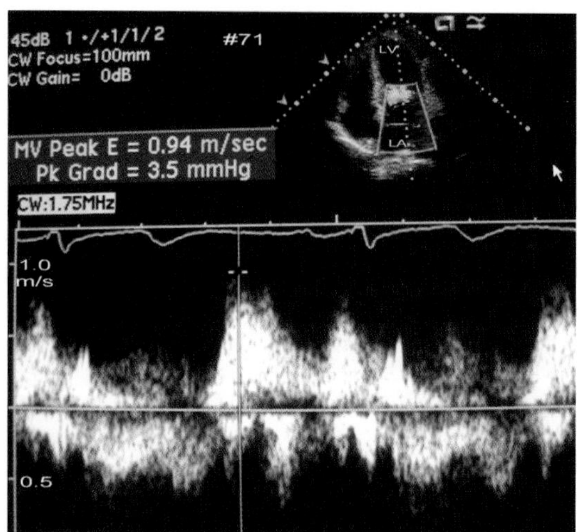

Figure 53.4 Doppler flow velocity studies in left heart.

Table 53.2 Echocardiographic dimensions and LV ejection fraction

Site	Measurement (cm)	Normal values
Aortic root	3.3	2.0–3.7
LA	3.4	1.9–3.6
LV septum (diastole)	0.87	0.7–1.2
LV post wall (diastole)	1.07	0.8–1.1
LV end-diastolic dimension	5.53	3.5–5.8
LV end-systolic dimension	3.27	3.1–4.6
RV end-diastolic dimension	<2.0	0.7–2.0

LV ejection fraction 70%

6 Diagnosis

What is the diagnosis?

7 Treatment

What is the treatment?

Answers and commentary

1 and 2 History and physical examination

The patient had palpitations but no arrhythmias were detected. The physical examination was unremarkable apart from her obesity.

3 ECG

Sinus rhythm. Rate 68/min. PR 0.17 s. QRS 0.08 s. QRS axis −15°.
Low voltage, otherwise normal ECG.

4 Chest X ray and stress echocardiogram report

Normal.

5 Echocardiograms

There is a membrane (x) dividing the LA into two parts, indicative of cor triatriatum (Figure 53.2).
The M mode shows the mitral valve (mv) and the membrane (m). The membrane divides the LA into two parts (Figure 53.3).
The Doppler flow velocity across the mitral valve is <1 m/s, which is normal (Figure 53.4).
Echocardiographic dimensions and LV systolic function are normal (Table 53.2).

6 Diagnosis

Non-obstructive cor triatriatum.

7 Treatment

Medical follow-up was recommended in 2006. No CVS symptoms as of 2012.
Echocardiogram in 2012 showed only borderline LA enlargement.

Discussion

Cor triatriatum occurs when the common pulmonary vein becomes poorly incorporated into the LA, leading to a fenestrated or stenotic membrane dividing the LA into a proximal and a distal chamber [1, 2]. The proximal chamber (true LA) contains the fossa ovalis and the left atrial appendage whereas the distal chamber (accessory LA) provides an inlet for the four pulmonary veins.

Cor triatriatum occurs in 0.1–0.4% of cases of congenital heart disease [1, 3]. Three types have been described by Marin-Garcia et al. [2] (see Figure 53.5). The opening in the membrane may be small, large, single, multiple, absent, central, or eccentric [3].

The most common type of cor triatriatum is the diaphragmatic type [2], as in this patient. There may be no symptoms in the non-obstructive type. The obstructive type of cor triatriatum is seldom diagnosed at the bedside. It may be misdiagnosed as mitral stenosis/regurgitation as there may be systolic or diastolic apical murmurs and evidence of pulmonary hypertension [1]. There may be an associated ASD [2, 3], VSD [2], or PDA [2].

An echocardiogram is essential to make the diagnosis of cor triatriatum [1, 3–5] as it will not only detect the membrane traversing the LA but also determine whether the lesion is causing obstruction or not [5]:

a) non obstructive: mitral valve peak flow velocity ≤1 m/s
b) obstructive: aliased high-velocity flow jet across the mitral valve (Figure 53.6).

The echocardiogram may also detect any associated cardiac anomalies.

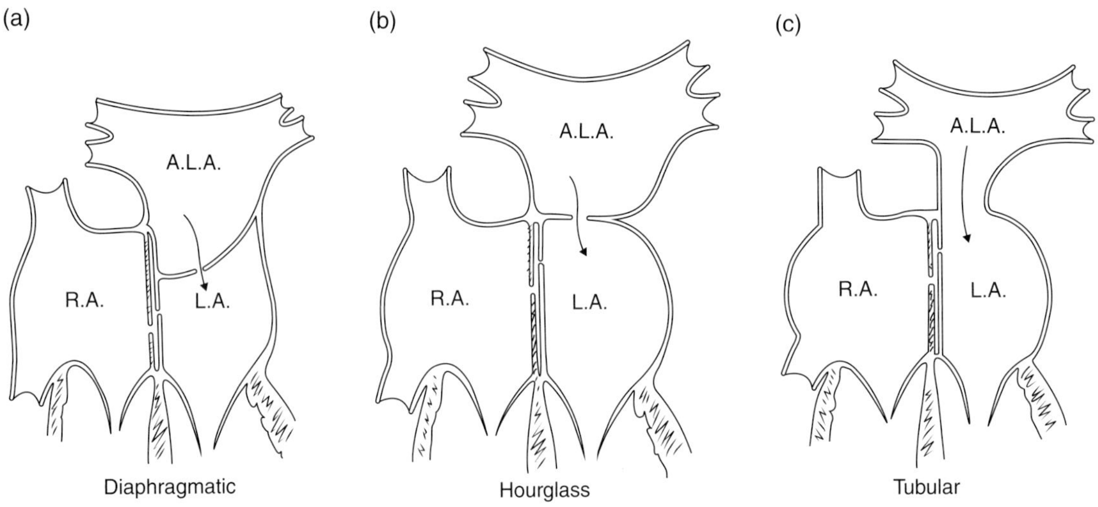

Figure 53.5 The three types of cor triatriatum. Source: Marin-Garcia J, Tandon R, Lucas RV, Edwards JE. (1975). Reproduced with permission of Elsevier. A.L.A = accessory left atrium.

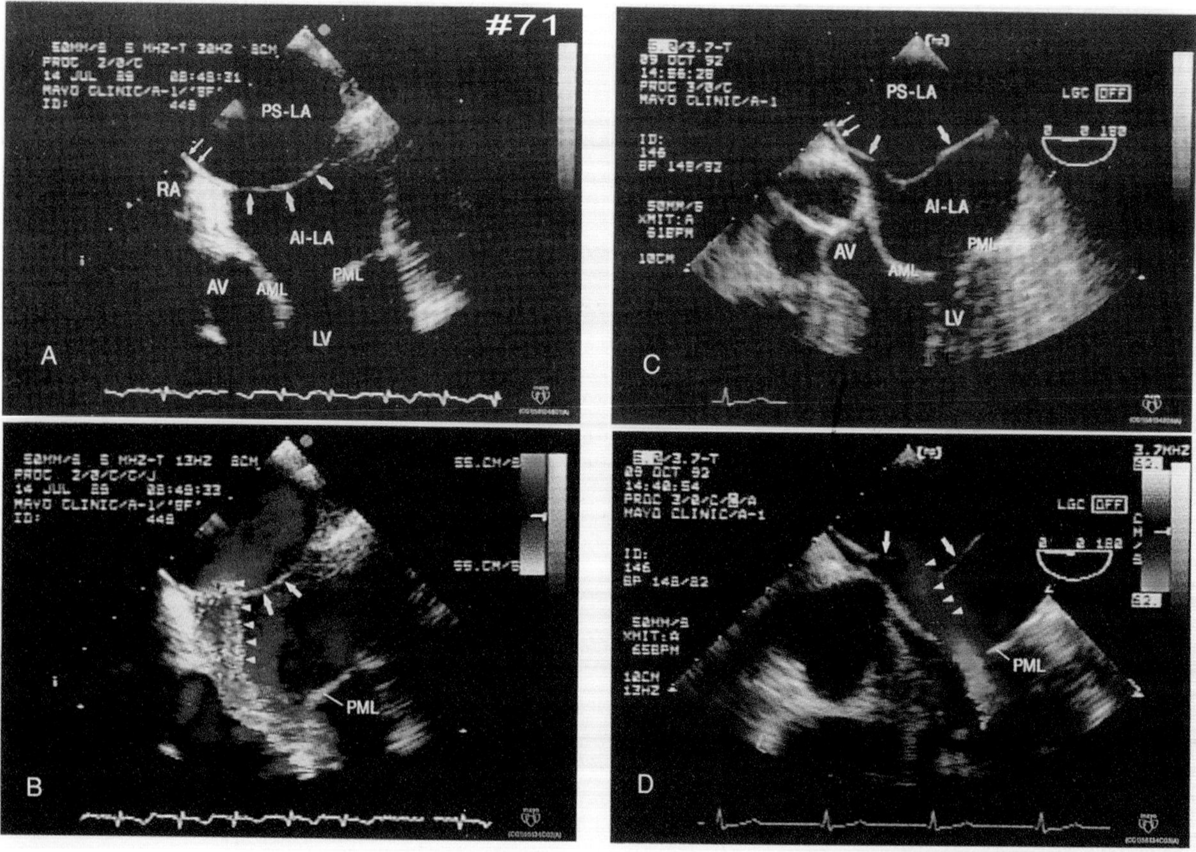

Figure 53.6 Panel A: obstructive form of cor triatriatum. Mean gradient across the membrane was 4 mmHg. Thick white arrows show the membrane. Thin white arrows show the attachment of the membrane to the atrial septum. PS-LA, postero superior LA; AI-LA, anteroinferior LA. Panel B: Doppler study showing high-velocity aliased jet across the membrane (white arrowheads). Thick white arrows show the membrane. Panel C: non-obstructive form of cor triatriatum. No significant gradient across the membrane. Thick white arrows show the membrane. Panel D: Doppler study showing a low velocity across the membrane (arrow heads). AML, anterior mitral valve leaflet; AV, aortic valve; PML, posterior mitral valve leaflet. Source: O'Murchu B, Seward JB. (1995). Reproduced with permission of Wolters Kluwer Health.

Key points

1. Cor triatriatum is a rare form of congenital heart disease consisting of a stenotic or fenestrated membrane that divides the LA into two parts.
2. In the adult it may be isolated or associated with an ASD.

3. The patient may be asymptomatic or have mitral valve obstructive symptoms.
4. Cor triatriatum is best detected by echocardiography and Doppler studies. The latter determine whether there is any significant obstruction to flow.

References

[1] Chen Q, Guhathakurta S, Vadalapali G et al. Cor triatriatum in adults. Three new cases and a brief review. *Tex Heart Inst J* 1999; 26: 206–210.

[2] Marin-Garcia J, Tandon R, Lucas RV, Edwards JE. Cor triatriatum: Study of 20 cases. *Am J Cardiol* 1975; 35: 59–66.

[3] Modi KA, Senthilkumar A, Kiel E, Reddy PC. Diagnosis and surgical correction of cor triatriatum in an adult: Combined use of transesophageal and contrast echocardiography, and a review of literature. *Echocardiography* 2006; 23: 506–509 (pooled data from 53 adult cases 1979–2004).

[4] O'Murchu B, Seward JB. Adult congenital heart disease. Obstructive and nonobstructive cor triatriatum. *Circulation* 1995; 92: 3574.

[5] Vick GW III, Murphy DJ Jr, Ludomirsky A et al. Pulmonary venous and systemic ventricular inflow obstruction in patients with congenital heart disease: detection by combined two-dimensional and Doppler echocardiography. *J Am Coll Cardiol* 1987; 9: 580–587.

54 PATIENT STUDY 54

Sequence of data presentation

1 Left foot examination
↓
2 X ray of left foot
↓
3 Doppler study of lower extremity 31 December 2007
↓
4 12-lead ECG on admission 29 December 2007
↓
5 History
↓
6 Physical examination
↓
7 Laboratory data
↓
8 Course

1 Left foot examination

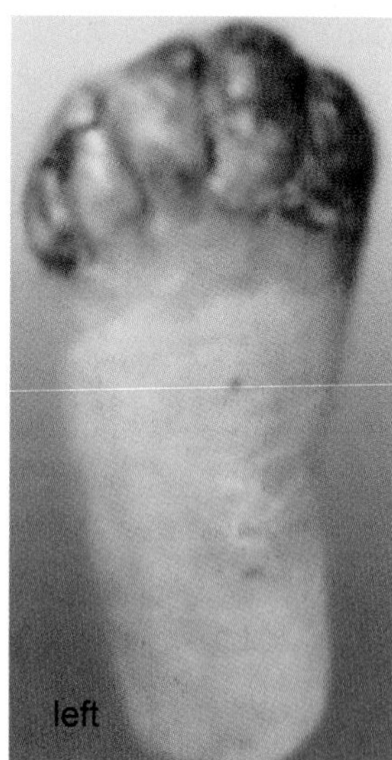

Figure 54.1 Dorsum of left foot 29 December 2007.

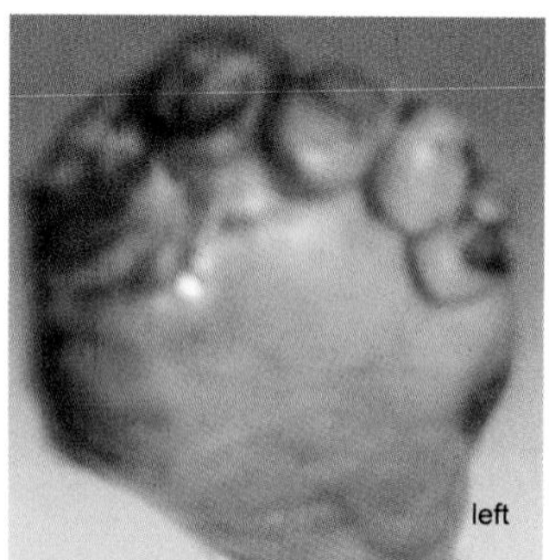

Figure 54.2 Plantar surface of left foot.

Patient Studies in Valvular, Congenital, and Rarer Forms of Cardiovascular Disease: An Integrative Approach, First Edition. Franklin B. Saksena.

Companion Website: www.wiley.com/go/saksena/patientstudies

2 X ray of left foot

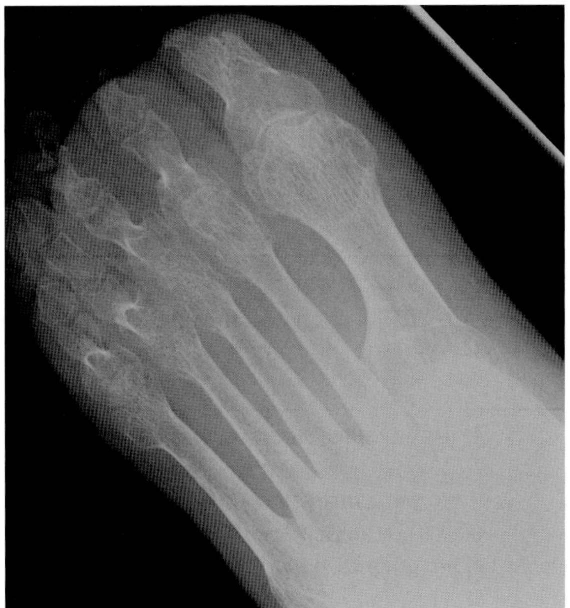

Figure 54.3 X ray of left foot.

3 Doppler study of lower extremity 31 December 2007

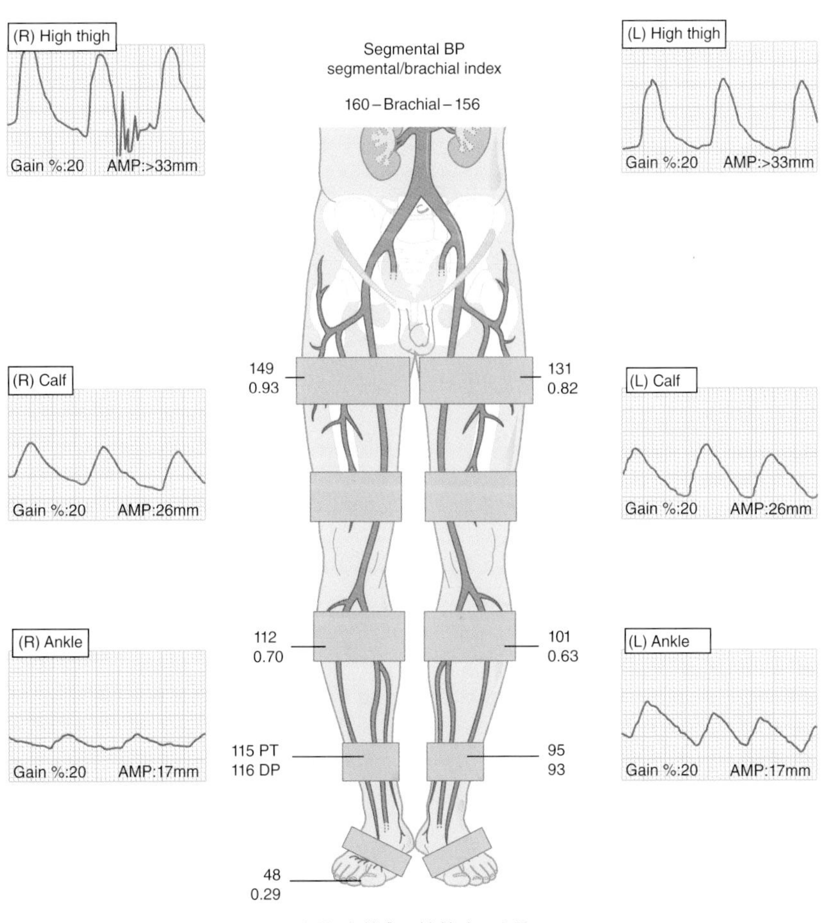

Figure 54.4 Doppler study of lower extremities showing pulse wave forms, pressures, and lower extremity/brachial artery indices at thigh, calf, ankle, and toe levels 31 December 2007.

4 12-lead ECG on admission 29 December 2007

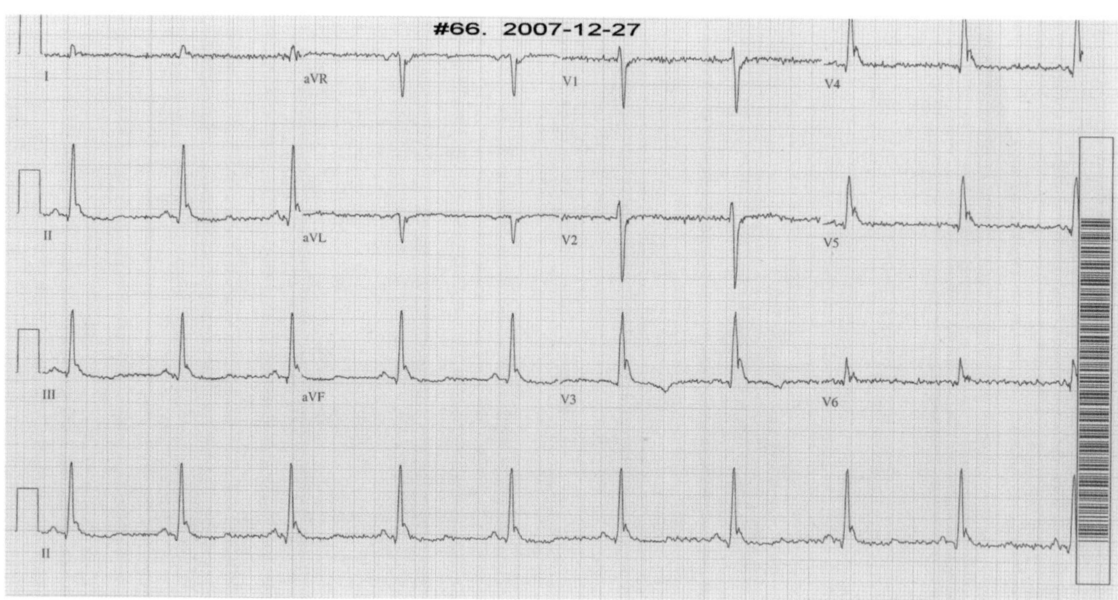

Figure 54.5 12-lead ECG on admission 27 December 2007.

5 History

53-year-old Polish speaking man found lying on the street in an alcoholic stupor. The ambient temperature was 30°F.

Subsequent history revealed that he had smoked for 30 pack years and drank one bottle of vodka a day. He had lived on the streets for the last few years. No history of diabetes, hypertension, myocardial infarction, or operations.

6 Physical examination

This revealed a malnourished, non-communicative man blind in the left eye.

BP 167/77. P 53/min. RR 18/min. Temperature 80.4°F.

No elevation of jugular venous pressure. Normal carotid upstroke.

Apex beat is in the 5th interspace, 7 cm from the mid-sternal line.

S1 and S2 are normal. No S3 or murmurs.

Lungs clear.

Femoral pulses are 4+/4+. Foot pulses 2+/4+.

He had wet gangrene of the first and second toes of the left foot with dry gangrene of the remaining toes. The right foot showed scattered areas of tissue necrosis.

7 Laboratory data

Hemoglobin 12 g%. WBC 5600/mm^3. Serum glucose level 118 mg%. BUN 8 mg%. The chest X ray was normal. Blood alcohol level 339 mg%. Lactate level 1.3 mmol/L.

8 Course

What is the diagnosis and treatment?

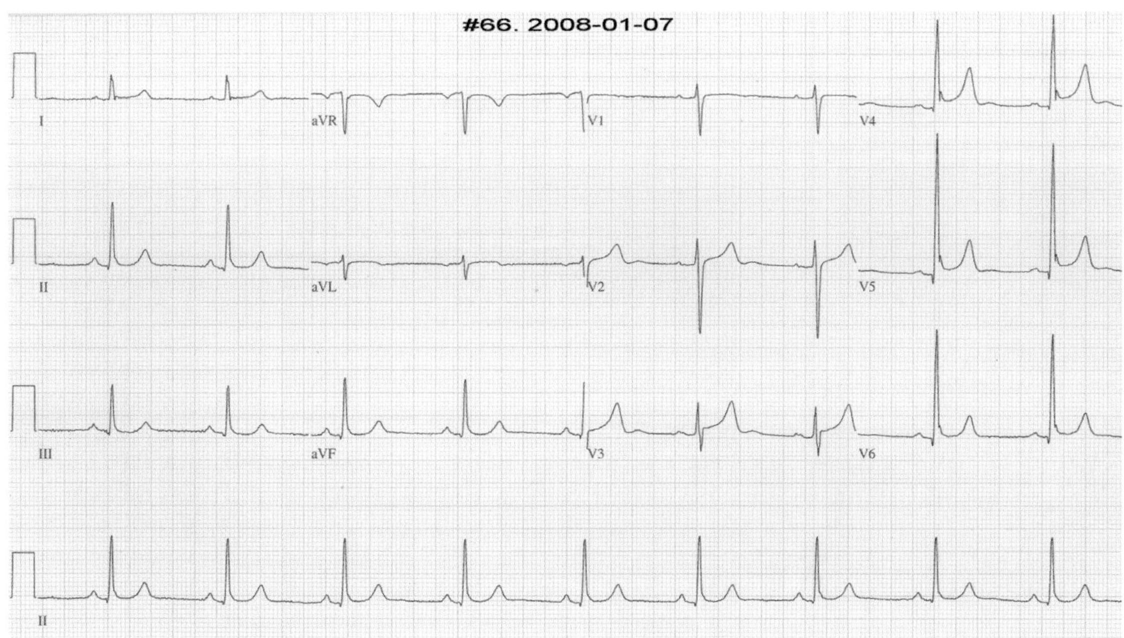

Figure 54.6 12-lead ECG 7 January 2008.

Answers and commentary

1 Left foot examination

The great toe is black with disappearance of the nail and distal pad. The second toe is also blackened.

2 X ray of left foot

Several of the distal phalanges have been destroyed especially of the great toe.

3 Doppler study of lower extremity 31 December 2007

There is marked reduction of the left ankle/brachial index to 0.59. The pressure in the left toe could not be measured because of gangrene.

In the right leg the ankle/brachial index is less severely reduced (0.73), but the right great toe pressure is very low, indicative of occlusive vascular disease of the small vessels of the foot.

There is also evidence of bilateral femoral artery disease as the thigh pressures exceed the calf pressures by 30 mmHg or more. At all levels in the lower extremities the pulse waveform is monophasic, which is another sign of severe peripheral vascular disease.

4 12-lead ECG on admission 29 December 2007

There is sinus bradycardia. Rate 56/min. PR 0.17 s. QRS 0.15 s. QRS axis +80°. QT_c 0.55 s.

Baseline tremor is seen. J waves are seen in V3–5 and 2, 3, F. While J waves may also be seen in early repolarization, hypercalcemia, and the Brugada syndrome [1], the combination of bradycardia, muscle tremors, and prominent J waves favors hypothermia [2] (Figure 54.7).

5 and 6 History and physical examination

Based on the history and physical examination he had:

1. frostbite of feet aggravated by peripheral vascular disease in a chronic alcoholic
2. hypothermia.

7 Laboratory data

The only abnormalities were borderline elevation of serum lactate and a very high blood alcohol level.

8 Course

The great toe and second toe were amputated. Some healing of the foot occurred over the next 2 weeks despite pre-existing femoral arterial disease. With gradual rewarming the patient's temperature returned to normal in 1–2 days. By day 18 he was able to walk 250 feet. He was then discharged to a shelter under social services supervision.

ECG on 7 January 2008 showed sinus bradycardia, rate 56/min, PR 0.17 s, QRS 0.11 s, QRS axis +70°, and QT_c 0.43 s. Minimal slurring of downslope of QRS complexes in V4–6. The QTc interval has now returned to normal. LVH by voltage criteria.

Discussion

Hypothermia

This is defined as a core (rectal, esophageal, tympanic) temperature below 95°F. It may be classified as follows [1, 3]:

mild hypothermia	90–95°F (32–35°C)
moderate hypothermia	82–90°F (28–32°C)
severe hypothermia	<82°F (<28°C)

Hypothermia occurred commonly in the UK in the elderly living in unheated houses in the early 1960s [4]. At that time frostbite was not considered a common accompaniment.

There are about 650 deaths per year in the USA [5] and about 100 deaths per year in Canada from environmental (accidental) hypothermia [3]. About half the patients are 65 years or older [5]. In the USA deaths are highest in those states that have milder climates associated with rapid temperature changes (e.g. North and South Carolina) and in those western states that have high daytime temperatures and often low night-time temperatures (e.g. Arizona) [5].

At ambient temperatures below 14°F (–10°C) wind speed increases the likelihood of cold-induced injuries [3]. With a wind chill index of –13°F (–25°C) there is a risk of frostbite and with a wind chill index of –49°F (–45°C) exposed skin will freeze within minutes [3].

In this patient the predisposing factors leading to cold injury included homelessness, alcoholism, and peripheral vascular disease. Other factors that increase the susceptibility to cold include sedative drugs, malnutrition, myxedema, hypoglycemia, and peripheral neuropathy [2, 3, 5].

Patients with severe hypothermia often have hypotension, bradycardia, pulmonary edema coma, ventricular fibrillation, and even cardiac arrest (core temperature <68°F or <20°) [6, 7]. This patient had severe hypothermia but fortunately only had a sinus bradycardia.

J wave

The J wave or Osborn wave is seen in patients with hypothermia [8, 9], occurring in about 80% of patients [6]. It may be seen when the core temperature falls below 91.4°F (33°C) as a slow positive deflection arising from the terminal portion of the QRS complex resembling a camel's hump. The amplitude and duration of the J wave increases in proportion to the severity of the hypothermia [6] but has no prognostic value [6, 8].

The J wave is best seen in leads V2–5. J waves may also be seen in early repolarization, hypercalcemia, and Brugada syndrome [1, 10]. Available software for ECG interpretation is unable to recognize Osborn waves and often misinterprets them as ischemic changes [1].

This patient had Osborn waves on admission, when his rectal temperature was 80°F. The computerized ECG interpreted these Osborn waves as a non-specific intraventricular block. Once the patient's temperature became normal the Osborn waves disappeared.

The mechanism of J waves has been discussed elsewhere [10]. Underlying acidosis may play a role in the appearance of J waves in hypothermia [11, 12] but does not seem to have been a factor in this patient as lactate levels were only slightly elevated to 1.3 mmol/L.

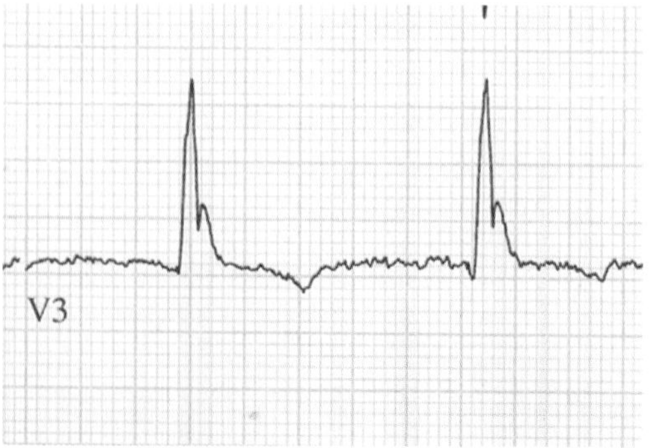

Figure 54.7 Enlarged view of QRS complex showing J waves 27 December 2007.

Key points

1. Hypothermia occurs when the core temperature is <95°F.
2. Common risk factors for hypothermia are homelessness, alcoholism, and malnutrition.
3. Hypothermia and frostbite may be seen in the USA where there are wide swings in the ambient temperature during the day.
4. Hypothermia can lead to bradycardia, hypotension, or ventricular fibrillation.
5. J waves occur when the core temperature is <95°F; their amplitude and duration increase the lower the core temperature. They have no prognostic value.
6. J waves may also be seen in repolarization abnormalities, hypercalcemia, or Brugada syndrome.

References

[1] Mechem CC, Danzl DF. *Accidental hypothermia in adults*. Uptodate 19.1 Jan 2011; pp 1–21 (www.uptodate.com).
[2] Reuler JB. Hypothermia: Pathophysiology, clinical settings and management. *Ann Int Med* 1978; 89: 519–527.
[3] Biem J, Koehncke N, Classen D et al. Out of the cold: management of hypothermia and frostbite. *CMAJ* 2003; 168: 305–311.
[4] McNicol MW, Smith R. Accidental hypothermia. *Br Med J* 1964; 1: 19–21.
[5] Jurkovich GJ. Environmental cold-induced injury. *Surg Clin N Am* 2007; 87: 247–267.
[6] Hanania NA, Zimmerman JL. Accidental hypothermia. *Crit Care Clin* 1999; 15: 236–249.
[7] O'Connell JJ, Petrella DA, Regan RF. The health care of homeless persons Part2: Accidental hypothermia and frostbite: Cold related conditions. In: The health care of homeless persons: A manual of communicable diseases and common problems in shelters and on the streets. *Boston Health Care for the Homeless Program*, pp 189–197. http://www..nhchc.org 2004.
[8] Emlsie-Smith D, Sladden GE, Stirling GR. The significance of changes in the electrocardiogram in hypothermia. *Br Heart J* 1959; 21: 343–351.
[9] Trevino A, Razi B, Beller BM. The characteristic electrocardiogram of accidental hypothermia. *Arch Intern Med* 1971; 127: 470–473.
[10] Antzelevitch C, Yan G. J wave syndromes. *Heart Rhythm* 2010; 7: 549–558.
[11] Edelman ER, Joynt K. J waves of Osborn revisited. *J Am Coll Cardiol* 2010; 55: 2287.
[12] Osborn JJ. Experimental hypothermic respiratory and blood pH changes in relation to cardiac function. *Am J Physiol* 1953; 175: 389–398.

Further reading

Brown DJA, Brugger H, Boyd J et al. Accidental hypothermia. *New Eng J Med* 2012; 367: 1930–1938 (good review of management).

55–56 PATIENT STUDIES 55 AND 56

Patients 55 and 56 had similar findings. Patient 55 is presented in detail and Patient 56 is mentioned in the discussion.

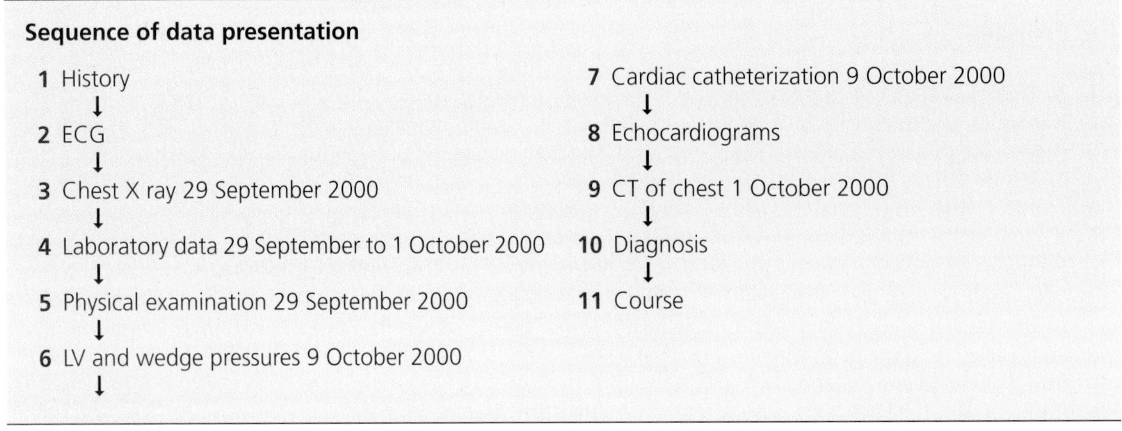

Sequence of data presentation

1 History
↓
2 ECG
↓
3 Chest X ray 29 September 2000
↓
4 Laboratory data 29 September to 1 October 2000
↓
5 Physical examination 29 September 2000
↓
6 LV and wedge pressures 9 October 2000
↓
7 Cardiac catheterization 9 October 2000
↓
8 Echocardiograms
↓
9 CT of chest 1 October 2000
↓
10 Diagnosis
↓
11 Course

1 History

90-year-old female admitted to hospital with hemoptysis for l day.
She has had a history of hypertension for the last 30 years.
She had smoked for 100 pack years and has had exertional dyspnea for the last 3 years.
3 days ago she had an increase in dyspnea and a cough productive of clear sputum. She had some chills but denied any fever. No history of chest pain or weight loss.

2 ECG

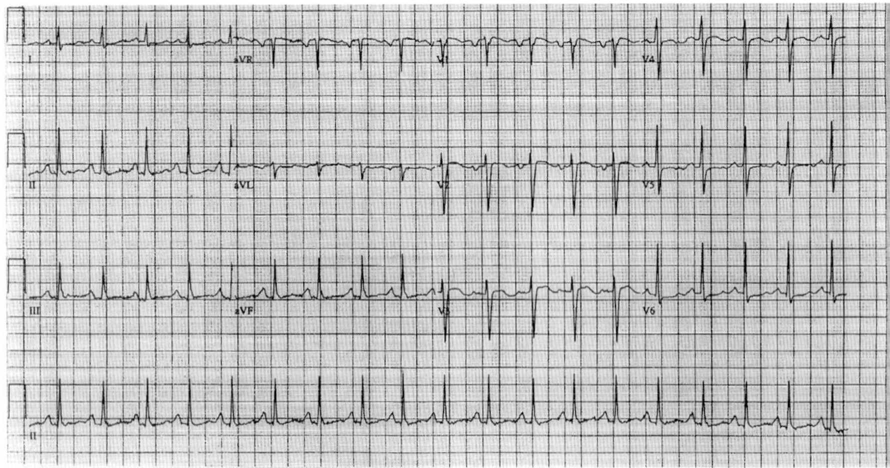

Figure 55.1 12-lead ECG 29 September 2000.

Patient Studies in Valvular, Congenital, and Rarer Forms of Cardiovascular Disease: An Integrative Approach, First Edition. Franklin B. Saksena.

Companion Website: www.wiley.com/go/saksena/patientstudies

3 Chest X ray 29 September 2000

There was LLL pneumonia. Lung fields were hyperinflated. No cardiomegaly.

4 Laboratory data 29 September to 1 October 2000

Hemoglobin 13.1 g%. WBC 19,4000/mm^3.
Arterial pCO_2 56 mmHg. Arterial pO_2 61 mmHg. Arterial saturation 91%.
A two-dimensional echocardiogram was done on 30 September 2000.
CT of the chest showed bullous emphysema (1 October 2000).

5 Physical examination 29 September 2000

60 inches tall female weighing 117 lb. BP 150/80. HR 115/min. Regular. R 37/min. T 97.7°F.
No elevation of jugular venous pressure.
Apex beat is in the 5th interspace, 8 cm from the mid-sternal line (i.e. no cardiomegaly).
S1 –1 decreased. S2 –1 decreased. S3 heard in epigastrium.
Grade 1/6 aortic systolic murmur.
Crepitations and decreased air entry in the left lower lobe. Diaphragms were lower than usual.
No edema, cyanosis, or clubbing .Good peripheral pulses.

6 LV and wedge pressures 9 October 2000

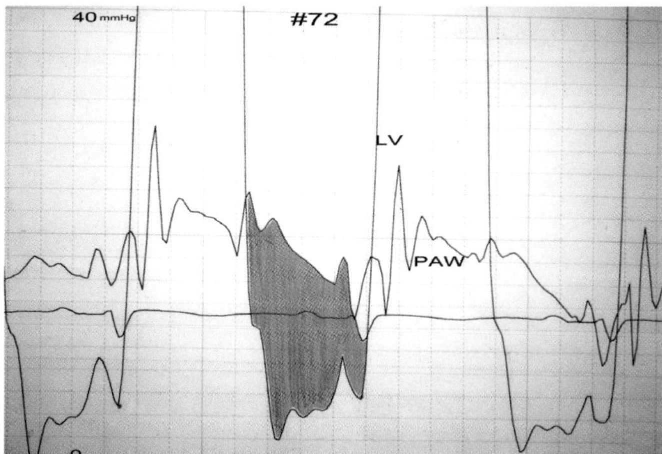

Figure 55.2 Simultaneous LV and PAW pressure. Simultaneous LV and PAW pressures. Scale 0–40 mm Hg. ECG tracing of V1 is second line from bottom. MDG shown in red. HR 75/min.

7 Cardiac catheterization 9 October 2000

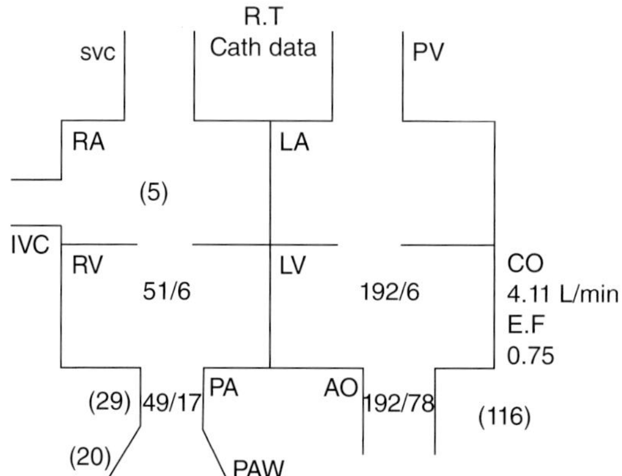

Figure 55.3 Right and left heart catheterization showing pressures, cardiac output, and LV ejection fraction. There was non-obstructive coronary artery disease on selective coronary angiography.

8 Echocardiograms

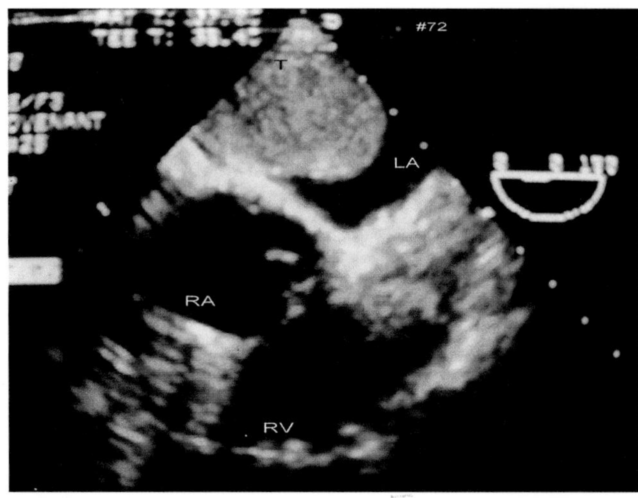

Figure 55.4 TEE showing a left atrial mass (T), 3–4 cm in diameter 6 October 2000.

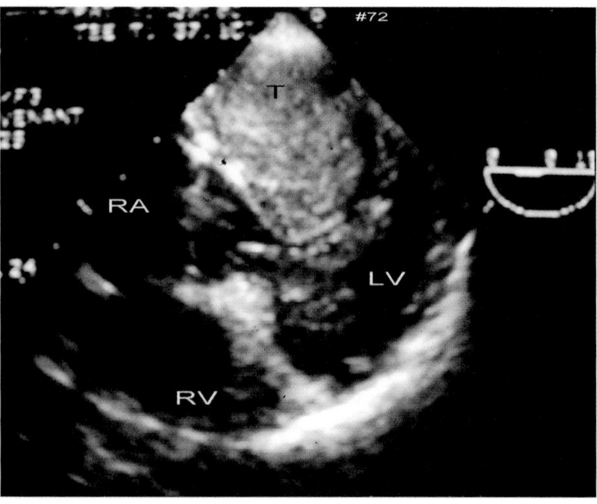

Figure 55.5 TEE showing a later frame in which the left atrial mass is impinging on the mitral valve.

9 CT of chest 1 October 2000

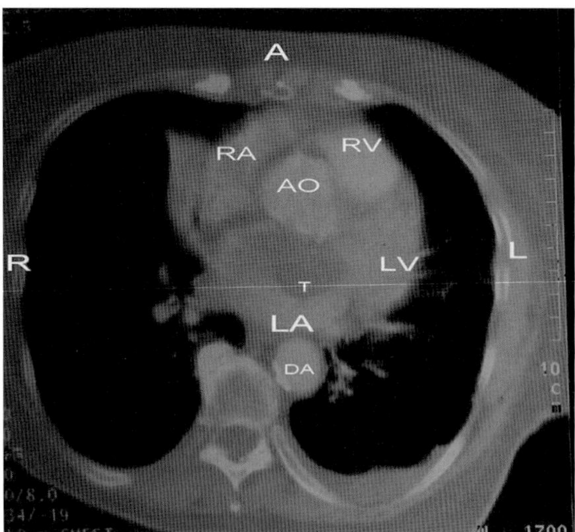

Figure 55.6 CT of chest 2 October 2000 showing a left atrial mass (T). AO, ascending aorta; DA, descending aorta. Orientation: A, anterior; L, left; R, right. A 0–10 cm scale is seen on the right-hand side.

10 Diagnosis

What is the diagnosis?

11 Course

What is the course and treatment?

Answers and commentary

1 History

The patient's symptoms of dyspnea and hemoptysis are suggestive of pneumonia. Her history of heavy smoking would imply she has underlying emphysema.

2 ECG

The rhythm is sinus tachycardia. Rate 114/min. PR interval 0.16 s. QRS 0.09 s. QRS axis +80°P wave is biphasic in V1. T waves are low or biphasic in inferolateral leads.

Impression: (i) LA enlargement, (ii) non-specific T wave abnormalities.

3 Chest X ray 29 September 2000

This confirmed the diagnosis of emphysema and pneumonia.

4 Laboratory data 29 September to 1 October 2000

The white count is elevated because of the pneumonia. Emphysema would account for the hypercapnia and hypoxemia. CT of the chest confirmed the presence of bullous emphysema.

5 Physical examination 29 September 2000

The patient had a left lower lobe pneumonia and chronic obstructive lung disease. The S3 in the epigastric area was attributed to RV dysfunction and hence a two-dimensional echocardiogram was ordered.

6 LV and wedge pressures 9 October 2000

The PAW pressure is elevated and shows a slow y descent.

There is a gradient in diastole between the wedge pressure and the LV pressure.

Such findings are commonly due to mitral stenosis, but this diagnosis is not supported by the physical findings (the first sound is not loud, there is no diastolic murmur, and the presence of an S3 is most unusual in pure mitral stenosis).

Other causes of a PAW–LV gradient are pulmonary vein stenosis, cor triatriatum, or a myxoma of the LA.

7 Cardiac catheterization 9 October 2000

There is mild pulmonary hypertension, a mean mitral diastolic gradient of 12.5 mmHg, and systolic hypertension. The patient had normal LV systolic function and non-obstructive coronary artery disease.

8 Echocardiograms

A mobile tumor 3–4 cm in diameter found in the LA, which periodically impinged on the mitral valve, was first seen on two-dimensional echocardiography on 30 September 2000 and was better delineated on TEE on 6 October 2000.

This tumor is most likely a myxoma and it would account for the mitral diastolic gradient. The S3 heard was probably a tumor plop sound.

9 CT of chest 1 October 2000

A 3–4 cm mass is seen in the LA, close to the mitral valve. The LA is enlarged. Areas of bullous emphysema were seen in other frames of the CT of the chest.

10 Diagnosis

1. Probable atrial myxoma obstructing the mitral valve.
2. Bullous emphysema.
3. Left-sided pneumonia.

11 Course

The patient was transferred to another hospital where she underwent successful surgical removal of a left atrial myxoma measuring 5 × 4 × 2.2 cm.

Microscopically spindle-shaped and stellate myxoma cells were seen.

Discussion

Atrial myxomas are the most common benign primary tumors of the heart [1], mostly involving the LA [1]. Atrial myxomas occur more commonly in females than males (2/1 to 3/1 ratio), between the ages of 30 and 60 [2], and with a range from 7 to 95 years of age [3].

This patient had a previously unsuspected left atrial myxoma. She did not have the characteristic triad of findings, namely obstruction to blood flow, embolic phenomenon, or constitutional symptoms [1–3]. About 10% of patients with myxoma will be asymptomatic [2].

A myxoma should be considered in the differential diagnosis of (i) a patient with mitral valve disease and heart failure who is also in sinus rhythm and (ii) unexplained embolism, especially in a young patient [2].

The diagnosis of a left atrial myxoma may be detected on two-dimensional echocardiography [3] as a mobile mass intermittently obstructing the mitral valve (see Figure 56.1).

TEE often provides additional information as to the tumor size and its atrial attachment [4] as well as the existence of any other cardiac tumors [3].

In this patient the echocardiogram was ordered to assess the significance of a third heart sound in a patient who was in sinus rhythm and not in heart failure.

The third sound in this case most likely occurred as a result of the tethered myxoma plunging through the mitral valve orifice in diastole and coming to a sudden halt. This produces a tumor plop sound resembling an S3 [5]. The tumor plop sound occurs 0.08–0.15 s after S2 [2].

A tumor plop sound is heard in about 15% of cases of myxomas [2]. Fifty-five per cent of patients with a left atrial myxoma have a diastolic apical rumble (that often varies with body position) due to intermittent mitral valve obstruction [2]. However, no diastolic apical rumble was heard in this patient, probably because she had bullous emphysema.

Atrial myxomas are on average 5–6 cm in diameter. They are friable, gelatinous, and may contain some areas of hemorrhage (see Figure 56.2). They are attached by a thin stalk to the atrial septum. Microscopically, these tumors have a myxoid matrix with polygonal cells arranged singly, often in a stellate shape and in small nests [1] (See Figure 56.3).

Pulmonary angiography with follow through to the LA may detect a mobile left atrial mass, later proven to be a myxoma on tissue diagnosis.

Coronary arteriography is carried out in patients over the age of 40 as part of pre-operative evaluation [2]. On rare occasions feeder vessels from the coronary arteries may be seen supplying a tumor (later shown to be a myxoma) showing a 'tumor blush' or a sea anemone appearance [3, 6, 7].

Prompt surgical resection of the tumor is recommended, even if the patient is asymptomatic, as myxomas have a propensity to embolize [2, 3] or cause sudden death (because of mitral valve obstruction). The surgical mortality is <5% [2, 3].

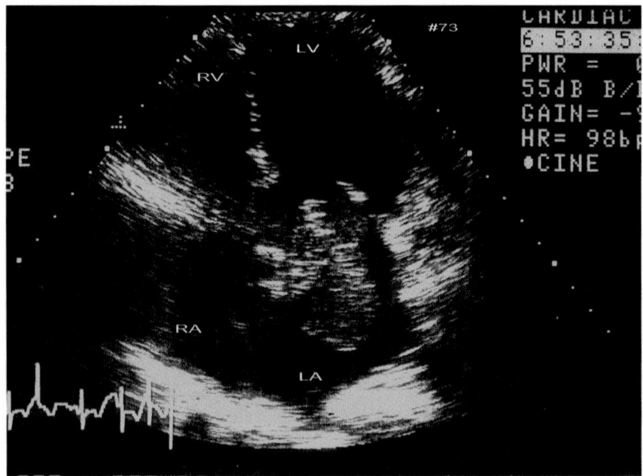

Figure 56.1 58-year-old female with dyspnea and syncope. Mean PA pressure 38 mmHg. The four-chamber view on two-dimensional echocardiography showed a left atrial tumor obstructing the mitral valve and entering the ventricle. Other views showed the tumor attached to the atrial septum via a long stalk (not shown).

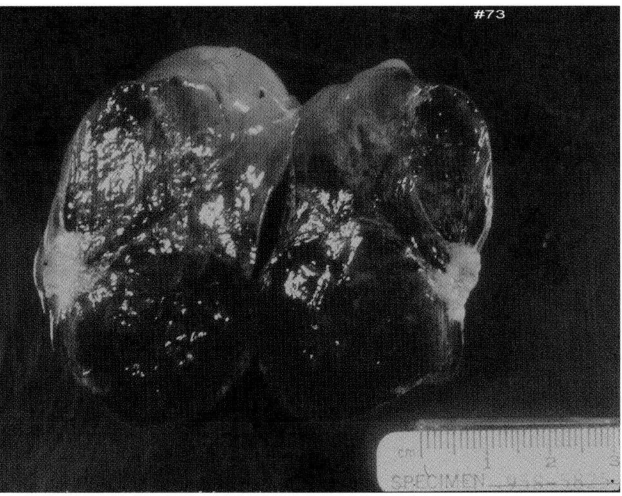

Figure 56.2 Gross appearance of the left atrial myxoma removed at surgery. It had a gelatinous consistency and showed areas of hemorrhage. Measurement: 5 cm × 4 cm (same patient as in Figure 56.1).

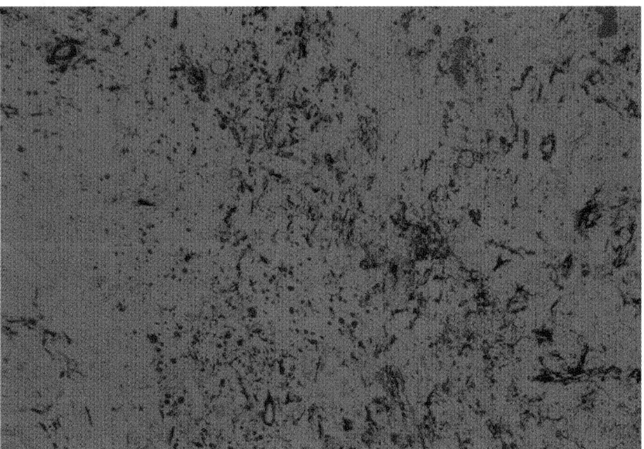

Figure 56.3 Microscopic appearance of myxoma. There are numerous stellate cells in a myxoid matrix (same patient as in Figures 56.1 and 56.2).

Key points

1. An atrial myxoma is the most common benign tumor of the heart.
2. Consider atrial myxoma if there is an unexplained systemic embolism in a young person or in a patient with mitral valve disease and heart failure who remains in sinus rhythm.
3. On physical examination there may be a diastolic apical murmur and a third sound (tumor plop).
4. Echocardiography will show a mobile mass in the LA impinging on the mitral valve.
5. Prompt removal is recommended as these tumors often embolize.

References

[1] McAllister Jr HA, Hall RJ, Cooley DA. Tumors of the heart and pericardium. *Curr Probl Cardiol* 1999; 24: 57–116.
[2] Pinede L, Duhaut P, Loire R. Clinical presentation of left atrial cardiac myxoma. A series of 112 consecutive cases. *Medicine* 2001; 80: 159–172.
[3] Salcedo EE, Cohen GI, White RD et al. Cardiac tumors: diagnosis and management. *Curr Probl Cardiol* 1992; 17: 77–137.
[4] Salustri A, Roelandt J. Left atrial myxoma visualized by transesophageal rotoplan echocardiographic computed tomography. *Circulation* 1995; 91: 2290.
[5] Ranganathan N, Sivaciyan V, Saksena FB. *The art and science of cardiac physical examination*. Humana Press, Totowa, NJ, 2006, p 195.
[6] Cleemput J van, Daenen W, Geest H. Coronary angiography in cardiac myxomas: Findings in 19 consecutive cases and review of the literature. *Cathet Cardiovasc Diagn* 1993; 29: 217–220.
[7] Huang C-Y, Yu W-C, Chen K-C et al. Coronary angiography of cardiac myxoma. *Clin Cardiol* 2005; 28: 505–509.

57 PATIENT STUDY 57

Sequence of data presentation

1 History and physical examination
↓
2 Echocardiogram
↓
3 Diagnosis

1 History and physical examination

A 1-month-old infant with a Shagreen patch and a pulmonic flow murmur.

2 Echocardiogram

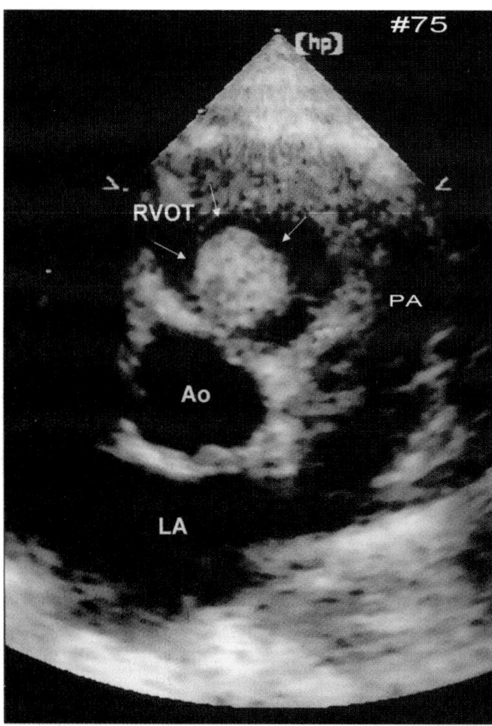

Figure 57.1 Two-dimensional echocardiogram in short axis view (courtesy of Dr Guerrero).

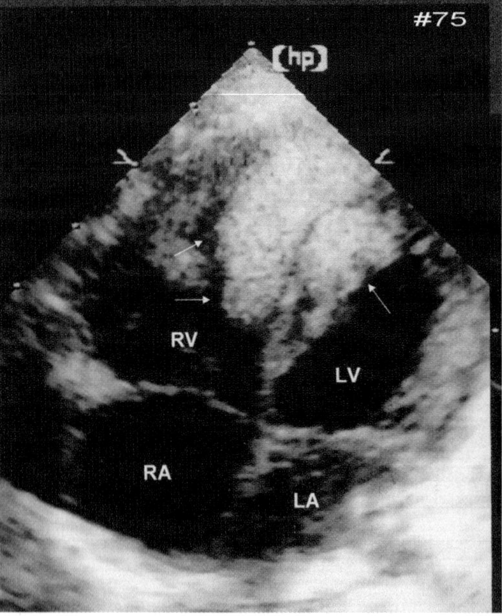

Figure 57.2 Two-dimensional echocardiogram in four-chamber view (courtesy of Dr Guerrero).

Patient Studies in Valvular, Congenital, and Rarer Forms of Cardiovascular Disease: An Integrative Approach, First Edition. Franklin B. Saksena.

Companion Website: www.wiley.com/go/saksena/patientstudies

3 Diagnosis

What is the diagnosis and what other clinical features might be present?

What is the treatment?

What is the course?

Answers and commentary

1 History and physical examination

The finding of a Shagreen patch or an ash leaf lesion is one of the major criterion in the diagnosis of tuberous sclerosis [1].

2 Echocardiograms

Figure 57.1 shows a rounded mass obstructing the RV outflow tract. A small stalk connects the mass to the pulmonary valve.

Figure 57.2 shows an oblong mass in the RV attached to the septum. The RV is enlarged. There is a wedged-shaped mass attached to the LV septum.

3 Diagnosis

The presence of a Shagreen patch (resembling the leaflet of a white ash tree) and multiple masses in the heart are major features in the diagnosis of tuberous sclerosis [1].

Discussion

A cardiac rhabdomyoma is a benign hamartoma [2, 3] that occurs in over 60% of cardiac tumors in the pediatric population [3].

They are associated with tuberous sclerosis in 80% of cases [2].

The tumors can cause outflow tract obstruction or arrhythmias but often regress by the age of 6 [1]. These tumors are often multiple and are usually found in the ventricles [1–3].

Very rarely a rhabdomyoma may be associated with other forms of congenital heart disease such as transposition of the great vessels or a VSD [2].

Unless the patient is severely symptomatic from outflow obstruction or intractable arrhythmias conservative treatment is recommended [1, 3].

Surgical intervention involves debulking the tumors and myocardial excision, and is not without risk [1].

Key points

1. Rhabdomyomas are benign tumors of the heart, usually seen in the pediatric population and often associated with tuberous sclerosis.
2. These tumors are often multiple and usually are seen in the ventr.icles. They can cause an outflow tract obstruction or arrhythmias.
3. Treatment is usually conservative. These tumors often regress by the age of 6.

References

[1] Madueme P, Hinton R. Tuberous sclerosis and cardiac rhabdomyomas: a case report and review of the literature. *Congenit Heart Dis* 2011; 6: 183–187.

[2] Burke A, Vermani R. Pediatric heart tumors. *Cardiovascular Pathology* 2008; 17: 193–198.

[3] Jain D, Maleszewski JJ, Halushka MK. Benign cardiac tumors and tumor-like condition. *Ann Diagn Path* 2010; 14: 215–230 (158 references).

58 PATIENT STUDY 58

Sequence of data presentation

1 Lower extremity appearance
↓
2 Laboratory data
↓
3 CT of abdomen
↓
4 MRI of abdomen
↓
5 Pathology
↓
6 History and physical examination
↓
7 Diagnosis and treatment

1 Lower extremity appearance

(a)

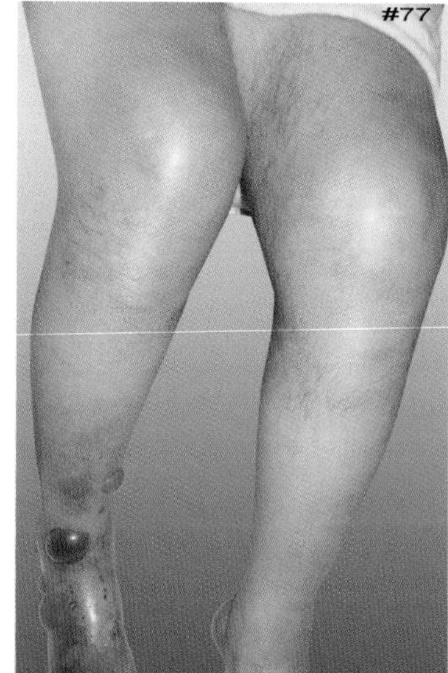

(b)

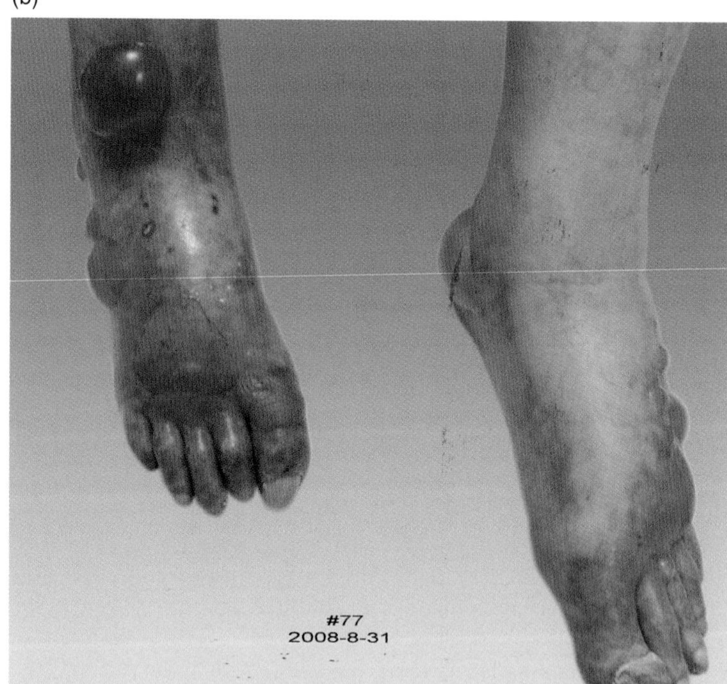

Figure 58.1 (a) Lower extremities while patient is sitting. (b) A close-up view of feet.

2 Laboratory data

Hb 7.5 g% rising to 10 g% after transfusion.
WBC 33,000. Serum albumin 3 g%.
Bacteroides septicemia.
Negative venous Doppler of lower extremity.

Patient Studies in Valvular, Congenital, and Rarer Forms of Cardiovascular Disease: An Integrative Approach, First Edition. Franklin B. Saksena.

Companion Website: www.wiley.com/go/saksena/patientstudies

3 CT of abdomen

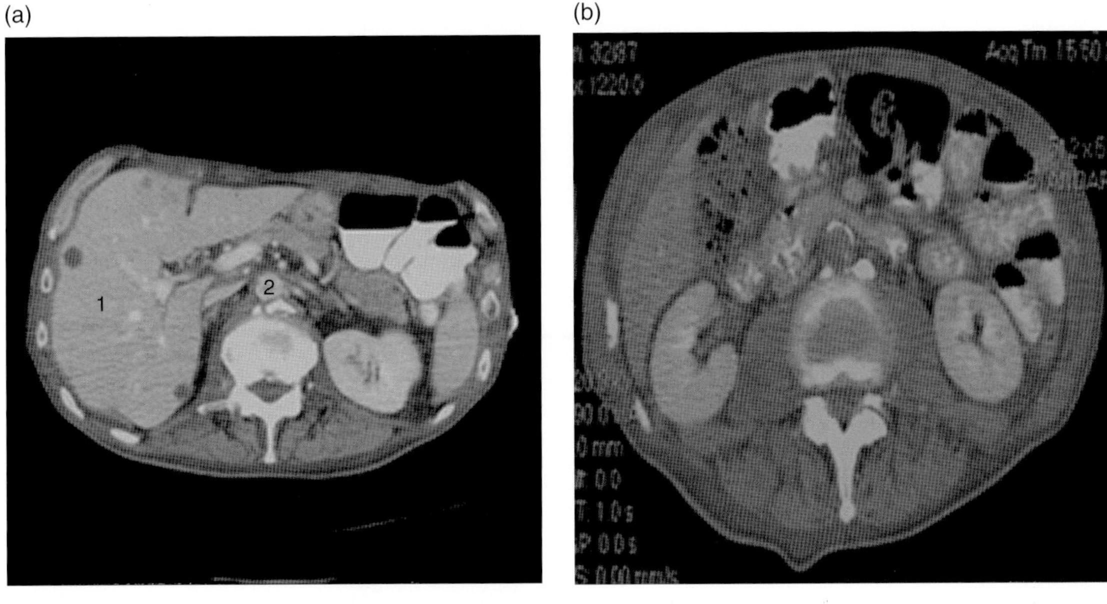

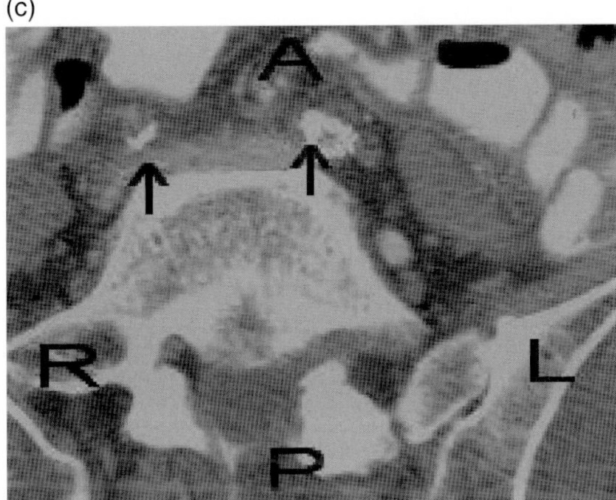

Figure 58.2 (a) CT of abdomen at level of liver. (b) CT of abdomen at renal level. (c) CT of abdomen at iliac level. Arrow heads point to right and left iliac arteries.

What are the structures labeled 1 and 2?

4 MRI of abdomen

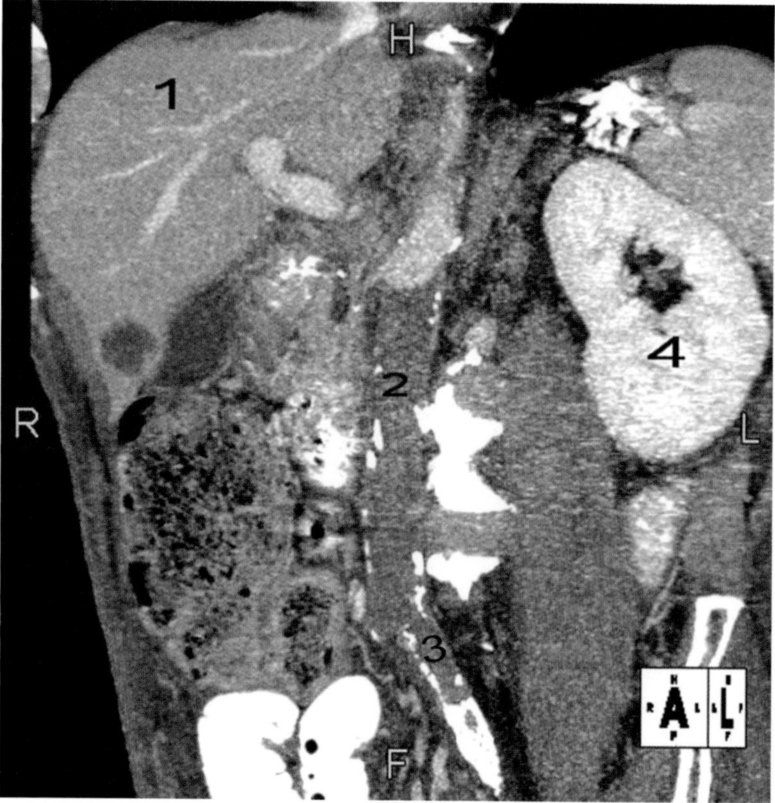

Figure 58.3 MRI of abdomen.
What are the structures labeled 1, 2, 3, and 4?

5 Pathology

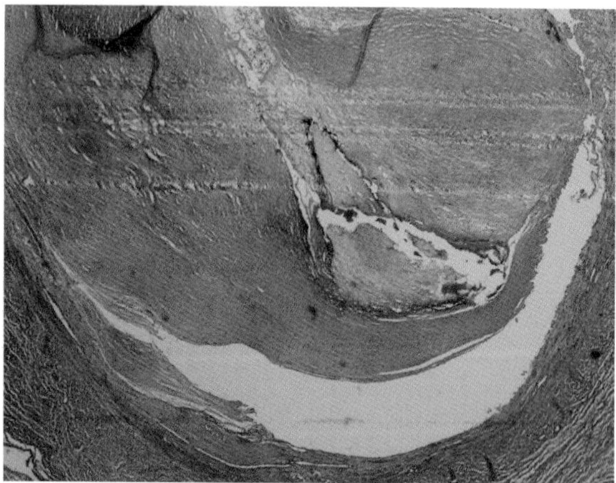

Figure 58.4 Microscopic appearance of popliteal artery in the amputated leg. H and E stain.

6 History and physical examination

History

69-year-old man, a former heavy smoker, underwent right femoral artery stenting and femoral–femoral bypass 20 years ago.

He had a CVA with right hemiparesis in March 2008 and rectal bleeding due to rectal cancer in August 2008. Colostomy done August 2008.

He had leg pain and inability to move his legs.

Physical examination

73 inches tall, 135 lb male. BP 115/64. HR 78/min irregular. R 20 /min. T 96.6°F.
Right leg spasticity with 3 out of 5 strength where 5 = normal.
He had difficulty in moving toes bilaterally.
He had no sensation below the knees.
Femoral pulses were 0–1+ where 4+ = normal.
2+ leg edema with bluish color to legs (Figure 58.1a and b). Right leg is cooler than the left.
Several bullae noted in legs.
Distal gangrene of toes of right foot.

7 Diagnosis and treatment

What is the diagnosis and treatment?

Answers and commentary

1 Lower extremity appearance

There is leg edema with a violaceous discoloration of the legs. Multiple bullae are seen on the dorsum of the feet and ankle areas. There is gangrene of both feet.

2 Laboratory data

The patient had septicemia. His anemia was corrected by blood transfusions.

3 CT of abdomen

(a) At the renal artery level the aorta (=2) is filled with intravenous contrast material: 1 = liver with two dark circular lesions due to metastatic disease. 2 = aorta.
(b) Below the renal artery the aorta is occluded as no contrast material is seen in the lumen.
(c) At the bifurcation of the aorta the left iliac (long arrow) and the right iliac arteries (short arrow) are similarly occluded.

4 MRI of abdomen

The MRI shows that the aorta was occluded just below the renal arteries. The distal aorta shows calcifications in several areas. The right common iliac artery is not seen. 1 = liver; 2 = abdominal aorta; 3 = left common iliac artery; 4= left kidney.

5 Pathology of amputated leg

Microscopically there is 90% stenosis of the popliteal artery.

6 History and physical examination

The patient has severe peripheral vascular disease complicated by septicemia and right hemiparesis.

7 Diagnosis and treatment

1. Occlusion of abdominal aorta at renal level.
2. Severe peripheral vascular disease of the lower extremities.
3. Rectal carcinoma with liver metastases.
4. Bacteroides septicemia.

He underwent bilateral above-knee amputation in September 2008. He died in January 2009 of rectal carcinoma with liver metastases.

Discussion

The patient had severe aorto-iliac disease and PVD, resulting in lower extremity cyanosis and gangrene of the feet. It is unusual for patients with arterial occlusive disease to have leg edema, especially with bullous formation [1]. The presence of leg edema means that there is a venous component to his vascular disease.
His leg edema could be due to (i) the tendency for patients with severe PVD to dangle their feet when in bed to relieve local pain or (ii) marked arterial occlusive disease compromising blood flow reaching the veins,

resulting in venous stasis and small vessel thrombosis. Other causes of leg edema such as heart failure, varicose veins with venous insufficiency, low serum albumin, lymphedema, and ilio-femoral thrombosis were not present in this patient. Phlegmasia cerulea dolens [1, 2] refers to extensive venous thrombosis of the ilio-femoral veins and is often associated with malignancies [1]. Phlegmasia cerulea dolens as defined above was excluded in this patient on the basis of a negative venous Doppler study of the ilio-femoral veins. However, a venous Doppler study cannot reliably exclude venous thrombosis of the legs [3, 4], which if present would further compromise arterial blood flow.

Edema with bullous formation is seen in elderly relatively immobile patients with an acute exacerbation of chronic edema [5], produced in this case by severe venous obstruction.

When there is severe venous obstruction the hydrostatic pressure on the venous side of the capillaries rises and exceeds the plasma oncotic pressure, and fluid seeps into the interstitium, producing edema and bullae [1]. These edema bullae usually occur on the dorsum of the foot and ankle, and over time will enlarge to several centimeters in diameter (see Figure 58.1b). The fluid in these bullae is sterile and usually clear [1,5].

Key points

1. Leg edema in a patient with severe arterial occlusive disease means that there is also a venous component.
2. Causes of leg edema include right heart failure, low serum albumin, venous insufficiency or thrombosis, and lymphatic obstruction.
3. A venous Doppler study of the lower extremity can detect ilio-femoral vein thrombosis but is not reliable in detecting thrombi in the legs.
4. Edema bullae are seen in elderly patients who are immobile and have severe venous obstruction.

References

[1] Brockman SK, Vasko J. Phlegmasia Cerulea Dolens. *Surg Gynecol Obstet* 1965; 121: 1347–1356.
[2] Mumoli N, Invernizzi C, Luschi R et al. Phlegmasia cerulea dolens. *Circulation* 2012; 125: 1056–1057.
[3] Fairbairn JF. *Clinical manifestations of peripheral vascular diseases.* In: Allen–Barker–Hines peripheral vascular disease, 5th edn, Juergens JL, Spittell JA, Fairbairn JF (eds). WB Saunders, Philadelphia, 1980, p 30.
[4] Pedersen OM, Aslaksen A, Vik-Mo H et al. Compression ultrasonography in hospitalized patients with suspected deep venous thrombosis. *Arch Intern Med* 1991; 151: 2217–2220 (A comparison of contrast venography with compression ultrasonography in 215 patients).
[5] Mascaro JM. *Edema bullae.* In: Dermatology, volume 1, Bolognia JL, Jorizzo JL, Rapini RP (eds), Mosby, Philadelphia, 2003, pp 506–508.

Further reading

Gibson CJ, Britton KA, Miller AL et al. Out of the blue. *New Engl J Med* 2014; 370: 1742–1748 (describes a patient with phlegmasia cerulea dolens).

59 PATIENT STUDY 59

Sequence of data presentation

1 History
↓
2 Facial examination
↓
3 Angiograms
↓
4 Physical examination and laboratory data
↓
5 Diagnosis
↓
6 Treatment and course

1 History

71-year-old man admitted to hospital with dizziness and weakness in 2010.

No visual symptoms, fever, or chest pain. No dyspnea on walking four blocks.

In 1993 he had a CVA with mild right-sided weakness with a full recovery subsequently.

He has had hypertension for 10 years, non-insulin dependant diabetes for 2 years and hypercholesterolemia for at least 1 year. He does not drink alcohol, smoke, or use drugs.

2 Facial examination

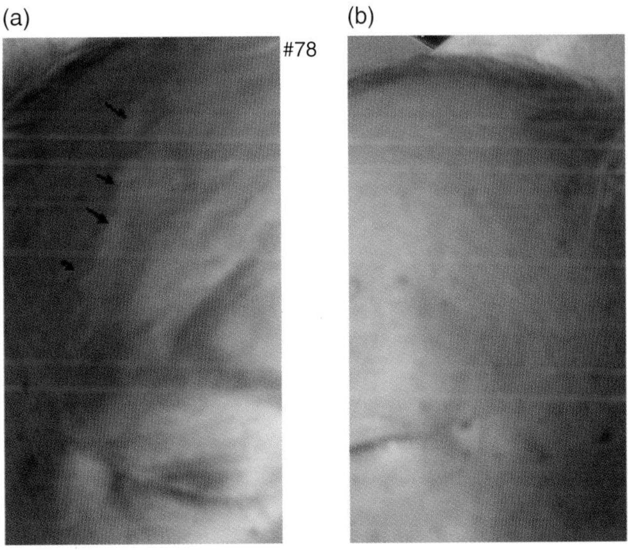

Figure 59.1 (a) Right temporal area. (b) Left temporal area.

What vessel do the arrows point to?

Patient Studies in Valvular, Congenital, and Rarer Forms of Cardiovascular Disease: An Integrative Approach, First Edition. Franklin B. Saksena.

Companion Website: www.wiley.com/go/saksena/patientstudies

3 Angiograms

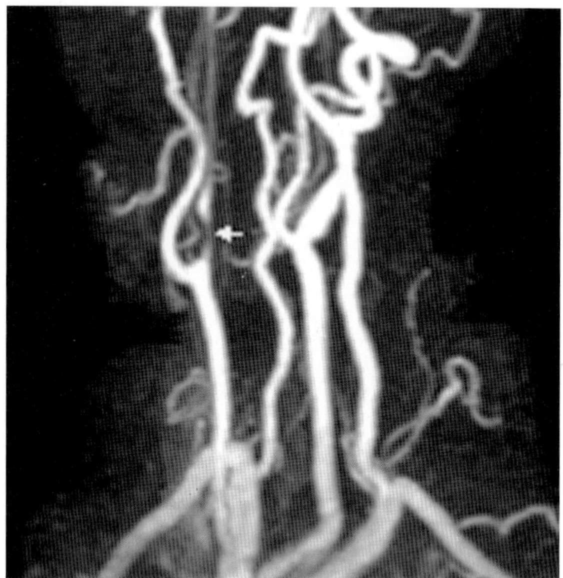

Figure 59.2 CT of neck with MRA of neck vessels RAO view.

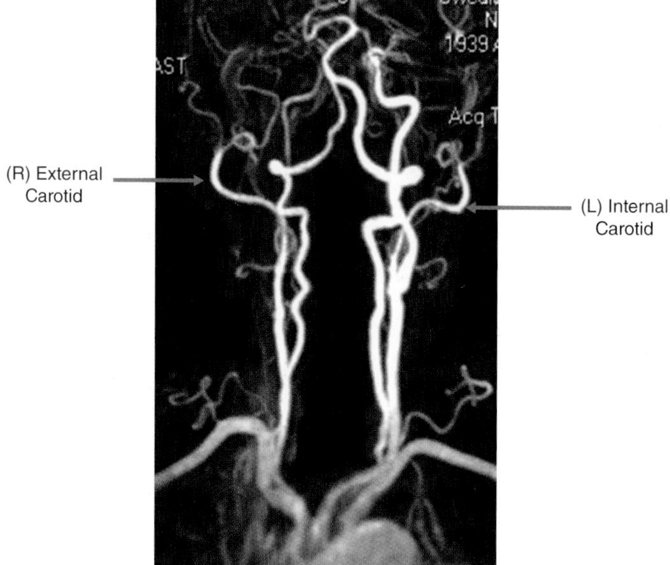

Figure 59.3 CT of neck comparing the size of the external carotid arteries AP view. R, right external carotid artery; L, left external carotid artery.

4 Physical examination and laboratory data

Physical examination

62 inches tall, 147 lb male. BP 130/80. HR 84/min regular.
Fundi showed normal optic discs. A/V ratio 1/3. No hemorrhages or exudates.
Xanthelasma bilaterally. A diagonal ear crease sign is present.
No carotid artery bruits. Right carotid pulse is diminished.
Biphasic Doppler sounds are diminished over right as compared to the left carotid artery.
External carotid sign seen on right side (Figure 59.1a).
No cardiomegaly. Grade 1/6 aortic systolic murmur.
Lungs clear.
Good peripheral pulses in lower extremity.
Reflexes and strength in arms and legs are equal. Normal gait.

Laboratory data

Hemoglobin 14.2 g%. WBC 6400/mm^3. HbA1C 5.8%. Serum cholesterol 214 mg%.

5 Diagnosis

What is the diagnosis?

6 Treatment and course

What is the treatment and likely course?

Answers and commentary

1 History

The patient has risk factors for development of atherosclerosis (brain, heart, and peripheral vessels). Dizziness and weakness are non-specific symptoms.

2 Facial examination

The right superficial temporal artery is more prominent on the right side as compared to the left side. This external carotid sign is seen in patients with ipsilateral internal carotid arterial disease [1]. Patients with internal carotid artery stenosis (>75% narrowing) will have some increase in blood flow in the external carotid artery on the same side so that the superficial temporal artery is more prominent on that side. The external carotid sign may be less useful if there is bilateral carotid arterial disease.

3 Angiograms

There is 99% stenosis of the cervical portion of the right internal carotid artery in the RAO view (Figure 59.2). In the AP view (Figure 59.3) the right external carotid artery (R) is slightly larger than the left external carotid artery (L), which gives some credence to the external carotid artery sign described above.

4 Physical examination and laboratory data

The external carotid sign was the only sign to suggest internal carotid arterial disease. The softer biphasic Doppler sounds over the right carotid artery as compared to the left merely suggest reduced flow in the common carotid artery or its branches. The absence of neck bruits [2,3] or a Hollenhorst plaque on funduscopic examination does not rule out carotid artery disease [4].

The laboratory data were normal except for an elevated serum cholesterol.

5 Diagnosis

99% stenosis of right internal carotid artery.

Non-specific CNS symptoms.

6 Course

The patient underwent successful carotid endarterectomy in 2010 and 9 months later continued to do well and was walking 10 blocks a day.

Discussion

Symptomatic carotid artery stenosis accounts for 15–30% of patients having an ischemic stroke [5]. Asymptomatic carotid artery stenosis occurs in 12.5% of men over the age of 70 [5].

This patient was 71 years old and had severe carotid artery stenosis that was essentially asymptomatic. He had three of the common risk factors for carotid atherosclerosis: hypertension, diabetes, and hypercholesterolemia [5].

Patients with internal carotid artery disease may have amaurosis fugax, carotid artery bruits, or Hollenhorst plaque [4]. None of these findings were present in this patient. The presence of a reduced carotid pulse, reduced Doppler flow to the carotid artery, and the external carotid sign were the only clues to the bedside diagnosis of carotid artery disease. CT of the neck with MRA is required to confirm this diagnosis as well as to guide the treatment plan [5].

Carotid endarterectomy was warranted in this patient to prevent an ipsilateral stroke [5] as he had 99% stenosis of the internal carotid artery.

Key points

1. The external carotid artery sign is useful in detecting ipsilateral internal carotid artery stenosis.
2. Risk factors for carotid artery disease are the same as for coronary artery disease: hypetension, diabetes, and hypercholesterolemia.
3. Carotid endarterectomy is the treatment of choice in patients with >75% internal carotid artery stenosis.

References

[1] Fisher CM. Facial pulses in internal carotid artery occlusion. *Neurology* 1970; 20: 476–478.

[2] Sandercock PAG, Kavvadia E. The carotid bruit. *Pract Neurol* 2002; 2: 221–224.

[3] Sauve JS, Laupacis A, Østbye T et al. Does this patient have a clinically important carotid bruit? *JAMA* 1993; 270: 2843–2845.

[4] Mohr JP, Gautier JC. *Internal carotid artery disease*. In: Stroke: pathophysiology, diagnosis, and management, 4th edn, Mohr JP, Choi DW, Grotta JC, Weir B, Wolf PA (eds). Churchill Livingstone, Philadelphia, 2004, pp 75–100.

[5] Kan P, Makin M, Dumont TM et al. Cervical carotid artery stenosis: Latest update on diagnosis and management. *Curr Probl Cardiol* 2012; 37: 127–169.

60 PATIENT STUDY 60

Sequence of data presentation

1 Chest X ray
↓
2 ECG 6 April 1996
↓
3 Laboratory data
↓
4 History and physical examination
↓
5 Hemodynamics
↓
6 RA angiogram and chest CT
↓
7 Diagnosis
↓
8 Surgical findings
↓
9 Course

1 Chest X ray

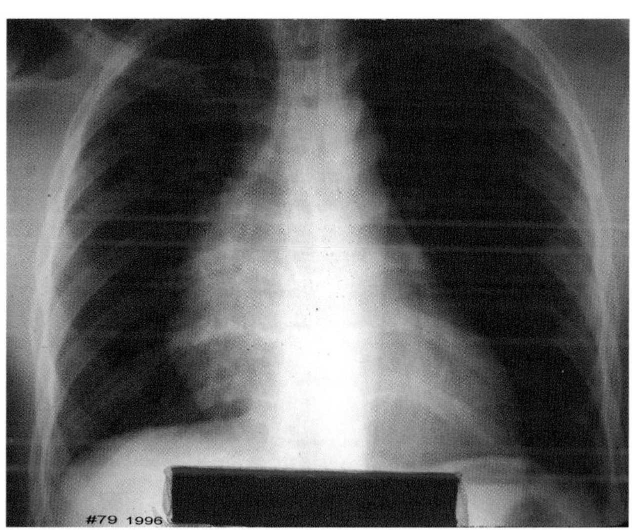

Figure 60.1 Chest X ray PA view 1996 (after thoracentesis).

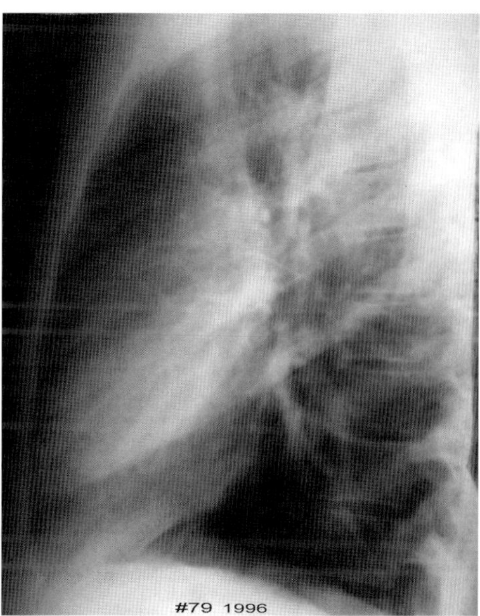

Figure 60.2 Chest X ray lateral view 1996.

Patient Studies in Valvular, Congenital, and Rarer Forms of Cardiovascular Disease: An Integrative Approach, First Edition. Franklin B. Saksena.

Companion Website: www.wiley.com/go/saksena/patientstudies

2 ECG 6 April 1996

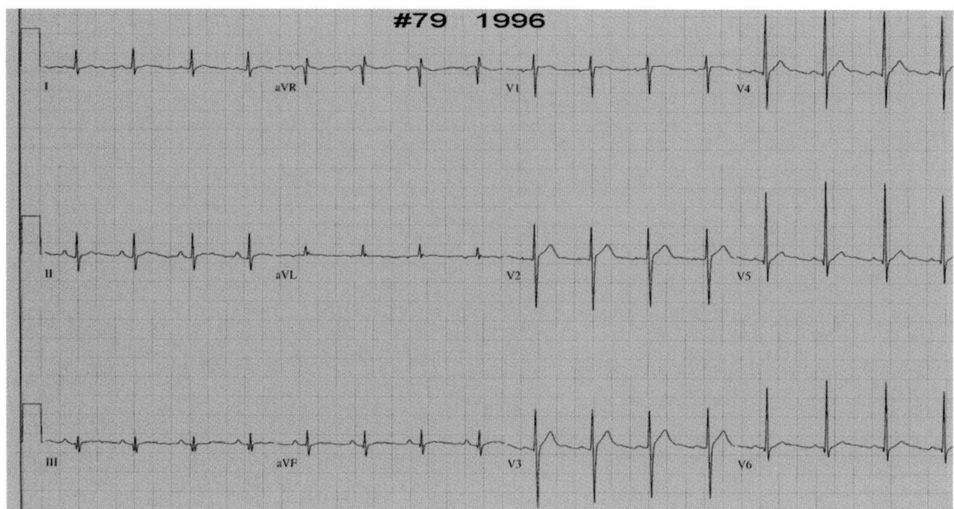

Figure 60.3 12-lead ECG 1996.

3 Laboratory data

Hb 14.5 g%. WBC 16,300/mm^3.
Normal echocardiogram.

4 History and physical exmination

History

20-year-old man with right shoulder pain and right-sided pleuritic chest pain for 2 days.

Physical examination

67 inches tall, 145 lb male. BP 92/57. HR 105/min. R 14/min. T 100.9°F.
RLL effusion. Apex is in the 5th interspace, 9 cm from the mid-sternal line.
Normal S1 and S2. No murmurs.

What is your diagnosis?

5 Hemodynamics

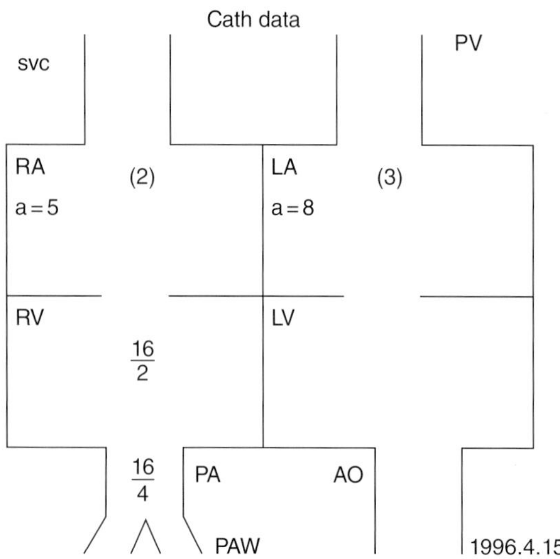

Figure 60.4 Intracardiac pressures 1996.

Table 60.1 Additional cardiac catheterization data

Normal oxygen saturation sample run
Normal arterial oxygen saturation
Normal pulmonary angiogram

6 RA angiogram and chest CT

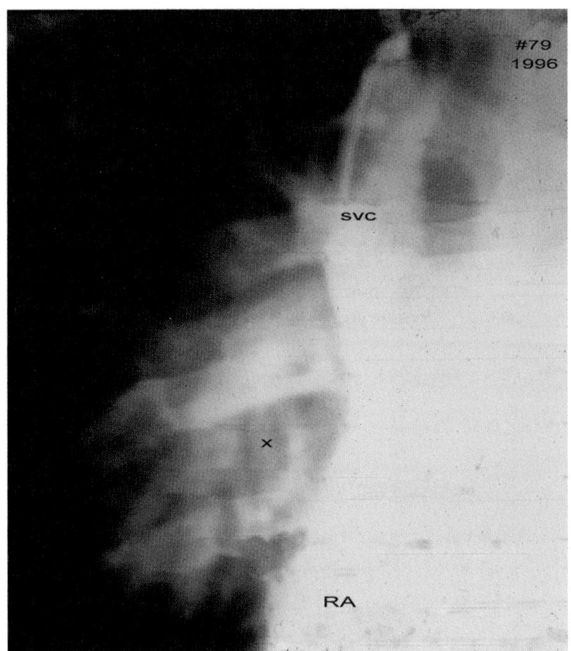

Figure 60.5 RA angiogram AP view.

What is x?

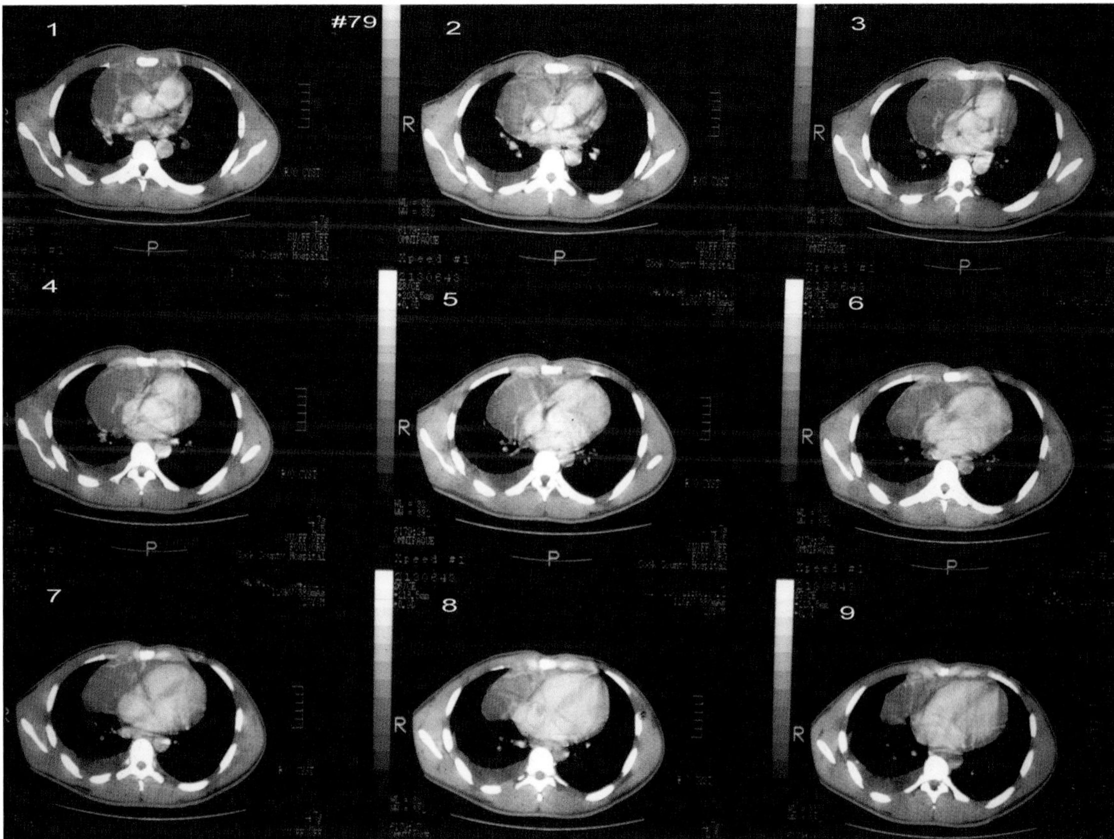

Figure 60.6 CT of chest taken in 1996 showing nine successive slices, arranged superiorly at slice 1 and ending at slice 9 inferiorly.

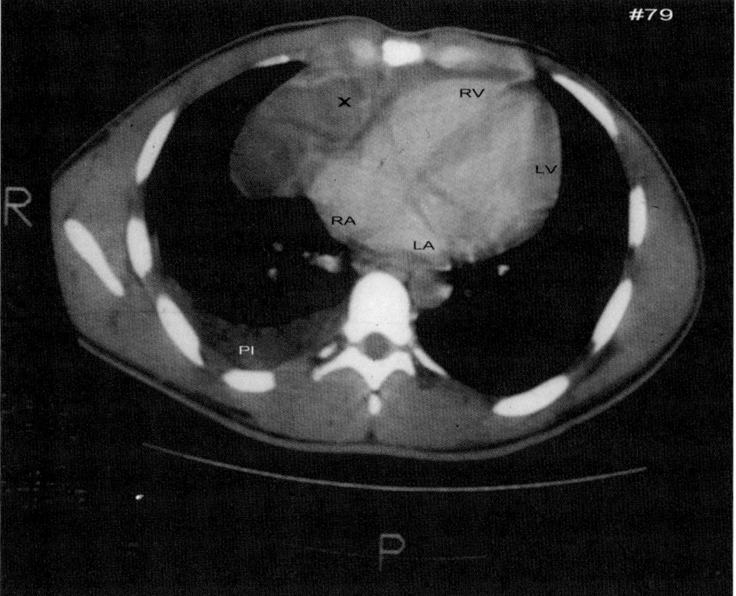

Figure 60.7 Enlargement of slice 8, depicted in Figure 60.6. PI, pleural fluid.
What is x?

7 Diagnosis

What is the diagnosis?

8 Surgical findings

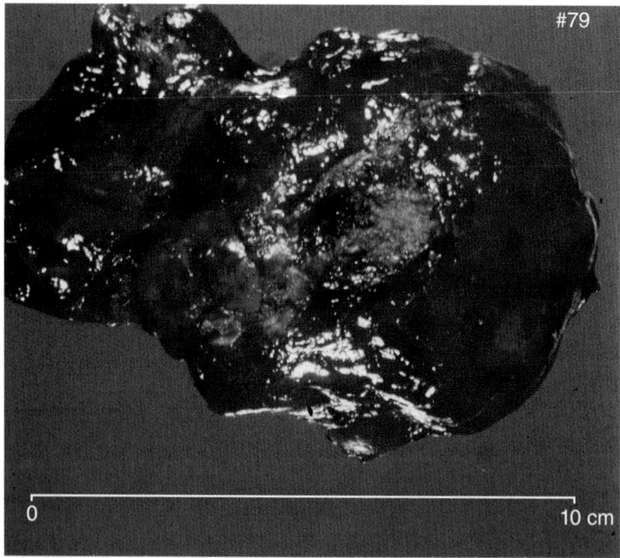

Figure 60.8 Gross appearance of tumor removed surgically in 1996.

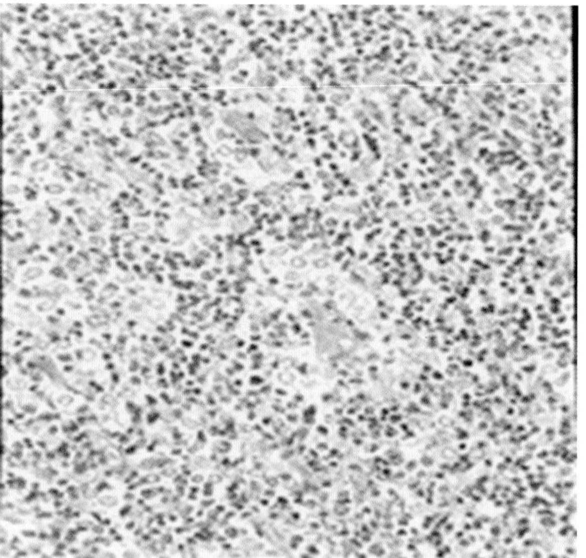

Figure 60.9 Microscopic appearance of tumor. Hematoxylin and eosin stain.

9 Course

Answers and commentary

1 Chest X ray

In Figure 60.1 there is an apparent enlargement of the right heart. The lateral border of the right heart appears slightly irregular.

In Figure 60.2 about two-thirds of the retrosternal space is almost completely filled by a dense structure that most likely represents a mass rather than RV enlargement, as it is much more dense than the cardiac shadow seen inferiorly.

No pleural fluid is seen as the patient had undergone thoracentesis prior to this X ray.

2 ECG 6 April 1996

The rhythm is sinus with a rate of 95/min. PR 0.13 s. QRS 0.07 s. QRS axis +30°. Non-specific T wave changes.

Impression: non-specific T wave changes.

A normal ECG makes it less likely that the dense structure seen on lateral chest X ray is due to RV enlargement or RVH.

3 Laboratory data

The WBC count is increased. A normal echocardiogram excludes RVH or RV enlargement, so that the dense structure must be a mass superimposed on the cardiac silhouette in the lateral X ray.

4 History and physical examination

The pleuritic chest pain, fever, and RLL effusion suggest a pneumonia but no infiltrates are seen on the PA chest X ray.

5 Hemodynamics

The right heart pressures are normal. LA pressure is normal.

The normal oxygen sample run excludes a significant left to right shunt.

The normal pulmonary angiogram excludes pulmonary vascular disease.

6 RA angiogram and chest CT

The RA angiogram shows a lobulated mass separate from the RA (Figure 60.5). PA angiogram was normal (not shown).

CT of chest confirmed a lobulated encapsulated mass separate from the heart and pressing on the RA and abutting against the pleura anteriorly (Figures 60.6 and 60.8).

There is a small right-sided pleural effusion (Pl).

7 Surgical findings

A fleshy mass measuring 5 × 10 cm was removed at thoracotomy. Microscopically the mass showed many uniformly sized lymphocytes with a few epithelial cells.

8 Final diagnosis

Thymoma.

9 Course

The patient did well after thymectomy. He was diagnosed with myasthenia gravis between 1996 and 1998 and responded well to mestenon and then steroid treatment. He was doing well as of 2012. His chest X ray in 2012 was normal (see Figures 60.10 and 60.11).

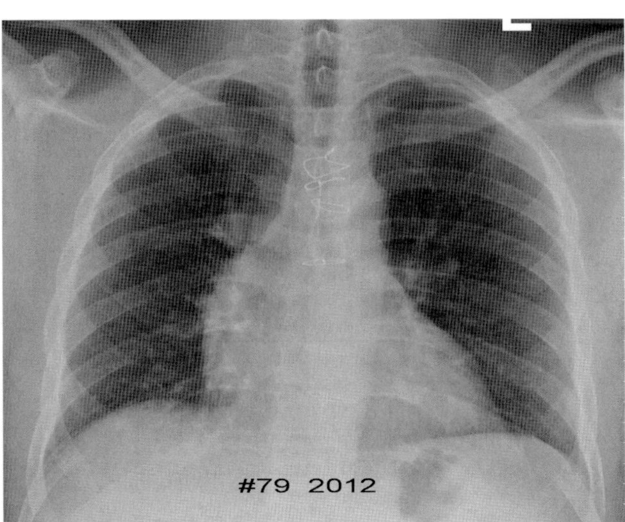

Figure 60.10 Chest X ray PA in 2012.

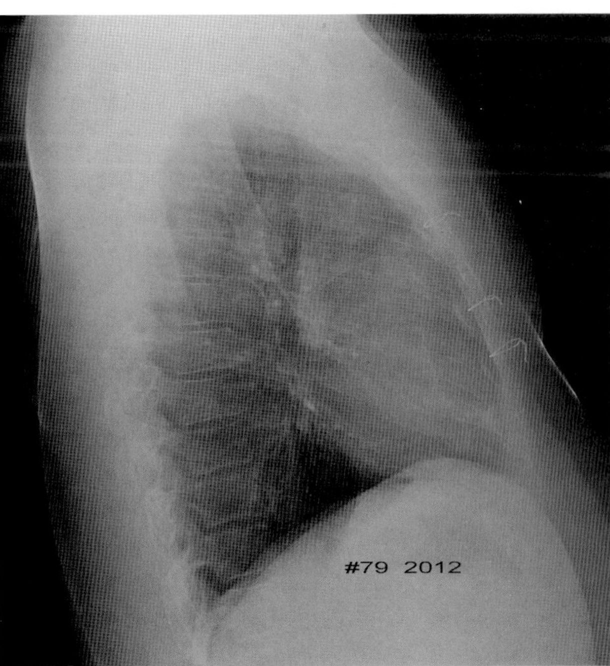

Figure 60.11 Lateral chest X ray in 2012.

Discussion

A thymoma is a neoplasm involving the epithelial cells of the thymus. It is usually encapsulated (75% of cases) but occasionally may invade other tissues (25% of cases) [1, 2].

A thymoma occurs with equal frequency in men and women in their fourth or fifth decades of life, but occasionally may be seen in younger patients, as in this patient [3, 4].

About one-third of patients have an asymptomatic mediastinal mass, one-third are symptomatic, and one-third have an autoimmune disease, usually myasthenia gravis [3, 4]. This patient had pleuritic chest pain as the tumor was abutting against the pleura anteriorly. He developed overt myasthenia gravis between 1996 and 1998 after thymectomy.

A thymoma is the most common tumor found in the anterior mediastinum and may be seen on chest X ray as a mass on either side of the heart [2]. The mass may be confluent with the cardiac shadow [2], as seen in this patient. In retrospect, the undulations of the right heart border and its position extending slightly more superior than usual for RV enlargement (Figure 60.1) may have provided a clue to the existence of a thymoma.

The lateral chest X ray was also highly suggestive of an anterior mediastinal mass superimposed on the cardiac silhouette.

RA angiography and CT of the chest (Figures 60.5–60.7) confirmed the presence of a mass separate from the heart.

MRI is also very useful in the detection of a mediastinal mass (such as a thymoma) as it does not require the use of intravenous contrast material and is also able to exclude cystic structures [1, 2].

This patient's tumor was encapsulated at surgery and would be classified as a Masaoka stage 1, which carries a 92.5% 5-year survival rate [2]. Surgical excision is recommended in patients with an encapsulated thymoma [4].

Key points

1. A thymoma is the most common anterior mediastinal tumor.
2. The thymoma is often confluent with the cardiac shadow and requires a CT of the chest or angiography to show that it is separate from the heart.
3. In one-third of cases it is associated with myasthenia gravis.
4. Thymectomy is the treatment of choice.

References

[1] Grasso AE, O'Hanlon R, Locca D et al. Cardiovascular magnetic resonance of thymoma. *Circulation* 2009; 120: 1453–1455.

[2] Rosado-de-Christenson ML, Galobardes J, Moran CA. Thymoma: Radiologic–pathologic correlation. *Radiographics* 1992; 12: 151–168 (X ray and pathological findings in 16 patients).

[3] Muller-Hermelink HK, Marx A. Thymoma. *Curr Opin Oncol* 2000; 12: 426–433 (discusses the WHO classification of thymoma).

[4] Thomas CR, Wright CD, Loehrer Sr PJ. Thymoma: State of the art. *J Clin Oncol* 1999; 17: 2280–2289 (lists paraneoplastic syndromes associated with thymoma and discusses chemoradiotherapy in advanced thymomas).

61 PATIENT STUDY 61

Sequence of data presentation

1 1 ECG
↓
2 Chest X ray 7 June 2008
↓
3 Laboratory data
↓
4 CT of facial bones
↓
5 History
↓
6 Physical examination
↓
7 Follow-up chest X ray 9 June 2008 and course
↓
8 Diagnosis

1 ECG

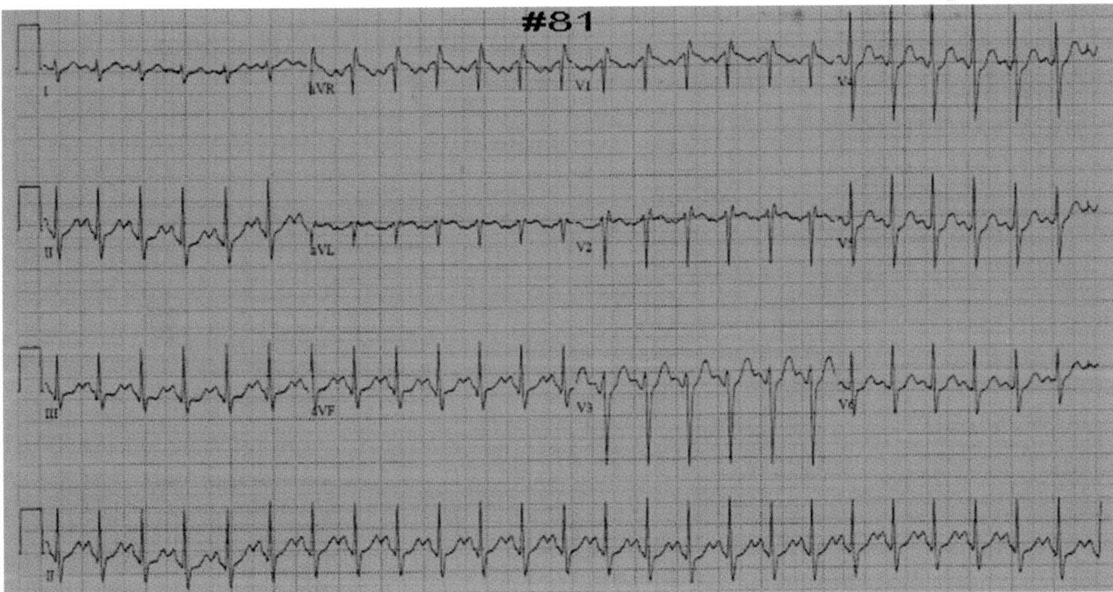

Figure 61.1 12-lead ECG.

Patient Studies in Valvular, Congenital, and Rarer Forms of Cardiovascular Disease: An Integrative Approach, First Edition. Franklin B. Saksena.

Companion Website: www.wiley.com/go/saksena/patientstudies

2 Chest X ray 7 June 2008

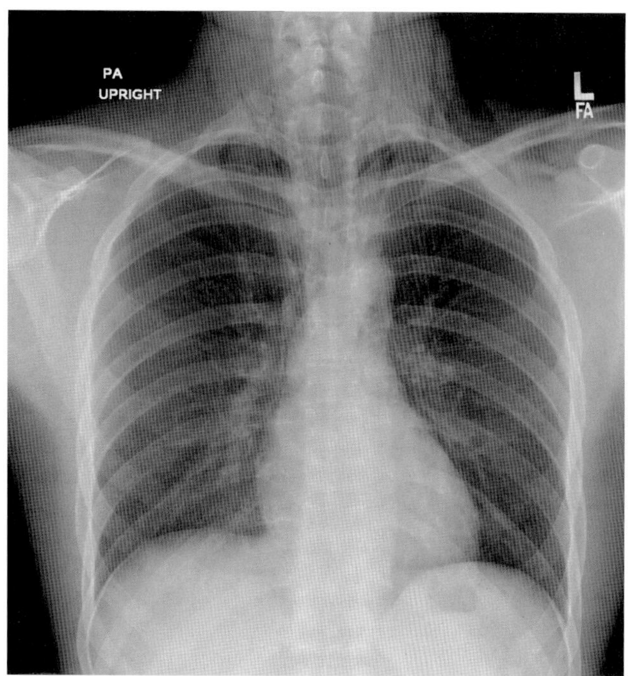

Figure 61.2 PA chest X ray 7 June 2008.

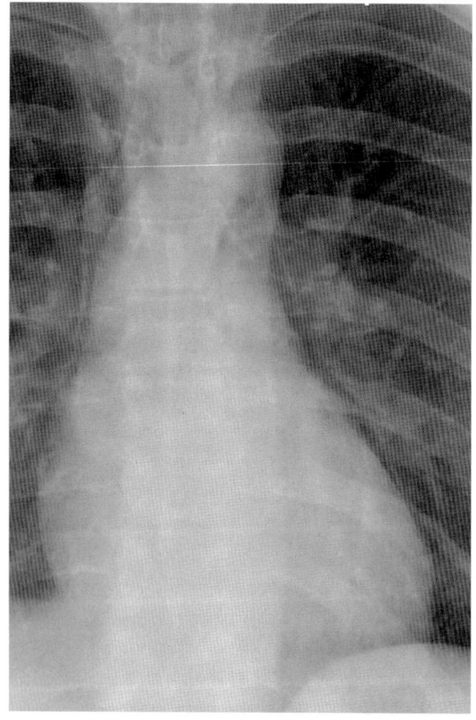

Figure 61.3 PA chest X ray 7 June 2008 (enlarged view of Figure 61.2).

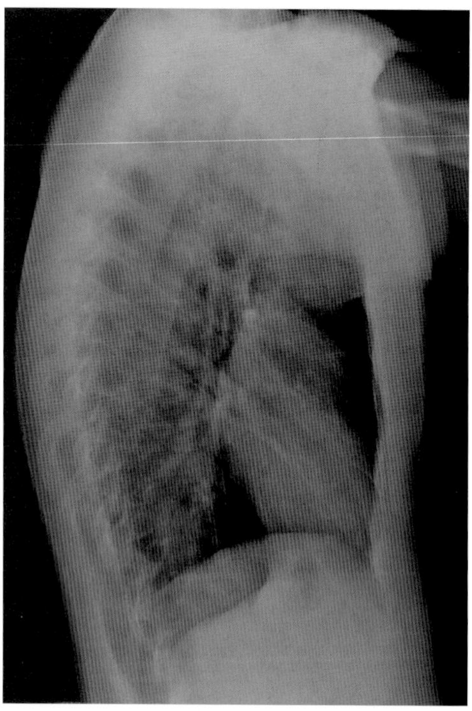

Figure 61.4 Lateral view of chest 7 June 2008.

3 Laboratory data

Hemoglobin 16.9 g%. WBC 14,800/mm^3. Platelets 223,000/mm^3.
Drug screen was positive for cocaine and opiates. Alcohol level <10 mg%. BUN 5 mg%.
Serum K 3.7 meg/L. Glucose 110 mg%.

4 CT of facial bones

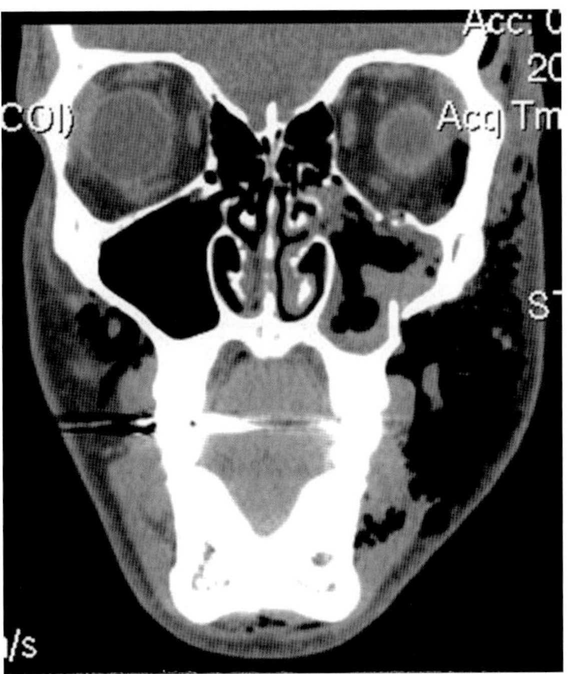

Figure 61.5 Frontal view of CT of skull 7 June 2008.

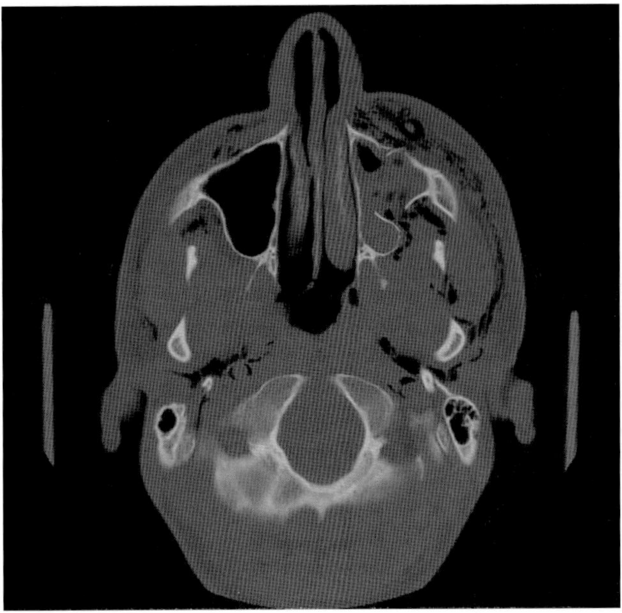

Figure 61.6 Cross-sectional view of skull 7 June 2008.

5 History

20-year-old former waiter admitted to hospital with a swollen painful face for 3 days and sharp bilateral chest pain on inspiration for 1 day.

3 days ago the patient was involved in an altercation and hit in the face multiple times after a bout of drinking. No loss of consciousness.

In the ER he had BP 150/102, HR 158/min, respiratory rate 24/min, and temperature 98°F.

There is a history of drug abuse, including cocaine, alcohol, LSD, and methamphetamine. No history of diabetes or hypertension.

6 Physical examination

70 inches tall, 148 lb male complaining of bilateral chest pain on inspiration.

HEENT

There is marked swelling and ecchymosis in the left periorbital area and a gash over the lower left eyebrow. The left eye is completely closed. Pupils are equal bilaterally.

Limited ability to open mouth.

Respiratory examination

There is crepitus over both supraclavicular fossae. Air entry is diminished bilaterally.

No basal crackles.

Cardiac examination

There is no elevation of jugular venous pressure. Apex beat is in the 5th interspace, 9 cm from the mid-sternal line. S1 normal. S2 physiologically split. No murmurs. Good peripheral pulses.

No edema, cyanosis, or clubbing.

Abdominal examination and CNS examination both normal.

7 Follow-up chest X ray 9 June 2008 and course

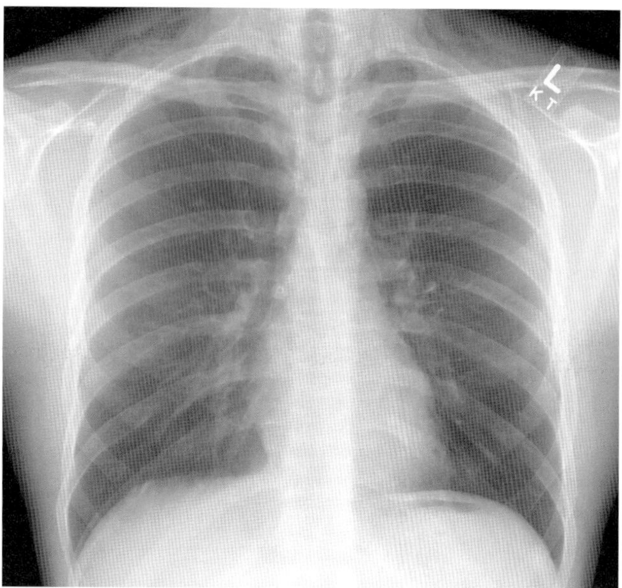

Figure 61.7 Chest X ray PA view 9 June 2008.

8 Diagnosis

What is the diagnosis?

Answers and commentary

1 ECG

Sinus tachycardia 152/min. PR 0.09 s. QRS 0.098 s. QRS axis +90°.

Impression: abnormal ECG because of rapid rate and rightward QRS axis.

2 Chest X ray 7 June 2008

There is subcutaneous emphysema in both supraclavicular fossae (Figure 61.2).

Figures 61.2 and 3 show a linear density lateral to the upper right cardiac border and a more extensive linear density paralleling the left heart border, representing the laterally displaced mediastinal pleura.

Figure 61.4 shows an air stripe anterior to the cardiac shadow in the lateral view.

These chest X ray findings are indicative of a pneumomediastinum as well as air in the subcutaneous tissues of the neck.

3 Laboratory data

The WBC count was increased because of the recent trauma. (It fell to normal 2 days later.) Drug screen confirmed his drug abuse.

4 CT of facial bones

Figures 61.5 and 61.6 show left orbital emphysema and subcutaneous emphysema of the neck. The left maxillary sinus contains a large amount of blood as well as an air fluid level. In addition, there are comminuted fractures of the left maxillary sinus and left orbit as well as a depressed but incomplete fracture of the left zygomatic arch.

5 and 6 History and physical examination

The history of facial trauma and chest pain aggravated by inspiration and subcutaneous emphysema should alert one to the possibility of pneumomediastinum. This diagnosis was confirmed by a PA and lateral chest X ray. The source of air entry was from the traumatised maxillary sinus.

7 Follow-up chest X ray 9 June 2008 and course

The follow-up chest X ray showed partial regression of pneumomediastinum and subcutaneous emphysema in the supraclavicular fossa.

The patient was placed on antibiotics and analgesics with symptomatic improvement. Conservative treatment was recommended by the ophthalmologist and ENT specialists.

He was discharged on the third hospital day but failed to keep his follow-up appointment.

8 Diagnosis

Subcutaneous emphysema and pneumomediastinum secondary to extensive facial injuries.

Discussion

Pneumomediastinum is rare in adults. Air in the mediastinum may originate from the lungs, mediastinal airways, esophagus, neck, and abdominal cavity [1, 2].

Pneumomediastinum may be spontaneous, i.e. without any obvious source, or secondary due to trauma, intrathoracic infections, or GI pathology [1,3].

Pneumomediastinum occurred in this patient following facial trauma. Pneumomediastinum occurred because air was forced into the parapharyngeal and retropharyngeal spaces, which then tracked down the prevertebral potential space and fascial planes, resulting in emphysema in the neck and mediastinum [4, 5]. This patient had subcutaneous emphysema in the neck but no Hamman's sign. Hamman's sign is seen in 30% of patients with a pneumomediastinum and consists of a crunchy systolic sound best heard in the left lateral decubitus position [6].

Spontaneous pneumomediastinum is a benign condition occurring in young patients exposed to a sudden pressure change in the intrathoracic cavity, as in another patient (Figure 61.8). As expected a CT of the chest is more sensitive than a plain chest X ray in detecting a pneumomediastinum and assessing other lung pathology [3].

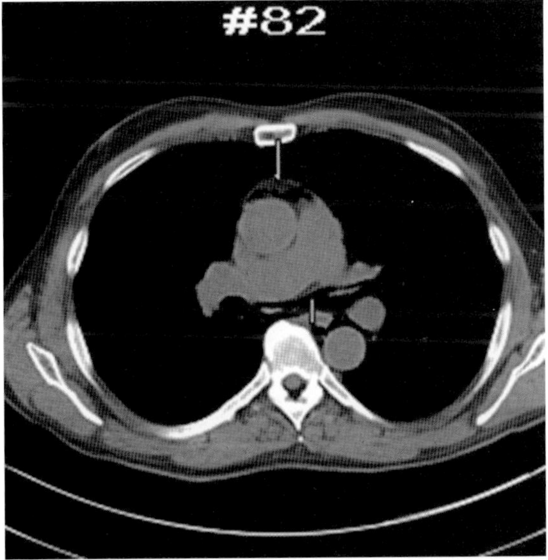

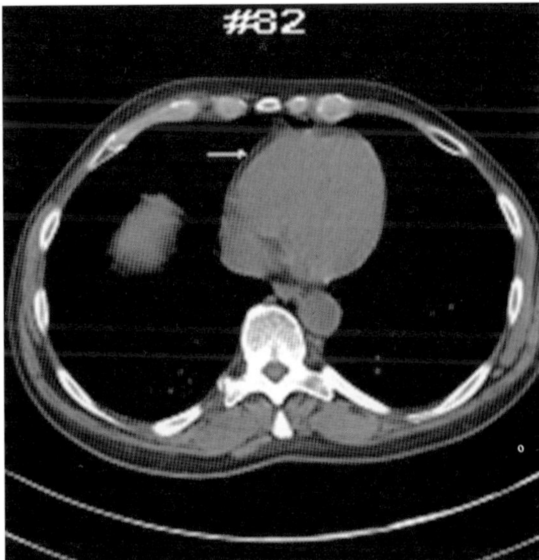

Figure 61.8 CT of chest 27 April 2013 in another patient, showing pneumomediastinum (see arrows). 55-year-old man who developed a retrosternal burning sensation after heavy lifting. No dyspnea or vomiting. A non-smoker who runs several times a week. Crunchy sensation felt in neck. Physical examination showed a 69 inches tall, 158 lb male with BP 140/85, HR 72, R 16, T 98.1°F. The CVS examination, CBC, ECG, and cardiac enzymes were normal. Chest X ray showed a pneumomediastinum and subcutaneous emphysema of the neck. The remainder of the chest CT was negative, i.e. there was no pneumothorax or lung blebs. Upper endoscopy on 29 April 2013 showed only reflux esophagitis and gastritis. CT of neck on 4 May 2013 showed partial resolution of his subcutaneous emphysema in the neck.

In most instances spontaneous pneumomediastinum resolves within a week and rarely recurs [2, 6]. Occasionally a pneumothorax may occur [3, 6] but to date no patients have developed a tension pneumomediastinum [5, 6].

Key points

1. Pneumomediastinum can be spontaneous or secondary to trauma, infections, or GI pathology.
2. Pneumomediastinum may be suspected if there is subcutaneous emphysema or Hamman's sign on physical examination.
3. A PA and lateral chest X ray can often detect a pneumomediastinum by the air stripe or a linear density adjacent to the cardiac shadow.
4. Most cases resolve spontaneously in about a week.

References

[1] Andrianov A, Nissenbaum MA. Pneumopericardium associated with a peptic ulcer. *New Engl J Med* 2011; 365: 2412.

[2] Fraser RS, Muller NL, Coleman N, Paré PD (eds). Fraser and Paré's Diagnosis of Diseases of the Chest, 4th edn, vol. 3. WB Saunders, Philadelphia, 1999, pp 2863–2870.

[3] Caceres M, Ali SZ, Braud R et al. Spontaneous pneumomediastinum: A comparative study and review of the literature. *Ann Thorac Surg* 2008; 86: 962–966.

[4] DeMers G, Camp JL, Bennett D. Pneumomediastinum caused by isolated oral-facial trauma. *Am J Emerg Med* 2011; 29: 841e3–841e8 (reviews the literature 1990–2010 and shows seven radiological signs of pneumomediastinum on chest X ray).

[5] Maunder R, Pierson DJ, Hudson LD. Subcutaneous and mediastinal emphysema: Pathophysiology, diagnosis and management. *Arch Intern Med* 1984; 144: 1447–1453 (contains a useful diagram of soft tissue compartments of the mediastinum, 73 references).

[6] Takada K, Matsumoto S, Hiramatsu T et al. Spontaneous pneumomediastinum: an algorithm for diagnosis and management. *Ther Adv Respir Dis* 2009; 3: 301–307.

62 PATIENT STUDY 62

Sequence of data presentation

1 ECG 2008 (for sports participation)
↓
2 Venous Doppler of left femoral vein 2012
↓
3 ECG 10 August 2013
↓
4 Laboratory data 2013
↓
5 Venous Doppler of left femoral vein 2013
↓
6 Echocardiogram 2013
↓
7 Cardiac catheterization 11 August 2013
↓
8 Coronary angiography 2013
↓
9 History and physical examination 2013
↓
10 Diagnosis and treatment

1 ECG 2008 (for sports participation)

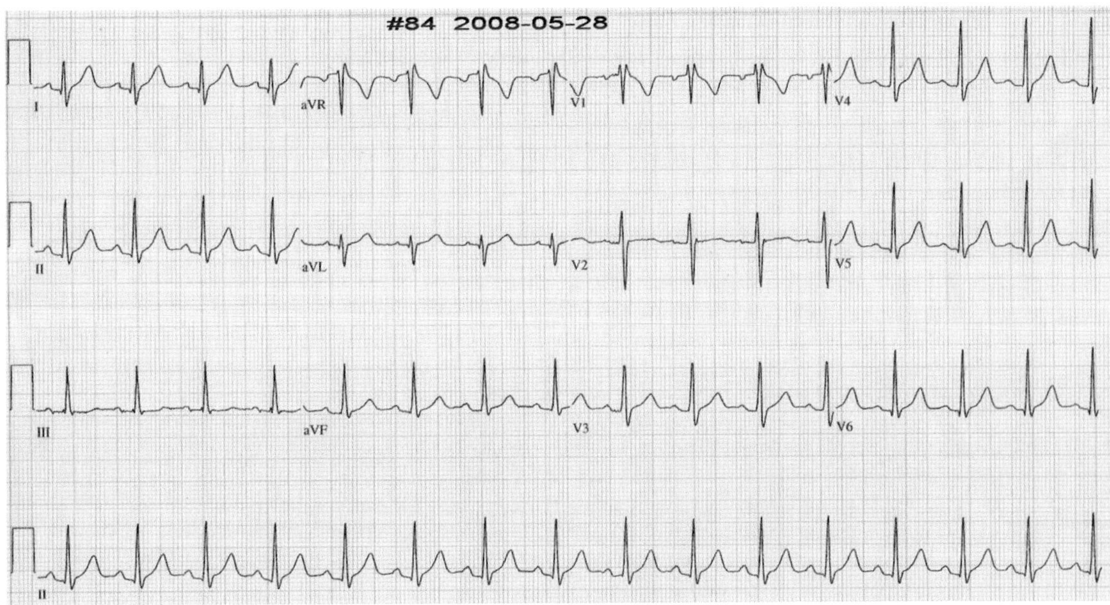

Figure 62.1 ECG 2008.

Patient Studies in Valvular, Congenital, and Rarer Forms of Cardiovascular Disease: An Integrative Approach, First Edition. Franklin B. Saksena.

Companion Website: www.wiley.com/go/saksena/patientstudies

2 Venous Doppler of left femoral vein 2012

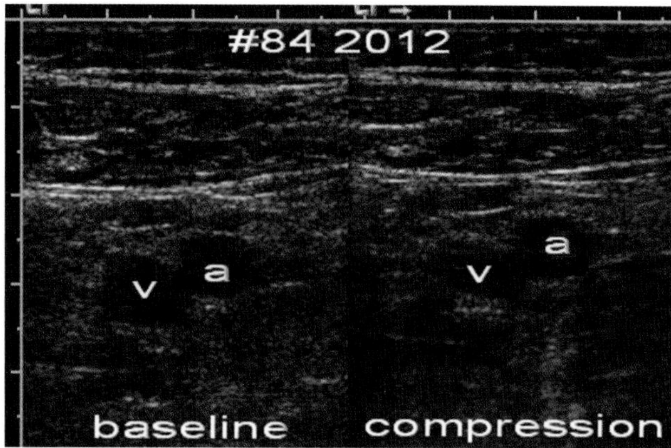

Figure 62.2 Venous Doppler of left femoral vein 2012, before and after compression. a, femoral artery; v, femoral vein.

3 ECG 10 August 2013

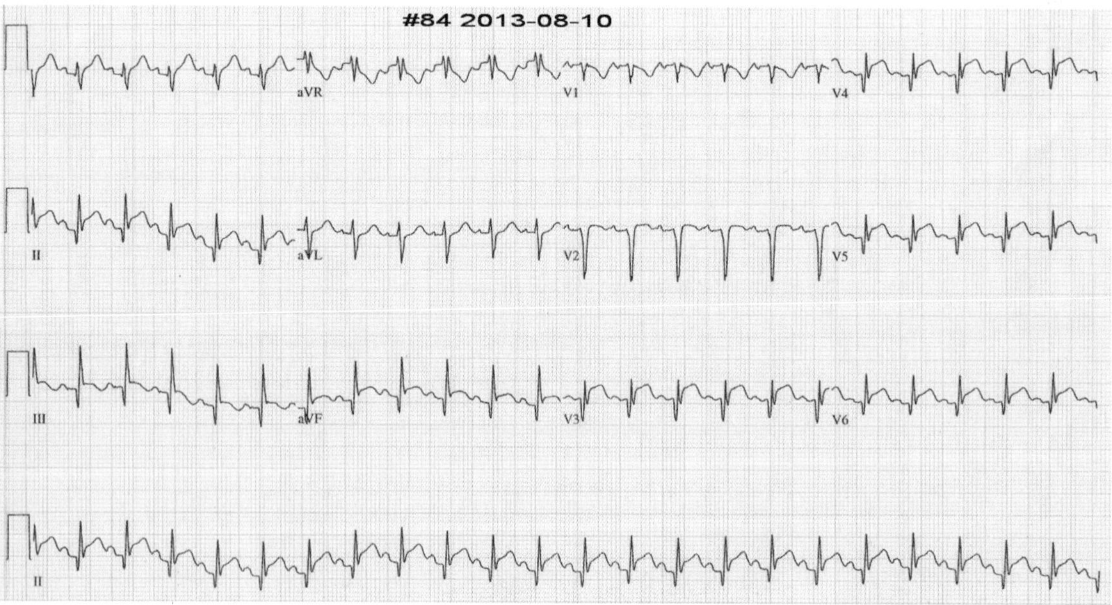

Figure 62.3 ECG 2013.

4 Laboratory data 2013

On admission (9 August 2013) Hb 12.9 g%, WBC 20,800/mm^3, platelet count 268,000/mm^3, ESR 98 mm/h, D dimer 1580 (normal <0.5 mcg/mL FEU), serum cholesterol 136 mg%.

Serum troponins on 10 August 2013 were 48 and 49 ng/mL.

CT of chest showed pneumonia but no pulmonary embolism.

CT of abdomen was normal.

5 Venous Doppler of left femoral vein 2013

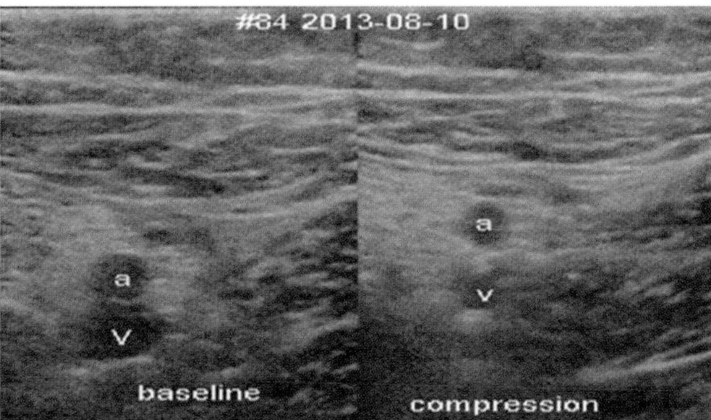

Figure 62.4 Venous Doppler of left femoral vein 9 August 2013, before and after compression. a, femoral artery; v, femoral vein.

6 Echocardiogram 2013

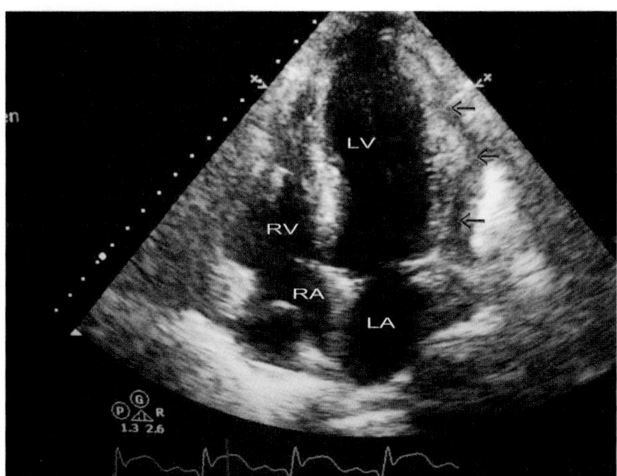

Figure 62.5 Echocardiogram 11 August 2013.

What are the arrows pointing to?

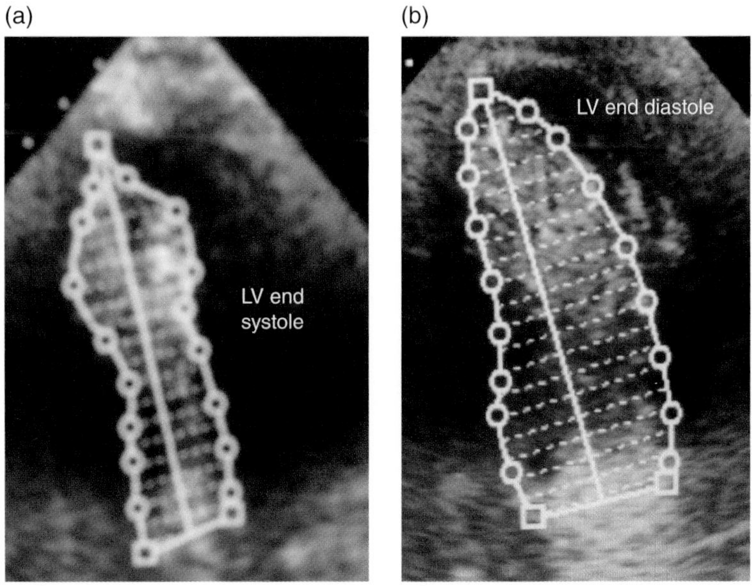

Figure 62.6 (a) Echocardiogram contrast study (end systole). (b) Echocardiogram contrast study (end diastole).

7 Cardiac catheterization 11 August 2013

LV 96/21. Aorta 80/54 (mean 68 mmHg).
LV angiogram: LV apical hypokinesia (not shown).

8 Coronary angiography 2013

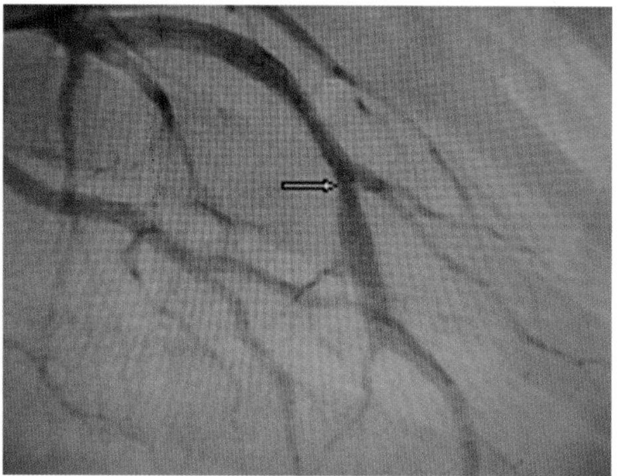

Figure 62.7 Left anterior descending coronary (LAD) angiography.

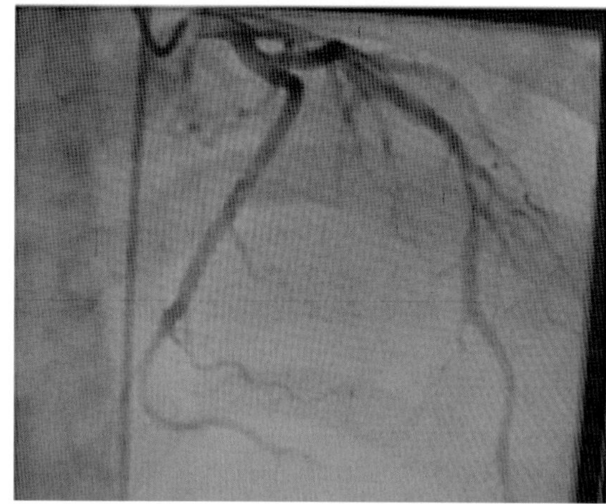

Figure 62.8 LAD and circumflex angiography.

9 History and physical examination 2013

History

The patient had an ECG at age 12 prior to participating in sports in 2009. She returned in October 2012 with left thigh pain caused by a deep vein thrombosis of the left femoral vein.

At that time she had a lupus-like anticoagulant antibody and Igg antibodies to cardiolipin exceeding 150 (normal 10–14 GPL u/mL). The levels of protein C, protein S, and antithrombin 3 were normal. She was treated with warfarin. In February 2013 the presence of a lupus-like anticoagulant antibody was again noted.

She stopped taking warfarin in June 2013 because of heavy menses.

She was admitted to hospital with upper right-sided abdominal and chest pain on 9 August 2013.

She does not drink, smoke, or use illicit drugs and is not on birth control pills.

No history of diabetes or hypertension. No family history of coronary artery disease.

Physical examination

65 inches tall female weighing 204 lb. BP 127/78. HR 130/min regular. T 102°F.
No elevation of jugular venous pressure.
No cardiomegaly. Normal heart sounds.
Bilateral basal crackles.
No abdominal masses. No pedal edema or lymphadenopathy.

10 Diagnosis and treatment

What is the diagnosis?

Answers and commentary

1 ECG 2008 (for sports participation)

Sinus rhythm. Rate 90/min. PR 0.17 s. QRS 0.11 s. QRS axis +80°. QTc 0.47 s.
Impression: incomplete RBBB with borderline prolongation of QTc.
She was cleared for sports participation.

2 Venous Doppler of left femoral vein 2012

There is a lack of compressibility of the femoral vein (v), implying the presence of femoral vein thrombosis. The femoral artery (a) was unaffected by external compression of the thigh.

3 ECG 10 August 2013

There is sinus tachycardia with a rate of 130/min. PR 0.14 s. QRS 0.10 s.

QRS axis + 100 degrees. q waves and ST elevation are seen in 2, 3, F and V3–6.

QS waves now seen in V1–2. q in V3–6.

Impression: anterolateral wall infarction with possible extension to inferior wall.

Coexisting pericarditis cannot be excluded.

An acute myocardial infarction in a 17-year-old female without known coronary risk factors should suggest a new onset of a vasculitis or a coagulopathy, especially since an ECG in 2008 was normal and there was no evidence of cocaine use.

4 Laboratory data 2013

There is marked elevation of the serum troponin levels, confirming the presence of an acute myocardial infarction. The right-sided upper abdominal pain was attributed to a pneumonia as there was no intra-abdominal pathology detected on CT of the abdomen.

The elevation of the D dimer is non-specific as there was no evidence of a pulmonary embolism on CT of the chest.

5 Venous Doppler of left femoral vein 2013

This showed normal compressibility of the femoral vein (v), i.e. there was no evidence of a deep vein thrombosis in August 2013 (compare Figure 62.2 with Figure 62.4).

6 Echocardiogram 2013

The four-chamber view showed normal chamber dimensions with a small pericardial effusion (arrows).

The echocardiogram with contrast material showed apical hypokinesia (Figures 62.6a and b).

7 Cardiac catheterization 11 August 2013

The LVEDP was elevated to 21 mmHg, indicative of LV dysfunction. The aortic systolic pressure was reduced, probably because of a low output state.

8 Coronary angiography 2013

The right coronary artery was non-dominant and free of disease (not shown).

The circumflex coronary artery was normal.

There was 50% stenosis of the mid left anterior descending artery just distal to its 2nd diagonal branch. There is a layered thrombus in the region of this stenosis. This implies that the left anterior descending artery had been occluded and has now partially recanalized over the last 2 days. This earlier occlusion of the left anterior descending artery would account for the patient's LV dysfunction.

9 History and physical examination 2013

The history of DVT and the detection of lupus-like antibodies pointed to antiphospholipid antibody syndrome and she was started on warfarin. She developed chest pain and incipient heart failure after stopping warfarin.

10 Diagnosis and treatment

1. Antiphospholipid antibody syndrome.
2. History of deep vein thrombosis of femoral vein.
3. Acute myocardial infarction associated with left anterior descending coronary artery thrombosis and LV apical hypokinesia.

The patient resumed taking warfarin. She will need to be on this treatment for life.

Discussion

The patient had evidence of the antiphospholipid antibody syndrome based on a positive lupus-like anticoagulant antibody (demonstrated on three separate occasions) and venous and arterial occlusive disease [1, 2].

The antiphospholipid antibody syndrome is a rare non-inflammatory autoimmune disease that usually affects women and is often associated with recurrent miscarriages. There may also be mitral or aortic valve dysfunction, thrombocytopenia, chorea, and livedo reticularis [1].

One hypothesis as to why thrombosis occurs in such patients is that the antibody to the phospholipid binding protein interferes with tissue factor pathway inhibitor. This means that factors 7 and 10 are no longer 'restrained' and the extrinsic pathway of coagulation is activated [1, 2].

When the patient stopped taking her anticoagulants she had a myocardial infarction.

Thus patients with the antiphospholipid antibody syndrome will probably need to be on anticoagulants for life.

Key points

1. Antiphospholipid antibody syndrome should be considered if there is a lupus-like anticoagulant antibody (verified on at least two occasions), and venous and arterial occlusive disease.
2. Patients need to be on anticoagulants for life.

References

[1] DeGroot PG, Derksen RHWM. Pathophysiology of the antiphospholipid syndrome. *J Thromb Haemost* 2005; 3: 1854–1860.

[2] Levine JS, Branch DW, Rauch J. The antiphospholipid syndrome. *New Eng J Med* 2002; 346: 752–763.

Further reading

Ruiz-Irastorza G, Crowther M, Branch W et al. Antiphospholipid syndrome. *Lancet* 2010; 376: 1498–1509 (detailed discussion of pathogenesis, clinical findings and treatment—124 references).

63 PATIENT STUDY 63

Sequence of data presentation

1 ECG 4 November 2008
↓
2 Chest X ray 2008
↓
3 Chest X ray 2009
↓
4 History and physical examination 2009
↓
5 Laboratory data 2008
↓
6 Diagnosis
↓
7 Surgery and course

1 ECG 4 November 2008

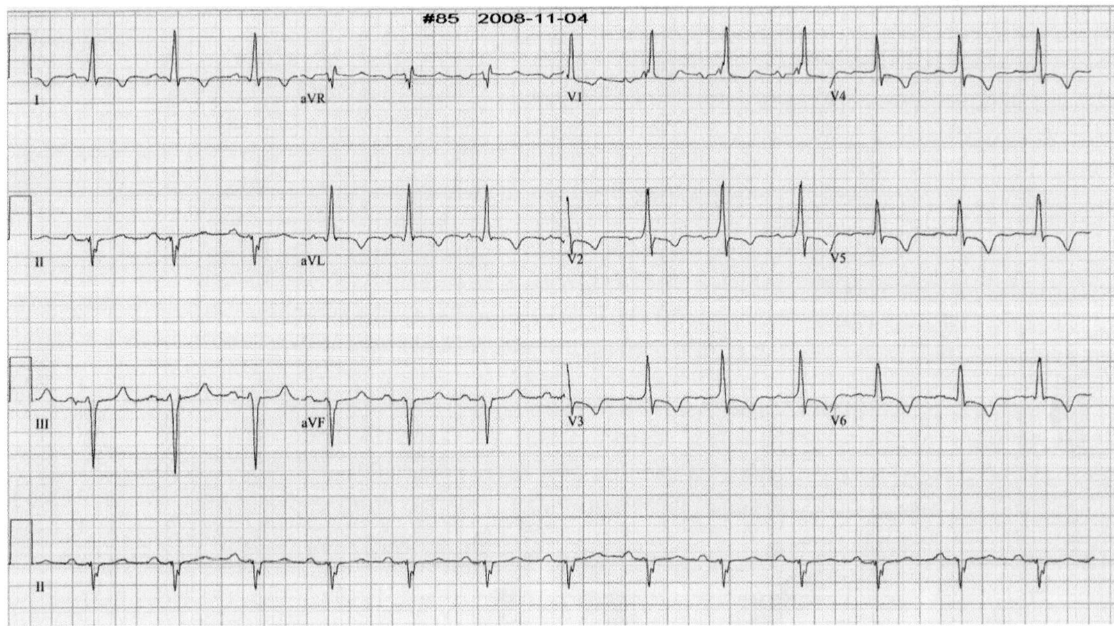

Figure 63.1 ECG 4 November 2008.

Patient Studies in Valvular, Congenital, and Rarer Forms of Cardiovascular Disease: An Integrative Approach, First Edition. Franklin B. Saksena.

Companion Website: www.wiley.com/go/saksena/patientstudies

2 Chest X ray 2008

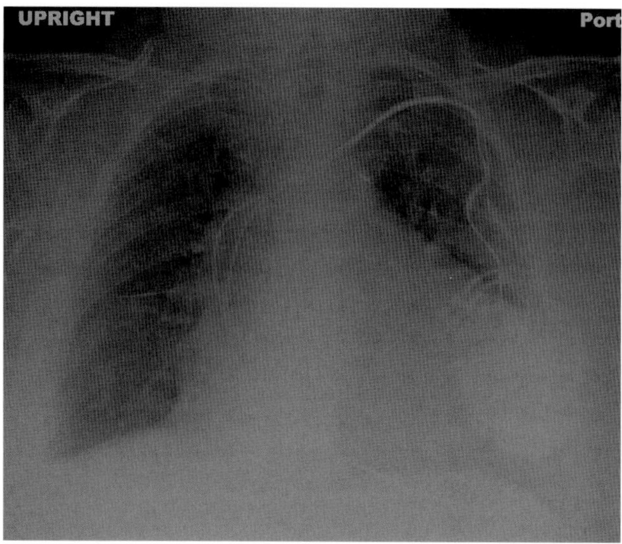

Figure 63.2 Chest X ray 2008 showing ICD in place. There is a lead in the RV (faintly seen) and one in the RA.

3 Chest X ray 2009

(a) (b)

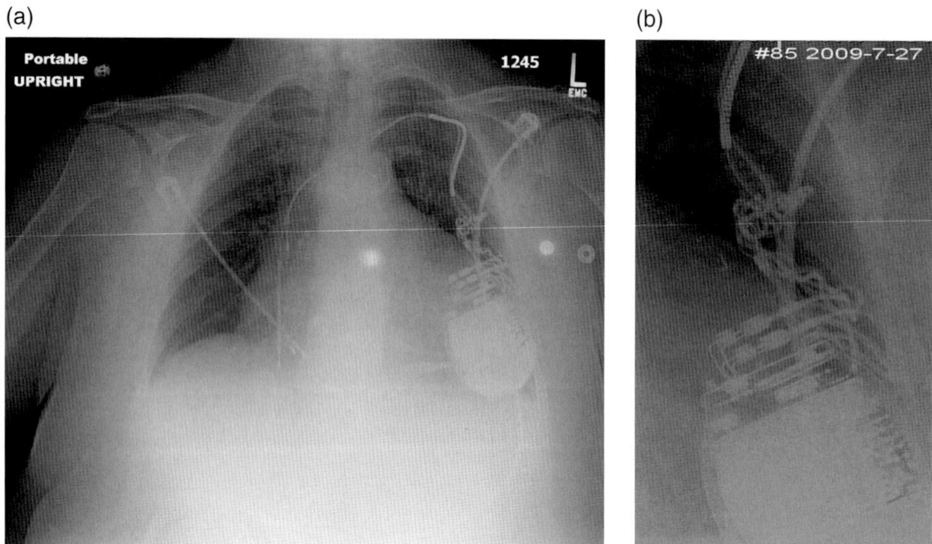

Figure 63.3 (a) Chest X ray 27 July 2009 taken after admission to hospital for multiple shocks. (b) Chest X ray 27 July 2009 showing an enlarged view of the leads just above the generator.

4 History and physical examination 2009

History

66-year-old diabetic female who underwent three-vessel coronary artery bypass surgery at another medical center in 2000. At that time the LV ejection fraction was 45%.

In 2004, two of her aorto-coronary vein grafts became occluded. The LIMA to the left anterior descending artery was still patent. Her LV ejection fraction was now only 20%. She underwent successful PTCA of her occluded vein graft to the right coronary artery. She was continued on digoxin, furosemide, metoprolol, statin, and insulin.

In 2006 the ECG showed a bifascicular block. Her LV ejection fraction remained at 20%.

In November 2008 she had cardiomegaly and a bifasicular block. An implantable cardioverter-defibrillator was inserted because of her low LV ejection fraction. The surgical pocket for the generator was made 4–5 cm below the left clavicle.

In July 2009 she was admitted to hospital having received 20 shocks to the heart in one hour.

Physical examination

Height 61 inches, weight 176 lb. BP 130/40. HR 40–60/min. T 98°F. There was cardiomegaly. Grade 1/6 aortic systolic murmur. Occasional crackles heard in the lower lung fields. No clubbing. Trace leg edema. Peripheral pulses are intact.

5 Laboratory data 2008

Hb 14.2 g%. WBC 8400/mm^3. BUN 32 mg%. Creatinine 1.1 mg%. Troponin 0.28 and 1.08 ng/mL. Glucose 102 mg%. Potassium 4 meq/L.

6 Diagnosis

What is your diagnosis and the patient's likely course?

7 Course

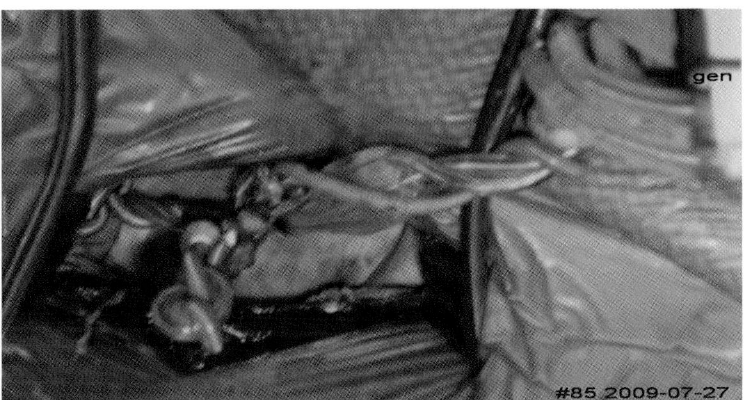

Figure 63.4 Operative view of pacing leads and generator (gen) 29 July 2009.

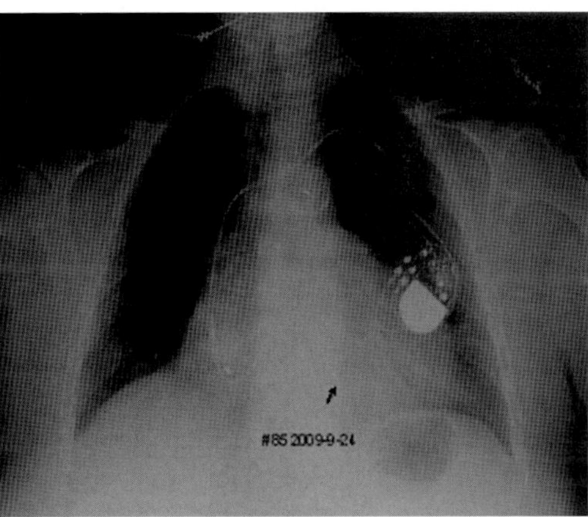

Figure 63.5 Postoperative chest X ray 2009 showing dual-chamber pacemaker in place. Arrow shows the position of the tip of the RV lead.

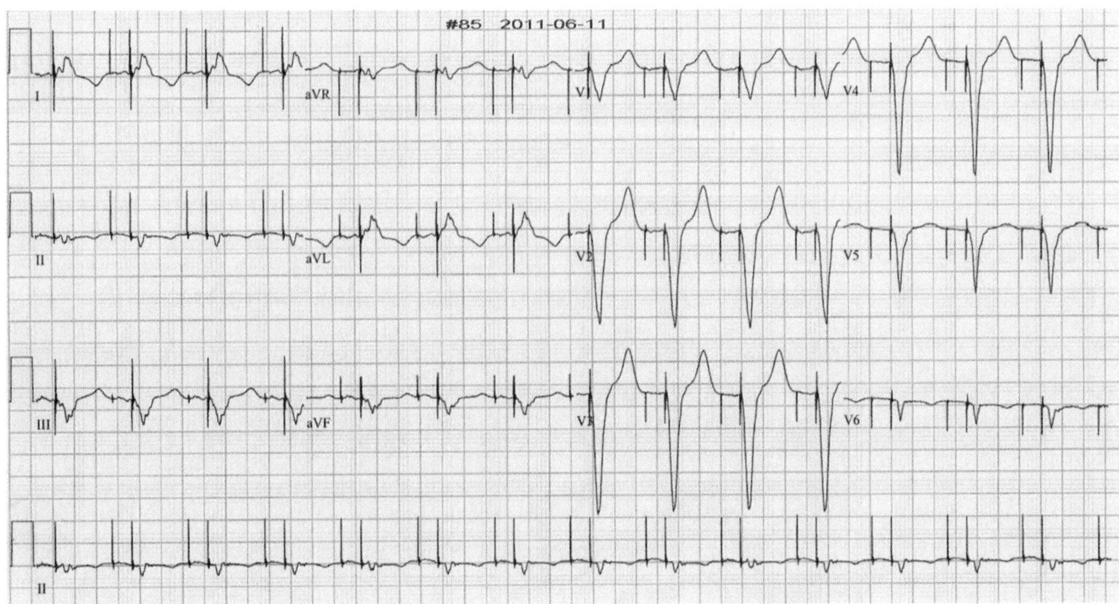

Figure 63.6 ECG 11 June 2011.

8 ECG 15 June 2011

Answers and commentary

1 ECG 4 November 2008

Sinus rhythm with first-degree heart block. Rate 80/min. PR 0.21 s. QRS 0.10 s. QRS axis –50°. QTc 0.47 s. rsR′ in V1. Q in 2, 3, F. T inversion 1, L, V2–6. R1+ S3 = 2.5 mv.

Lateral T wave abnormalities noted since 2000.

Impression: (i) bifascular block, (ii) old inferior wall infarction, (iii) anterolateral ischemia/necrosis, (iv) voltage criteria for LVH.

2 Chest X ray 2008

The heart is enlarged, with some pulmonary vascular congestion. A dual pacemaker defibrillator has been inserted. The position of the generator is lower than usual. An arrow shows the tip of the RV lead.

3 Chest X ray 2009

The heart remains enlarged. The leads above the generator are tangled up, causing retraction of the RV lead to the RA. The atrial lead is now in the SVC.

4 History and physical examination 2009

The patient received multiple inappropriate shocks from the ICD. Inappropriate shocks with an ICD occur in 20–25 % of cases, usually from supraventricular tachycardia, atrial fibrillation, sinus tachycardia, or non-sustained ventricular tachycardia [1]. Other causes include electrical noise, inappropriate sensing, ICD malfunction (such as lead fracture) [1] and RV displacement from the pacemaker-twiddler's syndrome.

She had bradycardia and was in mild LV failure on physical examination.

5 Laboratory data 2008

The CBC is normal with only borderline elevation of the BUN and troponin levels.

6 Diagnosis

Pacemaker-twiddler's syndrome.

7 Surgery and course

The ICD was turned off and the patient developed bradycardia. The patient refused to have a new ICD inserted but was agreeable to having a dual-chamber pacemaker inserted.

The patient was operated on by Dr Curran, who noted that the generator was loose in its pocket because the suture holding it to the pectoral fascia was torn off. He removed the ICD and the twisted wires. The patient then underwent successful implantation of a dual-chamber pacemaker. The new generator was placed in the subpectoral region to prevent any further twiddling of the leads.

The dual-chamber pacemaker continued to function (Figure 63.6) until the time of her death from congestive heart failure in 2011.

The ECG on 15 June 2011 showed functioning dual electronic pacemaker. Rate 85/min. QRS 0.17 s. QTc 0.58 s.

Discussion

Twiddling of the pacing leads may occur in patients who have undergone insertion of either a permanent pacemaker [2] or an ICD [3].

Pacemakers-twiddler's syndrome occurs in 0.07% of permanent pacemaker insertions [4], usually within the first year of implantation [3].

It occurs more commonly in obese patients (as this patient was) where the pectoral fascia is loose, making it difficult to secure the generator in one place, or it may occur if the pocket is too large for the size of the generator [5]. Patients may unconsciously twist the generator around and around, causing retraction of the RV pacing lead into the RA. The RV lead may then sense signals from both RA and RV, leading to a series of inappropriate shocks. Inappropriate shocks may also occur if one of the twisted leads above the surgical pocket has been damaged.

Other complications associated with the pacemaker-twiddler's syndrome are failure to pace, unilateral phrenic nerve, vagus nerve, pectoral muscle, or brachial plexus stimulation [3].

Key points

1. Pacemaker-twiddler's syndrome is an uncommon complication of permanent pacemaker or ICD implantation.
2. The patient with pacemaker-twiddler's syndrome may receive multiple inappropriate shocks to the heart if the RV lead is pulled back into the RA–RV junction.
3. The syndrome may be prevented if attention is paid to keeping the ICD surgical pocket small and firmly attaching the ICD to the pectoral fascia or in the subpectoral area.

References

[1] Ganz LI. *Implantable cardioverter–defibrillators: complications*. www.uptodate.com©2013 UpToDate, pp 1–19.

[2] Bayliss CE, Beanlands DS, Baird RJ. The pacemaker-twiddler's syndrome. A new complication of implantable transvenous pacemakers. *Canad Med Ass J* 1968; 99: 371–373.

[3] Mandal S, Pande A, Kahali D. A rare case of very early pacemaker twiddler's syndrome. *Heart Views* 2012; 13: 114–115.

[4] Williams JL, Stevenson RT. *Complications of pacemaker implantation*. http://dx.doi.org/10.5772/48682.2012 InTechchapter 6, pp 131–158.

[5] Nicholson WJ, Tuohy KA, Tilkemeier P. Twiddler's syndrome. *New Eng J Med* 2003; 348: 1726–1727.

Further reading

Thajudeen A, Shehata M, Wang X et al. In a twist: Reel Syndrome. *Am J Med*. 2014; 127: 1070–1071 (a variant of pacemaker–twiddler's syndrome in which the ICD lead became completely extravascular and wound around the pulse generator like a fishing reel).

64 PATIENT STUDY 64

Sequence of display data

1 History June–July 2011
↓
2 Laboratory data June–July 2011
↓
3 Course July–August 2011
↓
4 Diagnosis, treatment, and course August – September 2011

1 History June–July 2011

39-year-old man admitted to hospital on 29 June 2011 with recent cardiac arrest at home associated with ventricular fibrillation. He was placed on a hypothermia protocol for 36 hours [1, 2]. He became mentally alert 2 days after admission.

He also was treated for pulmonary embolism and pneumonia with anticoagulants and antibiotics, respectively

2 Laboratory data June–July 2011

Normal two-dimensional echocardiogram in 2011.

Cardiac catheterization on 13 July 2011 showed LV pressure 93/7, LV ejection fraction 60%, and normal coronary angiograms.

In electrophysiological studies on 14 July 2011 polymormphic ventricular tachycardia was readily inducible. Negative QT–epinephrine test, excluding congenital long QT syndrome [3].

3 Course July–August 2011

The patient underwent insertion of an ICD on 14 July 2011. He went swimming about 2 weeks post ICD implantation.

He was readmitted to hospital on 21 August 2011 with syncope and chest pain.

His ICD was interrogated and there was adequate capture and sensing thresholds of both RA and ventricular leads. His BP was 90 systolic.

Patient Studies in Valvular, Congenital, and Rarer Forms of Cardiovascular Disease: An Integrative Approach, First Edition. Franklin B. Saksena.

Companion Website: www.wiley.com/go/saksena/patientstudies

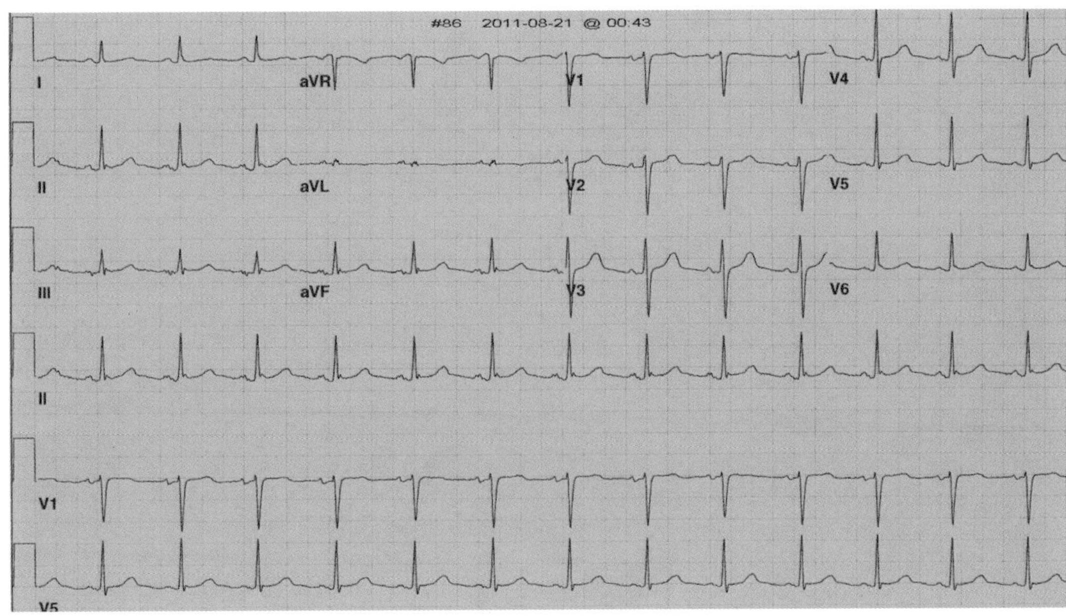

Figure 64.1 ECG 21 August 2011 taken at 00:43.

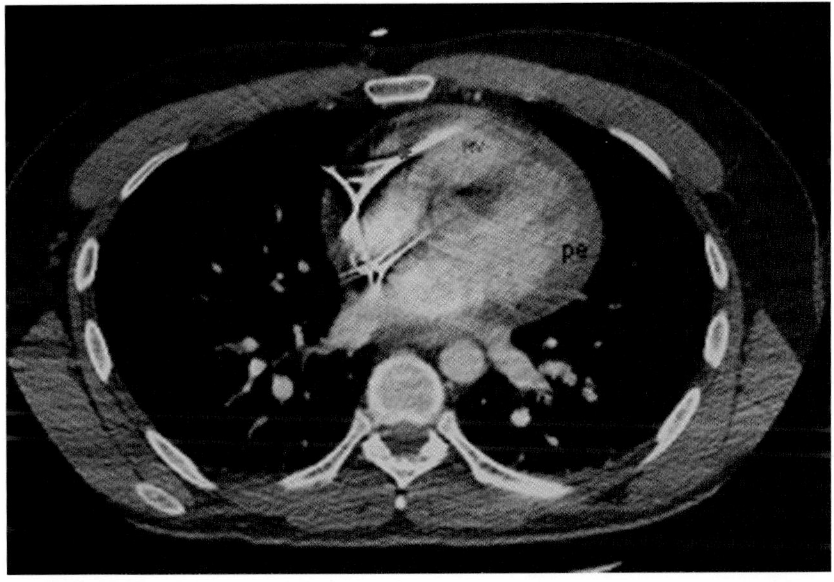

Figure 64.2 CT of chest 21 August 2011 taken at 03:03. Red star (*) shows position of ICD lead. pe, pericardial effusion.

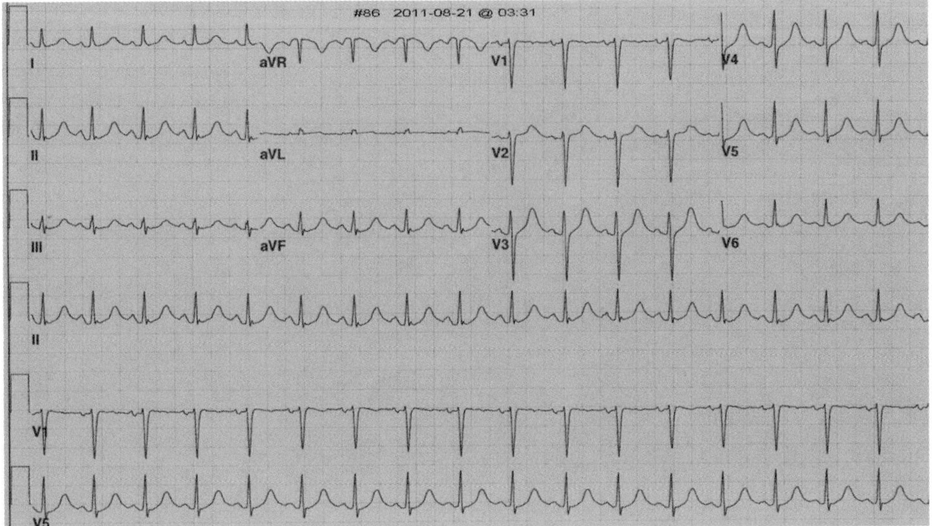

Figure 64.3 ECG 21 August 2011 taken at 03:31.

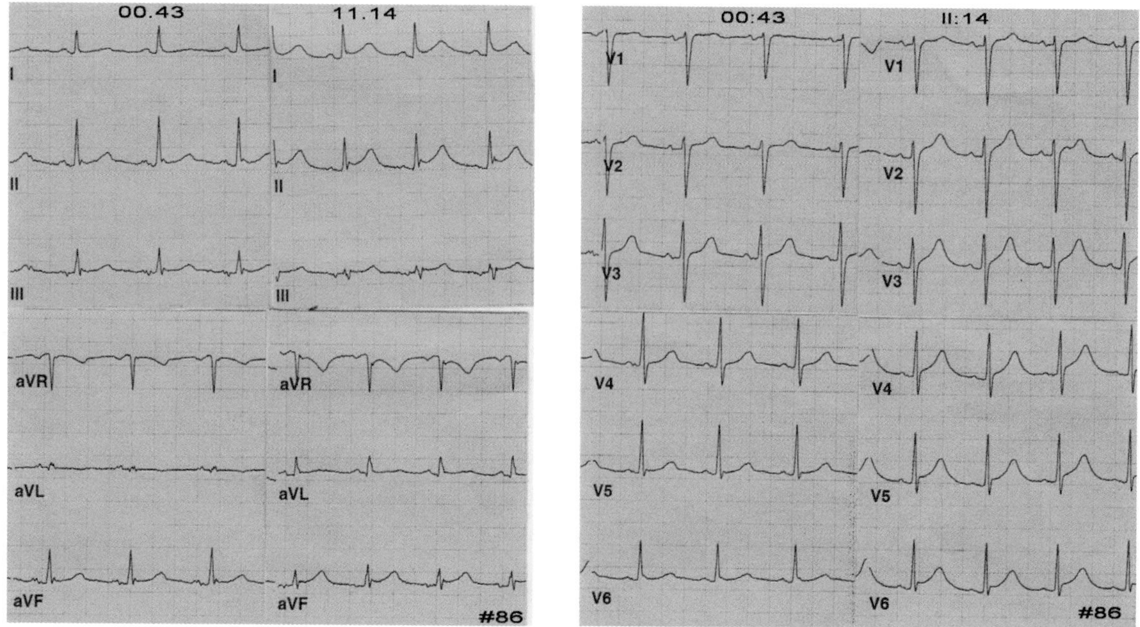

Figure 64.4 ECG 21 August 2011 taken at 11:14. (a) ECG comparison of 00:43 ECG with 11:14, limb leads. (b) ECG comparison of 00:43 ECG with 11:14, chest leads.

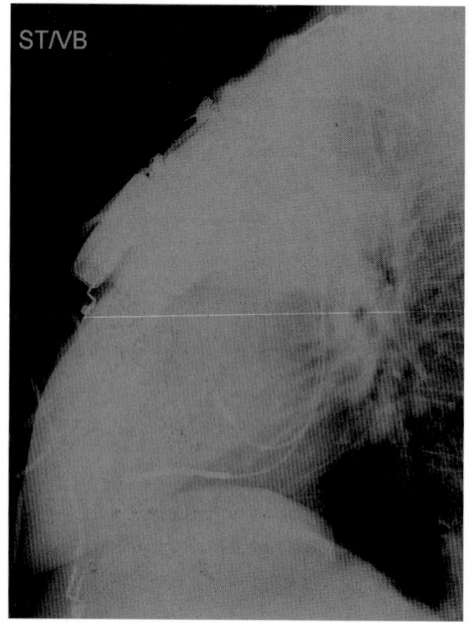

Figure 64.5 Chest X ray 21 August 2011 lateral view taken at 13:15.

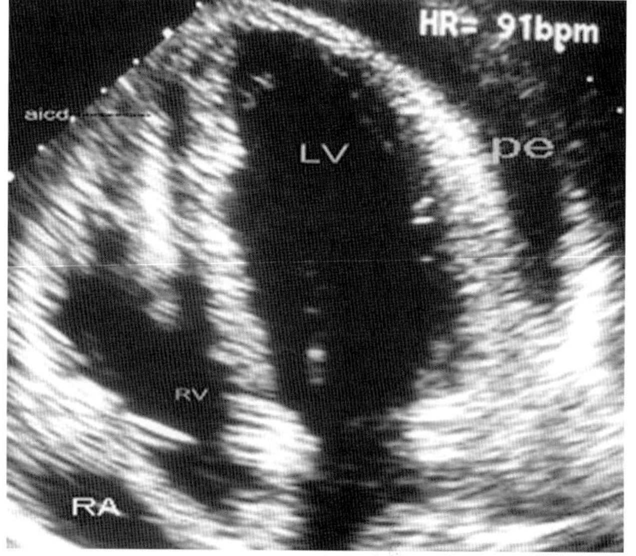

Figure 64.6 Echo 21 August 2011 taken at 13:32. Two-dimensional echocardiogram showing four-chamber view (RA is only partially seen). aicd, automatic implantable cardioverter defibrillator lead (aicd); pe, pericardial effusion.

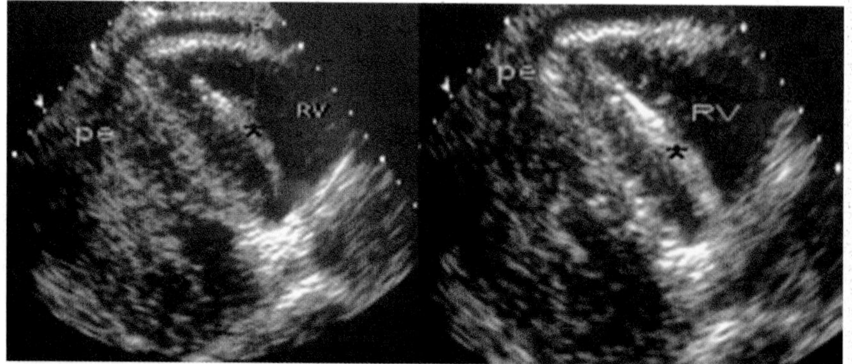

Figure 64.7 Echo 21 August 2011. Two-dimensional echocardiogram showing successive frames in the subcostal view. Red star (*) marks the ICD lead. pe, pericardial effusion.

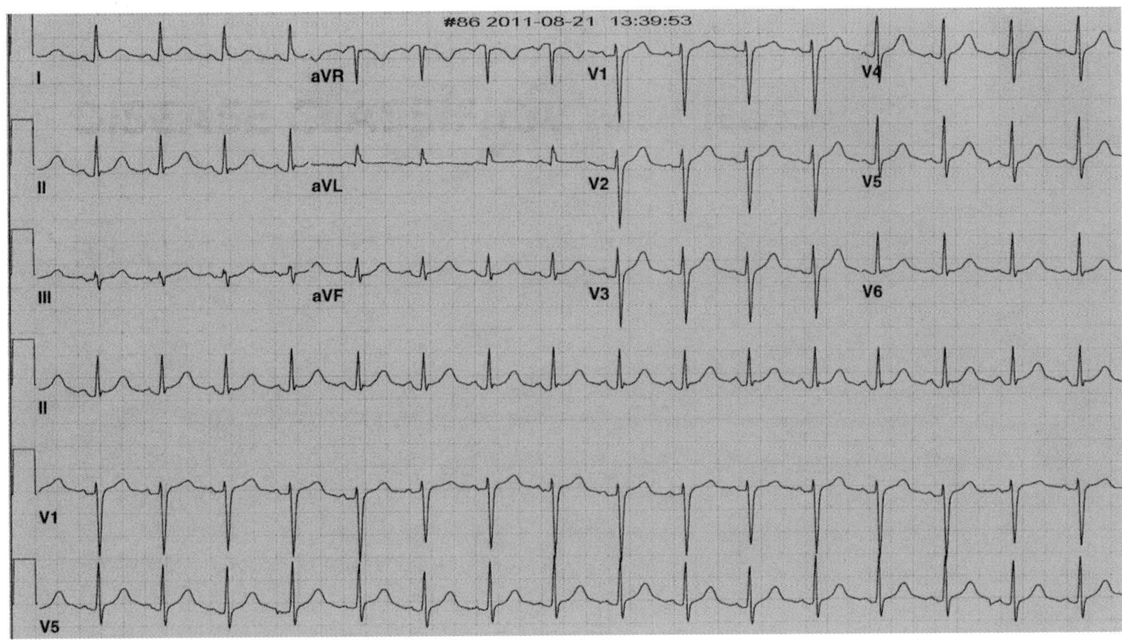

Figure 64.8 ECG 21 August 2011 taken at 13:39.

4 Diagnosis, treatment, and course August–September 2011

What is your diagnosis and treatment?

Answers and commentary

1 History June–July 2011

The patient had a cardiac arrest associated with idiopathic ventricular fibrillation. He did well after treatment with therapeutic hypothermia in which the body is cooled to 33°C for 36 hours. The latter is indicated in patients who re-establish a normal circulation after a cardiac arrest to minimize the deleterious effect of hypoxia on the brain [1,2].

2 Laboratory data June–July 2011

There was no underlying coronary artery disease and his LV function was normal.

3 Course July–August 2011

ECG 21 August 2011 taken at 00:43

Sinus rhythm. Rate 82/min. PR 0.13 s. QRS 0.09 s. QTc 0.44 s. QRS axis +60°.

Normal ECG unchanged from 30 July 2011.

CT of chest at about T5 level 21 August 2011 taken at 03:03

The CT of the chest shows the tip of the ICD (labeled with a red star) entering the pericardial space. There is a small pericardial effusion.

ECG 21 August 2011 taken at 03:31

The rhythm is sinus tachycardia. Rate 105/min. PR 0.14 s. QRS 0.09 s. QTc 0.52 s. QRS axis +50°.

The heart rate has increased, there is slight J point depression in 2, 3, F, V4–6, and QTc has increased since 00:43.

ECG 21 August 2011 taken at 11:14

Sinus rhythm. Rate 90/min. PR 0.13 s. QRS 0.08 s. QTc 0.52 s. QRS axis +30°.

ST elevation in the inferolateral wall has appeared since 21 August 2011 taken at 03:31, indicative of an epicardial injury pattern (see comparison of 03:03 ECG with 11:14 in Figures 64.4a and b).

Lateral chest X ray 21 August 2011 taken at 13:15

The upper lead is in its expected position in the RA. The lower lead is in the RV, whose tip is touching the RV apex.

Echocardiogram 21 August 2011 taken at 13:32

In the four-chamber view there is a pericardial effusion and collapse of the RA suggestive of pericardial tamponade. The tip of the ICD lead is touching the apex of the RV.

In the subcostal view the ICD is mobile as it is near the RV wall in one frame and in a later frame is touching the RV wall.

ECG 21 August 2011 taken at 13:39

Sinus tachycardia. Rate 100/min. PR 0.14 s. QRS 0.09 s. QTc 0.46 s. QRS axis +30°. Partial regression towards normal of ST elevation in inferolateral leads.

4 Diagnosis, treatment, and course August–September 2011

Diagnosis

Idiopathic ventricular fibrillation.

Perforation of the RV wall by tip of ICD lead associated with vigorous arm movements from swimming.

Treatment

He was started on dopamine and the effects of warfarin were reversed. He underwent pericardiocentesis in which 300 mL of non-clotted blood were removed. His systolic BP rose to 140 mmHg and dopamine was stopped.

Only the tip of the active fixation RV electrode, which was 1.05 mm in diameter, had penetrated the RV. The RV tip was retracted and repositioned. Echocardiography and the pericardial drainage catheter confirmed that no further accumulation of fluid had occurred during these catheter adjustments.

Subsequent ECGs (discussed below) showed regression to normal of the ST changes. As of 13 September 2013 he has remained asymptomatic.

Course

ECG 28 August 2011

Sinus rhythm. Rate 88/min. PR 0.15 s. QRS 0.09 s. QTc 0.45 s. QRS axis +40°.

Minimal evidence of J point depression in inferolateral leads noted as compared to 21 August 2011 taken at 13:39.

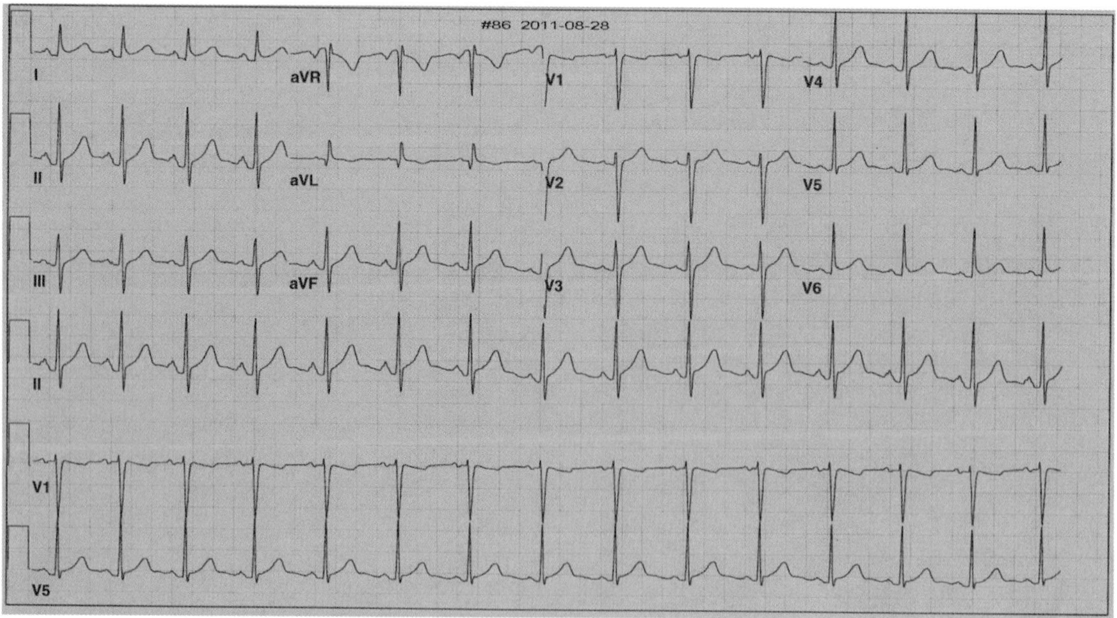

Figure 64.9 ECG 28 August 2011.

ECG 13 September 2011

Sinus rhythm. Rate72/min. PR 0.15 s. QRS 0.10 s. QTc 0.45 s. QRS axis +30°.

ECG is now within normal limits.

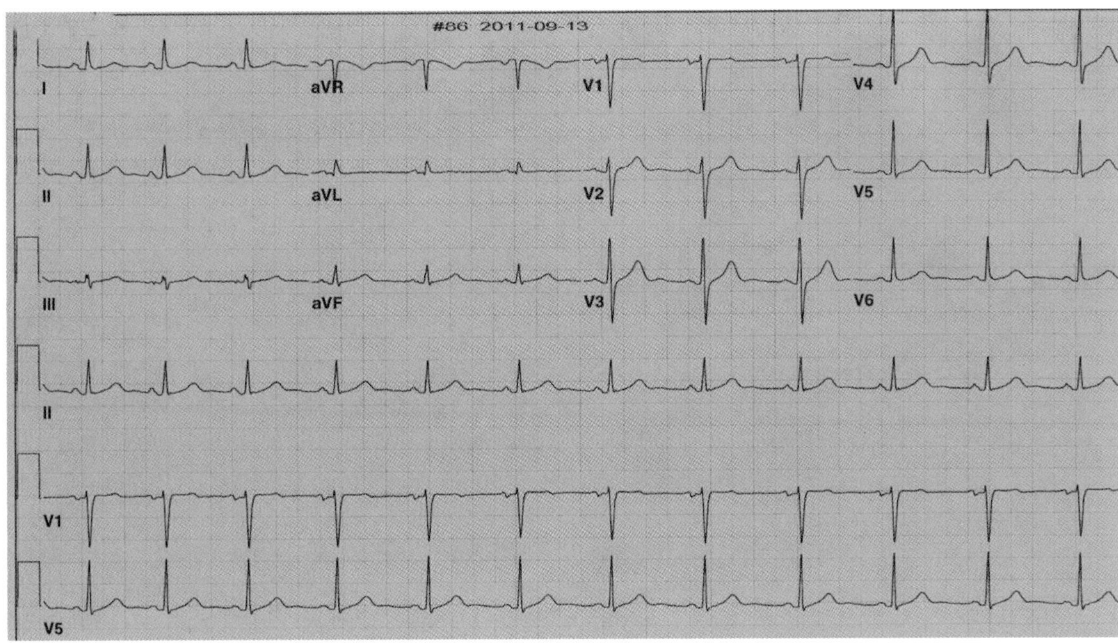

Figure 64.10 ECG 13 September 2011.

Discussion

Vigorous swimming after ICD implantation dislodged the RV electrode tip in this patient, which then perforated the RV wall at its thinnest part, i.e. the apex. The patient gradually developed an epicardial injury pattern on ECG over an 11-hour period, which could have been mistaken for a normal repolarization variant. Echocardiography and CT of the chest confirmed the RV perforation and the development of cardiac tamponade.

RV perforation by an ICD lead occurs in about 0.6–5.2% of cases [4]. It may occur when an excessive length of lead is left or there is chest trauma or frequent shocks [4]. Usually traction on the RV lead in the delayed case (>1 month post implantation) and repositioning the catheter is all that is needed. If there is a pericardial effusion or tamponade then surgical intervention may be required [4].

After implantation of an ICD at least a week should elapse to allow healing before the patient can resume ordinary (not race car) driving [5]. Competitive sports involving more than class 1A activities should be avoided. As swimming involves active arm motions, 4–6 weeks should elapse before recommending it to ICD patients.

Key points

1. Patients returning to hospital after ICD placement with chest pain, syncope, ST-T wave changes, and pericardial effusion may have had a myocardial lead perforation.
2. Patients with an ICD should avoid competitive sports more vigorous than class 1A activity (billiards, bowling, curling, golf, shooting).
3. Consider delaying swimming after ICD placement for at least 4–6 weeks.

References

[1] Brown DFM, Jaffer FA, Baker JN et al. Case 28-2013: A 52-year-old man with cardiac arrest after an acute myocardial infarction. *New Engl J Med* 2013; 369: 1047–1054 (good discussion of therapeutic hypothermia).

[2] Laish-Farkash A, Matetzky S, Oieru D et al. Usefulness of mild therapeutic hypothermia for hospitalized comatose patients having out-of-hospital cardiac arrest. *Am J Cardiol* 2011; 108: 173–178 (110 rescuscitated patients admitted to ICU after cardiac arrest treated with mild hypothermia).

[3] Vyas H, Hejlik J, Ackerman MJ. Epinephrine QT stress testing in the evaluation of congenital long-QT syndrome: diagnostic accuracy of the paradoxical QT response. *Circulation* 2006; 113: 1385–1392.
[4] Oh S. *Cardiac perforation associated with a pacemaker or ICD lead*. In: Modern Pacemakers – present and future. Das MR (ed.). InTech, 2011, pp 343–350 (www.intechopen.com).
[5] Lampert R. Managing with pacemakers and implantable cardioverter defibrillators. *Circulation* 2013; 128: 1576–1585 (extensive review article).

Further reading

Swerdlow CD, Ellenbogen KA. Implantable cardioverter–defibrillator leads design, diagnostics, and management. *Circulation* 2013; 128: 2062–2071.

65 PATIENT STUDY 65

Sequence of data presentation

1 Chest X ray
↓
2 12-lead ECG 30 May 2008
↓
3 Echocardiography
↓
4 MRI of heart 3 June 2008
↓
5 CT of abdomen 3 June 2008
↓
6 12-lead ECG 6 June 2008
↓
7 History
↓
8 Physical examination
↓
9 Laboratory data
↓
10 Diagnosis
↓
11 Course

1 Chest X ray

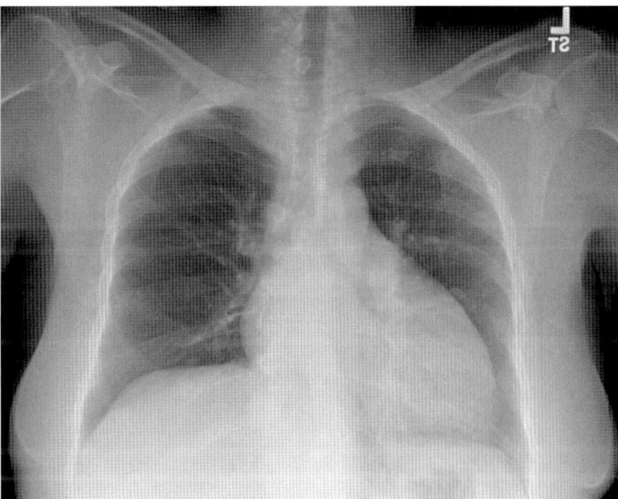

Figure 65.1 PA chest X ray 2008.

Patient Studies in Valvular, Congenital, and Rarer Forms of Cardiovascular Disease: An Integrative Approach, First Edition. Franklin B. Saksena.

Companion Website: www.wiley.com/go/saksena/patientstudies

2 12-lead ECG 30 May 2008

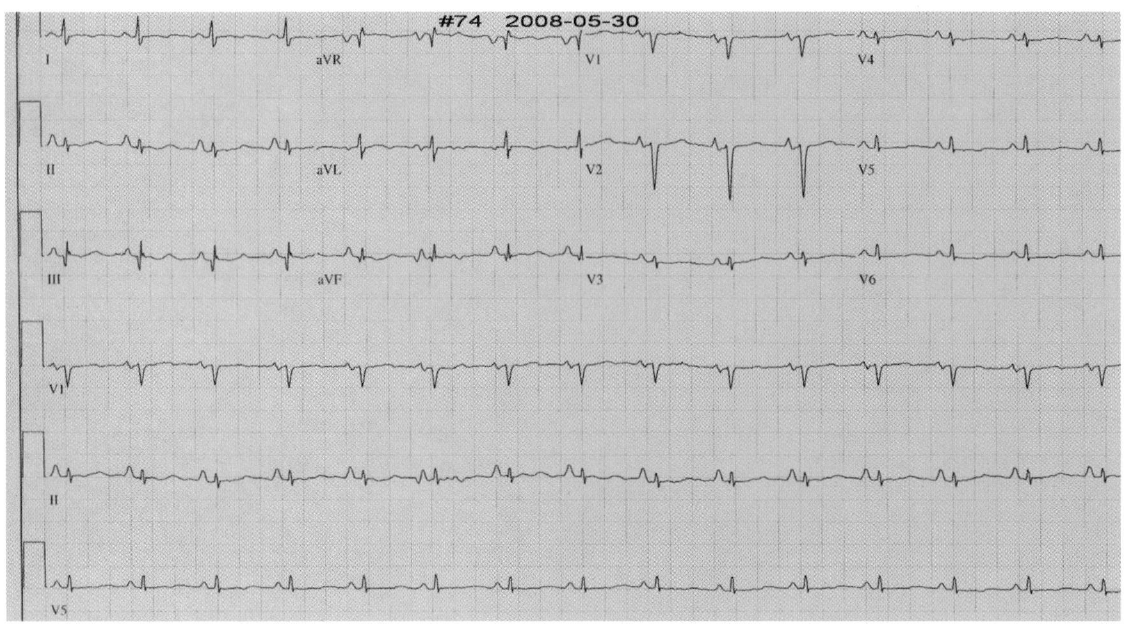

Figure 65.2 12-lead ECG 30 May 2008.

3 Echocardiography

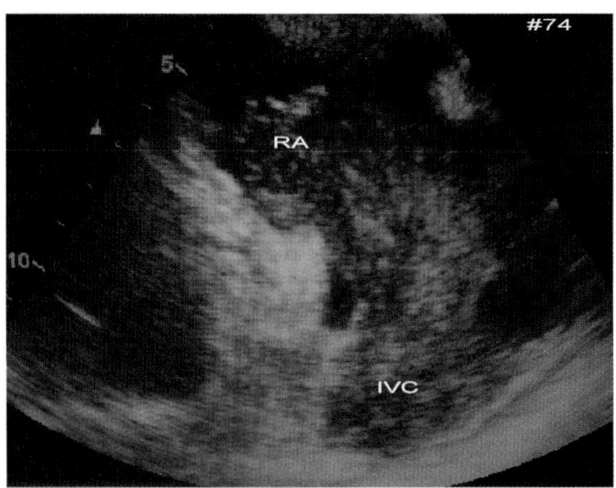

Figure 65.3 Echocardiogram showing RA and IVC (subcostal view).

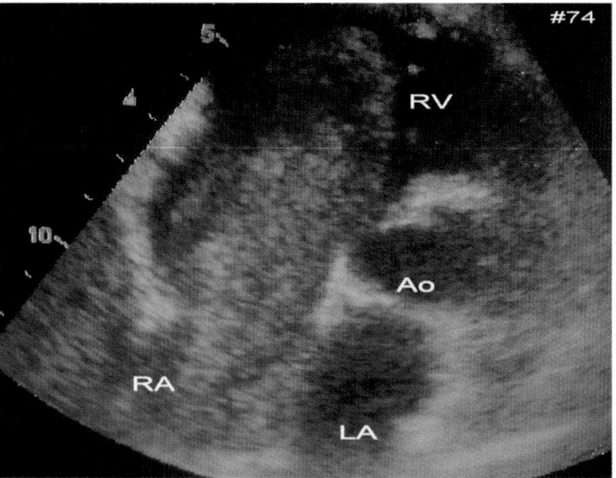

Figure 65.4 Two-dimensional echocardiography in short-axis view.

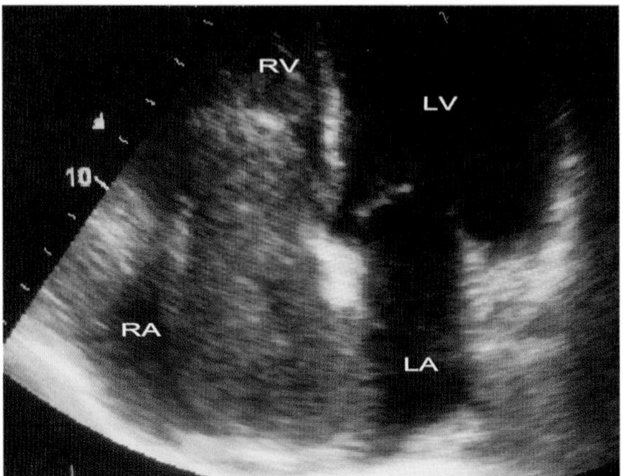

Figure 65.5 Two-dimensional echocardiogram in four-chamber view.

4 MRI of heart 3 June 2008

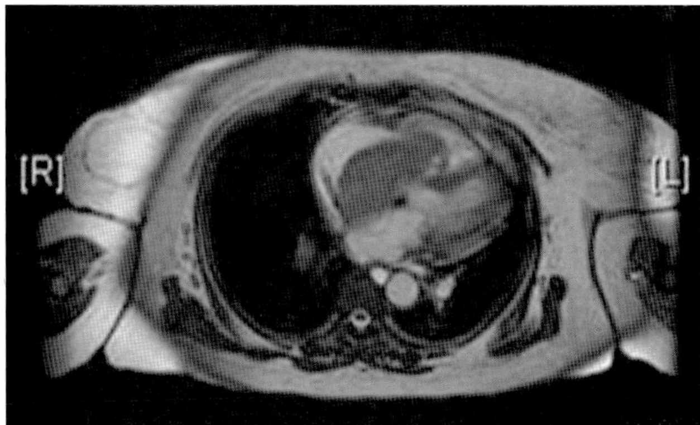

Figure 65.6 MRI of heart.

5 CT of abdomen 3 June 2008

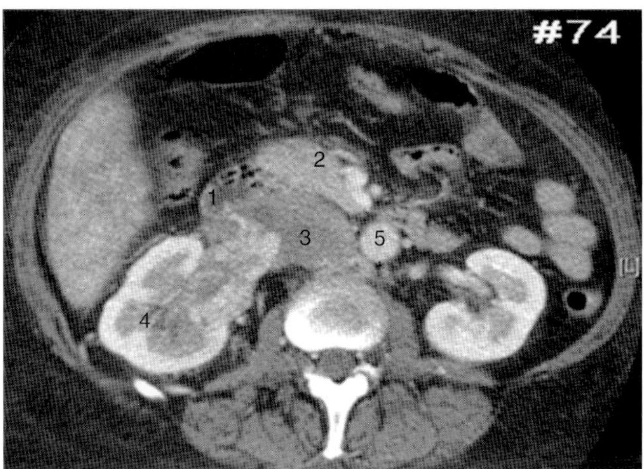

Figure 65.7 CT of abdomen.

Name the structures numbered 1–5.

6 12-lead ECG 6 June 2008

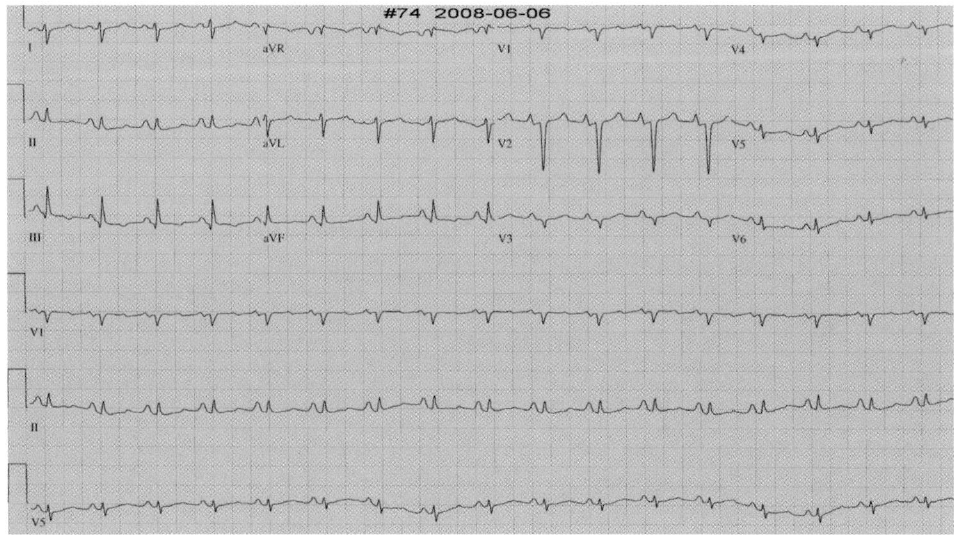

Figure 65.8 12-lead ECG 6 June 2008.

7 History

58-year-old female with half-block dyspnea for l month and hematuria for 1 day.
She had been hypertensive over the last year. No weight loss.

8 Physical examination

63 inches tall, 161 lb female. BP 110/70. HR 88/min regular.
Mild elevation of jugular venous pressure. Normal carotid upstroke.
Apex beat 5th interspace, 10 cm from the mid-sternal line.
S4 apex 1+. S1 1+ increased. Loud P2.
Grade 2/6 pulmonary systolic murmur.
Lungs clear.
Bilateral leg edema.
15 cm span liver.

9 Laboratory data

30 May 2008: hemoglobin 9.9 g%, WBC 11,600/mm^3, BUN 18 mg%, creatinine 1.4 mg%, LDH 784, d-dimer 1.94, urine 1+ blood 1+ protein, negative for sugar, bone scan was negative for metastases CT chest. Peripheral pulmonary emboli.
5 June 2008: BUN 45 mg%, creatinine 4.2 mg%.
6 June 2008: CT head without infusion was negative for intracranial bleeding, bilirubin 4.1 mg%, ammonia level 89 μ/dL (normal 19–60 μ/dL).
10 June 2008: ultrasound of the liver, spleen, and left kidney showed normal echo texture.

10 Diagnosis

What is the diagnosis?

11 Course

What is the course?

Answers and commentary

1 Chest X ray

There is mild cardiomegaly with probable LV enlargement (?hypertension a factor). Slight increase in pulmonary vasculature. Right diaphragm is slightly elevated. The latter is seen if there is hepatomegaly, phrenic nerve damage, or a subphrenic abscess.

2 12-lead ECG 30 May 2008

Sinus rhythm. Rate 90/min. PR 0.13 s. QRS 0.08 s. QRS axis +40°. QS in V1–2.
Impression: (i) possible old anteroseptal infarction, (ii) non-specific lateral T wave changes, (iii) right atrial enlargement.

3 Echocardiography

Figure 65.3 Two-dimensional echocardiogram showing a mass occupying the IVC and most of the RA (subcostal view).
Figure 65.4 Two-dimensional echocardiogram (short-axis view) showing the mass occupying the RA, the tricuspid valve orifice, and the RV. The mass measures 7 cm × 3 cm.
Figure 65.5 Four-chamber view showing the mass occupying most of the RA and RV. The LA and LV appear normal.

4 MRI of heart 3 June 2008

Figure 65.5 MRI of heart confirms the presence of a dense mass in the RA and RV without any left heart involvement.

5 CT of abdomen 3 June 2008

The left kidney is normal. An irregular mass appears to emanate from the right kidney (4), indicating spread of cancer (3) from the kidney and obliterating the IVC shadow (*). 1, duodenum; 2, pancreas; 3, cancer; 4, right kidney with distorted calcyceal structure; 5, aorta; *, IVC.

6 12-lead ECG 6 June 2008

Sinus tachycardia. HR 100/min. PR 0.14 s. QRS 0.07 s. QRS axis +120°.

QS in V1–3. Lateral T wave changes have resolved since 30 May 2008.

Impression: (i) old anteroseptal wall infarction, (ii) right atrial enlargement, (iii) right axis deviation has occurred since 30 May 2008.

7 History

Pulmonary congestion is one of several possibilities causing the patient's dyspnea.

Her hematuria suggests renal or bladder pathology.

8 Physical examination

The elevated jugular venous pressure and hepatomegaly could suggest some right heart failure. Hepatomegaly could also be due to metastatic disease from the kidney (later disproved by the normal liver ultrasound).

9 Laboratory data

The patient's anemia could be due to chronic renal disease and/or undetected long-standing hematuria. Borderline elevated d-dimer is a non-specific finding.

Subsequent laboratory data were consistent with a metabolic encephalopathy and progressive renal failure.

10 Diagnosis

Cancer of kidney.

Spread of tumor-thrombus to IVC, right heart, and lungs.

Mild right heart failure.

11 Course

The patient became confused and was diagnosed as having a metabolic encephalopathy and renal failure (BUN 45 mg%, Cr 4.5 mg%), making her an unsuitable candidate for surgery. Accordingly, MRI of brain to exclude metastatic disease was not carried out.

She was transferred to a hospice on 11 June 2008.

Discussion

Renal cell cancer may spread to the IVC in 3–10% of cases [1, 2], with involvement of the RA in <10% of cases [1].

In this patient the tumor-thrombus had spread from the IVC to the RA and RV with subsequent pulmonary embolization. Tumor obstruction of the right heart and pulmonary embolism would account for the right heart failure and the ECG changes of right-axis deviation. Bone and liver metastases were ruled out. However, brain metastases could not be excluded. She was not considered a good surgical candidate in view of her metabolic encephalopathy.

The spread of the renal cell cancer to the IVC does not always mean that there are distant metastases elsewhere. Thus, surgical removal of the kidney and the tumor clot can still be a consideration if the cancer has only spread to the IVC [1].

Key points

1. Renal cell cancer may spread via the IVC to the right heart. This is often best seen on echocardiography using the subcostal view.
2. Patients with renal cell carcinoma may then develop right heart failure and pulmonary embolism.
3. Surgical removal of the kidney and the tumor clot in the IVC is feasible provided there are no other metastases.

References

[1] Goldman A, Parmeswaran R, Kotler MN et al. Renal cell carcinoma and right atrial tumor diagnosed by echocardiography. *Am Heart J* 1985; 110: 183–186.

[2] Svane S. Tumor thrombus of the inferior vena cava resulting from renal carcinoma. A report of 12 autopsied cases. *Scand J Urol Nephrol* 1969; 3: 245–256.

CROSSWORD PUZZLE

Theme: Pediatric cardiology and other medical issues (clues marked with * refer to the theme of the crossword puzzle). Answers can be found on p. 427.

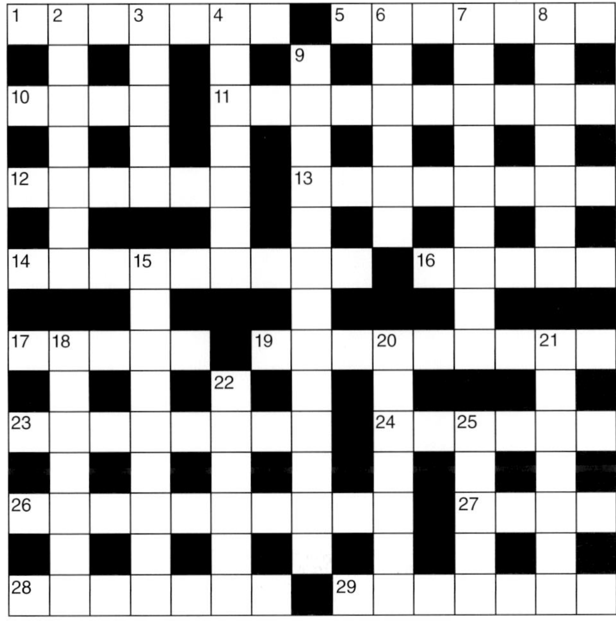

Across

1 and 5	Names associated with a subclavian artery to pulmonary artery anastomosis (7, 7)*.
10	A transaminase (abbreviated) (4).
11	An ______ ____ over 5 cm in diameter is an indication for surgery in Marfan syndrome (6, 4)*.
12	To take any substance into the body via the blood stream or lymphatics (6).
13	Describes dead tissue (8).
14	Morse's method of communication (9).
16	The cause of kyphoscoliosis is _____ unknown (5).
17	Informal term describing a GI examination (5).
19	The apical displacement of the tricuspid valve helps to _____ the diagnosis of Ebstein's anomaly (9)*.
23	One of the features that ____ ___ in Marfan syndrome is arachnodactyly (5, 3)*.
24	Crease found in Down syndrome (6)*.
26	Eye feature in dermatomyositis (10)*.
27	Name of surgeon who used a pulmonary autograft in the aortic position in patients with aortic stenosis (4)*.
28	Surgeon's name associated with an atrial switch procedure in which an intra-atrial baffle is made of atrial wall flaps (7)*.
29	Name of surgeon who replaced the ascending aorta and aortic valve with a composite graft-valve device and reimplanted the coronary arteries into the sides of the conduit (7)*.

Patient Studies in Valvular, Congenital, and Rarer Forms of Cardiovascular Disease: An Integrative Approach, First Edition. Franklin B. Saksena.

Companion Website: www.wiley.com/go/saksena/patientstudies

Down

2 Critics say that our handwriting is not always _____ (7).
3 Combining form for stone (5).
4 The four-________ view is useful in detecting an endocardial cushion defect (7)*.
6 For each one (6).
7 Sad (9).
8 Nucleoside formed by deamination of adenosine (7).
9 28 across operation was devised for this condition (13)*.
15 An abdominal aorta with an ______ rate of >1 cm/year may need to be operated on, especially if it is already over 4 cm in diameter (9)*.
18 A syndrome characterized by chromosomal abnormalities that is often associated with total anomalous pulmonary venous drainage (4, 3)*.
20 Morally strict (7).
21 One of the surgeons who devised the original operation for operating on patients with d loop transposition of the great vessels (the main PA is anastomosed to the ascending aorta and a valved conduit is placed between the RV and the main PA) (7)*.
22 Procedure involving anastomosis or conduit between RA and PA in patients with tricuspid atresia (6)*.
25 Deserve or earn (5).

Reference

Segar DS, A lexicon of commons surgical procedures for congenital heart disease. ACC Current Journal Review March/April 1996, p 46.

SUBJECT INDEX

Patient Studies in Valvular, Congenital, and Rarer Forms of Cardiovascular Disease: An Integrative Approach, First Edition. Franklin B. Saksena.

Companion Website: www.wiley.com/go/saksena/patientstudies

PATIENT STUDIES INDEX

Patient Studies in Valvular, Congenital, and Rarer Forms of Cardiovascular Disease: An Integrative Approach, First Edition. Franklin B. Saksena.

Companion Website: www.wiley.com/go/saksena/patientstudies

DISEASE CLASSIFICATION INDEX

Patient Studies in Valvular, Congenital, and Rarer Forms of Cardiovascular Disease: An Integrative Approach, First Edition. Franklin B. Saksena.

Companion Website: www.wiley.com/go/saksena/patientstudies

ANSWERS TO CROSSWORD PUZZLE

Across

1 Blalock
5 Taussig
10 SGOT
11 Aortic root
12 Absorb
13 Necrosis
14 Telegraph
16 Often
17 Scope
19 Establish
23 Stand out
24 Simian
26 Heliotrope
27 Ross
28 Senning
29 Bentall

Down

2 Legible
3 Litho
4 Chamber
6 Apiece
7 Sorrowful
8 Inosine
9 Transposition
15 Expansion
18 Cat's eye
20 Austere
21 Stansel
22 Fontan
25 Merit

Patient Studies in Valvular, Congenital, and Rarer Forms of Cardiovascular Disease: An Integrative Approach, First Edition. Franklin B. Saksena.

Companion Website: www.wiley.com/go/saksena/patientstudies